Heart Failure
A Combined Medical and Surgical Approach

We would like to dedicate this textbook to Linda H. and the late George M. Kaufman, who stimulated us, prodded us, encouraged us, and allowed us to accomplish a great deal. We would also like to dedicate it to our families, who encouraged us, understood us, and put up with us!

Heart Failure
A Combined Medical and Surgical Approach

EDITED BY

Patrick M. McCarthy, MD

Bluhm Cardiovascular Institute
Division of Cardiothoracic Surgery
Northwestern Memorial Hospital
Northwestern University School of Medicine
Chicago, IL, USA

James B. Young, MD

Division of Medicine and the Kaufman Center for Heart Failure
Cleveland Clinic Foundation
Cleveland, OH, USA

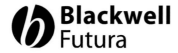
Blackwell
Futura

Futura, an imprint of Blackwell Publishing

© 2007 by Blackwell Publishing

Blackwell Futura is an imprint of Blackwell Publishing

Blackwell Publishing, Inc., 350 Main Street, Malden, Massachusetts 02148-5020, USA
Blackwell Publishing Ltd, 9600 Garsington Road, Oxford OX4 2DQ, UK
Blackwell Science Asia Pty Ltd, 550 Swanston Street, Carlton, Victoria 3053, Australia

First published 2007
1   2007

ISBN: 978-1-4051-2203-0

Library of Congress Cataloging-in-Publication Data

Heart failure : a combined medical and surgical approach / edited by
   Patrick M. McCarthy, James B. Young.
      p. ; cm.
   Includes bibliographical references and index.
   ISBN-13: 978-1-4051-2203-0 (alk. paper)
   ISBN-10: 1-4051-2203-X (alk. paper)
   1. Heart failure–Treatment.   I. McCarthy, Patrick M., 1955–
II. Young, James B.
   [DNLM: 1. Heart Failure, Congestive–therapy. 2. Cardiac Output,
Low–therapy. 3. Cardiac Surgical Procedures–methods.   WG 370
H436175 2007]
RC685.C53H4344 2007
616.1'2906–dc22

                                        2006027511

A catalogue record for this title is available from the British Library

Commissioning Editors: Steve Korn and Gina Almond
Editorial Assistant: Victoria Pittman
Development Editor: Beckie Brand
Production Controller: Debbie Wyer
Set in 9.5/12 Minion by Charon Tec Ltd (A Macmillan Company), Chennai, India
www.charontec.com
Printed and bound in Singapore by Fabulous Printers Pte Ltd.

For further information on Blackwell Publishing, visit our website:
www.blackwellcardiology.com

Contents

List of Contributors

Nancy M. Albert, MSN, RN, CCNS, CCRN, CAN
Director, Nursing Research and Clinical Nurse Specialist
Kaufman Center for Heart Failure
Cleveland Clinic Foundation
Cleveland, OH, USA

Arman T. Askari, MD
Departments of Cardiovascular Medicine and Cell Biology
Cleveland Clinic Foundation
Cleveland, OH, USA

Mandeep Bhargava, MD
Section of Cardiac Electrophysiology and Pacing
Department of Cardiovascular Medicine
Cleveland Clinic Foundation
Cleveland, OH, USA

Katrina A. Bramstedt, PhD
Bioethicist
Associate Staff
Cleveland Clinic Foundation
Cleveland, OH, USA

Tiffany Buda, BSN, RN
LVAD/Transplant Nurse Clinician
Department of Cardiovascular Surgery
Cleveland Clinic Foundation
Cleveland, OH, USA

Gary S. Francis, MD
Professor in Medicine
Cleveland Clinic Lerner College of Medicine of Case
Western Reserve University
Head, Section of Clinical Cardiology
Department of Cardiovascular Medicine
Cleveland Clinic Foundation
Cleveland, OH, USA

Bruce W. Lytle, MD
Chairman, Department of Thoracic and
Cardiovascular Surgery
Cleveland Clinic Foundation
Cleveland, OH, USA

Edwin C. McGee Jr., MD
Assistant Professor of Surgery
Feinberg School of Medicine at Northwestern University
Chicago, IL, USA

Raymond Q. Migrino, MD, FACC
Assistant Professor in Cardiovascular Medicine, Biophysics
and Radiology
Medical College of Wisconsin
Milwaukee, WI, USA

José Luis Navia, MD
Department of Thoracic and Cardiovascular Surgery
Cleveland Clinic Foundation
Cleveland, OH, USA

Marc S. Penn, MD, PhD, FACC
Director, Bakken Heart-Brain Institute
Medical Director, Coronary Intensive Care Unit
Director, Experimental Animal Laboratory
Associated Director, Cardiovascular Medicine Fellowship
Departments of Cardiovascular Medicine and Cell Biology
Cleveland Clinic Foundation
Cleveland, OH, USA

Randall C. Starling, MD, MPH, FACC
Director, Heart Transplant Medical Services
Director, Advanced Fellowship in Heart Failure and
Cardiac Transplant Medicine
Associate Professor of Internal Medicine
Section of Heart Failure and Cardiac Transplant Medicine
Department of Cardiovascular Medicine
Kaufman Center for Heart Failure
Cleveland Clinic Foundation
Cleveland, OH, USA

W. H. Wilson Tang, MD
Assistant Professor in Medicine
Cleveland Clinic Lerner College of Medicine of Case
Western Reserve University
Associate Staff
Section of Heart Failure and Cardiac Transplantation
Medicine
Department of Cardiovascular Medicine
Cleveland Clinic Foundation
Cleveland, OH, USA

David O. Taylor, MD
Director, Heart Failure Special Care Unit
Cleveland Clinic Foundation
Cleveland, OH, USA

Samuel Unzek, MD
Departments of Cardiovascular Medicine and Cell Biology
Cleveland Clinic Foundation
Cleveland, OH, USA

Richard D. White, MD, FACC, FAHA
Professor and Chairman
Department of Radiology
University of Florida College of Medicine – Jacksonville
Jacksonville, FL, USA

Bruce L. Wilkoff, MD
Section of Cardiac Electrophysiology and Pacing
Department of Cardiovascular Medicine
Cleveland Clinic Foundation
Cleveland, OH, USA

Mohamad H. Yamani, MD
Kaufman Center for Heart Failure
Cleveland Clinic Foundation
Cleveland, OH, USA

Preface

"To act as a unit". The motto of the Cleveland Clinic reflects the spirit of this textbook; cooperation among a multi-specialty group, and integration of care among the physicians, nursing staff, pharmacists, social workers, and consultants. Our patients with heart failure, in particular the patients with advanced heart failure, pose complex problems for the medical team. When we formed the George M. and Linda H. Kaufman Center for Heart Failure, we thought the only way to adequately address this challenge was to coordinate care among the many disciplines. This textbook is our effort to explain that process, and our thinking about how to approach patients with various stages of heart failure.

This model in medicine is not new. In many respects this process is very similar to the care of patients with congenital heart disease as employed in many children's hospitals across the world. Many of these centers have developed interdisciplinary teams of pediatric cardiologists, congenital heart surgeons, and affiliated consultants and support staff. The team works together to make the proper diagnosis, prevent the progression of disease, identify optimal medical therapy and the proper timing for interventional and surgical therapies. Centers of excellence evolved from this approach.

The care of heart failure patients has advanced along the same lines. The most common cause of systolic dysfunction in industrialized nations is ischemic cardiomyopathy. This requires a complex approach including proper diagnosis, medical therapy and then decision-making regarding percutaneous therapies, surgical therapies, potentially electrical therapies such as biventricular pacing and implantable cardioverter defibrillators, and a variety of mechanical circulatory support devices and transplantation. All are potential therapies. Various chapters in this book reflect our thinking about the proper role for these therapies. Whenever possible, we use the most up-to-date evidence-based medicine. This is inherently easier to study in drug trials. Surgical trials are more difficult to accomplish, especially when the surgical decision-making and techniques may be very complex. For instance, a patient with ischemic cardiomyopathy may be well served by coronary artery bypass, mitral and/or tricuspid valve repair, left ventricular reconstruction, and possibly additional therapies for surgical ablation of atrial fibrillation, and placement of left ventricular epicardial pacing wires for perioperative and postoperative biventricular synchronous pacing. Drug trials study one drug at a time and therefore, there are fewer confounding variables. Despite these limitations, the surgical trials recently include the REMATCH trial, the randomized trial of the Acorn CorCap Device, the ongoing STICH trial, and the Myocor Coapsys RESTOR-MV trial. Since surgery and medical therapy work on different targets, and in different fashions, we think optimal patient care is derived by doing the most complete surgery that is practical, and then continuing medical therapy for patients with severe left ventricular dysfunction.

Each chapter of this textbook is written around one aspect of the treatment for heart failure, because it is easiest to organize the topics that way. When it comes to an individual patient, however, the strategy has to adapt a variety of different therapies together. We hope that our attempt to clarify our thinking is clear. Much of what we do is based on sound scientific evidence, and in other instances the art of medicine has to be applied. We have tried to explain which part of care is science, and which is the art, in each chapter.

When we began this textbook we were Medical and Surgical Directors of the Kaufman Center for Heart Failure. By the time of the textbook's publication however, both of us had evolved, Jim Young to be the Chair of Medicine at the Cleveland Clinic, and

Patrick McCarthy to be the Chief of Cardiothoracic Surgery Division and Co-Director of the Bluhm Cardiovascular Institute at Northwestern Memorial Hospital. The "transplant" of the multidisciplinary team to Northwestern to create centers in heart failure, valve disease, and atrial fibrillation among others, has been an interesting and enlightening broadening of the concept of the Kaufman Center for Heart Failure. It appears to be a mindset of ideal patient care that can be easily transferred and broadened to other medical centers. We hope that this textbook serves as a stimulus for others to employ this patient care model.

Patrick M. McCarthy, MD
James B. Young, MD

Acknowledgements

The authors would like to acknowledge the extensive help and support preparing this text by Linda Huerta, Michele Langenfeld, and Barbara Garren at Northwestern Memorial's Bluhm Cardiovascular Institute and Katherine Hoercher from The Cleveland Clinic's Kaufman Center for Heart Failure.

CHAPTER 1

Epidemiology of heart failure: progression to pandemic?

Randall C. Starling

Introduction

Congestive heart failure (CHF), traditionally considered an edematous disorder, was described hundreds of years ago. Hypertension and valvular heart disease were the most frequent co-morbidities [1]. Physicians could only attempt to control pulmonary and peripheral congestion with diuretic therapy. Heart failure was a progressive disease culminating in biventricular dysfunction, anasarca, and finally organ failure due to hypoperfusion. Symptomatic heart failure in the 21st century is most often characterized by effort intolerance (dyspnea) and fatigue. CHF is growing at epidemic proportions, particularly in the elderly, consuming significant health-care dollars and resulting in disability and premature death. Common illnesses, including coronary artery disease, hypertension, and diabetes mellitus, are the major etiologic risk factors. In the United States, heart failure incidence is twice as common in hypertensives and five times greater in persons who have had a myocardial infarction (http://www.nhlbi.nih.gov/health/public/heart/other/CHF.htm) [2]. The National Heart, Lung and Blood Institute (NHLBI) estimates that 75% of heart failure cases have antecedent hypertension. Major advances in the treatment of coronary artery disease and acute ischemic syndromes that have saved countless lives have resulted in a growing population of chronic patients with left ventricular dysfunction that may develop clinical heart failure. The NHLBI estimates that 22% of male and 46% of female myocardial infarction victims will develop heart failure within 6 years (Figure 1.1). Heart failure is the most common indication for hospitalization in the United States in patients over 65 years of age. It is estimated that about one-half of patients with heart failure are greater than or equal to 65 years old. Finally, it is now recognized that the syndrome of heart failure may also occur as a consequence of diastolic dysfunction. Recent reports have shown that 40–50% of patients hospitalized with heart failure have normal ejection fractions.

The mainstay of heart failure therapy today is "treatment" for established and symptomatic diseases. The public health impact of heart failure for our society will continue to grow until effective primary and secondary prevention strategies are adopted and employed. The recent heart failure guidelines now define patients at risk of heart failure (ACC Stage A) as a high priority for preemptive therapy. Patients with advanced heart failure, ACC Stage D (www.acc.org/guidelines/heart failure) represents almost 10% of the total heart failure population, have the highest short-term mortality and consume the greatest percentage of resources [3]. The cost of treating advanced symptomatic heart failure is a growing economic burden for industrialized nations. An analysis of six countries revealed that 1–2% of total health-care expenditures were for heart failure and about 70% of the total heart failure cost was consumed for hospital costs [4]. The rapidly increasing prevalence of heart failure clearly represents the most important public health problem in cardiovascular medicine [1,4,5].

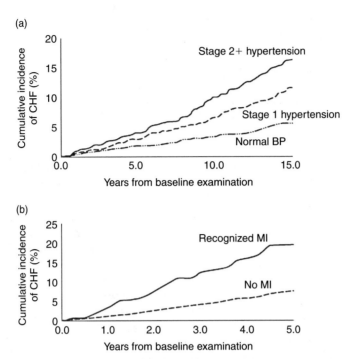

Figure 1.1 (a) Incidence of heart failure in men and women age 50–79 years by hypertension status. Stage 1 hypertension is defined as a systolic BP of 140–159 mmHg or diastolic BP of 90–99 mmHg in people not receiving antihypertensive medication; Stage 2 or greater is defined as systolic BP of 160 mmHg or greater, diastolic BP of 100 mmHg or greater, or current use of antihypertensive medication (adapted from [2]). *Source*: Framingham Heart Study, National Heart, Lung, and Blood Institute. **(b)** Incidence of heart failure by myocardial infarction status (adapted from [2]). *Source*: Cardiovascular Heart Study, National Heart, Lung, and Blood Institute.
CHF: congestive heart failure; BP: blood pressure; MI: myocardial infarction.

Epidemiology

An epidemic is described as affecting or tending to affect a disproportionately large number of individuals within a population, community, or region at the same time (excessively prevalent). Pandemic refers to a disease occurring over a wide geographic area and affecting an exceptionally high proportion of the population. Heart failure is a worldwide phenomenon that is indeed pandemic. Heart failure affects approximately 2–4 million Americans and over 15 million people worldwide [5]. The American Heart Association estimates there are 4.9 million Americans alive in 2002 with CHF (http://www.americanheart.org). Based on the 44-year follow-up of the NHLBI's Framingham Health Study, heart failure incidence approaches 10 per 1000 population after 65 years of age. Despite declining mortality rates for cardiovascular disease in the United States, hospitalizations for heart failure have increased substantially. Hospital discharges for CHF in the United States rose from 377,000 in 1979 to 999,000 in 2000, a 165% increase (http://www.americanheart.org).

The criteria for the diagnosis of the syndrome of CHF are not standardized, hence population estimates may underestimate the extent of heart failure. Measures used in population-based studies and cardiovascular drug research rely on a composite of signs, symptoms, and diagnostic findings. Attempts to validate the Framingham Clinical Heart Failure Score against a measure of ejection fraction showed that, in patients with a low left ventricular ejection fraction (LVEF <0.40), 20% met none of the criteria for CHF. A cohort of 2000 persons aged 25–74 years living in Scotland underwent a detailed assessment of cardiac status including echocardiography [4]. The overall prevalence of left ventricular systolic dysfunction (ejection fraction 30%) was 2.9%;

concurrent symptoms of heart failure were found in 1.5%, while the remaining 1.4% were asymptomatic. Prevalence was greater with age and in men, reaching 6.4% in men aged 65–74 years. Therefore, population estimates of heart failure have many pitfalls, and utilization of death rates and hospitalizations likely grossly underestimate the true magnitude of the heart failure pandemic. An analysis using administrative data sets to create a definition of heart failure using diagnosis codes (REACH Study) confirmed the heart failure epidemic in the United States [6]. The authors concluded that International Classification of Diseases, Clinical Modification (ICD-9-CM) codes and automated sources of data can be used within health systems to describe the epidemiology of heart failure. Newer modalities such as the brain natriuretic peptide assay may enable investigators to interrogate populations to determine the incidence of subclinical ventricular dysfunction, hence diagnosing and perhaps treating asymptomatic patients and ultimately improving long-term outcomes.

Incidence and prevalence

Incidence refers to the number of new cases observed in a year in a defined population. Prevalence refers to the number of cases observed at a specified point in time in a defined population. The crude incidence of heart failure (unadjusted for age) ranges from one to five cases per 1000 population per year, and increases sharply with advancing age to as high as 40 cases per 1000 population over 75 years in some studies [7]. A reflection of the incidence of heart failure in the US is made from the Framingham Study and the Framingham Offspring Study, representing a population of over 10,000 [8]. The incidence of heart failure raises with age in both men and women as shown in Figure 1.2. The incidence of CHF after adjustment for age is one-third lower in women than in men. Based on the increasing age of the US population and improved survival, it is estimated that the CHF prevalence will nearly double to 5.7 million cases by the year 2030 [9].

A recent analysis of the Framingham Heart Study cohort demonstrated over the past 50 years that the incidence of heart failure has declined among women, but not men; however, survival after the onset of heart failure has improved in both sexes [10].

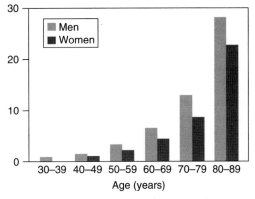

Figure 1.2 The annual incidence of congestive heart failure is shown by population age/decade in men and women among The Framingham Heart Study subjects (adapted from [8], with permission from the American College of Cardiology Foundation).

When established clinical criteria are used to define heart failure, the lifetime risk for heart failure is one in five for both men and women [11]. Both hypertension and antecedent myocardial infarction significantly impact the lifetime risk for heart failure between ages 40 and 80 years in both men and women. These findings highlight the importance of risk factor modification to reduce ischemic heart disease and the potential impact of antihypertensive therapy to reduce the development of overt clinical heart failure.

Mortality

Since 1968, heart failure as the primary cause of death has increased fourfold [8]. The most dismal prognosis for patients with severe symptoms (New York Heart Association Class IV) and coronary artery disease was a 43% and 18% survival rate at 1 and 3 years, respectively [12]. Symptomatic patients with dilated nonischemic cardiomyopathy who are with medical therapy have a better prognosis compared to patients with underlying coronary artery disease [12].

Survival in patients with heart failure has improved over the past 50 years. The 30-day, 1-year, and 5-year age-adjusted mortality among men declined from 12%, 30%, and 70% from 1950 through 1969 to 11%, 28%, and 59% in the period from 1990 through 1999. In women, the corresponding rates were 18%, 28%, and 57% for the period 1950 through 1969, and 10%, 24%, and 45% from 1990 through 1999 [10].

Overall there was an improvement in survival rate after the onset of heart failure of 12% per decade, a significant reduction in both men ($P = 0.01$) and women ($P = 0.02$). The explanation for this is purely speculative; however, the improved survival was temporally associated with the use of both angiotensin-converting enzyme inhibitors (ACEIs) and beta blockers. Another analysis examined the short- and long-term mortality of patients after initial hospitalizations for heart failure using a cohort of 38,702 consecutive patients from April 1994 through March 1997 in Ontario, Canada. The crude 30-day and 1-year mortality rates were 11.6% and 33.1%, respectively [13]. Complex interactions among age, sex, and co-morbidities impacted short- and long-term survival. In the oldest co-morbidity-laden subgroup, 30-day and 1-year mortality were 23.8% and 60.7%, respectively. A subgroup analysis from the Digitalis Investigation Group (DIG) study showed that, in ambulatory patients with CHF, estimated creatinine clearance predicts all-cause mortality independently of established prognostic variables [14]. In Cox regression analyses, independent predictors of mortality were estimated creatinine clearance, 6-min walk distance ≤ 262 m, ejection fraction, recent hospitalization for worsening heart failure, and need for diuretic treatment. It is obvious that, as a population ages, heart failure becomes more prevalent and the

mortality raises, especially in patients with compromised renal function and co-morbidities. It has been recognized that elderly persons have a substantial risk for death after a diagnosis of heart failure with normal left ventricular systolic function. A longitudinal population based in 5888 persons of at least 65 years of age revealed that 4.9% had CHF, and ejection fraction was normal in 63%, borderline decreased 15% or impaired in 22%, and determined by a core echocardiographic laboratory [15]; 45% of those with heart failure and 16% without heart failure died within 6–7 years [15]. A cross-sectional survey was performed in Olmsted County, Minnesota to determine the prevalence of diastolic and systolic dysfunction, and if diastolic dysfunction was predictive of all-cause mortality [16]. A cohort of 2042 randomly selected residents of Olmsted County aged 45 years or older were surveyed between June 1997 and September 2000. The prevalence of heart failure was 2.2% with 44% having an ejection fraction $>50\%$. Among those with moderate or severe diastolic or systolic dysfunction, $<50\%$ had recognized heart failure. Both mild and moderate or severe diastolic dysfunction were predictive of all-cause mortality (hazard ratio for severe diastolic dysfunction: 10.17; $P < 0.001$).

Despite medical advances, heart failure remains a lethal illness. Heart failure in the elderly has the

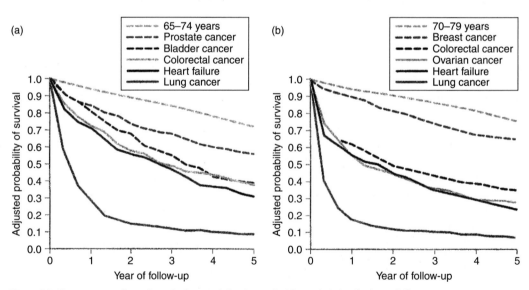

Figure 1.3 Five-year age-adjusted, survival curves following an incident admission for heart failure versus common types of cancer in age-matched patients. (a) Scottish men and (b) Scottish women (adapted from [17] with permission from the European Society of Cardiology). *Source:* Adapted with permission from [32].

highest mortality. Heart failure with preserved systolic function is a growing concern and carries an ominous prognosis. Mortality from heart failure is high, and most patients and families are uninformed and unprepared for the risk of death and need to make end-of-life decisions. A recent Scottish analysis showed that the 5-year age- and sex-adjusted mortality for heart failure is worse than common forms of cancer [17] as depicted in Figure 1.3.

Reasons for increasing prevalence

The prevalence of heart failure increases with age. Furthermore, advances in the pharmacologic and surgical management of coronary artery disease, arrhythmias, valvular heart disease, and hypertension have resulted in an ever-enlarging aging pool of patients who are likely to develop worsening systolic or diastolic function and pathologic ventricular remodeling leading to irreversible heart failure. Effective medical and surgical interventions have resulted in a reduction in mortality. However, the prevalence of heart failure is rising because predisposing conditions (coronary artery disease and diabetes mellitus) are palliated but not cured. The use of implantable cardiac defibrillators (ICDs) will reduce the incidence of sudden cardiac death but does not change the natural history of heart failure/pump dysfunction.

Economics of heart failure

Recent estimates of total annual health-care expenditures for heart failure in Americans have ranged from $10.3 to $37.8 billion [18,19]. The disparity of these figures demonstrates the lack of available accurate economic data, but the cost to American society per year is at least $10 billion and may be as high as $40 billion. The American Heart Association estimates $21.0 billion for direct and indirect costs of CHF in the United States in 2001 [20]. The breakdown includes: $14.3 billion hospitals/nursing homes, $1.5 billion physicians/professionals, $1.6 billion medications, $1.5 billion home health care, and $1.6 billion for lost productivity/mortality. Hence, 68% of the total expense is for inpatient care, very similar to the estimates consumed on inpatient

care (73% and 62%) in the other two reports [18,19]. Considering the rates of hospitalization (including readmissions) for heart failure, it is not surprising that 1–2% of the total health-care expenditures is consumed for heart failure in a number of industrialized countries [4].

The frequency of hospitalizations for CHF accounts for much of the economic burden. A conservative estimate of cumulative care costs during hospitalization ranges from $6000 to $12,000 per admission. Approximately, 35% of the diagnosed heart failure population become hospitalized on an annual basis [5]. Multiple hospitalizations, particularly of elderly patients with multiple co-morbid conditions (50% have three or more), are especially common. Indeed, it has been found that the 3-month readmission rate after an index hospitalization for CHF was as high as 47% of discharges [21]. Many factors are related to the high rates of hospitalization for heart failure, including progression of underlying disease, inappropriate treatment plans, lack of patient compliance with prescribed regimens or diet or both, and use of detrimental drug therapy in certain heart failure settings. There are many patient- and physician-specific issues that contribute to "heart failure decompensation" which are potentially reversible [22]. An analysis in Germany of 179 patients admitted to the hospital with acute decompensation of pre-existing heart failure concluded that 54% of admissions could be regarded as preventable [23]. Noncompliance with drugs or diet was the leading cause of acute decompensation, present in 42%. Practitioners should utilize pharmacologic agents, proven to be effective in multicenter clinical trials, at target doses when managing chronic heart failure.

Interventions to reduce the high frequency and acuity of hospitalization, prolonged length of hospital stays and frequent emergency room visits are essential to attenuate costs. Outpatient care is less costly. Thus, the costs to intensify the outpatient delivery of care are trivial and are offset by the major reduction in total health-care costs if hospital days are reduced. One goal should be to improve the "effectiveness" of inpatient stays such that the readmission rate declines. Up to 25% of Medicare expenditures for hospitalizations are for readmissions [24]. Thus, in heart failure, improving the "quality of the hospitalization" may be most cost-effective. Reduction in length of stay initiatives are important but should not compromise efforts to decrease the risk of hospital readmission.

Severity of heart failure and resource utilization

Patients with advanced heart failure represent about 10% of the total heart failure population, experience the highest short-term mortality and consume tremendous resources. With improved pharmacotherapy and management, an increasing pool of patients are expected to survive with severe left ventricular dysfunction who will ultimately die from refractory heart failure. Patients with refractory heart failure are the consumers of expensive technologic-sophisticated therapies, including cardiac transplantation, mechanical circulatory assist devices, automatic ICDs, biventricular pacemakers, outpatient intravenous inotropic therapy, and frequent high-acuity admissions (intensive care unit stays and hemodynamic monitoring). A European analysis has shown that it is more expensive to treat severe heart failure than mild heart failure, primarily due to the high rate and costs of hospitalization over a 6–12-month period prior to dying [25]. An admission for cardiac transplantation and postoperative care averages $303,400. Cost for implantation and care associated with a left ventricular assist device averages $175,000, and implantation of a cardiac defibrillator $50,000. Specialized regional heart failure centers will play a critical role in the delivery of cost-effective high-quality care to this group of patients. The proper use of sophisticated therapies, including ventricular assist devices, biventricular pacemakers/ICDs, outpatient infusion therapies, and high-risk surgical procedures (coronary artery bypass grafting (CABG), mitral valve repair, and Dor procedure) can improve outcomes and reduce costs.

Heart failure guidelines

Clinical practice guidelines have been developed by carefully evaluating the world's literature with emphasis on well-controlled randomized clinical trials of solid scientific validity and expert opinion from prominent clinicians. Consensus guideline documents for the evaluation and management of heart failure have been published [3,26]. Heart failure experts believe that the pharmacologic treatment of patients remains suboptimal and that both beta blockers and ACEI are underutilized. The guidelines emphasize the importance of appropriate pharmacologic therapy (target doses and ACEI use for asymptomatic left ventricular dysfunction) and nonpharmacologic treatment (counseling, education, and lifestyle modifications) in the management of heart failure. The economic and quality of care ramifications related to the adoption and improved adherence of heart failure guidelines are enormous. The advent of published guidelines has led to the development of disease care management algorithms that can be implemented within healthcare systems [27,28].

Educational programs can improve quality of life for the patient and reduce hospitalization. Multidisciplinary interventions designed to improve dietary compliance and reduce hospital admissions in heart failure patients have been found to be highly effective. A multidisciplinary heart failure disease management program is employed at the Cleveland Clinic Health System [27]. The cornerstone of a heart failure disease management program is to employ pharmacologic therapy in compliance with evidence-based heart failure guidelines and to develop a mechanism to monitor compliance both for patients and physicians. Elderly, socially deprived, recently hospitalized heart failure patients are at increased high risk for readmission and likely will derive the greatest benefit from disease management programs [29,30].

The future and the heart failure epidemic

Many heart failure patients are treated suboptimally with pharmacotherapy [26,31,32]. A US survey showed that cardiologists are more likely to prescribe ACEIs than are general practitioners and internists [38]. A survey comparing the practice patterns between cardiologists and heart failure specialists showed general conformity but concluded that a portion of heart failure patients may be better managed by heart failure specialists [33]. Few data are currently available to prove that heart failure specialists provide superior care for heart failure patients. Perhaps the greatest impact of heart failure specialists is to evaluate patients with cryptogenic heart failure with the goal to find treatable components that have precipitated the heart failure syndrome (i.e. surgical coronary and/or valvular disease, dysynchrony responding to resynchronization therapy, ablation for tachycardia-induced cardiomyopathy). A recent study concluded that cardiology participation in outpatients with new-onset heart failure was associated with improved guideline adherence and a reduction in the composite endpoint of death plus cardiovascular hospitalization [34]. Specialized centers for heart failure can treat severe decompensated patients, often resulting in prolonged stabilization and improved quality of life in patients originally referred expecting cardiac transplantation was the only option [35].

Strategies to attack the epidemic of heart failure should include the following initiatives:

(a) reduction of inpatient costs;
(b) investment in outpatient care and development of chronic disease management programs;
(c) reduce admissions (more important than reduction in length of stay);
(d) focus efforts/resources on the "high-risk" patient (history of frequent readmissions);
(e) utilization of specialized "heart failure providers" (physicians, nurses, dietitians, rehabilitation specialists);
(f) extensive patient education.

Dedicated "specialized heart failure centers" should include the following mandates to help achieve these initiatives:

(a) detailed patient evaluation to "stage" disease and ensure appropriate diagnosis and treatment;
(b) close patient monitoring at intervals tailored to the individual patient's needs;
(c) immediate access to "heart failure team" staff and timely responses to patient needs;
(d) patient education concerning heart failure.

Specialized heart failure centers can provide expertise in the medical and surgical management of heart failure [36]. Surgical therapy for heart failure (high-risk standard cardiac surgical procedures, transplantation, mechanical circulatory assist devices, ventricular remodeling procedures (partial left ventriculectomy, Dor procedure, Acorn device®, Myosplint®), transmyocardial laser revascularization,

etc.) has become an essential component and now extends far beyond transplantation [37]. Many high-risk patients will benefit from standard surgical procedures with a safety net of mechanical support and transplantation available at specialized heart failure centers.

Primary prevention is the solution to heart failure. However, secondary prevention strategies to alleviate morbidity and reduce mortality are the immediate focus to reduce the burden of this global pandemic.

References

1 Garg R, Packer M, Pitt B, Yusaf S. Heart failure in the 1990s: evolution of a major public health problem in cardiovascular medicine. *J Am Coll Cardiol* 1993; **22(Suppl A)**: 3A–5A.

2 National Heart Lung and Blood Institute. *Congestive Heart Failure in the United States: A New Epidemic.* US Department of Health and Human Services, Bethesda, MD, 1996.

3 Hunt SA, Baker DW, Chin MH *et al.* ACC/AHA guidelines for the evaluation and management of chronic heart failure in the adult: executive summary a report of the American College of Cardiology/American Heart Association Task Force on practice guidelines (Committee to revise the 1995 guidelines for the evaluation and management of heart failure). Developed in collaboration with the International Society for Heart and Lung Transplantation; endorsed by the Heart Failure Society of America. *Circulation* 2001; **104(24)**: 2996–3007.

4 McMurray JJ, Stewart S. Epidemiology, aetiology, and prognosis of heart failure. *Heart* 2000; **83**: 596–602.

5 Eriksson H. Heart failure: a growing public health problem. *J Intern Med* 1995; **237**: 135–141.

6 McCullough PA, Philbin EF, Spertus JA *et al.* Confirmation of a heart failure epidemic: findings from the resource utilization among congestive heart failure (REACH) study. *J Am Coll Cardiol* 2002; **39**: 60–69.

7 Cowie MR, Mosterd A, Wood DA *et al.* The epidemiology of heart failure. *Eur Heart J* 1997; **18**: 208–225.

8 Ho KKL, Pinsky JL, Kannel WB, Levy D. The epidemiology of heart failure: The Framingham Study. *J Am Coll Cardiol* 1993; **22(Suppl A)**: 6A–13A.

9 Field JL. *Beyond Four Walls: Research Summary for Clinicians and Administrators on CHF Management.* Cardiology Preeminence Round Table, Advisory Board Company, Washington, DC, 1994.

10 Levy D, Kenchaiah S, Larson MG *et al.* Long-term trends in the incidence of and survival with heart failure. *N Engl J Med* 2002; **347**: 1397–1402.

11 Lloyd-Jones DM, Larson MG, Leip EP *et al.* Lifetime risk for developing congestive heart failure: The Framingham Heart Study. *Circulation* 2002; **106**: 3068–3072.

12 Smith WM. Epidemiology of congestive heart failure. *Am J Cardiol* 1985; **55**(Suppl A): 3A–8A.

13 Jong P, Vowinckel E, Liu PP *et al.* Prognosis and determinants of survival in patients newly hospitalized for heart failure. *Arch Intern Med* 2002; **162**: 1689–1694.

14 Mahon NG, Blackstone EH, Francis GS *et al.* The prognostic value of estimated creatinine clearance alongside functional capacity in ambulatory patients with chronic congestive heart failure. *J Am Coll Cardiol* 2002; **40**(6): 1106–1113.

15 Gottdiener JS, McClelland RL, Marshall R *et al.* Outcome of congestive heart failure in elderly persons: influence of left ventricular systolic function. *Ann Intern Med* 2002; **137**: 631–639.

16 Redfield MM, Jacobsen SJ, Burnett JC *et al.* Burden of systolic and diastolic ventricular dysfunction in the community; appreciating the scope of the heart failure epidemic. *J Am Med Assoc* 2003; **289**: 194–202.

17 Stewart S. Prognosis of patients with heart failure compared with common types of cancer. *Heart Fail Monit* 2003; **3**: 87–94.

18 O'Connell JB, Bristow MR. Economic impact of heart failure in the United States: time for a different approach. *J Heart Lung Transplant* 1993; **13**: S107–S112.

19 Parmley WW. Cost-effective cardiology: cost-effective management of heart failure. *Clin Cardiol* 1996; **19**: 240–242.

20 American Heart Association. *Heart and Stroke Statistical Update: Economic Cost of Cardiovascular Diseases.* American Heart Association, Dallas, TX, 2001.

21 Rich MW, Beckham V, Wittenberg C, Leven C, Freedland K, Carney R. A multidisciplinary intervention to prevent the readmission of elderly patients with congestive heart failure. *N Engl J Med* 1995; **333**: 1190–1195.

22 Mudge GH, Goldstein S, Addonizio LJ *et al.* 24th Bethesda Conference: cardiac transplantation. Task Force 3: Recipient guidelines/prioritization. *J Am Coll Cardiol* 1993; **22**: 21–31.

23 Michalsen A, Konig MA, Thimme W. Preventable causative factors leading to hospital admission with decompensated heart failure. *Heart* 1998; **80**: 437–441.

24 Anderson GF, Steinberg EP. Hospital readmission in the Medicare population. *N Engl J Med* 1984; **311**: 1349–1353.

25 Cleland JGF. Health economic consequences of the pharmacological treatment of heart failure. *Eur Heart J* 1998; **19**(Suppl P): 32–39.

26 Heart Failure Society of America Practice Guidelines. HFSA guidelines for the management of patients with heart failure due to left ventricular systolic dysfunction: pharmacological approaches. *Conges Heart Fail* 2000; **4**: 11–39.

27 Albert NM, Young JB. Heart failure disease management: a team approach. *Clev Clin J Med* 2001; **68**(1): 53–62.

28 Starling RC. The heart failure pandemic: changing patterns, costs, and treatment strategies. *Cleve Clin J Med* 1998; **65**: 351–358.

29 Kornowski R, Zeeli D, Averbuch M *et al.* Intensive homecare surveillance prevents hospitalization and improves morbidity rates among elderly patients with severe congestive heart failure. *Am Heart J* 1995; **129**: 762–766.

30 Rich MW, Nease RF. Cost-effectiveness analysis in clinical practice; the case of heart failure. *Arch Int Med* 1999; **159**: 1690–1700.

31 Baker DW, Konstam MA, Bottorff M, Pitt B. Management of heart failure I. Pharmacologic treatment. *J Am Med Assoc* 1994; **272**: 1361–1366.

32 Jessup M, Brozena S. Heart failure. *N Engl J Med* 2003; **348**: 2007–2018.

33 Bello D, Shah NB, Edep ME, Tateo IM, Massie BM. Self-reported differences between cardiologists and heart failure specialists in the management of chronic heart failure. *Am Heart J* 1999; **138**: 100–107.

34 Ansari M, Alexander M, Tutar A *et al.* Cardiology participation improves outcomes in patients with new-onset heart failure in the outpatient setting. *J Am Coll Cardiol* 2003; **41**: 62–68.

35 Nohria A, Lewis E, Stevenson LW. Medical management of advanced heart failure. *J Am Med Assoc* 2002; **287**: 628–640.

36 Abraham WT, Bristow MR. Specialized centers for heart failure management. *Circulation* 1997; **96**(9): 2755–2757.

37 O'Neill JO, Starling RC. Surgical remodeling in ischemic cardiomyopathy. *Curr Treat Option Cardiovasc Med* 2003; **5**: 311–319.

CHAPTER 2

Heart failure clinical trials: shaping the evidence for treatment guidelines

James B. Young

Introduction and overview

As has been abundantly documented, heart failure in the year 2006 remains the only cardiovascular disease or syndrome with an increasing prevalence and extraordinary morbidity and mortality [1–3]. Arguably, the syndrome has become the most important inpatient medical challenge in the United States, particularly from the economic perspective. As Figure 2.1 demonstrates, survival rates in patients with the diagnosis of congestive heart failure are improving somewhat as medical, interventional, and surgical therapies advance, but outcomes are still far from ideal. There has been a stepwise increase in the 5-year survival for both men and women diagnosed with congestive heart failure and followed in the Framingham Study between 1950 and 1999 [3]. A decade-by-decade analysis plotted in Figure 2.1 demonstrates that the 5-year survival rate for men has improved from about 30% to 40% over time. Still, the fact that the 5-year survival rate for men is only 40% (and women only about 55%) emphasizes the extraordinary challenge at hand. Certainly, a better understanding of the pathophysiology and molecular biodynamic difficulties which cause, and then perpetuate, the heart failure syndrome has led to new therapies. Perhaps longer-term outcomes will be improved with greater insight and understanding while more definitive therapeutic interventions directed at the molecular basis of remodeling and cardiac failure emerge. Ultimately, however, our goal should be prevention of heart failure in a

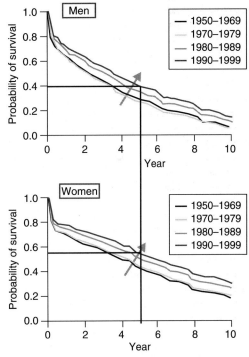

Figure 2.1 Patient survival curves for men and women followed in the Framingham study and segregated by decade of diagnosis [3]. Though there has been some improvement over time with outcomes, the 5-year survival rates for both men and women with congestive heart failure remain dismal.

fashion similar to successful prevention of infectious scourges, such as smallpox, polio, and tuberculosis. Unfortunately, unlike those communicable diseases, the pathophysiology of the heart failure syndrome is more multi-faceted and the syndrome far less well understood.

Nonetheless, over the past 25 years clinical trials have played an important and unparalleled role in shaping the evidence we now use for guiding interventions in the heart failure patient. Indeed, the emergence of "guidelines" over the past decade detailing best treatment practices have been made possible, for the most part, because of outcomes well defined and characterized by clinical trial evidence. In fact, one of the more robust arenas for practice of so-called "evidenced-based" medicine has been in patients with heart failure, and this is because of the successful completion of well over 120 clinical trials of varying size, design, and complexity [2].

Clinical trials and evidence-based medical practice

As can be seen in Figure 2.2, clinical trials play a key role in the ever cycling evidence-based medical practice. Initial clinical experience and observation of ill patients drive a desire to treat patients who have significant suffering and disability from heart failure or, for that matter, any disease. Initially, rudimentary interventions are developed that are generally based on limited understanding of disease pathophysiology and the potential for beneficial response. In the best of circumstances, research and experimentation emerge which are focused both on basic science and clinical questions, such that pathophysiologic processes, and perturbed molecular biodynamics associated with disease, become better understood. Disease paradigms can be evaluated and extrapolation then made to humans. In patients with heart failure, two excellent examples of this are the characterization of ventricular remodeling linked to disturbance of cardiac cell molecular maintenance resulting in hypertrophy and clinical heart failure in patients with chronic, poorly controlled hypertension. Another example is our present insight into how the renin–angiotensin–aldosterone system modulates molecular dynamics such that ventricular hypertrophy develops. Basic observations must be intimately linked to clinical experimentation, with therapies developed that can be subjected to individual human experimentation and randomized trials, with systematic overviews of data occasionally

done to generate hypotheses which can be studied in subsequent clinical trials.

Usually, early clinical experimentation, often limited to only a few patients, generates rudimentary treatment strategies. This leads to more carefully done, long-term, prospective, randomized, and controlled clinical trials which allow a more robust consensus to emerge and this is what sets the stage for development of treatment guidelines. A challenge is, then, to educate health care providers, patients, and the public with the knowledge gained from these clinical experiments, such that health care providers and health care systems can implement best medical practices.

Obviously, the clinical trial is key to developing guidelines as well as implementation strategies. It is within a singular clinical practice that individual patient treatment occurs, but, hopefully, utilizing guidelines that have been developed from clinical trial observations. One can then continue to objectively assess patient responses, public health issues, and implement quality improvement strategies such that the clinical outcome is improved. Obviously, observation will be cyclical with the research and experimentation chain begun again and again.

With respect to heart failure syndromes, one of the more frustrating issues is that many patients, if not most, in clinical trials do not respond to the therapeutic ministrations tested. Indeed, most "positive" randomized clinical trials done in patients with systolic left ventricular dysfunction show a reduction in mortality at 1 or 2 years of 15–30% which is usually statistically significant. This means, however, that many patients do not see benefit from intervention. Understanding why that occurs is challenging and should drive the continued cycle of repetitive clinical experimentation and trials. Unlike treating an infectious disease, we are hampered in our heart failure clinics because the syndrome is vastly more heterogeneous than lobar pneumonia caused by pneumococcal bacterium. We are further fettered by not having a "sensitivity and susceptibility" test for a specific treatment as we do for antibiotic therapy of many bacterial infections. Clinical trials would obviously be much easier to do if we could exactly determine which heart failure patient will, in fact, respond to blockade of angiotensin II receptors, for example.

Figure 2.3 summarizes the different methods of obtaining evidence that ultimately impact decision

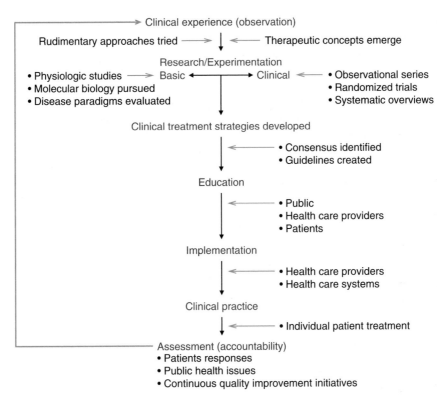

Figure 2.2 The cycle of clinical observation, experimental trial, and subsequent clinical trial that shapes the evidence supporting "evidence-based medical practice". This process is a never ending cycle.

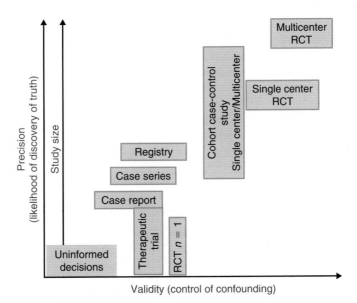

Figure 2.3 Methods of obtaining evidence with a subjective ranking of an efforts complexity, ability to control for confounding and precision (the likelihood of discovery of truth) (modified from [4]).

making in any clinical environment [4]. Of course, as can be seen in the lower left-hand corner of this figure, the least precise and most invalid method of addressing patients with heart failure is to treat them based on simple whim, prejudice, and uninformed decisions. On the other hand, the greatest control of confounding in studies, which will lead to the most precise and valid observation, is the large-scale, multi-center, randomized, properly controlled, clinical trial. Indeed, the likelihood of discovery of truth, or the precision of a trial, is often directly related to the size or power of the study. Arguably, best control of confounding is reached when one has a double-blind, placebo controlled, randomized clinical trial design, sized with statistical power enough to definitively address the hypothesis. Obviously, this can neither occur in all clinical settings, nor can every relevant question to the practice of medicine be answered in such fashion. Certainly other ways of gaining evidence can be helpful and should never be ignored. Indeed, it is the totality of evidence that is most important. Single center randomized trials, cohort case control studies, registry analysis, case series, and case reports (even with a therapeutic trial of $N = 1$) can all provide, depending on the circumstance, valuable information. Simply remember the clinical story of heart transplantation. Nonetheless, it has been multi-center, large-scale, randomized, clinical trials in patients with heart failure that has best shaped our clinical treatment guidelines.

There are some disadvantages to clinical trials. Table 2.1 puts the advantages and disadvantages of these efforts into perspective. Knowing the limitations of clinical trials can help temper interpretation of the evidence and prompt development of new clinical trial approaches. Certainly, clinical trials have a difficult time evaluating the "Art of Medicine". Medicine is, after all, still an art with respect to both professionalism and patient care. We must remember that we have an extraordinarily incomplete understanding of many disease states, including heart failure. Still, clinical trials in heart failure can only address a limited number of questions and the lengthy duration of most large-scale multi-center, heart failure trials causes inflexibility in patient management and they generally ignore advances made while the trial is ongoing. Anyone involved with design, implementation, and management of a clinical trial knows the fear of a "blockbuster" observation coming out of another trial before yours is

Table 2.1 Clinical trial advantages and problems.

Issues

Advantages
- Most precise and valid study of treatment outcomes
- Best characterization of risk/benefit ratios
- Quantify precisely outcomes
- Define adverse events

Disadvantages
- Hard to evaluate the "Art of Medicine"
- Limited number of questions can be answered
- Lengthy duration causes inflexibility and ignores intercurrent advances
- Study populations are highly biased
- Large sample size usually required
- Costs are enormous
- Generally only study "add-on" therapies in rote sequence
- Focus on observations that can easily be quantified (death)
- Ignore important issues that cannot easily be quantified (quality of life)
- Driven largely by health care industry need for regulatory approval of therapies
- Difficult to perform surgical trials

completed, particularly if it suggests that an important therapy was absent in your trial. Also problematic with clinical trials is that study populations are highly biased and large sample size is usually required. This is best illustrated by the fact that women, racial minorities, the elderly, and patients with significant co-morbidities are underrepresented in most major heart failure trials that have been done to date. Due to the complexities of study design, and number of patients required in a multi-center clinical trial, the costs of doing these studies are staggering and largely borne by the medical–industrial complex which is, for the most part, motivated by the need for regulatory approval of therapies. Obviously, this limits significantly the questions that can be studied. Clinical trials also seem to focus more on observations that can be easily quantified, such as death or hospitalization. These endpoints can be readily determined, however, adjudication of finer distinctions become problematic. For example, did a patient die because of an arrhythmia (sudden cardiac death) or was death due to progressive systemic congestion and organ malfunction? On the other hand, most clinical trials generally ignore important issues that cannot easily be quantified, such as quality of life and neurocognitive function. We have also backed ourselves into a difficult polypharmacy corner because clinical trials usually just "add on" one therapy after another, so that at the end of the day, "standard therapies" in patients with heart failure require utilization of many different drugs including an angiotensin-converting enzyme (ACE) inhibitor, an angiotensin II receptor blocker, a beta-adrenergic blocker, and an aldosterone antagonist, in addition to diuretics, digoxin, and mineral supplements. Unfortunately, when the trials are lined up, it is difficult to determine if truly additive effects are apparent. Clinical trials in the future likely will compare one overall treatment paradigm against a second. Finally, it is possible, but vastly more difficult to perform trials of surgical interventions in heart failure patients and, though some have been done, better methods need to be developed to clarify risk/benefit of these procedures.

Heart failure clinical trial focus

Table 2.2 paints a broad picture of the heart failure clinical trial evolution and should be coupled to Figure 2.3, Panels (a) and (b). In the 1960s, heart failure was largely considered a "dropsical" syndrome with fluid retention creating peripheral edema, organ congestion and malfunction, and dyspnea syndromes. Rudimentary understanding of the pathophysiology of heart failure created a desire to improve cardiac contractility and relieve congestion. Limited therapies were available, however, but in the mid-1960s the loop diuretic furosemide greatly changed management strategies. Digitalis preparations, usually digoxin, were used to treat the contractility impairment. It is fascinating to review the literature which emerged in the 1950s and 1960s regarding loop diuretics and digitalis preparations. No large-scale, randomized, well-controlled clinical trials with meaningful outcomes were done. Interestingly, an extraordinary literature emerged addressing the most effective way to "digitalize" a patient and effect best blood levels, based on organ function and dose. Sadly, only more recently, has it been realized that out-comes were likely worsened with historic approaches because individuals were being overdosed! It has only been a new analysis of the seminal Digitalis Investigation Group (DIG) trial, which was originally completed

Table 2.2 Heart failure clinical trial focus.

Time period	Focus	Issues
1960–1970s	• Congestion • Blood pressure	• New diuretics • New anti-hypertensive's
1970–1990s 1985–2000s	• Hemodynamics • Neurohumors	• "Vasodilation" • RAAS modulation
2000s–present	• Biomechanical remodeling	• Surgery • CRT
Future	• Pharmacogenomics	• "Designer" drugs

RAAS: renin–aldosterone–angiotensin systems; CRT: cardiac resynchronization therapy.

and presented in 1997, that the proper dose and best therapeutic level of digoxin have finally been agreed upon [5]. In the 1960s and 1970s observational studies and a few randomized clinical trials began in earnest. It was in this environment that design considerations for heart failure studies emerged. Early clinical efforts focused on hemodynamic manipulation, particularly arterial and venous vasodilation with blood pressure lowering. Indeed, early studies in the 1950s with hexamethonium, hydralazine, and nitroglycerin characterized the beneficial clinical and hemodynamic responses that could be seen with vasodilation. At that time, proposing such studies was a radical departure from "common wisdom" because vasodilation would generally be associated with a falling blood pressure. Indeed, though that did occur, this was associated with falling pulmonary artery pressures, relief of dyspnea, and generalized clinical improvement. Interestingly, these observations led directly to a study of nitroproside in acute myocardial infarction patients which, for the most part, was a negative clinical trial. Nonetheless the first Vasodilator in Heart Failure Patient Trial (V-HeFT) reported in 1986 (Table 2.3), the reduction in morbidity and mortality that occurred when the vasodilators hydralazine and isosorbide nitrate were given together and compared to placebo in the first large-scale, randomized, clinical trial of congestive heart patients to be reported. Another control agent, prazosin, though a balanced arterial and venous dilator, was of no benefit and suggests that vasodilator actions alone could not explain observed beneficial outcomes. Another, arguably,

Table 2.3 Clinical trials shaping our therapeutic approaches.

Trial acronym (intervention tested; year published)

ACE inhibitors/angiotensin receptor blockers post-MI/CHF
- CATS (captopril) 1992
- AIRE (ramipril) 1993
- SMILE (zofenopril) 1995
- TRACE (trandolapril) 1995
- CATS (captopril) 1996
- VALIANT (valsartan) 2003

ACE inhibitors in CHF
- CONSENSUS (enalapril) 1987
- SOLVD (enalapril) 1991–1992
- V-HeFT-II (enalapril) 1991
- MHFT (captopril) 1992
- ATLAS (lisinopril) 1999
- APRES (ramipril) 2000
- OVERTURE (omapatrilat) 2001

Angiotensin receptor blockers in CHF
- ELITE (losartan) 1997
- RESOLVD (candesartan) 1999
- SPICE Trial (candesartan) 1999
- STRETCH (candesartan) 1999
- ELITE-II (losartan) 2000
- RESOLVD: B-Blocker Study (candesartan/metoprolol) 2000
- Val-HeFT (valsartan) 2000
- CHARM (candesartan) 2003

Anti-arrhythmics in CHF
- BASIS (amiodarone) 1990
- CHF-STAT (amiodarone) 1993
- GESICA (amiodarone) 1994
- SWORD (d-sotalol) 1996
- CAMIAT (amiodarone) 1997
- EMIAT (amiodarone) 1997
- DIAMOND-MI (dofetilide) 1999
- AMIOVERT (amiodarone) 2000
- DIAMOND-CHF (dofetilide) 2000
- MUSTT (variable) 2000
- PIAF (diltiazem/amiodarone) 2000

Beta-Blockers in CHF
- MDC (metoprolol) 1993
- CIBIS (bisoprolol) 1994
- MEXIS (metoprolol) 1995
- PRECISE (carvedilol) 1996
- MOCHA (carvedilol) 1996
- CIBIS-II (bisoprolol) 1999
- MERIT-HF (metoprolol cr/xl) 2000

- BEST (bucindolol) 2001
- CAPRICORN (carvedilol) 2001
- COMET (carvedilol) 2003

Calcium channel blockers in CHF
- PRAISE (amlodipine) 1996
- V-HeFT-III (felodipine) 1997
- MACH-I (mibefradil) 2000
- PRAISE II (amlodipine) 2000

Inotropes in CHF
- Enoximone: oral enoximone in moderately severe CHF (enoximone) 1990
- Xamoterol (xamoterol) 1990
- PROMISE (milrinone) 1991
- DIMT (ibopamine) 1993
- PROVED (digoxin) 1993
- RADIANCE (digoxin) 1993
- VEST (vesnarinone) 1993
- PICO (pimobendan) 1996
- DIG (digoxin) 1997
- PRIME-II (ibopamine) 1997
- LIDO (levosimendan) 2002
- OPTIME-CHF (milrinone) 2002
- ESSENTIAL (enoximone) 2005
- SURVIVE (levosimendan) 2005
- REVIVE (levosimendan) 2005

Other treatments in CHF
- RALES (spironolactone) 1999
- IMPRESS (omapatrilat) 2000
- ATTACH (infliximab) 2001
- IMAC (IVIG) 2001
- RENAISSANCE (etanercept) 2002
- EPHESUS (eplerenone) 2003
- OPT-CHF (oxypurinol) 2005
- ACCLAIM (immune modulation) 2006

Vasodilators in CHF
- V-HeFT-I (hydralazine/isosorbide dinitrate) 1986
- Hy-C (hydrazaline) 1992
- PROFILE (flosequinan) 1993
- REFLECT (flosequinan) 1993
- FIRST (prostacyclin) 1997
- MOXCON (moxonidine) 1999
- ENABLE I & II (bosentan) 2001
- RITZ (tezosentan) 2001
- EARTH (darosentan) 2002
- VMAC (nesiritide) 2002
- A-HeFT (bidil) 2004

ACE: angiotensin-converting enzyme; CHF: congestive heart failure; IVIG: intravenous immunoglobulin; MI: myocardial infarction; acronyms for clinical trials not listed. For complete list of trials see [1].

more interesting and even earlier study, the Beta-Blocker Heart Attack Trial (BHAT), reported in 1982 (Table 2.3) on a large subset of heart failure patients post-myocardial infarction who received inderal in a randomized, multi-center, placebo controlled clinical trial and demonstrated that the patients gaining the most benefit were those significantly ill in the peri-infarct setting having congestive heart failure! It is hard to recall now, but giving a beta-blocker to a patient of this sort in the late 1970s and early 1980s was believed to be irresponsible.

The original V-HeFT Trial lead to the "vasodilator in heart failure" hypothesis which was pursued for many years. Interestingly, the ACE inhibitor trials were developed because this agents were believed to be effective "vasodilators" and anti-hypertensive agents not because they were significant modulators of the renin–angiotensin system. The successes of heart failure trials with ACE inhibitors did, once the importance of the renin–angiotensin–aldosterone system was identified, usher in the "neurohumoral modulation" hypothesis for heart failure therapies.

Table 2.3 and Figure 2.4 (a) and (b) list the acronyms of seminal trials that emerged after the original vasodilator studies were performed [5]. These trials have focused largely on ACE inhibitors, angiotensin receptor blockers, anti-arrhythmics, beta-adrenergic receptor blockers, calcium channel blockers, a variety of inotropes and "inodilators" (agents with varying degrees of inotropic effects and vasodilators), and a variety of other more direct-acting atrial and venous vasodilators, and other therapies in heart failure. It is less important to know the acronym definition than the intervention studied and the year observations were presented. More detailed descriptions of the studies can be found in the Clinical Trials Database maintained by the American College of Cardiology [5]. In summary, it has been these trials, along with the defibrillator and cardiac resynchronization studies detailed in Table 2.4, that created our therapeutic knowledge base in heart failure and upon which the heart failure treatment guidelines summarized in Figure 2.5 rest.

Simply stated, ACE inhibitors are clearly indicated to reduce morbidity and mortality after a myocardial infarction when significant left ventricular dysfunction and heart failure are present. The angiotensin receptor blocking agent valsartan has been studied in this setting as well, and compared to an ACE inhibitor, arguably, has equivalent benefit. ACE inhibitors have also been demonstrated to be the underpinning therapeutic agent in all patients with symptomatic left ventricular systolic dysfunction and many believe these drugs can prevent the development of symptomatic heart failure in individuals at risk or with asymptomatic left ventricular systolic dysfunction. More recently, angiotensin receptor blockers, particularly candesartan and valsartan, have also been demonstrated to be effective in patients with symptomatic left ventricular systolic dysfunction. Some believe that angiotensin receptor blockers produce benefit of equivalent magnitude compared to ACE inhibitors. Interestingly, a combination of candesartan and an ACE inhibitor can achieve added improvement, at least as noted in one of the CHARM Trials [5]. Beta-adrenergic blockers represent another group of drugs quite beneficial in heart failure patients. Carvedilol, sustained release metoprolol, and biosoprolol all have demonstrated impressive results in heart failure patient populations. Indeed, it is the combination of beta-adrenergic blockers and ACE inhibitors (or angiotensin receptor blockers) that, today, remains the basic approach for heart failure patient management. Interestingly, anti-arrhythmic agents and calcium channel blockers have not lived up to original expectations with respect to morbidity and mortality reduction in heart failure populations. As heart failure patients have a very high risk of sudden cardiac death, one would have thought that anti-arrhythmic drugs would be helpful. Most anti-arrhythmic agents have not been associated with benefit and, indeed, some such as pronestyl and quinidine, among others, are linked to worse outcomes in individuals with heart failure. Amiodarone is the one anti-arrhythmic drug which, arguably, has demonstrated some benefit in highly select patients studied in clinical trials, but when this approach is compared to implantation of a defibrillator or cardiac resynchronization device the benefits pale in comparison. Calcium channel blockers, once thought ideal agents for heart failure because of their excellent tolerability and effectiveness as anti-hypertensive agents (secondary to vasodilation), have not demonstrated benefit in the clinical trials listed in Table 2.3.

One of the more contentious questions is related to the role of inotropes in patients with heart failure. Obviously, when patients are identified as having

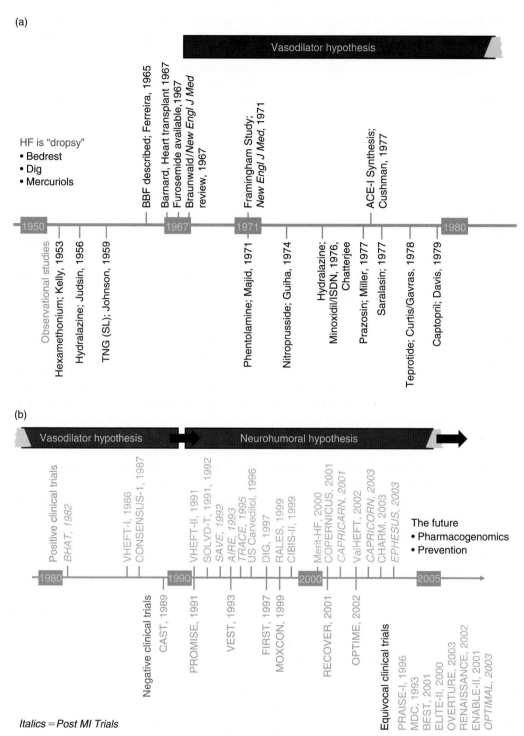

Figure 2.4 Parts (a) and (b) comprise a timeline of observational and randomized clinical trials performed over the last half century that have guided our heart failure treatment practices and provided the evidence for clinical treatment guidelines [2,5].

HF: heart failure; MI: myocardial infarction.

Table 2.4 Defibrilator and cardiac resynchronization trials.

Trial acronym (intervention tested; year published)

Implantable cardioverter defibrillators in CHF
- MADIT 1996
- CABG Patch 1997
- AMIOVERT (ICD/amiodarone) 2000
- CASH 2000
- MADIT-II 2002
- MIRACLE ICD (ICD/CQT) 2003
- COMPANION (ICD/CRT) 2004
- SCD-HeFT 2005

Cardiac resynchronization therapy
- MUSIC (CRT) 2001
- MIRACLE (CRT) 2002
- COMPANION (CRT/ICD) 2002
- MIRACLE-ICD (CRT-ICD) 2003
- CARE-HP (CRT) 2005

decreased systolic left ventricular function one would think an inotrope is beneficial. This has not, however, proven the case with a variety of drugs ranging from phosphodiesterase inhibitors to calcium sensitizers and digoxin. Digoxin is the one agent which seems more clearly associated with morbidity reduction (hospitalization for heart failure), however. Whether levosimendan will prove beneficial in the long run is going to rest with final analyses of two large clinical trials, SURVIVE and REVIVE, presented at the 2005 annual American Heart Association meeting. There was some suggestion in the REVIVE Trial that acute administration of intravenous levosimendan beneficially affected a quality of life and re-hospitalization endpoint. The SURVIVE Trials suggested that dobutamine and levosimendan with respect to long-term morbidity had similar outcomes. Many other treatments for heart failure have been studied with variable results. Blocking the aldosterone pathways with spironolactone or eplerenone has proven effective in heart failure patients with left ventricular systolic dysfunction generally (RALES) and in postmyocardial infarction heart failure more specifically (EPHESUS). On the other hand, omapatrilat and oxypurinol did not prove efficacious in heart failure clinical trials. Immune modulation with antitumor necrosis factor (TNF) antibodies also did not benefit patients and there was some suggestion that infliximab could actually be harmful in this patient population. We are awaiting additional clinical trials of immune-modulation efforts to determine if this is a viable strategy for heart failure patients.

Vasodilators also have been somewhat disappointing in heart failure patients with a few exceptions. The previously mentioned hydralazine and isosorbide nitrate combination studied in the V-HeFT Trial led to an interesting clinical trial of a proprietary combination of these drugs in African Americans, the A-HEF Trial which demonstrated rather profound effects on mortality and morbidity in patients of African American heritage. Centrally blocking the alpha-adrenergic pathways with moxonidine seemed to create detriment as was also seen with studies of flosequinan and prostacycline. Vasodilators operating by blocking endothelin (bosentan, tezosentan, and darosentan) have also been disappointing, and these agents likely will no longer be pursued in patients with congestive heart failure.

Finally, as listed in Table 2.4 several clinical trials have definitively addressed the question of automatic implantable cardioverter defibrillators and cardiac resynchronization devices in patients with symptomatic systolic left ventricular dysfunction. Clearly, in individuals similar to those studied in the clinical trials, these devices are extraordinarily important. Indeed, in some individuals with wide QRS complexes, mitral regurgitation, and ischemic heart disease predisposing them to a sudden cardiac death risk, the impact has been rather dramatic and far superior to treatment with pharmaco-therapeutic strategies only.

Clinical trial-based therapeutic guidelines

Figure 2.5 summarizes the most recent (2005) American College of Cardiology and American Heart Association "stages" in the development of heart failure and recommended therapies. Therapeutic recommendations are linked to the clinical trials with the compendium of evidence available determining the strength of the recommendation. Stage A patients are individuals at high risk for the development of heart failure but without structural heart disease or symptoms of heart failure. These are represented by patients with hypertension, atherosclerotic cardiovascular disease, diabetes, obesity, the metabolic syndrome, or patients undergoing therapy

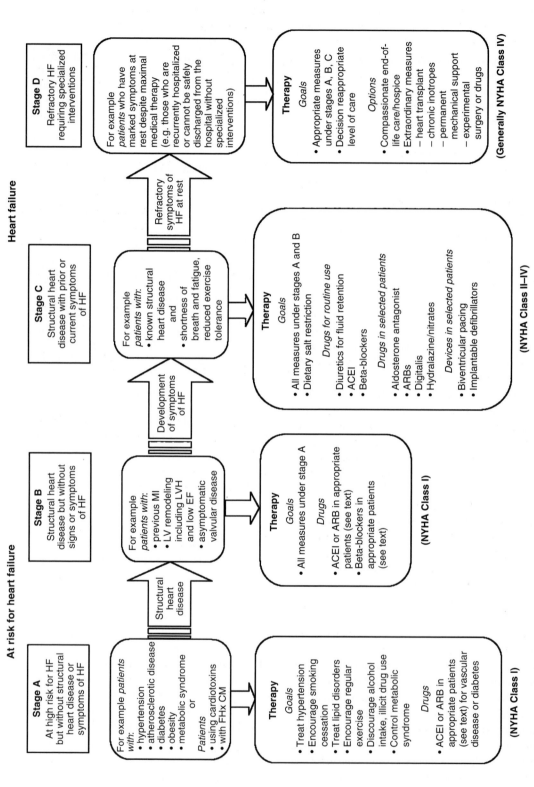

Figure 2.5 American College of Cardiology and American Heart Association "Stages" in the development of heart failure and treatment guidelines [2]. NYHA: New York Heart Association; ARB: angiotensin receptor blockers; HF: heart failure; ACEI: angiotensin converting enzyme inhibitor.

with cardiotoxins, such as adriamycin and those with a familial history of cardiomyopathy. Therapeutic recommendations based on clinical (largely studies in hypertensive and diabetic patients) suggest that one should treat the hypertension, control atherosclerotic risk factors, and consider prescription of an ACE inhibitor or angiotensin receptor blocker in appropriate patients having vascular disease and diabetes. Stage B heart failure includes those with structural heart disease but without signs or symptoms of heart failure and, like Stage A patients, are generally New York Heart Association functional Class I. These are characterized by individuals having a previous myocardial infarction or demonstrating left ventricular hypertrophy with systolic or diastolic dysfunction. An individual with asymptomatic valvular heart disease would also be correctly classified as having Stage B heart failure. In these patients, all measures detailed under Stage A are appropriate and, in addition, prescription of an ACE inhibitor or angiotensin receptor blocker and beta-adrenergic blocker is generally appropriate. When a Stage B heart failure patient develops symptoms, the transition is made to Stage C which characterizes individuals having structural heart disease and prior or current symptoms. These patients present with shortness of breath, fatigue, and reduced exercise tolerance. Therapy begins with all measures for Stages A and B patients, dietary salt restriction, diuretics for fluid retention, and ACE inhibitors with beta-adrenergic blockers. Other drugs in sub-select patients would be aldosterone antagonists, angiotensin receptor blockers, digitalis preparations, and the combination of hydralazine and isosorbide nitrate. It is also in these patients who, despite best medical therapy, remain symptomatic that cardiac resynchronization with a biventricular pacemaker would be appropriate. These Stage C patients are generally New York Heart Association Class II–IV. Also certain patients in this group could benefit with an implantable defibrillator. Finally, Stage D represents refractory heart failure requiring specialized interventions and frequent hospitalizations. Compassionate end of life care may be most appropriate but some are candidates for cardiac transplantation, chronic inotropic infusion, permanent mechanical circulatory support, or experimental surgery or drugs. These patients are generally New York Heart Association functional Class IV.

Future directions for heart failure clinical trials

In the future, it is likely that heart failure clinical trials will continue with great vigor because of the challenge outlined at the beginning of this chapter. Certainly, polypharmacy is daunting and hopefully we will see fewer "add-on" trials. Polypharmacy limits patient compliance and since most agents studied to-date lower blood pressure and worsen renal function, there are limitations we have with the intensity of vaso-active medications we can give. Furthermore, blocking individual receptor sites may not be adequate to force a de-remodeling process as drivers for this pathologic event are heterogeneous and redundant. Future clinical trials, in all likelihood, will delve a bit deeper into determining clinical predictors of beneficial outcomes. Indeed, as alluded to, perhaps only 30% of a study population responds to any intervention. By gaining more insight into heart failure pathophysiology, we likely will be able to define more specifically which patients will benefit from which specific therapy. Clinical trials will also explore pharmacogenetic and genomic

Table 2.5 Future directions for heart failure clinical trials.

Emerging principals

- Polypharmacy daunting
  - Limits of patient compliance
  - Only so much blood pressure/renal function to work with
  - Remodeling drivers heterogeneous and redundant
- Clinical predictors of beneficial outcomes limited
  - Perhaps 30% of study population respond favorably
  - Incomplete insight into heart failure pathophysiology still exists
- Pharmacogenomics largely ignored today
  - Genetic links to heart failure ill characterized
  - Environmental modifiers of genetic predisposition to heart failure is plastic
- Better definitions of patient populations needed
  - "Systolic" versus "diastolic" heart failure
  - "Congestive" versus "non-congestive" states better recognized
  - Co-morbidities deserve better attention (diabetes, renal insufficiency, anemia, etc.)
- Clinical trials must better represent "real world clinical practice"

issues, perhaps better defining environmental modifiers of genetic predisposition to heart failure. We
also need to do a better job of defining heart failure
patient populations in our clinical trials and focus
more on "diastolic" heart failure, though representing
half of the patients admitted to the hospital with
congestive heart failure have yet to be studied
intensely. Clinical trials will also have to better characterize co-morbidities in the heart failure setting,
particularly diabetes, renal insufficiency, and anemia. Finally, heart failure clinical trials in the future
must better represent a real world clinical practice and have patient entry specifically linked to
older, female, and multi-co-morbidity populations
(Table 2.5).

References

1   Young JB, Mills RM. *Clinical Management of Heart Failure*,
    2nd edn. Professional Communications, Caddo, OK, 2004.
2   Hunt SA, Abraham WT, Chin MH *et al.* ACC/AHA 2005
    Guideline update for the diagnosis and management of
    chronic heart failure in the adult: summary article.
    Circulation 2005; **112**: 105–167.
3   Levi D, Kenchaiah S, Larson MG, Benjamin EJ, Kopka MJ,
    Ho KK *et al.* Long term trends in the incidence of and sur-
    vival of heart failure. *N Engl J Med* 2002; **347**: 1397–1402.
4   Engels EA, Spitz MR. Pace-setting research. *Lancet* 1997;
    350: 677–678.
5   Lewis RP, O'Gara PT, Freezinger GC, Hirsch GA. *Adult
    Clinical Cardiology Self Assessment Program.* Version 6.
    ACC Foundation, 2005. Clinical Trials Database.

CHAPTER 3

Standard medical therapy of heart failure

Mohamad H. Yamani

Heart failure continues to emerge as a rapidly growing clinical problem with an immense socio-economic burden that is associated with a rising incidence and prevalence driven by the aging of the world population [1,2]. It represents the most frequent cause of hospitalization in the Medicare population. It is estimated that 10% of patients over the age of 75 years have heart failure. In 2001, 4.7 million Americans were alive with CHF spending an estimated $21.0 billion for direct and indirect costs on this devastating disease [3].

Despite major advances in the pathophysiologic understanding of heart failure, the morbidity and mortality rates of these patients continue to rise reflecting thus, the complexity and heterogeneity of this lethal disease. The last two decades have witnessed an evolution of therapeutic strategies and an intense investigation of novel pharmacotherapy that resulted in improved survival and quality of life for patients with this syndrome. Unfortunately, many patients remain suboptimally treated because many of these advances have not been translated into clinical practice use [4].

The goal of this chapter is to provide an integrated approach to the medical management of chronic heart failure directed towards symptom control, preventing progression of left ventricular dysfunction, and improving survival (Table 3.1). Standard medical therapy comprises five classes of drugs: digitalis, diuretics, direct-acting vasodilators, neurohumoral antagonists, and beta-adrenergic receptor blockers. Guidelines for medical therapy are linked to staging the severity of the heart failure

Table 3.1 Standard medical therapy of heart failure.

Class	Improve symptoms	Reversal of LV remodeling	Improve survival
Digitalis	+	0	0
Diuretics	+	0	0
Spironolactone	+	+	+
ACE inhibitors	+	+	+
ARBs	+	+	+
Vasodilators			
Hydralazine + nitrates	+	0	+
Amlodipine	+	0	0
Beta-blockers	+	+	+
Inotropes	+	0	0

LV: left ventricle; ACE: angiotensin converting enzyme; ARBS: angiotensin receptor blockers.

syndrome with angiotensin-converting enzyme (ACE) inhibitors and beta-blockers as the cornerstones of pharmacological therapy.

Digitalis glycosides

The Digitalis Investigation Group trial (DIG-trial) has shed light on the 200-year-old controversy surrounding the use of digoxin in heart failure [5]. Several prior minor clinical trials and two large withdrawal studies, PROVED (Prospective Randomized Study of Ventricular Function and

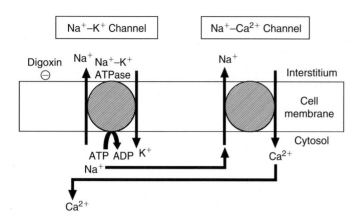

Figure 3.1 Sodium pump inhibition by Digoxin. The sodium pump is responsible for the active (ATP consuming) transport of the monovalent cations Na^+ and K^+. The sodium–calcium channel exchanges $3\,Na^+$ ions for every Ca^{2+} ion during cellular depolarization. Digoxin inhibits the Na^+–K^+-ATPase pump, which increases the intracellular Na^+ concentration that in turn activates the Na^+–Ca^{2+} exchange mechanism, which leads to an increase in intracellular Ca^{2+} resulting in a positive inotropic effect.

Efficacy of Digoxin) [6] and RADIANCE (Randomized Assessment of Digoxin and Inhibitors of Angiotensin-Converting Enzyme) [7], have demonstrated efficacy of digoxin in the symptomatic treatment of systolic heart failure. Digoxin withdrawal has been consistently associated with clinical deterioration. When patients were randomly assigned to either continue active digoxin therapy or to withdraw from active therapy and receive a matching placebo, 40% of patients in the PROVED trial and 28% of patients in the RADIANCE trial who received placebo noted a significant worsening of heart failure symptoms compared with 20% and 6%, respectively, in patients who continued to receive digoxin. Deterioration was noted irrespective of whether patients were receiving background therapy with diuretics alone or diuretics plus ACE inhibitors. Recently, the data from PROVED and RADIANCE were further analyzed to determine whether there was a relationship between serum digoxin concentration and clinical efficacy related to digoxin in patients with symptomatic left ventricular dysfunction [8]. It was noted that the beneficial effects of digoxin on common clinical end points in patients with heart failure were similar, regardless of serum digoxin concentration. Although the withdrawal design may be biased in favor of the drug and cannot establish safety, the DIG trial has resolved these issues [5]. In that study with nearly 8000 randomized patients with New York Heart Association (NYHA) class I–III CHF, digoxin treatment had neither a beneficial nor an adverse effect on all-cause mortality. There was a significant decrease in deaths due to CHF but a counterbalancing trend toward an increase in deaths ascribed

to arrhythmias and acute myocardial infarction (MI). The DIG trial, like previous studies, found that digoxin therapy was associated with a 28% reduction in patients hospitalized for CHF (from 32.5% to 25.1%, $P < 0.001$). This benefit tended to be greater in patients with lower ejection fractions, non-ischemic cardiomyopathy, more severe symptoms and larger cardiothoracic ratios on radiography.

All major clinical practice guidelines and consensus recommendations (ACC/AHA) [9] for heart failure has recommended digoxin for patients who continue to be symptomatic despite adequate treatment with an ACE inhibitor and a diuretic.

Digoxin is an inhibitor of the Na^+/K^+-ATPase pump (Figure 3.1), which increases the intracellular sodium concentration that in turn activates the Na^+/Ca^{2+} exchange mechanism, which leads to an increase in intracellular Ca^{2+} [10]. Activation of cardiac ryanodine receptors has also been described [11]. These processes serve as the underlying mechanisms for digoxin's inotropic activity, although the clinical benefits of digoxin are thought to be primarily related to its modulating neurohormonal effects [12]. These effects result in a decrease in serum norepinephrine concentration [13], improved baroreceptor function [14], and a decrease in sympathetic nerve activity [15]. Digoxin also has important electrophysiologic effects that result in a decrease in atrioventricular node conduction [16]. These electrophysiologic effects may sound like an attractive therapeutic strategy for the control of the ventricular rate in patients with atrial fibrillation. However, the clinical efficacy of digoxin in this group of patients is controversial. This controversy has been fueled recently by the finding that digoxin potentiates the shortening of atrial effective refractory period, and hence, its use may in fact facilitate short-term recurrences and predisposes toward further episodes of atrial fibrillation [17].

Although clinical data has firmly established a role for digoxin therapy in patients who have symptomatic CHF with reduced systolic function, debate will continue concerning its use in patients with dilated cardiomyopathy and few symptoms and when it should be initiated in relation to other medications. Further, little is known about the role of digoxin in the presence of diastolic dysfunction. It has recently been argued that digoxin may have a potential benefit in patients with preserved left ventricular systolic function based on a subgroup analysis of the DIG trial which showed a similar reduction in heart failure hospitalization endpoint in such patients as was achieved in patients with ejection fraction less than 45% [18]. Whether a future study would be conducted to address this specific issue is unlikely, and therefore, the controversy over the use of digoxin may not come to an end.

Diuretics

Salt and water retention comprises one of the hallmarks of chronic heart failure. It results from the activation of neurohormonal system and although it is usually apparent on physical examination, it may be subclinical or even absent. Even when there is no evidence of fluid retention, normal intravascular volumes may be associated with elevated ventricular filling pressures during physical activity. The predominant impact of diuretic therapy is to reduce left ventricular filling pressure and relieve congestion as illustrated by the Frank–Starling curve in Figure 3.2 (from point A to B). Diuretics have also been reported to improve cardiac performance at rest and during exercise shifting the curve upward and to the left (Figure 3.2, new point D) [19,20]. Some of these hemodynamic benefits are likely due to the release of vasodilatory prostaglandins with secondary reduction in systemic vascular resistance, improvement in neurohormonal system and resultant vasodilatation [21,22]. A decrease in chamber radius results with reduction in wall stress (Laplace effect) and hence, improvement in myocardial oxygen demands [19]. Diuretic-induced volume reduction also decreases secondary mitral regurgitation

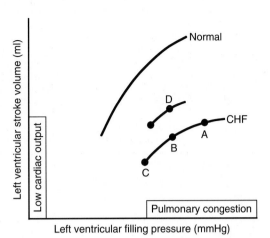

Figure 3.2 Frank–Starling curve in normal subject and heart failure patients.

and thereby improves cardiac output [23]. Thus, diuretics produce rapid hemodynamic and clinical improvement in most symptomatic patients. Despite these initial improvements, which may be sustained during chronic treatment [24], diuretics have not been subjected to rigorous mortality trials with clinical endpoints. Of course, it would be ethically challenging to conduct such a trial in patients with advanced and overt heart failure symptoms where the need for diuresis is essential to alleviate the fluid overload status.

Diuretic therapy is usually initiated with restriction of daily salt intake (1.5–2.0 g). However, judicious use of diuretics is required since over-diuresis may in fact lead to reduction in cardiac output as the patient may move from the flat segment to the ascending portion (Figure 3.2, new point C) of the Starling curve. Aggressive diuresis is associated with further activation of the renin–angiotensin–aldosterone system and the sympathetic nervous system, as well as with electrolyte imbalances, so it is preferable to combine these agents with ACE inhibitors in most cases. Some patients with mild symptoms obtain adequate symptom relief from ACE inhibitors alone, but they are the exception rather than the rule. In contrast, asymptomatic patients with left ventricular dysfunction usually do not require diuretic therapy.

Diuretics comprise a group of four classes [25] that act on different sites in the nephron (Figure 3.3,

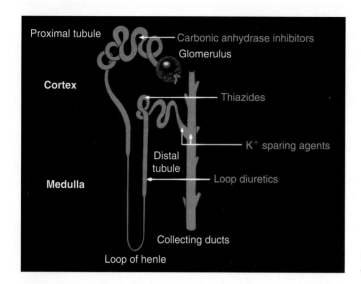

Proximal tubule — Carbonic anhydrase inhibitors
Glomerulus

Cortex

Thiazides

K⁺ sparing agents

Distal
tubule

Medulla

Loop diuretics

Collecting ducts

Loop of henle

Figure 3.3 Sites of action of different diuretics on the nephron.

Table 3.2). Acetazolamide, a carbonic anhydrase inhibitor, acts on the proximal tubule. The "loop" diuretics consist of sulfonamide derivatives (bumetanide, furosemide) and non-sulfonamide derivatives (ethacrynic acid, torsemide), which act on the ascending loop of Henle, and are considered to be most potent. Thiazides, indapamide, and metolazone act on the early portion of the distal convoluted tubule, and are moderately potent. The "potassium-sparing" spironolactone, amiloride, and triamterene are mildly potent and act on the late portion of the distal tubule and in the collecting duct.

Thiazide diuretics may be sufficient in patients with mild symptoms and are preferable in hypertensive individuals, as they provide more prolonged blood pressure control [26]. Loop diuretics are required in most patients with moderate-to-severe symptoms [27]. Because an intraluminal threshold must be exceeded to obtain the desired effect, greater diuresis is best achieved by increasing the amount of each dose. Divided doses are appropriate to prolong the period of diuresis. When it is difficult to obtain and adequate diuresis or if the total daily dose becomes high (above 320 mg of furosemide), a useful strategy is to combine diuretics with different sites of action [28]. Metolazone, because it is effective even in patients with substantial reductions in glomerular filtration rate, is often used in this setting [29], and the combination of metolazone and a loop diuretic is the most effective approach to stabilizing refractory patients [30]. Several factors

Table 3.2 Select diuretics in heart failure.

Agent	Initial dose (mg)	Recommended maximum dose (mg)
Hydrochlorothiazide	25 qd	50 qd
Metolazone	2.5 qd	10 bid
Furosemide	20 qd	240 bid
Torsemide	10 qd	200 qd
Bumetanide	0.5 qd	10 qd
Spironolactone	25 qd	100 bid

contribute to the appearance of diuretic resistance, a phenomenon seen in as many as 1 in 3 patients with CHF [31]. Renal blood flow and glomerular filtration rate are reduced. Increased neuroendocrine activity increases the proximal tubular absorption of sodium. Loop diuretics flood the distal nephron with sodium, which induces hypertrophy of the tubular cells, thereby increasing their reabsorptive capacity for sodium. Together, these developments result in a reduction of the fractional excretion of sodium and the development of resistance to the natriuretic activity of diuretic monotherapy. Further, bowel edema, which impairs drug absorption, and use of non-steroidal anti-inflammatory agents, which impair the natriuretic effects of loop diuretics, also contribute to the diuretic resistance phenomenon. The combination of a loop diuretic and thiazide may achieve a significantly greater diuresis than doubling the doses of either alone. However, caution must be exercised to avoid severe electrolyte disturbances, and intermittent metolazone administration is preferred. The addition of low doses of spironolactone (12.5–50.0 mg a day) may also be helpful, even in patients receiving ACE inhibitors, although careful monitoring of K^+ is essential.

Because of the impressive results of the ACE inhibitor trial and the desire to avoid hypotension and renal dysfunction while administering these agents, many physicians are under-utilizing diuretics. A noteworthy diuretic withdrawal trial demonstrated that a large number of heart failure patients require diuretic treatment, and that substitution of an ACE inhibitor is not usually sufficient [32].

Important side effects of diuretics include electrolyte and metabolic abnormalities, such as hyponatremia, hypokalemia, metabolic alkalosis, increased uric acid, hyperglycemia, and insulin resistance. The use of potassium-sparing diuretics may be helpful to reduce the severity of hypokalemia. Other specific side effects include ototoxicity of furosemide, and gynecomastia and galactorrhea associated with spironolactone.

Interest in spironolactone in the management of heart failure has resurged since the inception of the Randomized Aldactone Evaluation Study (RALES), which showed 30% reduction in the risk of death, 35% reduction in hospitalizations related to worsening heart failure and a significant improvement in heart failure symptoms among patients treated with Aldactone [33]. Spironolactone has been shown to attenuate the process of myocardial fibrosis [34,35], and induce a favorable sympathovagal response with improved heart rate variability [35,36]. Other studies have also shown that spironolactone improves endothelial dysfunction, increases nitric oxide bioactivity, and inhibits vascular angiotensin I (AI)/ angiotensin II (AII) conversion in patients with heart failure, providing thus, novel mechanisms for its beneficial impact on cardiovascular mortality [37]. The role of aldosterone antagonism was further examined in post-infarction heart failure in the Eplerenone Post-Acute Myocardial Infarction Heart Failure Efficacy and Survival (EPHESUS) study [38]. During a mean follow-up of 16 months, the use of eplerenone, a selective aldosterone antagonist, was associated with a relative risk reduction of 15% in total mortality ($P = 0.008$). The rate of the other

primary end point, death from cardiovascular causes or hospitalization for cardiovascular events, was reduced by eplerenone (relative risk: 0.87, $P = 0.002$), as was the rate of sudden death from cardiac causes (relative risk: 0.79, $P = 0.03$). The results of both RALES [33] and EPHESUS [38] provide strong evidence for the addition of an aldosterone antagonist to optimal conventional therapy in patients with CHF and reduced left ventricular systolic function.

Direct-acting vasodilators

The rationale for vasodilator therapy has evolved from the recognition that cardiac performance could be modulated by altering loading conditions. A wide variety of vasoactive medications have been investigated, and most have been found to produce acute, and in some cases sustained, hemodynamic improvement. Among the non-parenteral direct-acting vasodilators, only hydralazine and nitrates have been shown to positively affect clinical endpoints. However, several other vasodilators, such as prazosin, minoxidil, flosequinan, epoprostenol and some calcium channel blockers have been found to be ineffective or even resulted in adverse effects.

The best evidence for a beneficial effect of direct-acting vasodilators comes from the Vasodilator-Heart Failure Trial (V-HeFT) studies [39,40], which showed that chronic therapy with hydralazine 300 mg a day and isosorbide 160 mg a day increased exercise tolerance and prolonged survival. Symptom and exercise improvement were at least as great as with enalapril, but the latter agent was associated with better survival. Because of the latter finding and the better side effect profile of ACE inhibitors, direct-acting vasodilators are used primarily in patients who are not candidates for ACE inhibitors or who do not tolerate them. Nitrates and hydralazine are also reasonable agents to add for patients who remain symptom-limited on optimal therapy with diuretics, ACE inhibitors, and beta-blockers. Recently, the addition of a fixed dose of isosorbide dinitrate plus hydralazine to standard therapy for heart failure including neurohormonal blockers was found to be efficacious and improve survival among African American patients with advanced heart failure [41]. The study was terminated early due to a significantly higher mortality rate in the placebo group than in the group given isosorbide dinitrate plus hydralazine (10.2% versus 6.2%, $P = 0.02$). The results of this study does not however preclude the possibility of survival benefit in other ethnic groups. It might have been ideal to compare this combination to conventional therapy (which by present standards includes an ACE inhibitor and a beta-blocker) for all patients with heart failure, regardless of race. Because mitral regurgitation is frequent in severe heart failure and is afterload-dependent, hydralazine may be particularly useful when regurgitation is substantial [42]. Nitrate tolerance limits the efficacy of these agents. However, the concomitant use of hydralazine may prevent tolerance to the hemodynamic effects of nitrates by scavenging free oxygen radicals [43].

Calcium channel blockers have fueled some interest to treat heart failure, as these agents are both potent vasodilators and effective for other cardiovascular conditions. However, the first-generation calcium channel blockers, including the dihydropyridine nifedipine, showed disappointing results in patients with symptomatic heart failure or severe left ventricular dysfunction [44–46].The second-generation dihydropyridines were expected to be of more value, and of all the calcium channel blockers, these drugs were the ones most studied in patients with heart failure. Amlodipine, which improved exercise capacity, had a neutral effect on mortality in a large morbidity and mortality trial known as the Prospective Randomized Amlodipine Survival Evaluation (PRAISE) trial [47]. This trial enrolled 1153 patients with severe NYHA class III and IV heart failure and ejection fractions of less than 30%. Overall there was no difference in mortality between the amlodipine and placebo-treated patients, establishing for the first time the safety of a calcium channel blocker in patients with heart failure. Amlodipine has higher selectivity for the pulmonary and coronary vasculature than do the first-generation calcium channel antagonists, and it lacks the negative inotropic properties associated with diltiazem and verapamil. These pharmacologic features may explain its neutral effect on mortality in this trial. An interesting finding, was that the patients clinically classified as having non-ischemic cardiomyopathy had 45% lower mortality on amlodipine. However, this survival benefit has not been reproduced by the subsequent randomized PRAISE II

trial [48]. The neutral effects of amlodipine suggest safety and thus, make it possible to recommend amlodipine for the treatment of angina and hypertension in patients with reduced ejection fractions or symptomatic heart failure.

Felodipine (another new calcium channel blocker) in the Vasodilator-Heart Failure Trial III (V-HeFT-III), exerted a well-tolerated additional sustained vasodilator effect in patients with heart failure treated with enalapril, but the only possible long-term benefit was a trend for better exercise tolerance [49]. However, no survival benefit was noted with this agent.

Mibefradil, a T-type calcium channel blocker, had no significant effect on morbidity or mortality in patients with moderate-to-severe heart failure in the Mortality Assessment in CHF Trial (MACH-1 study) [50]. In fact, there was a trend for increased mortality with mibefradil in the first 3 months in patients with severe heart failure especially those who were receiving amiodarone.

The above studies, therefore, do not support the concept that a dihydropyridine calcium antagonist can strikingly augment the favorable clinical response to ACE inhibitors in heart failure. Nonetheless, amlodipine and felodipine can be used safely in patients with heart failure if used for another indication requiring vasodilatation as in patients with hypertension or valvular regurgitation.

Neurohumoral antagonists

ACE inhibitors
The discovery of ACE inhibitors has significantly altered the natural history of CHF over the past two decades. Although the use of these agents stem from the fact that plasma renin activity and other components of the renin–angiotensin system are elevated in CHF, it is now clear that ACE inhibitors are effective even in patients with normal circulating levels of these hormones [51]. This discordance is likely explained by the importance of the tissue renin–angiotensin system, the inhibition of bradykinin degradation, and resulting increase in prostaglandin levels and endothelial release of nitric oxide (Figure 3.4). ACE inhibitors inhibit the conversion of AI to AII in the vasculature by blocking the ACE enzyme. They enhance the actions of kinins and augment kinin-mediated prostaglandin

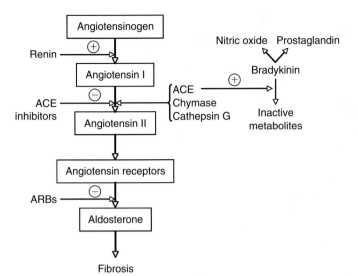

Figure 3.4 The effect of ACE inhibitors and ARBs on the renin–angiotensin system. ACE inhibitors by blocking ACE cause an increase in bradykinin, which results in an increase in nitric oxide and prostaglandins.

synthesis. ACE inhibitors decrease both preload and afterload, and improve cardiac function with significant and sustained hemodynamic benefits [52].

ACE inhibitors have been shown to improve exercise tolerance over a period of weeks to months in patients with mild-to-moderate heart failure [53]. Chronic therapy has been associated with improved peripheral vasodilation and enhanced tissue oxygen extraction [54]. The benefits of ACE inhibitors also included improvement in endothelial function [55], reduction of cardiac fibrosis [56], reversal of ventricular remodeling [57] and favorable effects on coronary vascular events [58].

The clinical benefits of ACE inhibitors on symptoms and survival have been demonstrated in several trials in patients with severe heart failure (Cooperative New Scandinavian Enalapril Survival Study, CONSENSUS) [59], mild-to-moderate heart failure (the original Captopril Multicenter Study, Studies of Left Ventricular Dysfunction (SOLVD) treatment trial, and V-HeFT-II) [40,60,61], and chronic or post-MI asymptomatic left ventricular systolic dysfunction (SOLVD prevention trial, Survival and Ventricular Enlargement (SAVE), Acute Infarction Ramipril Efficacy (AIRE) and others) [62–65]. These results indicate that ACE inhibitors should be used in all patients with low ejection fractions, regardless of symptoms. Six ACE inhibitors are approved for heart failure treatment: captopril, enalapril, lisinopril, fosinopril, quinapril, and trandolapril. It is recommended to up titrate dosage to

achieve desirable clinical benefit (Table 3.2). ACE inhibitors were found to be more effective in reducing mortality in the NYHA class IV patients as noted in CONSENSUS trial [59] with a reported mortality reduction of 40% compared to 8% mortality reduction in less severe heart failure, NYHA class I–II, reported in the SOLVD prevention trial [60]. Their efficacy was greatest in patients with the worst left ventricular ejection fraction [60,62]. Pooled analysis of the SOLVD prevention and treatment trials has shown that the effect of ACE inhibitors on the risk of heart failure hospitalization was less in the Africa-American population [66]. Further research is required to elucidate these ethnic differences. The SOLVD echocardiography substudy provided clear evidence that ACE inhibitors prevent the progressive increase in left ventricular mass and volume [67], suggesting thus, that the clinical benefits are related to their favorable impact on the remodeling process. However, these benefits may be attenuated with concomitant administration of aspirin [68,69]. Further, the addition of aspirin to ACE inhibitors has been noted to be associated with increased heart failure hospitalization rates suggesting the presence of a significant negative interaction between these agents [70].

The preventive use of ACE inhibitors in patients at high risk of cardiovascular events has been well illustrated in the Heart Outcomes Prevention Evaluation (HOPE) study [71] where the use of ramipril was associated with a relative risk reduction of 22%

($P < 0.001$) in the combined primary endpoint of cardiovascular death, non-fatal myocardial infarct and non-fatal stroke. The results of European trial On reduction of cardiac events with Perindopril in stable coronary artery disease (EUROPA) study were very much in accord with the results of HOPE, and extended the administration of perindopril to a wider population with coronary artery disease [72]. Treatment with perindopril was associated with 20% relative risk reduction ($P = 0.0003$) in the primary endpoint of cardiovascular death, MI and cardiac arrest. However, such a vasculoprotective effect has not been substantiated in the Prevention of Events with Angiotensin-Converting Enzyme Inhibition (PEACE) Trial, where the addition of trandolapril, in patients with stable coronary heart disease and preserved left ventricular function, to "current standard" therapy did not confer further benefit in terms of death from cardiovascular causes, MI, or coronary revascularization [73].

The absolute contraindications to the use of ACE inhibitors include pregnancy, hypersensitivity or life-threatening angioedema, acute renal failure, and hyperkalemia (serum K^+ greater than 5.5 mmol/L). Moderate hyperkalemia or renal insufficiency with serum creatinine concentrations up to 3.0 mg/dl mandates the need for careful monitoring and does not preclude the use of ACE inhibitors. ACE inhibitors are not recommended in patients with significant bilateral renal artery stenosis. There is a 10–30% incidence of ACE intolerance manifested by hyperkalemia, hypotension, azotemia, dysgeusia, cough, angioedema, or agranulocytosis.

ACE inhibitors can be initiated without difficulty in most patients (Table 3.3), although the occasional acute drop in blood pressure or occurrence of renal dysfunction or hyperkalemia mandates low dosage administration with careful monitoring. Patients at higher risk for these adverse effects are those with low baseline blood pressure (systolic pressure less than 100 mmHg), intravascular volume depletion, hyponatremia (serum Na^+ less than 135 mmol/L), baseline K^+ more than 5.0 mmol/L, and diabetes. In such patients, an initial captopril dose of 6.25 mg may be administered, and the blood pressure should be observed 1–2 h after the dose. In other patients the initial doses can be higher (captopril 12.5 mg tid or enalapril 2.5 mg bid). Telephone

Table 3.3 Select ACE inhibitors in heart failure.

Agent	Initial dose (mg)	Target dose (mg)	Recommended maximum dose (mg)
Captopril	6.25 tid	50 tid	100 tid
Lisinopril	5 qd	20 qd	40 qd
Enalapril	2.5 bid	10 bid	20 bid
Ramipril	5 qd	10 qd	20 qd
Quinapril	5 qd	20 qd	40 qd
Trandolapril	1 qd	4 qd	4 qd

follow-up to determine whether symptoms of hypotension have occurred is advisable and renal function and K^+ should be reassessed within a week. The doses should be gradually titrated to captopril 50 mg tid or enalapril 10 mg bid as tolerated, even if the patient has improved at lower dosages. Although ACE inhibitor usage is increasing, even among primary care physicians [4], most physicians prescribe doses well below those shown to be effective in clinical trials. There continues to be debate on the optimal ACE inhibitor dose to be used. The Assessment of Treatment with Lisinopril on Survival (ATLAS) study compared the effects of low (2.5–5 mg) and high (32.5–35 mg) doses of lisinopril on morbidity and mortality rates in patients with NYHA class II–IV heart failure [74]. Although the all-cause mortality was similar in both dose groups, the combined end point of mortality and worsening heart failure favored the use of a high dose. Further, a *post-hoc* investigation of the ATLAS database has shown that the high dose was associated with a reduction in vascular and arrhythmic events, as well as benefits on ventricular remodeling which could have accounted for the decrease in death or hospitalization noted in the high-dose group [75]. A recent study characterizing vascular tissue AI/AII conversion changes in heart failure patients on chronic lisinopril therapy has shown that vascular ACE inhibition was significantly reduced, suggesting gradual reactivation of vascular ACE in CHF over time [76]. This reactivation process was suppressed by increasing the dose of the ACE inhibitor. It is concluded that ACE inhibitor therapy in most patients with CHF can be successfully titrated to and maintained at high doses, and that more aggressive use of these agents is warranted.

Angiotensin receptor blockers

These agents block the cell surface receptor for AII at the tissue level (Table 3.4) and therefore, they block the effects of AII produced not only through the classical ACE pathway but also by the chymase pathway [77]. Since some of the side effects of ACE inhibitors such as cough and angioedema are bradykinin related, these agents are better tolerated than ACE inhibitors with fewer side effects since they are not associated with bradykinin release.

Angiotensin receptor blockers (ARBs) have similar beneficial hemodynamic effects to ACE inhibitors in reducing preload, afterload, and increasing cardiac output while improving exercise performance [78,79]. However, ACE inhibitors remain the therapy of choice for all levels of heart failure and left ventricular dysfunction. Currently, there are no data to support using ARBs as first-line agents except in patients who are intolerant to ACE inhibitors (usually due to angioedema, rashes or intolerable cough).

There is no evidence that ARBs produce less renal dysfunction than ACE inhibitors. The Evaluation of Losartan in the Elderly (ELITE) study compared losartan and captopril in elderly patients with heart failure. No significant differences were observed in the primary end point, incidence of renal dysfunction (10.5%), between the two groups [80]. However, the secondary mortality end point demonstrated less all-cause mortality in the losartan group (4.8% versus 8.7%, $P = 0.035$). These interesting survival benefits, however, were not reproduced in the subsequent ELITE II (the Evaluation of Losartan in the Elderly II) trial, a larger clinical trial that showed no significant differences in the primary end point, all-cause mortality, between the two groups [81].

ARBs have a favorable profile on morbidity including decreasing symptoms and hospitalizations while improving quality of life, ejection fraction, and NYHA functional class.

Whether a more complete blockade of the tissue ACE, by combining ACE inhibitors and ARBs, is a more effective therapeutic strategy has been studied recently by several pilot trials. The Randomized evaluation of Strategies for Left Ventricular Dysfunction (RESOLVD) pilot study compared candesartan, enalapril, and their combination in CHF [82]. Although the combination therapy had a favorable effect on ventricular remodeling, no significant differences were noted in exercise, functional class, or

Table 3.4 Select ARBs in heart failure.

Agent	Initial dose (mg)	Target dose (mg)	Recommended maximum dose (mg)
Losartan	25 qd	50 qd	100 qd
Candesartan	16 qd	32 qd	32 qd
Valsartan	80 qd	160 qd	320 qd

quality of life. A second RESOLVD pilot study evaluated the addition of long-acting metoprolol to enalapril and candesartan [83] with the main objective to determine tolerability of extensive neurohormonal blockade with the combination of an ACE inhibitor, AII receptor blocker, and beta-blocker. Again, no differences in exercise, functional class, or quality of life were noted between any of the groups, but significant improvement of left ventricular systolic function and attenuation of remodeling with a greater decrease of AII and renin levels was noted when metoprolol was added.

The results of the Valsartan Heart Failure trial, the largest AII receptor antagonist trial, indicated a lack of effect of valsartan on all-cause mortality when added to ACE inhibitor therapy [84]. Further lessons derived from a subgroup analysis indicated that the addition of Valsartan to an ACE inhibitor and a beta-blocker baseline therapy resulted in a significant increase in mortality. These unexpected findings raised a huge concern suggesting that extensive blockade of the renin–angiotensin system may in fact be lethal rather than beneficial.

The impact of candesartan, a recently Food and Drug Administration (FDA) approved agent, on morbidity and mortality in patients with heart failure has been evaluated in Candesartan in Heart Failure Assessment of Reduction in Mortality and Morbidity (CHARM) [85]. CHARM comprised three parallel ongoing trials, patients with left ventricular dysfunction and intolerant to ACE inhibitors (CHARM-Alternative) [86], patients with left ventricular dysfunction taking ACE inhibitors (CHARM-Added) [87], and patients with preserved left ventricular function, left ventricular ejection fraction exceeding 40% (CHARM-Preserved) [88]. The primary outcome of the overall program was all-cause mortality, and for all the component trials was cardiovascular death or hospital admission for

CHF. Overall, candesartan was well tolerated and significantly reduced all-cause mortality (adjusted hazard ratio: 0.90, $P = 0.032$) [85]. The primary outcome was significantly reduced in each of the CHARM-Alternative [86] (adjusted hazard ratio: 0.70, $P < 0.0001$) and CHARM-Added [87] (adjusted hazard ratio: 0.85, $P = 0.01$) trials with moderate impact in the CHARM-Preserved trial [88] (adjusted hazard ratio: 0.86, $P = 0.051$).

A recent meta-analysis could not confirm that ARBs are superior in reducing all-cause mortality or heart failure hospitalization in patients with symptomatic heart failure when compared to ACE inhibitors [89]. Therefore, ACE inhibitors still remain the therapy of choice. Further, two major studies were designed to address the issue whether losartan in the Optimal Trial in Myocardial Infarction with Angiotensin II Antagonist Losartan (OPTIMAL) study [90] or valsartan in the Valsartan In Acute Myocardial Infarction (VALIANT) study [91] are considered to be superior or as good as the proven ACE inhibitor captopril in improving survival in high-risk post-MI patients. In the OPTIMAL study [90], Losartan was significantly better tolerated than captopril, with fewer patients discontinuing study medication. However, a non-significant difference in total mortality in favor of captopril was noted (relative risk: 1.13, $P = 0.07$) suggesting that ACE inhibitors should remain first-choice treatment in patients after complicated acute MI unless if the patient is ACE intolerant, then losartan might be considered as a substitute. Valsartan was found to be equally effective as captopril in reducing all-cause mortality (hazard ratio: 1.00, $P = 0.98$) in the VALIANT study [91]. Combining valsartan with captopril increased the rate of adverse events without improving survival. VALIANT added another evidence that ACE inhibitors should be considered as first-line therapy for such patients.

Beta-adrenergic receptor blockers

Beta-blockers constitute a promising new avenue for the treatment of CHF. The increased sympathetic activity noted in CHF plays an important role in the progression of the cardiac dysfunction and correlates with severity of the syndrome [92]. Such activated adrenergic response is associated with down-regulation of beta-adrenergic receptors,

myocyte apoptosis, augmented renin release, and increased arrhythmias [93–96].

Three generations of β-blockers are available (Figure 3.5). First-generation agents are non-selective antagonists (i.e., they block both β1- and β2-adrenergic receptors). Second-generation agents are selective agents. Third-generation agents are non-selective and they posses ancillary properties such as vasodilation. Carvedilol has moderate alpha-adrenergic receptor antagonist effect and moderate vasodilating effects [97]. Bucindolol has a weak alpha-adrenergic receptor antagonist effect and mild vasodilating effects [98]. Both carvedilol and bucindolol lower cardiac norepinephrine spill over without causing up-regulation of the beta-receptors [99,100]. By contrast, metoprolol has been shown to be associated with up-regulation of the beta-1 receptors without significant effect on cardiac norepinephrine [99,101]. A unique feature of carvedilol is its protective effect against *in vivo* low-density lipoprotein oxidation [102]. The antioxidant activity of carvedilol is approximately 10 times greater than that of vitamin E. It also prevents leukocyte adhesion to smooth muscle cells, and protects against reactive oxygen species-induced damage [103]. Whether these pharmacologic differences translate into differences in clinical outcome is yet to be determined. Multiple mechanisms of action of beta-blockade have been described including sympathetic modulation, reversal of remodeling, improved beta-receptor pathway function, modulation of calcium handling and reduced apoptosis [104–106]. Recently, beta-blockers have been shown to reverse protein kinase A hyper phosphorylation of the ryanodine receptor (RyR2), a key calcium release channel present on the sarcoplasmic reticulum which is required for excitation–contraction coupling [107]. The resulting attenuation of intracellular Ca^{2+} overload may prevent the development of left ventricular remodeling and may, in part, explain the improved cardiac function observed in heart failure patients treated with beta-adrenergic receptor blockers [108]. In addition to the favorable effects on myocardial function and structure, the general mechanisms through which beta-blocking agents reduce mortality likely involve their established anti-arrhythmic and anti-ischemic properties [109]. In contrast to ACE inhibitors, beta-blocking agents have consistently lowered the sudden death rate in heart failure trials,

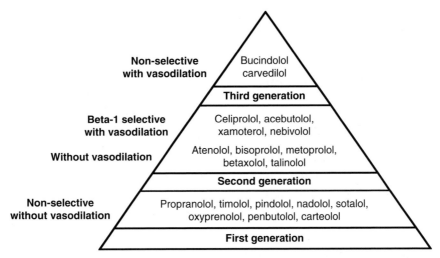

Figure 3.5 Beta-adrenergic receptor antagonists.

which suggests an anti-arrhythmic contribution to mortality reduction.

The use of beta-blockers in CHF, although counterintuitive, is not new. However, only recently have trials provided evidence of clinical benefit. Experience with three highly different agents has now shown that chronic therapy consistently improves left ventricular function, as assessed by the ejection fraction, and prevents progression and hospitalizations [110–112]. Several studies have suggested that beta-blockade may be more effective in patients with non-ischemic cardiomyopathy [111,112], but it has not been a consistent finding [110].

Seven mortality trials evaluated the impact of second- and third-generation beta-blockers on patients with chronic heart failure (Table 3.5). No mortality benefit was noted with metoprolol in "Metoprolol in Dilated Cardiomyopathy" (MDC) [111], bisoprolol in "Cardiac Insufficiency Bisoprolol Studies" (CIBIS I) [112], carvedilol in the "Australia–New Zealand" (ANZ) [113], or bucindolol in "Beta-blocker Estimation of survival trial" (BEST) [114]. However, significant reduction in all-cause mortality was associated with metoprolol CR/XL in the "MEtoprolol CR/XL Randomized Intervention Trial in Heart Failure" (MERIT-HF) [115], bisoprolol in "Cardiac Insufficiency Bisoprolol Studies II" (CIBIS II) [116], and carvedilol in both, the "United States Carvedilol Clinical Trial Program" [110] and the "Carvedilol Prospective Randomized

Cumulative Survival Trial" (COPERNICUS) [117]. Several meta-analyses of beta-blocker trials have conclusively shown that beta-blocker use is associated with a consistent 30% reduction in mortality, 40% reduction in hospitalizations, and 38% reduction in sudden death in patients with chronic heart failure [118,119]. It was estimated that 26 patients would need to be treated to avoid one death [120].

The data is persuasive that these drugs are effective in preventing progressive symptoms and left ventricular remodeling in moderate-to-severe heart failure. There is also evidence that these beneficial effects are also seen during early mild heart failure [121]. Patients with decompensated heart failure or volume overload, however, are not candidates, as early deterioration is frequent. It is also uncertain whether all beta-blockers produce comparable effects. Whether one agent is superior remains to be determined. This controversy has been substantially advanced by the results of The Carvedilol or Metoprolol European Study (COMET) [122], a European trial that compared all-cause mortality between carvedilol and metoprolol over a 4-year period. Carvedilol reduced mortality by 17% when compared with metoprolol ($P = 0.0017$). However, questions have been raised about the interpretation of these findings since the trial did not use the metoprolol-controlled release formulation that was shown to prolong survival in MERIT-HF [115].

Table 3.5 Mortality trials of beta-blockers.

Trial	Beta-blocker	NYHA	Mortality risk reduction	P-value
MDC (1993)	Metoprolol	II–IV (dilated cardiomyopathy)	9%	NS
MERIT-HF (1999)	Metoprolol CR/XL	II–IV	35%	0.0062
CIBIS-I (1994)	Bisoprolol	III–IV	20%	NS
CIBIS-II (1999)	Bisoprolol	III–IV	34%	<0.0001
ANZ	Carvedilol	II–III (ischemic cardiomyopathy)	28%	NS
US Carvedilol (1996)	Carvedilol	II–IV	65%	<0.001
COPERNICUS (2001)	Carvedilol	IV	35%	0.0014
BEST (2001)	Bucindolol	III–IV	10%	NS

NS: not significant; NYHA: New York Heart Association.

The benefits of beta-blockers are seen in patients already receiving ACE inhibitors, suggesting that combined blockade of two neurohormonal systems (renin–angiotensin system and sympathetic nervous system) can produce additive effects. The CAPRI-CORN study examined the addition of carvedilol to background ACE inhibitor therapy in patients with post-infarction left ventricular systolic dysfunction [123]. Significant reductions in all-cause mortality (23%, $P = 0.031$), cardiovascular mortality (25%, $P = 0.024$), and non-fatal MI (40%, $P = 0.041$) were noted in the carvedilol group compared to placebo providing thus, additional benefit to ACE inhibitor background therapy. However, extensive blockade of multiple neurohormonal systems in patients with heart failure could be deleterious as is evidenced from the subgroup analysis of the Valsartan Heart Failure Trial (Val-HeFT) where a significant increase in mortality was noted in the subgroup that was receiving valsartan in addition to both beta-blockers and ACE inhibitors [84]. Whether a beta-blocker is superior to an ACE inhibitor is yet to be determined. The Carvedilol and ACE-inhibitor remodeling mild heart failure evaluation (CARMEN) trial evaluated the need for combined treatment for remodeling and order of introduction by comparing enalapril against carvedilol and their combination [124]. Left ventricular end-systolic volume index was reduced by 5.4 ml/m^2 ($P = 0.0015$) in favor of combination therapy compared to enalapril. CARMEN was the first study to demonstrate that early combination of ACE-I and carvedilol significantly reverses LV remodeling in patients with mild-to-moderate CHF suggesting thus, the need for early institution of beta-blockade.

Table 3.6 Select beta-blockers in heart failure.

Agent	Initial dose (mg)	Target dose (mg)	Recommended maximum dose (mg)
Metoprolol	12.5 bid	100 bid	100 bid
Metoprolol CR/XL	12.5 qd	200 qd	200 qd
Bisoprolol	1.25 bid	5 qd (<85 kg) 10 qd (>85 kg)	20 qd
Carvedilol	3.125 bid	25 bid (<85 kg) 50 bid (>80 kg)	25 bid (<85 kg) 50 bid (>80 kg)

As the use of beta-blockers in heart failure expands, caution must be exercised and hence, several points must be emphasized. First, these agents should be administered to stable patients in the absence of refractory hemodynamic compromise. Second, the initial dosages should be small (Table 3.6). Third, 10% or more of the patients deteriorate early, but many of these patients can be gradually titrated to target doses. In patients with severe symptoms and elevated filling pressures, a useful strategy is to increase the diuretic dosage at the time of initiating beta-blockers.

Suggested approach to the pharmacologic therapy of congestive heart failure secondary to systolic dysfunction

The severity of heart failure symptoms is the driving force for selecting the appropriate pharmacologic approach (Figure 3.6) for the treatment of CHF and

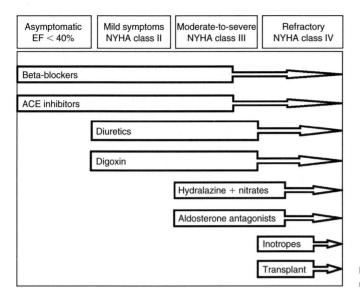

Figure 3.6 Suggested approach to treatment of congestive heart failure.

left ventricular dysfunction, based on published guidelines [125].

Asymptomatic left ventricular dysfunction

The recognition of benefits of neurohormonal antagonists in the early asymptomatic stage of heart failure has revolutionized the philosophy of heart failure therapy that has evolved from symptom treatment to prevention strategy. Hence, the importance of early detection of left ventricular dysfunction with the ultimate goal to prevent further deterioration in left ventricular function before the appearance of heart failure symptoms. It has been suggested that neurohumoral activation precedes the development of symptoms. A *post-hoc* analysis of the SOLVD trial has shown that increased plasma norepinephrine levels in patients with asymptomatic left ventricular dysfunction appear to predict all-cause and cardiovascular mortalities and development of clinical events related to the onset of heart failure or acute ischemic syndromes [126]. Plasma norepinephrine levels above the median of 393 pg/mL were associated with a relative risk of 2.59 ($P = 0.002$) for all-cause mortality and 1.88 ($P = 0.002$) for development of heart failure. It has also been shown that coronary endothelial function is abnormal in patients with asymptomatic left ventricular dysfunction highlighting thus, the potential importance of the endothelium in the early development of heart failure [127].

In patients who are identified as having left ventricular systolic dysfunction (ejection fractions of less than 35–40%) without symptoms, the proved therapy is an ACE inhibitor, which should be initiated in all such individuals. Three clinical trials, SAVE [63], AIRE [64], and Trandolapril Cardiac Evaluation (TRACE) [128] have clearly indicated that in MI survivors with asymptomatic left ventricular dysfunction, ACE inhibitor use has been associated with 19–27% reduction in all-cause mortality and 22–29% reduction in the development of heart failure.

Data from the post-MI beta-blocker trials have also suggested that this class of agents may have an important role in such patients as well. A *post-hoc* analysis of the SAVE study has shown that treatment with a beta-adrenergic blocking agent in addition to the use of the ACE inhibitor, captopril decreases cardiovascular mortality and morbidity in patients with asymptomatic left ventricular dysfunction after MI [129]. Beta-blocker use was associated with a 30% reduction in risk of cardiovascular death and 21% reduction in the development of heart failure. The beneficial effects of beta-blocker use in patients with asymptomatic left ventricular dysfunction after MI appear to be additive to those of ACE inhibitor. A synergistic reduction in the risk of death was also noted in the SOLVD Prevention trial with the combination of a beta-blocker and enalapril [130]. These data therefore, clearly show an important role for beta-blockers in patients with asymptomatic left ventricular dysfunction. At this point it might be prudent to use a combination strategy of ACE inhibitor and beta-blocker with the goal of reversing remodeling and preventing the development of heart failure.

Symptomatic left ventricular dysfunction

In symptomatic patients, initial therapy usually consists of a combination of diuretics and ACE inhibitors, started together or in sequence. A few patients with mild symptoms and no evidence of fluid retention may be managed with ACE inhibitors alone. Beta-blockers should be instituted early with mild-to-moderate symptoms and aldosterone antagonists should be added with moderate-to-severe symptoms. Digoxin is recommended if the patient remains symptomatic. Patients who continue to be symptomatic on all these drugs may respond to increasing doses of diuretics or to the addition of a direct-acting vasodilator, such as a nitrate. With increasing symptoms (NYHA class III), more aggressive use of diuretics and vasodilators, including hydralazine particularly in patients with substantial mitral regurgitation, is appropriate. Advanced class III and class IV patients often require combination diuretic regimens, with loop diuretics supplemented by metolazone. Patients refractory to all of these approaches may benefit from intermittent or chronic intravenous inotropic therapy with dobutamine or milrinone.

There is enough evidence to support the use of beta-blockers in patients with mild-to-moderate symptoms with the objective of preventing progression. Their role in severely symptomatic patients has also been recently confirmed but they should be initiated after achieving euvolemic status and full hemodynamic stabilization of the patient.

The A-II blockers are logical alternatives to ACE inhibitors in intolerant individuals, but they should be considered a second choice.

Amlodipine is promising for patients with non-ischemic cardiomyopathy and might be considered an alternative to hydralazine and nitrates as a fourth line of therapy in these patients, but the data for beta-blockers is more robust.

Intravenous inotropic agents such as dobutamine and milrinone can be helpful in patients with acute decompensation and refractory heart failure to achieve hemodynamic stabilization [131,132]. However, the recent results of The Outcomes of a Prospective Trial of Intravenous Milrinone for Exacerbations of Chronic Heart Failure (OPTIME-CHF) trial [133] do not support the routine use of intravenous milrinone as an adjunct to standard therapy in the treatment of patients hospitalized for an exacerbation of chronic heart failure. In fact, sustained hypotension requiring intervention and new atrial arrhythmias occurred more frequently in patients who received milrinone. Though questions regarding safety of these agents have been raised, a reasonable compendium of data supports the contention that the use of outpatient intermittent or continuous inotropic therapy ameliorates symptoms [134,135]. However, the use of intermittent infusion of these agents has no proven mortality benefit [136] and other studies have shown increased risk of mortality [137].

Cardiac assist devices and transplantation have an important role in the management of patients with refractory heart failure. The selection of candidates and appropriate timing of transplantation are important issues but are beyond the scope of this chapter.

Management of the patient with heart failure and preserved systolic function

It is estimated that 20–40 % of patients with heart failure have preserved left ventricular systolic function (ejection fractions of more than 45%), and this percentage rises among the elderly [138–141]. However, other comorbidities such as anemia, thyroid abnormalities and pulmonary disease should be excluded before the clinical picture is attributed to heart failure. Valvular abnormalities must also be ruled out. Intermittent ischemia often induces episodic symptoms and signs of heart failure without accompanying chest pain, particularly when underlying left ventricular hypertrophy or diabetes is present. Stress testing may be helpful when planning therapy for these patients, even if revascularization is not being considered. If all these explanations are excluded, amyloidosis should also be considered, albeit specific therapy is not available. However, after complete evaluation, most patients are not found to have a specific etiology but, rather, to have multiple contributory causes, including hypertension, left ventricular hypertrophy, diabetes and coronary disease; and the symptoms are ascribed to diastolic dysfunction. The clinical presentation of heart failure due to diastolic dysfunction overlaps considerably with that of systolic dysfunction.

Unfortunately, but not surprisingly, in view of its multifactorial nature, heart failure due to diastolic dysfunction is often difficult to treat, even though it tends to carry a more benign prognosis [141,142]. There is no specific therapy for diastolic heart failure, although calcium channel blockers have been advocated [143]. In the absence of specific therapy, there are three primary goals of treatment: to reduce symptoms, to control hypertension and reverse consequent left ventricular hypertrophy and to prevent myocardial ischemia.

Diuretics provide the most symptom relief if fluid retention is a feature. Thiazide diuretics are among the most effective therapy for isolated systolic hypertension [144], and chronic diuretic therapy tend to produce the greatest regression of left ventricular hypertrophy [145,146], which is an important mechanism of diastolic dysfunction. Hypertension is not only the main stimulus to left ventricular hypertrophy in these patients; it is also a frequent precipitant of ischemia and therefore should be aggressively controlled. Beta-blockers and ACE inhibitors complement diuretics well and calcium channel blockers are another effective alternative. Central sympatholytics may also mitigate episodic hypertensive episodes. Beta-blockers and calcium channel blockers can also be used to treat ischemia. Because tachycardia is often poorly tolerated in these patients, the former agents should be used when the basal or exercise heart rate is excessive.

Ancillary therapy in heart failure patients

CHF is usually accompanied by a number of medical illnesses or conditions that may complicate its management, some of which are briefly discussed below.

Treatment of hypertension

The increased afterload effect of hypertension contributes to the worsening of heart failure and hence, an aggressive treatment is warranted to achieve a desirable clinical effect. At least two large studies, Systolic Hypertension in the Elderly Program (SHEP) [147] and Swedish Trial in Old Patients (STOP) with Hypertension [148], reported reduction in the incidence of heart failure and other cardiovascular events with optimal treatment of hypertension. Indeed, patients with CHF often perform better when their pressures are at the low end of normal. Unless the patient becomes symptomatic from hypotension or develops renal dysfunction or angina due to renal or coronary hypoperfusion, systolic blood pressures of 90 mmHg or even lower should be accepted. Agents such as diuretics, ACE inhibitors, beta-blockers and vasodilators, form the cornerstone of therapy for CHF and are usually sufficient to control blood pressure. Central sympatholytics are effective; but given the most recent data on beta-blockers (initiated at low doses) and amlodipine, they are the more preferable choices.

Treatment of angina

When angina persists in patients with heart failure, revascularization is the favored approach in select candidates who demonstrate evidence of myocardial viability and this issue is discussed elsewhere in this text. The use of nitrates as an initial therapeutic approach is reasonable and the cautious use of beta-blockers and amlodipine are additional options.

Treatment of arrhythmias

Both supraventricular and ventricular arrhythmias are common in patients with heart failure and often pose challenging management problems [149]. In patients who develop atrial fibrillation, it is desirable but not always possible to restore and maintain sinus rhythm [150]. Poor rate control may exacerbate cardiac dysfunction and a coordinated atrial contraction may improve cardiac output. The main medication likely to be helpful in this setting is amiodarone. Digoxin, directly or indirectly by improving the heart failure, appears to maintain sinus rhythm. There were significantly fewer hospitalizations for supraventricular tachycardia with digoxin in the DIG trial [5].

Because sudden, presumably arrhythmic, deaths account for 40–50% of deaths in heart failure patients and because ventricular arrhythmias are an indicator of worse prognosis, the finding of symptomatic and even asymptomatic ventricular ectopy is often considered ominous [149]. Patients with symptoms suggestive of an arrhythmia, such as syncope or near-syncope, require careful evaluation. Those with demonstrated sustained or symptomatic ventricular tachycardia on monitoring should be considered for implantable defibrillator placement [151,152]. The role of implantable cardioverter-defibrillators in heart failure has recently been addressed by The Sudden Cardiac Death in Heart Failure Trial (SCD-HeFT) which is discussed elsewhere in this text.

Patients with asymptomatic ventricular ectopy, including moderately long burst of ventricular tachycardia, present a dilemma [149]. Two trials have evaluated amiodarone in such individuals but unfortunately reached opposite conclusions. The Grupo de Estudio de la Sobravida en la Insuficiencia Cardiaca en Argentina (GESICA) study found that amiodarone 300 mg daily prolonged survival and prevented both sudden and non-sudden death in a group of patients with severe CHF primarily due to non-ischemic cardiomyopathy [153]. In contrast, a Veterans Administration cooperative study using a 400 mg daily dosage in patients with predominantly NYHA class II CHF due in most cases to coronary artery disease found no benefit despite a significant rise in ejection fraction and successful suppression of asymptomatic ventricular arrhythmias [154]. The most likely explanation for these discordant findings is that the benefits of amiodarone may be conveyed by its beta-blocking activity and be limited to non-ischemic cardiomyopathy [155]. In any case, pharmacologic therapy for asymptomatic ventricular arrhythmias is not encouraged.

Anticoagulation

Patients with heart failure are at increased risk of thromboembolism [156]. Several markers of platelet activity have been found to be increased in CHF patients, including beta-thromboglobulin, platelet factor 4, osteonectin, and cellular adhesion molecules [157–159]. Patients with atrial fibrillation are at particularly high risk and should receive warfarin anticoagulation. Anticoagulation is also recommended for patients with a history of thromboembolism and those with mobile intracardiac thrombi. However, the rate of arterial thromboembolism in

patients who are in sinus rhythm is low, 2.0–2.4% in large studies. Though a cohort analysis from the SOLVD study indicates that anticoagulation may improve survival in patients with heart failure [160], two randomized trials, The Warfarin and Antiplatelet Therapy in Heart Failure (WATCH) trial [161] and the Warfarin versus Aspirin in Reduced Cardiac Ejection Fraction (WARCEF) trial [162] were designed to evaluate the optimal antithrombotic agent for heart failure patients with a composite primary end point of death and stroke. Unfortunately, the WATCH trial was terminated prematurely by the Veterans Affairs (VA) Cooperative Study Program because of poor enrollment with a resulting reduction of its power to achieve its original objective though no significant differences in primary outcome were seen among the different agents, warfarin, aspirin or clopidogrel in this underpowered study. The results of the ongoing WARCEF trial may provide further information regarding the role of anticoagulation and/or antiplatelet therapy in the heart failure population.

The use of aspirin in heart failure patients is also controversial. Most of these patients have underlying coronary artery disease, for which aspirin is often administered but for which evidence of efficacy for long-term therapy is limited. What makes this problematic is that there is a suggestion that aspirin may interfere with the benefit of ACE inhibitor therapy.

Important drug interactions

Unfortunately, the management of CHF is a challenging problem and requires a polypharmacy. Because of its effects on renal and hepatic function, drug metabolism is likely to be abnormal. Thus care must be taken to avoid drug interactions and excessive dosing. The most obvious drug interactions are those that involve digoxin (quinidine and amiodarone) and warfarin (amiodarone). A more frequent problem is the interaction of ACE inhibitors with aspirin. A significant benefit of ACE inhibitor is mediated by the increased bradykinin levels, which result in enhanced synthesis of vasodilatory prostaglandins. In contrast, aspirin inhibits cyclooxygenase, and thereby suppresses prostaglandin production. Thus, these counteracting effects may result in antagonism between ACE inhibitor and aspirin therapy in heart failure patients [163,164]. A recent subgroup analysis of the CONSENSUS II has shown that the survival benefit of enalapril was less favorable among patients taking aspirin than among patients not taking aspirin at baseline [165]. Another adverse interaction has been recorded in the Multicenter Oral Carvedilol Heart Failure Assessment (MOCHA) trial where aspirin was noted to alter the beneficial effects of beta-blockers on left ventricular ejection fraction in patients with CHF and therefore, it was suggested that it may impair reverse remodeling [166].

Follow-up of patients with heart failure

It is recommended that patients be followed primarily by clinical assessments, including a quantitative assessment of the patient's activity tolerance and symptoms and careful physical examination. Serial testing procedures are discouraged because they are poorly reproducible and are insensitive to either deterioration or improvement. Exceptions to this recommendation include assessments for transplantation and the evaluation of findings such as new heart murmurs or abrupt changes in clinical course.

Conclusion

CHF is a lethal disorder with a growing social and economic burden. There have been seminal advances in the diagnosis and management of heart failure, but several have not been adequately incorporated into practice. Guidelines have attempted to rectify this deficiency by providing evidence-based medicine supported by clinical trials. The pharmacological treatment of heart failure entails a combined preventive and symptomatic management strategy. ACE inhibitors and beta-blockers have strengthened the armamentarium to improve quality of life and survival. Yet, there is always a critical need for further research efforts to develop novel therapeutic strategies to improve clinical outcome in this gloomy syndrome.

References

1 Massie BM, Shah NB. The heart failure epidemic. Magnitude of the problem and potential mitigating approaches. *Curr Opin Cardiol* 1996; **11**: 221–226.

2 Cleland JG, Khand A, Clark A. The heart failure epidemic: Exactly how big is it? *Eur Heart J* 2001; **22**: 623–626.

3 American Heart Association. *2001 Heart and Stroke Statistical Update: Economic Cost of Cardiovascular Diseases.* American Heart Association, Dallas, TX, 2001: 19–21.

4 Ansari M, Alexander M, Tutar A, Bello D, Massie BM. Cardiology participation improves outcomes in patients with new-onset heart failure in the outpatient setting. *J Am Coll Cardiol* 2003; **41(1)**: 62–68.

5 The Digitalis Investigation Group. The effect of digoxin on mortality and morbidity in patients with heart failure. *N Engl J Med* 1997; **336**: 525–533.

6 Uretsky BF, Young JB, Shahidi FE *et al.* Randomized study assessing the effect of digoxin withdrawal in patients with mild to moderate chronic CHF: results of the PROVED trial. *J Am Coll Cardiol* 1993; **22**: 955–962.

7 Packer M, Gheorghiade M, Young JB *et al.* Withdrawal of digoxin from patients with chronic heart failure treated with angiotensin-converting-enzyme inhibitors: RADIANCE Study. *N Engl J Med* 1993; **329**: 1–7.

8 Adams Jr KF, Gheorghiade M, Uretsky BF *et al.* Clinical benefits of low serum digoxin concentrations in heart failure. *J Am Coll Cardiol* 2002; **39(6)**: 946–953.

9 Guidelines for the evaluation and management of heart failure. Report of the American College of Cardiology/American Heart Association Task Force on Practice Guidelines (Committee on Evaluation and Management of Heart Failure). *Circulation* 2001; **104**: 2996–3007.

10 Arnold SB, Byrd RC, Meister W *et al.* Long-term digitalis therapy improves left ventricular function in heart failure. *N Engl J Med* 1980; **303**: 1443–1448.

11 Sagawa T, Sagawa K, Kelly JE *et al.* Activation of cardiac ryanodine receptors by cardiac glycosides. *Am J Physiol Heart Circul Physiol* 2002; **282(3)**: H1118–H1126.

12 Gheorghiade M, Ferguson D. Digoxin: a neurohormonal modulator in heart failure? *Circulation* 1991; **84**: 2181–2186.

13 Krum H, Bigger JT, Goldsmith RL, Packer M. Effect of long-term digoxin therapy on autonomic function in patients with chronic heart failure. *J Am Coll Cardiol* 1995; **25**: 289–294.

14 Brouwer J, Van Veldhuisen DJ, Man in't Veld AJ *et al.*, for the Dutch Ibopamine Multicenter Trial (DIMT) Study Group. Heart rate variability in patients with mild to moderate heart failure: effects of neurohumoral modulation by digoxin and ibopamine. *J Am Coll Cardiol* 1995; **26**: 283–290.

15 Ferguson DW, Berg WJ, Sanders JS *et al.* Sympathoinhibitory responses to digitalis glycosides in heart failure patients: direct evidence from sympathetic neural recordings. *Circulation* 1989; **80**: 65–77.

16 Redfors A. The effect of different digoxin doses on subjective symptoms and physical working capacity in patients with atrial fibrillation. *Act Med Scand* 1971; **190**: 307–320.

17 Sticherling C, Oral H, Horrocks J *et al.* Effects of digoxin on acute, atrial fibrillation-induced changes in atrial refractoriness. *Circulation* 2000; **102**: 2503–2508.

18 Massie BM, Abdalla I. Heart failure in patients with preserved left ventricular systolic function: do digitalis glycosides have a role? *Prog Cardiovasc Dis* 1998; **98**: 1184–1191.

19 Stampfer M, Epstein SE, Beiser GD, Brauwald E. Hemodynamic effects of diuresis at rest and during intense upright exercise in patients with impaired cardiac function. *Circulation* 1968; **37**: 900–911.

20 Wilson JR, Reicheck N, Dunkman WB *et al.* Effects of diuresis on the performance of the failing left ventricle in man. *Am J Med* 1981; **70**: 234–239.

21 Biddle TL, Yu PN. Effect of furosemide on hemodynamics and lung water in acute pulmonary edema secondary to myocardial infarction. *Am J Cardiol* 1979; **43**: 86–90.

22 Johnston GD, Hiatt WR, Nies AS *et al.* Factors modifying the early non-diuretic vascular effects of furosemide in man. The possible role of renal prostaglandins. *Circ Res* 1983; **53**: 630–635.

23 Stevenson LW, Brunken RC, Belil D *et al.* Afterload reduction with vasodilators and diuretics decreases mitral regurgitation during upright exercise in advanced heart failure. *J Am Coll Cardiol* 1990; **15**: 174–180.

24 Silke B. Hemodynamic impact of diuretic therapy in chronic heart failure. *Cardiology* 1994; **84(Suppl 2)**: 115–123.

25 Puschette JB. Pharmacologic classification and renal actions of diuretics. *Cardiology* 1994; **84(Suppl 2)**: 4–13.

26 Baker DW, Konstam MA, Bottorf M, Pitt B. Management of heart failure. I. Pharmacologic treatment. *J Am Med Assoc* 1994; **272**: 1361–1366.

27 Brater DC. Diuretic therapy. *N Eng J Med* 1998; **339**: 387–395.

28 Ghose RR, Gupta SK. Synergistic actions of metolazone with loop diuretics. *Br Med J* 1981; **812**: 1432–1433.

29 Ellison DH. The physiologic basis of diuretic synergism. Its role in treating diuretic resistance. *Ann Intern Med* 1991; **114**: 886–894.

30 Kiyingi A, Mield MJ, Pawsey CC *et al.* Metolazone and the treatment of severe refractory CHF. *Lancet* 1990; **335**: 29–31.

31 Taylor SH. Diuretic therapy in CHF. *Cardiology in Review* 2000; **8(2)**: 104–114.

32 Grinstead WC, Francis MJ, Marks GF *et al.* Discontinuation of chronic diuretic therapy in stable CHF secondary to coronary artery disease or to idiopathic dilated cardiomyopathy. *Am J Cardiol* 1994; **73**: 881–886.

33 Pitt B, Zannad F, Remme WJ *et al.* The effect of spironolactone on morbidity and mortality in patients with severe heart failure. Randomized Aldactone Evaluation Study Investigators. *N Eng J Med* 1999; **341(10)**: 709–717.

34 Brilla CG. Aldosterone and myocardial fibrosis in heart failure. *Herz* 2000; **25(3)**: 299–306.

35 MacFadyen RJ. Barr CS. Struthers AD. Aldosterone blockade reduces vascular collagen turnover, improves heart rate variability and reduces early morning rise in heart rate in heart failure patients. *Cardiovasc Res* 1997; **35(1)**: 30–34.

36 Korkmaz ME, Muderrisoglu H, Ulucam M, Ozin B. Effects of spironolactone on heart rate variability and left ventricular systolic function in severe ischemic heart failure. *Am J Cardiol* 2000; **86(6)**: 649–653.

37 Farquharson CA, Struthers AD. Spironolactone increases nitric oxide bioactivity, improves endothelial vasodilator dysfunction, and suppresses vascular angiotensin I/ angiotensin II conversion in patients with chronic heart failure. *Circulation* 2000; **101(6)**: 594–597.

38 Pitt B, Remme W, Zannad F *et al.* Eplerenone Post-Acute Myocardial Infarction Heart Failure Efficacy and Survival Study Investigators. Eplerenone, a selective aldosterone blocker, in patients with left ventricular dysfunction after myocardial infarction. *N Engl J Med* 2003; **348(14)**: 1309–1321.

39 Cohn JN, Archibald DG, Ziesche S *et al.* Effect of vasodilator therapy on mortality in chronic CHF. Results of a Veterans Administration cooperative study. *N Engl J Med* 1986; **314**: 1547–1552.

40 Cohn JN, Johnson G, Ziesche S *et al.* A comparison of enalapril with hydralazine-isosorbide dinitrate in the treatment of chronic CHF. *N Engl J Med* 1991; **325**: 303–310.

41 Taylor AL, Ziesche S, Yancy C *et al.* Combination of isosorbide dinitrate and hydralazine in blacks with heart failure. *N Engl J Med* 2004; **351(20)**: 2049–2057.

42 Haeusslein EA, Greenberg BH, Massie BM. The influence of mitral regurgitation on the hemodynamic response to vasodilators in chronic CHF. *Chest* 1991; **100**: 1312–1315.

43 Gorgia H, Mehra A, Parekh S *et al.* Prevention of tolerance to hemodynamic effects of nitrates with concomitant use of hydralazine in patients with chronic heart failure. *J Am Coll Cardiol* 1995; **26**: 1575–1580.

44 Packer M. Pathophysiologic mechanisms underlying the adverse effects of calcium channel blocking drugs in patients with chronic heart failure. *Circulation* 1989; **80(Suppl IV)**: 59–67.

45 Elkayam U, Amin J, Mehra A *et al.* A prospective, randomized, double-blind, crossover study to compare the efficacy and safety of chronic nifedipine therapy with that of isosorbide dinitrate and their combination in the treatment of chronic CHF. *Circulation* 1990; **82**: 1954–1961.

46 Goldstein RE, Boccuzzi SJ, Cruess D, Nattel S. Diltiazem increase late-onset CHF in post-infarction patients with early reduction in ejection fraction. *Circulation* 1991; **83**: 52–60.

47 Packer M, O'Connor CM, Ghali JK *et al.*, for the Prospective Randomized Amlodipine Survival Evaluation Study Group.

Effect of amlodipine on morbidity and mortality in severe chronic heart failure. *N Engl J Med* 1996; **335**: 1107–1114.

48 Thackray S, Witte K, Clark AL, Cleland JG. Clinical trials update: OPTIME-CHF, PRAISE-2, ALL-HAT. *Eur J Heart Fail* 2000; **2(2)**: 209–212.

49 Cohn JN, Ziesche S, Smith R *et al*. Effect of the calcium antagonist felodipine as supplementary vasodilator therapy in patients with chronic heart failure treated with enalapril: V-HeFT III. Vasodilator-Heart Failure Trial (V-HeFT) Study Group. *Circulation* 1997; **96(3)**: 856–863.

50 Levine TB, Bernink PJ, Caspi A *et al*. Effect of mibefradil, a T-type calcium channel blocker, on morbidity and mortality in moderate to severe CHF: the MACH-1 study. Mortality Assessment in CHF Trial. *Circulation* 2000; **101(7)**: 758–764.

51 Massie BM, Amidon T. Angiotensin converting enzyme inhibitor therapy for CHF. Rationale, results and current recommendations. In: Hosenpud JD & Greenberg BH, eds. *CHF*. Springer-Verlag, New York, 1993: 380–399.

52 Fault JM, Tavolaro O, Antony I, Nitenberg A. Direct myocardial and coronary effects of enalaprilat in patients with dilated cardiomyopathy: assessment by a bilateral intracoronary infusion technique. *Circulation* 1988; **77**: 337–344.

53 Levin TB, Franciosa JA, Cohn JN. Acute and long-term response to an oral converting enzyme inhibitor, captopril in chronic heart failure: a rest and exercise hemodynamic study. *Circulation* 1983; **67**: 807–816.

54 Mancini DM, Davis L, Wexler JP *et al*. Dependence of enhanced maximal exercise performance on increased peak skeletal muscle perfusion during long-term captopril therapy in heart failure. *J Am Coll Cardiol* 1987; **10**: 845–850.

55 Mancini GBJ, Henry GC, Macaya C *et al*. Angiotensin-converting enzyme inhibition with quinapril improves endothelial vasomotor dysfunction in patients with coronary artery disease. The TREND (Trial on Reversing Endothelial dysfunction) Study. *Circulation* 1996; **94**: 258–265.

56 Yoshida H, Takahashi M, Tanonaka K *et al*. Effects of ACE inhibition and angiotensin II type 1 receptor blockade on cardiac function and G proteins in rats with chronic heart failure. *Br J Pharmacol* 2001; **134(1)**: 150–160.

57 Pfeffer MA, Lamas GA, Vaughan DE *et al*. Effect of captopril on progressive ventricular dilation after anterior myocardial infarction. *N Engl J Med* 1988; **319**: 80–86.

58 Lonn EM, Yusuf S, Jha P *et al*. Emerging role of angiotensin-converting enzyme inhibitors in cardiac and vascular protection. *Circulation* 1994; **90**: 2056–2069.

59 CONSENSUS Trial Study Group. Effects of enalapril on mortality in severe CHF. Results of the Cooperative North Scandinavian Enalapril Survival Study (CONSENSUS). *N Engl J Med* 1987; **316**: 1429–1435.

60 SOLVD Investigators. Effect of enalapril on mortality and the development of heart failure in asymptomatic patients with reduced left ventricular ejection fractions. *N Engl J Med* 1992; **327**: 685–61.

61 Captopril Multicenter Research Group. A placebo controlled trial of captopril in refractory chronic CHF. *J Am Coll Cardiol* 1983; **2**: 755–763.

62 SOLVD Investigators. Effect of enalapril on survival in patients with reduced left ventricular ejection fractions and CHF. *N Engl J Med* 1991; **325**: 293–302.

63 Pfeffer MA, Braunwald E, Moye LA *et al*. Effect of captopril on mortality and morbidity in patients with left ventricular dysfunction after myocardial infarction. Results of the survival and ventricular enlargement trial. *N Engl J Med* 1992; **327**: 669–677.

64 Acute Infarction Ramipril Efficacy (AIRE) Study Investigators. Effects of ramipril on mortality and morbidity of survivors of acute myocardial infarction with clinical evidence of heart failure. *Lancet* 1993; **342**: 821–828.

65 Ambrosioni E, Borghi C, Magnani B. The effect of the angiotensin-converting-enzyme inhibitor zofenopril on mortality and morbidity after anterior myocardial infarction. *N Engl J Med* 1995; **332**: 80–85.

66 Exner DV, Dries DL, Domanski MJ, Cohn JN. Lesser response to angiotensin-converting-enzyme inhibitor therapy in black as compared with white patients with left ventricular dysfunction. *N Engl J Med* 2001; **344(18)**: 1351–1357.

67 Greenberg B, Quinones MA, Koilpillai C *et al*. Effects of long-term enalapril therapy on patients with left ventricular dysfunction: results of the SOLVD echocardiography substudy. *Circulation* 1995; **91**: 2573–2581.

68 Hall D, Zeitler M, Rudolf W. Counteraction of the vasodilator effects of enalapril by aspirin in severe heart failure. *J Am Coll Cardiol* 1992; **20**: 1549–1555.

69 Spaulding C, Charbonnier B, Cohen-Solal A *et al*. Acute hemodynamic interaction of aspirin and ticlopidine with enalapril: results of a double-blind, randomized comparative trial. *Circulation* 1998; **98**: 757–765.

70 Harjai KJ, Nunez E, Turgut T, Newman J. Effect of combined aspirin and angiotensin-converting enzyme inhibitor therapy versus angiotensin-converting enzyme inhibitor therapy alone on readmission rates in heart failure. *Am J Cardiol* 2001; **87(4)**: 483–487.

71 Yusuf S, Sleight P, Pogue J *et al*. Effects of an angiotensin-converting-enzyme inhibitor, ramipril, on cardiovascular events in high-risk patients. The Heart Outcomes Prevention Evaluation Study Investigators. *N Engl J Med* 2000; **342(3)**: 145–153.

72 Fox KM. EURopean trial On reduction of cardiac events with Perindopril in stable coronary Artery disease. Efficacy of perindopril in reduction of cardiovascular events among patients with stable coronary artery disease: randomised,

double-blind, placebo-controlled, multicentre trial (the EUROPA Study). *Lancet* 2003; **362(9386):** 782–788.

73 Braunwald E, Domanski MJ, Fowler SE *et al.* Angiotensin-converting-enzyme inhibition in stable coronary artery disease. *N Eng J Med* 2004; **351(20):** 2058–2068.

74 Packer M, Poole-Wilson PA, Armstrong PW *et al.* Comparative effects of low and high doses of the angiotensin-converting enzyme inhibitor, lisinopril, on morbidity and mortality in chronic heart failure. ATLAS Study Group. *Circulation* 1999; **100(23):** 2312–2318.

75 Cleland JG, Thygesen K, Uretsky BF, Armstrong P, Horowitz JD, Massie B, Packer M, Poole-Wilson PA, Ryden L, ATLAS Investigators. Cardiovascular critical event pathways for the progression of heart failure; a report from the ATLAS study. *Eur Heart J* 2001; **22(17):** 1601–1612.

76 Farquharson CA, Struthers AD. Gradual reactivation over time of vascular tissue angiotensin I to angiotensin II conversion during chronic lisinopril therapy in chronic heart failure. *J Am Coll Cardiol* 2002; **39(5):** 767–775.

77 Goodfriend TL, Elliot ME, Catt KJ *et al.* Angiotensin receptors and their antagonists. *N Eng J Med* 1996; **334:** 1649–1654.

78 Crozier I, Ikram H, Awan N *et al.*, for the Losartan Hemodynamic Study Group. Losartan in heart failure: hemodynamics effects and tolerability. *Circulation* 1995; **91:** 691–697.

79 Dickstein K, Chang P, Willinheimer R *et al.* Comparison of the effects of losartan and enalapril on clinical status and exercise performance in patients with moderate or severe chronic heart failure. *J Am Coll Cardiol* 1995; **26:** 438–445.

80 Pitt B, Segal R, Martinez FA *et al.* Randomized trial of losartan versus captopril in patients over 65 with heart failure (Evaluation of Losartan in the Elderly Study, ELITE). *Lancet* 1997; **349:** 747–752.

81 Pitt B, Poole-Wilson PA, Segal R *et al.* Effect of losartan compared with captopril on mortality in patients with symptomatic heart failure: randomized trial – the Losartan Heart Failure Survival Study ELITE II. *Lancet* 2000; **355(9215):** 1582–1587.

82 McKelvie RS, Yusuf S, Pericak D *et al.* Comparison of candesartan, enalapril, and their combination in CHF: Randomized evaluation of Strategies for Left Ventricular Dysfunction (RESOLVD) pilot Study. *Circulation* 1999; **100:** 1056–1064.

83 The RESOLVED Investigators. Effects of metoprolol CR in patients with ischemic and dilated cardiomyopathy. The Randomized Evaluation of Strategies for Left Ventricular Dysfunction Pilot Study. *Circulation* 2000; **101:** 378–384.

84 Cohn JN, Tognoni G. A randomized trial of the angiotensin receptor blocker valsartan in chronic heart failure. *N Engl J Med* 2001; **345(23):** 1667–1675.

85 Pfeffer MA, Swedberg K, Granger CB *et al.* Effects of candesartan on mortality and morbidity in patients with chronic heart failure: the CHARM-Overall programme. *Lancet* 2003; **362(9386):** 759–766.

86 Granger CB, McMurray JJ, Yusuf S *et al.* Effects of candesartan in patients with chronic heart failure and reduced left-ventricular systolic function intolerant to angiotensin-converting-enzyme inhibitors: the CHARM-Alternative trial. *Lancet* 2003; **362(9386):** 772–776.

87 McMurray JJ, Ostergren J, Swedberg K *et al.* Effects of candesartan in patients with chronic heart failure and reduced left-ventricular systolic function taking angiotensin-converting-enzyme inhibitors: the CHARM-Added trial. *Lancet* 2003; **362(9386):** 767–771.

88 Yusuf S, Pfeffer MA, Swedberg K *et al.* Effects of candesartan in patients with chronic heart failure and preserved left-ventricular ejection fraction: the CHARM-Preserved Trial. *Lancet* 2003; **362(9386):** 777–781.

89 Jong P, Demers C, McKelvie RS, Liu PP. Angiotensin receptor blockers in heart failure: meta-analysis of randomized controlled trials. *J Am Coll Cardiol* 2002; **39(3):** 463–470.

90 Dickstein K, Kjekshus J. OPTIMAAL Steering Committee of the OPTIMAAL Study Group. Effects of losartan and captopril on mortality and morbidity in high-risk patients after acute myocardial infarction: the OPTIMAAL randomised trial. Optimal Trial in Myocardial Infarction with Angiotensin II Antagonist Losartan. *Lancet* 2002; **360(9335):** 752–760.

91 Pfeffer MA, McMurray JJ, Velazquez EJ *et al.* Valsartan in Acute Myocardial Infarction Trial Investigators. Valsartan, captopril, or both in myocardial infarction complicated by heart failure, left ventricular dysfunction, or both. *N Eng J Med* 2003; **349(20):** 1893–1906.

92 Francis GS, Benedict C, Johnstone DE *et al.* Comparison of neuroendocrine activation in patients with left ventricular dysfunction with and without CHF: a sub-study of the Studies of Left Ventricular Dysfunction (SOLVD). *Circulation* 1990; **82:** 1724–1729.

93 Mann DL, Kent RL, Parsons B, Cooper G III. Adrenergic effects on the biology of the adult mammalian cardiomyocyte. *Circulation* 1992; **85:** 790–804.

94 Muntz KH, Zhao M, Miller JC. Down-regulation of myocardial β-adrenergic receptors: receptor subtype selectivity. *Circ Res* 1994; **74:** 369–375.

94 Kaye DM, Lefkovits J, Jennings GL *et al.* Adverse consequences of high sympathetic nervous activity in the failing human heart. *J Am Coll Cardiol* 1995; **26:** 1257–1263.

96 Communal C, Singh K, Pimental DR, Colucci WS. Norepinephrine stimulates apoptosis in adult rat ventricular myocytes by activation of the β-adrenergic pathway. *Circulation* 1998; **98:** 1329–1334.

97 Bristow MR, Larrabee P, Minobe W *et al.* Receptor pharmacology of carvedilol in the human heart. *J Cardiovasc Pharmacol* 1992; **19**: S68–S80.

98 Hershberger RE, Wynn JR, Sundberg L, Bristow MR. Mechanism of action of bucindolol in human ventricular myocardium. *J Cardiovasc Pharmacol* 1990; **15**: 959–967.

99 Gilbert EM, Abraham WT, Olsen S *et al.* Comparative hemodynamic, left ventricular functional, and antiadrenergic effects of chronic treatment with metoprolol versus carvedilol in the failing heart. *Circulation* 1996; **94**: 2817–2825.

100 Bristow MR. Mechanism of action of bet-blocking agents in heart failure. *Am J Cardiol* 1997; **80(Suppl L)**: 26L–40L.

101 Eichhorn EJ, Heesch CM, Barnett JH *et al.* Effect of metoprolol on myocardial function and energetics in patients with non-ischemic dilated cardiomyopathy: a randomized, double-blind, placebo-controlled study. *J Am Coll Cardiol* 1994; **24**: 1310–1320.

102 Maggi E, Marchesi E, Covini D *et al.* Protective effects of carvedilol, a vasodilating beta-adrenoceptor blocker, against *in vivo* low density lipoprotein oxidation in essential hypertension. *J Cardiovasc Pharmacol* 1996; **27(4)**: 532–538.

103 Cheng J, Kamiya K, Kodama I. Carvedilol: molecular and cellular basis for its multifaceted therapeutic potential. *Cardiovasc Drug Rev* 2001; **19(2)**: 152–171.

104 Sabbah HN, Sharov VG, Gupta RC *et al.* Chronic therapy with metoprolol attenuates cardiomyocyte apoptosis in dogs with heart failure. *J Am Coll Cardiol* 2000; **36**: 1698–1705.

105 Ruffolo Jr RR, Feuerstein GZ. Carvedilol: preclinical profile and mechanisms of action in preventing the progression of CHF. *Eur Heart J* 1998; **19(Suppl B)**: B19–B24.

106 Sabbah HN. The cellular and physiologic effects of beta-blockers in heart failure. *Clin Cardiol* 1999; **22(Suppl V)**: V16–V20.

107 Reiken S, Gaburjakova M, Gaburjakova J *et al.* Beta-adrenergic receptor blockers restore cardiac calcium release channel (ryanodine receptor) structure and function in heart failure. *Circulation* 2001; **104(23)**: 2843–2848.

108 Doi M, Yano M, Kobayashi S *et al.* Propranolol prevents the development of heart failure by restoring FKBP12.6-mediated stabilization of ryanodine receptor. *Circulation* 2002; **105(11)**: 1374–1379.

109 Bristow MR. Beta-adrenergic receptor blockade in chronic heart failure. *Circulation* 2000; **101**: 558–569.

110 Packer M, Bristow MR, Cohn JN *et al.* The effect of carvedilol on morbidity and mortality in patients with chronic heart failure. *N Engl J Med* 1996; **334**: 1349–1355.

111 Waagstein F, Bristow MR, Swedberg K *et al.* Beneficial effects of metoprolol in idiopathic dilated cardiomyopathy. *Lancet* 1993; **342**: 1441–1446.

112 CIBIS Investigators and Committees. A randomized trial of β-blockade in heart failure. The Cardiac Insufficiency Bisoprolol Study (CIBIS). *Circulation* 1994; **90**: 1765–1773.

113 Australia–New Zealand Heart Failure Research Collaborative Group. Randomized, placebo-controlled trial of carvedilol in patients with CHF due to ischemic heart disease. *Lancet* 1997; **349**: 375–380.

114 BEST Investigators. A trial of the beta-blocker bucindolol in patients with chronic heart failure. *N Eng J Med* 2001; **344**: 1659–1667.

115 MERIT-HF. Effect of metoprolol CR/XL in chronic heart failure: Metoprolol CR/XL Randomized Intervention Trial in CHF (MERIT-HF). *Lancet* 1999; **353**: 2001–2007.

116 CIBIS-II Investigators and Committees: The Cardiac Insufficiency Bisoprolol Study II (CIBIS-II). *Lancet* 1999; **353**: 9–13.

117 Packer M, Coats AJS, Fowler MB *et al.* Effect of carvedilol in severe chronic heart failure. *N Engl J Med* 2001; **344**: 1651–1658.

118 Foody JM, Farrell MH, Krumholz HM. β-Blocker therapy in heart failure. Scientific review. *J Am Med Assoc* 2002; **287(7)**: 883–889.

119 Teerlink JR, Massie BM. The role of β-blockers in preventing sudden death in heart failure. *J Cardiac Fail* 2000; **6(2)**: 25–33.

120 Brophy JM, Joseph L, Rouleau JL. Beta-blockers in CHF: a Bayesian meta analysis. *Ann Int Med* 2001; **134**: 550–560.

121 Colucci WS, Packer M, Bristow MR *et al.* Carvedilol inhibits clinical progression in patients with mild symptoms of heart failure. US Carvedilol Heart Failure Study Group. *Circulation* 1996; **94**: 2807–2816.

122 Poole-Wilson PA, Swedberg K, Cleland JG *et al.* Carvedilol Or Metoprolol European Trial Investigators. Comparison of carvedilol and metoprolol on clinical outcomes in patients with chronic heart failure in the Carvedilol Or Metoprolol European Trial (COMET): randomised controlled trial. *Lancet* 2003; **362(9377)**: 7–13.

123 The CAPRICORN Investigators. Effect of carvedilol on outcome after myocardial infarction in patients with left ventricular dysfunction: the CAPRICORN randomized trial. *Lancet* 2001; **357**: 1385–1390.

124 Remme WJ, Riegger G, Hildebrandt P *et al.* The benefits of early combination treatment of carvedilol and an ACE-inhibitor in mild heart failure and left ventricular systolic dysfunction. The carvedilol and ACE-inhibitor remodelling mild heart failure evaluation trial (CARMEN). *Cardiovas Drugs Ther* 2004; **18(1)**: 57–66.

125 Hunt SA, Baker DW, Chin MH *et al.* American College of Cardiology/American Heart Association. ACC/AHA guidelines for the evaluation and management of chronic heart failure in the adult: executive summary. A

report of the American College of Cardiology/American Heart Association Task Force on Practice Guidelines (Committee to revise the 1995 Guidelines for the Evaluation and Management of Heart Failure). *J Am Coll Cardiol* 2001; **38(7)**: 2101–2113.

126 Benedict CR, Shelton B, Johnstone DE *et al*. Prognostic significance of plasma norepinephrine in patients with asymptomatic left ventricular dysfunction. SOLVD Investigators. *Circulation* 1996; **94(4)**: 690–697.

127 Cannan CR, McGoon MD, Holmes Jr DR, Lerman A. Altered coronary endothelial function in a patient with asymptomatic left ventricular dysfunction. *Int J Cardiol* 1996; **53(2)**: 147–151.

128 Kober L, Torp-Pedersen C, Carlsen J *et al*., for the Trandolapril Cardiac Evaluation (TRACE) Study Group. A clinical trial of the angiotensin-converting-enzyme inhibitor trandolapril in patients with left ventricular dysfunction after myocardial infarction. *N Engl J Med* 1995; **333**: 1670–1676.

129 Vantrimpont P, Rouleau JL, Wun CC *et al*. Additive beneficial effects of beta-blockers to angiotensin-converting enzyme inhibitors in the Survival and Ventricular Enlargement (SAVE) Study. *J Am Coll Cardiol* 1997; **29(2)**: 229–236.

130 Exner DV, Dries DL, Waclawiw MA *et al*. Beta-adrenergic blocking agent use and mortality in patients with asymptomatic and symptomatic left ventricular systolic dysfunction: a *post hoc* analysis of the Studies of Left Ventricular Dysfunction. *J Am Coll Cardiol* 1999; **33(4)**: 916–923.

131 Stevenson LW, Massie BM, Francis GS. Optimizing therapy for complex or refractory heart failure: a management algorithm. *Am Heart J* 1998; **135(Suppl)**: 293–309.

132 Steimle AE, Stevenson LW, Chelimsky-Fallick C *et al*. Sustained hemodynamic efficacy of therapy tailored to reduce filling pressures in survivors with advanced heart failure. *Circulation* 1997; **30**: 725–732.

133 Cuffe MS, Califf RM, Adams Jr KF *et al*. The Outcomes of a Prospective Trial of Intravenous Milrinone for Exacerbations of Chronic Heart Failure (OPTIME-CHF) Investigators. Short-term intravenous milrinone for acute exacerbation of chronic heart failure: a randomized controlled trial. *J Am Med Assoc* 2002; **287(12)**: 1541–1547.

134 Young JB. Moen EK. Outpatient parenteral inotropic therapy for advanced heart failure. *J Heart Lung Transplant* 2000; **19(8 Suppl)**:S49–S57.

135 Collins JA, Skidmore MA, Melvin DB, Engel PJ. Home intravenous dobutamine therapy in patients awaiting heart transplantation. *J Heart Transplant* 1990; **9**: 205–208.

136 Elis A, Bental T, Kimchi O *et al*. Intermittent dobutamine treatment in patients with chronic heart failure: a randomized, double-blind, placebo-controlled study. *Clin Pharmacol Ther* 1998; **63**: 682–685.

137 O'Connor CM, Gattis WA, Uretsky BF *et al*. Continuous intravenous dobutamine is associated with an increased risk of death in patients with advanced heart failure: insights from the Flolan International Randomized Survival Trial (FIRST). *Am Heart J* 1999; **138**: 78–86.

138 Grossman W. Diastolic dysfunction in CHF. *N Engl J Med* 1991; **325**: 1557–1564.

139 Goldsmith SR, Dick C. Differentiating systolic from diastolic heart failure. Pathophysiologic and therapeutic considerations. *Am J Med* 1993; **95**: 645–655.

140 Bonow RO, Udelson JE. Left ventricular diastolic dysfunction as a cause of CHF. Mechanisms and management. *Ann Intern Med* 1992; **117**: 502–510.

141 Vasan RS, Benjamin EJ, Levy D. Prevalence, clinical features and prognosis of diastolic heart failure. An epidemiologic perspective. *J Am Coll Cardiol* 1995; **26**: 1565–1574.

142 Cohn JN, Johnson GR, Shabetai R *et al*. Ejection fraction, peak exercise oxygen consumption, cardiothoracic ratio, ventricular arrhythmias and plasma norepinephrine as determinants of prognosis in heart failure. The V-HeFT VA Cooperative Studies Group. *Circulation* 1993; **87(Suppl VI)**: V15–V16.

143 Setaro JF, Zaret BL, Schulman DS, Black HR, Soufer R. Usefulness of verapamil for CHF associated with abnormal left ventricular diastolic filling and normal left ventricular systolic performance. *Am J Cardiol* 1990; **66**: 981–986.

144 MRC Working Party. Medical Research Council trial of treatment of hypertension in older adults. Principal results. *Br Med J* 1992; **304**: 405–412.

145 Liebson PR, Grindits GA, Dianzumba S *et al*. Comparison of five antihypertensive monotherapies and placebo for change in left ventricular mass in patients receiving nutritional-hygienic therapy in the Treatment of Mild Hypertension Study (TOMHS). *Circulation* 1995; **91**: 698–706.

146 Gottdiener JS, Reda DJ, Massie BM *et al*. Effect of single-drug therapy on reduction of left ventricular mass in mild to moderate hypertension. Comparison of 6 antihypertensive agents with placebo. *Circulation* 1997; **95(8)**: 2007–2014.

147 SHEP Cooperative Research Group. Prevention of stroke by antihypertensive treatment in older persons with isolated systolic hypertension. Final results of the Systolic Hypertension in the Elderly Program (SHEP). *J Am Med Assoc* 1991; **265**: 3255–3264.

148 Dahlöf B, Lindholm LH, Hannson L *et al*. Morbidity and mortality in the Swedish Trial in Old Patients with Hypertension (STOP Hypertension). *Lancet* 1991; **338**: 1281–1285.

149 Stevenson WG. Mechanism and management of arrhythmias in heart failure. *Curr Opin Cardiol* 1995; **10**: 274–281.

150 Chun SH, Sager PT, Stevenson WG *et al.* Long-term efficacy of amiodarone for the maintenance of normal sinus rhythm in patients with refractory atrial fibrillation or flutter. *Am J Cardiol* 1995; **76**: 47–50.

151 Stevenson WG, Stevenson LW, Middlekauff HR, Saxon LA. Sudden death prevention in patients with advanced ventricular dysfunction. *Circulation* 1993; **88**: 2953–2961.

152 Saxon LA, Wiener I, DeLurgio DB *et al.* Implantable defibrillators for high-risk patients with heart failure who are awaiting cardiac transplantation. *Am Heart J* 1995; **130**: 501–506.

153 Doval HC, Nul DR, Grancelli HO *et al.* Randomized trial of low-dose amiodarone in severe CHF. Grupo de Estudio de la Sobravida en la Insuficiencia Cardiaca en Argentina (GESICA). *Lancet* 1994; **344**: 493–498.

154 Singh SN, Fletcher RD, Fisher SG *et al.* Amiodarone in patients with CHF and asymptomatic ventricular arrhythmia. Survival Trial of Antiarrhythmic Therapy in CHF. *N Engl J Med* 1995; **333**: 77–82.

155 Massie BM, Fisher SG, Radford M *et al.* Effect of amiodarone on clinical status and left ventricular function in patients with CHF. *Circulation* 1996; **93**: 2318–2334.

156 Baker DW, Wright RF. Management of heart failure. IV. Anticoagulation for patients with heart failure due to left ventricular systolic dysfunction. *J Am Med Assoc* 1994; **272**: 1614–1618.

157 Weidinger F, Glogar D, Sochor H, Sinzinger H. Platelet survival in patients with dilated cardiomyopathy. *Thromb Haemost* 1991; **66(4)**: 400–405.

158 O'Connor CM, Gurbel PA, Serebruany VL. Usefulness of soluble and surface-bound P-selectin in detecting heightened platelet activity in patients with CHF. *Am J Cardiol* 1999; **83**: 1345–1349.

159 Serebruany VL, Murugesan SR, Pothula A *et al.* Increased Soluble Platelet/Endothelial Cellular Adhesion Molecule-1 and Osteonectin Levels in Patients with Severe CHF. Independence of Disease Etiology, and Antecedent Aspirin Therapy. *Eur J Heart Fail* 1999; **1**: 243–249.

160 Al-Khadra AS, Salem DN, Rand WM *et al.* Warfarin anticoagulation and survival: a cohort analysis from the Studies of left ventricular dysfunction. *J Am Coll Cardiol* 1998; **31**: 749–753.

161 Massie BM, Krol WF, Ammon SE *et al.* The Warfarin and Antiplatelet Therapy in Heart Failure trial (WATCH): rationale, design, and baseline patient characteristics. *J Card Failure* 2004; **10(2)**: 101–112.

162 Scardi S, Mazzone C. Antithrombotic prophylaxis in patients with ventricular dysfunction: critical review of the literature and new perspectives. *Italian Heart J Suppl* 2003; **4(3)**: 201–209.

163 Packer M. Interaction of prostaglandins and angiotensin II in the modulation of renal function in CHF. *Circulation* 1988; **77(Suppl I)**:64–73.

164 Moskowitz R. The angiotensin-converting enzyme inhibitor and aspirin interaction in CHF: fear or reality? *Curr Cardiol Rep* 2001; **3**: 247–253.

165 Nguyen KN, Aursnes I, Kjekshus J. Interaction between enalapril and aspirin on mortality after acute myocardial infarction: subgroup analysis of the Cooperative New Scandinavian Enalapril Survival Study II (CONSENSUS II). *Am J Cardiol* 1997; **79**: 115–119.

166 Lindenfeld J, Robertson AD, Lowers BD, Bristow MR. Aspirin impairs reverse myocardial remodeling in patients with heart failure treated with beta-blockers. *J Am Coll Cardiol* 2001; **38**: 1950–1956.

CHAPTER 4

Novel therapies in heart failure

W.H. Wilson Tang & Gary S. Francis

Introduction

Although there has been substantial progress in recent years in the development of pharmacologic therapies for heart failure, on average these drugs increase lifespan by a few months or years at most [1]. The therapies that are currently in vogue, including renin–angiotensin–aldosterone inhibitors and β-adrenergic blockers, simply delay the inexorable progression of disease. There are no existing drugs that "cure" heart failure. Therefore, there is an ongoing need to develop effective new therapies for the management of this condition that might slow further progression of heart failure.

The marketplace largely drives the development of new and innovative therapies. Heart failure is now the single most common reason for patients over the age of 65 years to be admitted to the hospital [2], and data from the Framingham Heart Study suggest that the lifetime risk of developing heart failure is about 20% in both men and women [3]. Contemporary therapies are not wholly satisfactory, leading pharmaceutical and biotechnology companies to invest millions of dollars into the development of new drugs. Regulatory agencies maintain very high standards for the approval of new pharmaceutical therapies. Relative to other specialties, development of new drugs for cardiovascular disease has been a successful enterprise, but remains challenging [4]. This has led to the current industry concept that heart failure is a "niche market."

This chapter provides a brief overview of several "up and coming" developmental strategies of medical therapy for patients with heart failure, (some with preliminary data and others only preclinical data), recognizing that many of these therapies will never come to market. We will briefly discuss several

approved drug classes that are extending their current heart failure indications, several drug classes that have tried in large-scale clinical trials without success, and several promising drug classes that are currently under investigation.

Approved drugs classes with extended indications

Selective aldosterone receptor antagonists

It is now clear that aldosterone plays a far more important role in cardiovascular disease than originally envisioned. Aldosterone promotes collagen deposition and structural remodeling in the heart and the blood vessels in response to altered loading conditions and various forms of tissue injury [5]. Angiotensin-converting enzyme (ACE) inhibitors, though widely and successfully used in the treatment of hypertension and heart failure, do not consistently suppress the release of aldosterone. This "escape" of aldosterone and its action on the heart and blood vessels may account for some of the organ damage that occurs in patients with hypertension and heart failure [6]. Aldosterone receptors are largely nuclear receptors. That is, they are activated in the cytosol by aldosterone and carry their message to the nucleus where they activate the transcription of numerous genes. Therefore, much of the pharmacologic activity of aldosterone is delayed for hours to days. There are also non-nuclear aldosterone receptors on external cell membranes that subserve non-genomically regulated functions such as the transport of cations (sodium and potassium) across cell membranes. Blocking these receptors can cause immediate pharmacologic effects. The "proof of concept" here is that aldosterone antagonism favorably alters the natural history of heart failure as pointed out in the Randomized Aldactone Evaluation Study (RALES) trial [7]. Despite RALES, widespread use of spironolactone has been limited because of adverse effects including hyperkalemia, renal insufficiency, painful gynecomastia, impotence, and menstrual irregularities, in some instances even have harmful consequences if not carefully utilized [8].

Eplerenone (Inspra, Pfizer) is a new, highly selective aldosterone receptor antagonist that has demonstrated efficacy in patients with hypertension [9]. Several studies have demonstrated that eplerenone has effective blood-pressure-lowering effects in patients with hypertension [10,11]. The recent EPHESUS (Eplerenone Post-AMI (Acute Myocardial Infarction) Heart Failure Efficacy and Survival) Study involved 6200 subjects with left ventricular ejection fraction (LVEF) <40% plus clinical heart failure, and randomized them 3–10 days post-myocardial infarction (post-MI) to eplerenone versus placebo. The EPHESUS study has confirmed mortality and morbidity benefits of eplerenone in patients with post-infarction heart failure [12]. The drug appears to be much more selective for the mineralo-corticoid receptor than spironolactone, thus reducing the troublesome side effects of painful gynecomastia [13]. A large multicenter study is currently underway to establish the efficacy of eplerenone in reverse left ventricular (LV) remodeling in patients with mild-to-moderate heart failure. As with all aldosterone antagonists, hyperkalemia (especially in the setting of renal insufficiency and diabetes mellitus) remain a potential problem. Therefore, careful patient selection and close monitoring of electrolytes and renal function will be essential with eplerenone use, as it now is with spironolactone.

One of the more dramatic effects of aldosterone antagonism is the regression of established LV hypertrophy and reversal of LV remodeling. This effect is magnified when eplerenone is used with ACE inhibition as demonstrated by the recent 4E (Efficacy and Safety of Eplerenone, Enalapril, and Eplerenone/Enalapril Combination Therapy in Patients With Left Ventricular Hypertrophy) study [14]. In this study, the effects of eplerenone plus enalapril were synergistic and additive. Inhibition of the aldosterone receptors also abrogates vascular and myocardial remodeling [15,16]. Spironolactone reduces collagen

deposition and remodeling of injured myocardial tissue [17] thereby improving diastolic heart function [18,19]. It is likely that aldosterone receptor antagonists will be helpful even in less ill patients, but such indications will only be justified if results from the upcoming European EMPHASIS (Eplerenone in Mild Patients Hospitalization and Survival Study in Heart Failure) trial are positive. Several studies are also currently underway to explore the role of eplerenone in reverse remodeling in the setting of valvular diseases and in diastolic dysfunction. In addition, a large international mortality trial, TOPCAT (Treatment Of Preserved Cardiac Function Heart Failure with an Aldosterone Antagonist) is also ongoing to determine if treating patients with diastolic heart failure with spironolactone is beneficial or not.

Natriuretic peptides

B-type natriuretic peptide (BNP) is an endogenous circulating natriuretic peptide that is synthesized constitutively by cardiac myocytes and released into the circulation in the setting of cardiac dysfunction, such as heart failure [20]. As a counter-regulatory peptide, BNP has multiple functions. It mediates vasodilation via a vascular cyclic guanosine monophosphate (cGMP) receptor pathway, promotes a modest natriuresis, is anti-trophic and suppresses vasoconstrictor neurohormonal actions to a modest extent. Plasma levels of BNP progressively rise in heart failure as symptoms worsen [21]. Therefore, it would seem natural to consider exogenous BNP as a form of therapy, particularly in patients with acute heart failure who require an intravenous agent.

Recombinant human BNP has been synthesized and developed for intravenous use [22]. Intravenous BNP, known as nesiritide (Natrecor, Scios), has been approved for short-term intravenous use in patients with acute heart failure syndrome (AHFS). In the VMAC (Vasodilation in the Management of Acute Congestive Heart Failure) trial, nesiritide was found to be at least as effective as intravenous nitroglycerin [23]. It has the added advantage of promoting a rather smooth decline in central filling pressures while providing a synergistic diuretic effect when used in conjunction with loop diuretic therapy. However, patients who demonstrate a substantial diuresis in response to nesiritide and diuretics may develop volume depletion hypotension, which can persist for several hours unless volume is replaced. Data from the PRECEDENT (Prospective Randomized Evaluation of Cardiac Ectopy with Dobutamine or Nesiritide Therapy) trial suggested that nesiritide is not proarrhythmic [24]. Nesiritide is often given as a bolus followed by an infusion drip, but recent experience have limited to just low-dose infusions. The duration of the infusion is usually determined by the clinical and hemodynamic response to the drug. Most patients are maintained on nesiritide for 24–48 h. Nesiritide is currently being investigated in the European registration trial, ENTA (Evaluating Treatment with Nesiritide in Acute Decompensated Heart Failure), and a large international mortality mega-trial of 7000 subjects is in the planning stages to refute recent concerns regarding the association of the use of nesiritide and worsening renal function and late mortality[25,26]. Meanwhile, further investigations into the role of nesiritide regarding renal preservation or deterioration will be explored several smaller studies.

Similar approaches using recombinant atrial natriuretic peptide (carperitide, Daiichi/Fujisawa)[27] and recombinant urodilatin (ularitide, Protein Design Labs, Inc)[28], are currently undergoing clinical trials in the United States. Other "endogenous vasodilators" such as urocortin II (Neurocrine Biosciences)[29] as well as "chimeric" peptides like the eel ventricular natriuretic peptide (VNP) are also in early clinical phase development. The concepts of all these compounds are similar to that of nesiritide, except that each compound boasts to have its unique properties or different-half-lives at different sites of action that will require further research validation.

Another active area of investigation is the role of intermittent infusion of nesiritide. The pilot FUSION (Follow-Up Serial Infusions Of Nesiritide) study evaluated 210 patients at high risk of hospitalization for heart failure, who were randomized to one of three treatment arms: standard care or serial infusions of either 0.005 or 0.01 mcg/kg/min of nesiritide. During a 12-week period, more patients in the standard-treatment group died or were hospitalized than in the nesiritide-treated groups (58% versus 48%, $P = 0.185$), without a significantly different incidence of serious adverse events. The effects of long-term intermittent (1–2 times per week) nesiritide outpatient infusion in advanced heart

failure will be examined in the 24-week, 900-patient FUSION-II study that has recently completed enrollment. The objective of this approach is to reduce hospitalizations for acute decompensated heart failure episodes with intermittent nesiritide infusions. Long-term nesiritide infusion for advanced heart failure patients waiting for cardiac transplantation will also be tested in the TMAC (Nesiritide in Transplant – Eligible Management of Congestive Heart Failure) study.

Statin therapy

Statin therapy has been widely used in patients with hypercholesterolemia and coronary artery disease. Pleiotropic properties of statins may include non-specific anti-inflammatory effects, improvements in endothelial dysfunction, inhibition of cardiac hypertrophy pathways, restore autonomic balance, reduction in oxidative stress, and increase in nitric oxide bioavailability [30–35]. The idea that statins may be beneficial in patients with heart failure stem from several *post-hoc* analyses on the utilization of lipid-lowering agents in heart failure clinical trials and observational clinical series [36–39]. Recent mechanistic data are also pointed to improvements in LV remodeling in a prospective randomized-controlled trial [43], but preliminary results from the UNIVERSE (Rosuvastatin Impact on Ventricular Remodeling lipids and cytokines) trial in Australia did not show any additional benefits in improving cardiac remodeling with resuvastating therapy [44]. Several upcoming heart failure trials using rosuvastatin (Crestor, AstraZeneca) are ongoing. These included the Italian GISSI (Gruppo Italiano per lo Studio della Sopravvivenza nell'Infarto Miocardico) Prevenzione trial that investigates whether treatment with rosuvastatin or fish oil improves mortality and morbidity of people with symptomatic heart failure of any etiology already receiving standard treatment [45]. The multicenter CORONA (COntrolled ROsuvastatin multiNAtional trial) is a long-term, randomized, double-blind, placebo-controlled, multi-national study to evaluate rosuvastatin 10 mg on cardiovascular mortality and morbidity and overall survival in 4950 patients with chronic ischemic cardiomyopathy (NYHA II–IV). Until these results are available, the role of statin therapy in patients with heart failure should still be confined to the treatment of dyslipidemia or secondary prevention following ischemic events.

Erythropoietin analogues

Anemia has been more widely recognized in patients with heart failure, and may contribute to the classic signs and symptoms [46]. The exact mechanisms are unclear, but may simple relate to chronicity of the heart failure states, nutritional deficiencies, or dilutional effects due to hypervolemia. The overall prevalence of anemia in the general heart failure population is estimated to be about 15%, while patients with more advanced heart failure have a higher prevalence of anemia, (estimated to be about 25%) [47,48]. The anemia of heart failure is associated with worsening symptoms, greater impairment in functional capacity, higher mortality, and poorer prognosis in both systolic and diastolic dysfunction [49]. Critically ill patients, including those in the intensive care unit with heart failure, typically require multiple red blood cell transfusions [50]. Although the cause of anemia in heart failure is multifactorial [51], the risks and benefits of intervening specific targets in the vicious cycle of anemia, chronic renal failure and exacerbation of heart failure is unclear.

It is well known that anemia contributes to the morbidity and mortality of patients with another disease of end-organ dysfunction – end-stage renal failure (ESRD) [52]. Patients with ESRD are now routinely treated with recombinant human erythropoietin (rHuEPO) and intravenous iron. A large proportion of patients with heart failure and anemia have normal or even elevated serum levels of erythropoietin, suggesting that the response to erythropoietin in the setting of anemia rather than the lack of erythropoietin may be abnormal in this population. A study by Silverberg and colleagues showed that when anemia in patients with heart failure was corrected by treatment with rHuEPO, there was marked improvement in cardiac and patient function associated with fewer hospitalizations and decreased diuretic requirements [53,54]. A novel erythropoiesis stimulating protein (NESP, or darbepoetin alpha), a hyperglycosylated analog of rHuEPO with 3 times longer half-life.

Although the concept of using rHuEPO to treat patients with heart failure is rational, the selection of patients, the appropriate dosing, and the therapeutic target hematocrit level remain problematic.

There is a theoretical concern that raising blood viscosity and plasma volume could contribute to additional afterload stress, worsening fluid overload and hypertension, and further impairing cardiac function. Additionally, the "anemia" of heart failure may be, in part, a dilutional problem caused by fluid retention, rather than an actual decrease in red blood cell mass. Despite these uncertainties, it is reasonable to consider rHuEPO as a management strategy for patients with anemia and heart failure. Preliminary results from two Phase II studies showed that treatment with darbepoetin alfa in anemic patients with symptomatic heart failure was well-tolerated, effectively raised hemoglobin, and improved patients' symptoms [44,55]. This hypothesis is currently being tested in large, international randomized-controlled trial called RED-HF (Reduction of Events with Darbepoetin alfa in Heart Failure) using darbepoeting alpha injections.

Drug classes that faltered in clinical trials

Endothelin receptor antagonists

Endothelin is a family of 21-amino acid peptides (ET-1, ET-2, and ET-3) that have potent vasoconstriction and growth properties in both the pulmonary and systemic vascular circulations [56,57]. Endothelin-1 (ET-1) is synthesized in the vascular endothelial cells from its precursor, big-ET-1. The large molecule is cleaved by endothelin-converting enzymes (ECE-1 and ECE-2) or other less specific proteases such as neutral endopeptideases (NEPs) to release active ET-1. Synthesis of ET-1 is regulated by many factors, including neurohormones (angiotensin-II, norepinephrine, vasopressin), cytokines (tumor necrosis factor-alpha (TNF-α), transforming growth factor beta, bradykinin), thrombin and mechanical stress. Plasma ET-1 levels correlate with disease severity and prognosis in patients with heart failure [58]. Like angiotensin-II, endothelin may have an important role in the pathophysiology of heart failure progression, including remodeling.

Since the original report by Yanagisawa and colleagues in 1988 [59], there has been an explosive growth of information regarding endothelin and its role in the progression of cardiovascular disease. Recognizing its huge potential, pharmaceutical laboratories quickly developed a series of endothelin receptor antagonists and ECE inhibitors designed to block the detrimental effects of endothelin [60]. However, it was soon recognized that there were at least two endothelin receptors, including A (ET_A) and B (ET_B), that subserve somewhat different functions. ET_A receptors bind ET-1 and ET-2 with much higher affinity than ET-3 [61]. ET_A stimulation leads to vasoconstriction. In contrast, ET_B receptors bind all three endothelins with relatively equal affinities, and mediate vasorelaxation as well as clearance of circulating ET-1. Of interest, infusion of ET-3 (relatively selective to ET_B receptors) results in vasoconstriction [62]. Both receptors may mediate pathologic hypertrophy and fibrosis.

The first widely studied endothelin receptor antagonist was the dual endothelin receptor antagonist, bosentan (Tracleer, Actelion). Bosentan demonstrated an acute, highly favorable hemodynamic effect in patients with chronic heart failure [63]. Cardiac output was improved and LV filling pressure was reduced. However, bosentan also increased plasma levels of ET-1, probably by inhibiting the clearance of ET-1 by ET_B receptors. The consequences of this observation are not certain. Preliminary animal and human studies suggested that there are short-term benefits of bosentan in patients with heart failure. This was followed by the REACH-1 (Research on Endothelin Antagonism in Chronic Heart Failure) trial – a multi-center, randomized controlled trial comparing bosentan (target dose 500 mg twice daily) to placebo in patients with advanced heart failure (NYHA IIIb–IV, LVEF ≤ 35%, $n = 370$). The study showed an initial worsening in the bosentan group (especially with worsening heart failure during the fast titration group in the first 20 days) and was terminated prematurely as a result of an unexpectedly high incidence of dose-dependent liver function abnormalities (15.6% in the bosentan group) [64]. Clinical benefits were observed in patients who received the full 6 months of randomized treatment with bosentan. The REACH-1 data suggested the hypothesis that despite a potential early adverse effect profile over time, bosentan may improve morbidity and mortality. As a result, the ENABLE (Endothelin Antagonist Bosentan for Lowering Cardiac Events in Heart Failure) trials (NYHA IIIb–IV, LVEF <35%, $n = 1613$) were conducted to compare bosentan (target dose 125 mg twice daily) with placebo in patients with advanced heart failure. These two parallel trials, ENABLE-1 (Europe, $n = 750$) and ENABLE-2 (North America, $n = 750$), either combined or analyzed separately, indicated no overall mortality benefit with bosentan therapy [65]. The survival curves again crossed over, as was seen in REACH-1. The study demonstrated that patients randomly assigned to bosentan developed weight gain from edema. The mechanism of salt and water retention with bosentan is not well understood.

Other endothelin receptor antagonists that have been tested in clinical trials include the dual ET_A/ET_B antagonist enrasentan (SB 217242, GlaxoSmithKline) and J-104132 (Banyu/Merck). Also, selective ET_A receptor antagonists, sitaxsentan (TBC-11251, ICOS-Texas Biotechnology), darusentan (LU-135252, Abbott), edonentan (BMS-207940, Bristol-Myers Squibb), and ambrisentan (BSF-208075, Myogen) have all been tried as potential drug therapy for heart failure. However, disappointing results from Phase II/III studies on enrasentan (ENCOR [66]) and darusentan (EARTH [67]) indicate no clinical benefit. In the case of darusentan, there was a strong trend for the drug to increase morbidity, and cardiac remodeling was not prevented at any dose within the 6 months of therapy. The reason for the failure of this drug class as heart failure therapy in unclear, although dosing has often been the concern [68]. Furthermore, tezosantan (Veletri, Actelion), an intravenous ET_A/ET_B antagonist, has demonstrated potential favorable hemodynamic effects in a series of Phase II studies (Randomized Intravenous Tezosentan Studies, RITZ 1–5). However, disappointing results from VERITAS (Value of Endothelin Receptor Inhibition with Tezosentan in Acute Heart Failure Study)[69] reported no statistically significant differences in changes in dyspnea at 24 h, death or worsening heart failure at 7 or 30 days, or overall mortality at 6 months between those receiving Tezosentan versus placebo [70].

On the other hand, there are substantial data to support the use of bosentan in patients with pulmonary hypertension (PH) [71]. Bosentan significantly improves exercise capacity, symptoms, and functional status in patients with PH. Results from large-scale studies of bosentan in patients with primary pulmonary hypertension (PPH) have established its long-term safety and tolerability profiles. Bosentan has been approved in November 2001 by the US Food and Drug Administrations and registered for this indication. Sitaxentan (Thelin, Encysive Pharmaceuticals) is also undergoing approval process as PH therapy, but a Phase II study is currently underway to evaluate its potential use in the setting of diastolic heart failure.

Neutral endopeptidase and vasopeptidase inhibitors

NEPs are ubiquitous enzymes that are responsible for degrading numerous peptides, including bradykinin and the counter-regulatory natriuretic peptides [72]. Natriuretic peptides are cleared from the body by NEPs and by c-receptors (clearance), primarily located in the brush borders of the kidney. Pharmacologists have reasoned that since endogenous natriuretic peptides have a favorable profile in hypertension and heart failure, delaying their degradation by inhibition of NEPs should result in higher plasma levels of these peptides and reduced blood pressure with a modest natriuresis and diuresis. Prototype compounds such as ecadotril and candoxatril (UK-79300) were studied in the early 1990s and provided proof of concept.

Vasopeptidase inhibitors (VPI) are single hybrid, molecular compounds that inhibit two distinct zinc metalloproteases: NEP and ACE. Vasopeptidase inhibitors attenuate the formation of angiotensin-II while increasing endogenous levels of natriuretic peptides and bradykinin. The initial experience with vasopeptidase inhibitors was generally positive in that they significantly lowered blood pressure and promoted a modest diuretic and natriuretic effect. The development of omapatrilat (Vanlev, Bristol-Myers Squibb) was an attempt to eventually market a hybrid compound to inhibit both ACE and NEPs. The added benefit of prolonging counter-regulatory natriuretic peptides, in addition to a further reduction in high blood pressure, and a modest natriuresis and diuresis, includes the inhibition of the sympathetic and renin–angiotensin–aldosterone systems [73,74]. Preliminary data from IMPRESS (Inhibition of Metalloproteases by Omapatrilat in a Randomized Exercise and Symptoms Study) [75] suggested a very favorable hemodynamic and neurohormonal effect in patients with heart failure. Based on a large dataset that demonstrated both safety and efficacy, two additional large studies were

conducted: the OVERTURE (Omapatrilat Versus Enalapril Randomized Trial of Utility in Reducing Events) trial for heart failure (NYHA II–IV, LVEF <30%, $n = 5770$) [76], and the OCTAVE (Omapatrilat Cardiovascular Treatment Assessment Versus Enalapril) [77] trial for hypertension. Omapatrilat was associated with a lower rate of worsening heart failure and renal impairment in OVERTURE [76], but showed an increased rate of hypotension and dizziness. Mortality was not favorably influenced by omapatrilat. Although omapatrilat was superior to enalapril in systolic blood pressure reduction in OCTAVE, angioedema was increased in patients assigned to omapatrilat (2.2%), particularly in African-Americans (5.5%) and in smokers (3.9%) [78]. The OPERA (Omapatrilat in Persons with Enhanced Risk of Atherosclerotic events) trial was a large study designed to examine the safety and efficacy of omapatrilat in older patients with Stage I isolated systolic hypertension [79], and was discontinued due to poor enrollment. Omapatrilat and other VPIs [80] are unlikely going to be approved for hypertension or heart failure. Meanwhile, a unique dual ECE/ NEP inhibitor, daglutril (SLV306, Solvay) is reportedly still undergoing Phase II trial called REMODELED (Reduce Myocardial Dilatation and Enlargement by the Enzyme-inhibitor Daglutril) to determine its potential benefits in reverse remodeling in patients with heart failure.

Novel anti-adrenergic therapies

Moxonidine (Physiotens/Moxon, Eli Lilly/Solvay) and rilmenidine are imidazoline-1 (I_1) receptor agonists that powerfully inhibit sympathetic traffic from the central nervous system to the periphery [81,82]. Short-acting moxonidine is widely used in Europe as an anti-hypertensive agent. Unlike clonidine, a mixed agonist that stimulates both α_1 and α_2 receptors, moxonidine is a relatively selective I_1 agonist. Therefore, some of the side effects of clonidine, such as dry mouth and somnolence, can be avoided with moxonidine. The overly active sympathetic nervous system in patients with heart failure was a logical target for the use of moxonidine. In order to test the hypothesis that moxonidine would have a favorable effect on morbidity and mortality in patients with heart failure, the MOXCON (Effect of Sustained-Release Moxonidine on

Mortality and Morbidity in Patients with Congestive Heart Failure) trial was designed and conducted [83]. The new sustained-release moxonidine preparation was compared to placebo in patients on receiving conventional therapy for heart failure. The trial was stopped early when the Data Safety Monitoring Board noted an early excessive number of deaths in the moxonidine arm of the trial. Subsequent data analysis indicated that moxonidine SR, the preparation used in the MOXCON trial, was associated with a very substantial fall in plasma norepinephrine levels, sometimes up to 50% from baseline [84,85]. There is the possibility that sustained-release moxonidine was detrimental because of its propensity to over-inhibit the sympathetic nervous system. The observations from MOXCON provided a first glimpse into the possibility that there may be limits to the concept of comprehensive neurohormonal blockade. Based on the results of MOXCON and a concomitant safety and efficacy study, MOXSE (Moxonidine Safety and Efficacy) [86], investigators have recommended that for patients not receiving moxonidine for hypertension, the drug should not be abruptly stopped, but that it should be tapered over several days to avoid a rebound hypertensive phenomenon. The future of centrally acting sympatholytics drugs for the treatment of heart failure remains uncertain.

There have been other efforts to develop anti-adrenergic agents with novel targets. Early studies on dopamine analogs such as ibopamine have raised hopes that these drugs may reduce catecholamine release via the inhibition of postganglionic sym-pathetic nerves and sympathetic ganglia [87]. Bromocriptine and its vascular dopaminergic effects have also been studied in the 1980s [88]. Nolomirole (CHF1035, Chiesi), an esterified amino-tetraline derivative, is an oral selective dual agonist of DA_2 dopaminergic presynaptic receptors and α_2 adrenergic receptors. This novel vasodilator produced improvement in symptoms and exercise capacity without arrhythmogenic side effects in Phase II studies [89]. However, the ECHOS (Echocardiography and Heart Outcomes Study) showed no significant difference between nolomirole and placebo in hospitalizations, NYHA class, mortality, or 6-min walk test between the groups[55], dampening the early enthusiasm for this drug.

Cytokine antagonists

The failing heart has been known to express the inflammatory cytokine TNF-α, which likely contributes to hypertrophy, remodeling and development of cardiomyopathy. There is a body of literature suggesting that TNF-α is important in the pathogenesis of heart failure [90]. Patients with heart failure develop progressively higher levels of TNF-α as their conditions worsens [91,92]. There is growing interest in the development of novel drugs that inhibit cytokines, important mediators of inflammation [90]. Infliximab (Remicade, Centocor), a chimeric (mouse/human) immunoglobulin G_1 monoclonal antibody against TNF-α, is widely used to treat patients with Crohn's disease and rheumatoid arthritis. Etanercept (Embrel, Immunex/Amgen) is a fusion protein that is widely used in patients with rheumatoid arthritis. Etanercept is designed to inhibit the effects of TNF-α by binding to circulating TNF-α, thus limiting its interaction with its cognate membrane-bound receptor. Preliminary data with etanercept in both experimental models and in patients with heart failure were strongly supportive of the concept that TNF-α contributes to the development of heart failure. In small, observational studies, antagonism of TNF-α with etanercept was associated with objective myocardial and clinical improvement. Based on these observations, two related randomized control trials; RENAISSANCE (in the United States and Canada) and RECOVER (in Europe and Australia) were conducted. The studies, whether analyzed separately or combined (as RENEWAL, or Randomized Etanercept Worldwide Evaluation), did not show a morbidity or mortality benefit of etanercept over placebo in patients receiving conventional therapy [93,94]. The Phase II ATTACH (Anti-TNF-α Therapy Against CHF) study using intermittent intravenous infusion of infliximab also demonstrated worsening clinical endpoints especially at high doses [93,94]. The reasons for the lack of efficacy in TNF-α antagonism strategies have been widely debated, but are not entirely clear. The lack of benefit may be related to inappropriate dosing, partial agonist activity of drug-bound TNF-α, or flawed trial designs [95]. New analogs of thalidomide [96] (a potent TNF-α inhibitor) and pentoxifylline [97] (a widely used xanthine derivative that blocks TNF-α) are being considered as potential therapeutic agents.

Sodium–hydrogen exchange

Sodium–hydrogen exchange (NHE) has been considered a key target for the treatment of heart failure [98]. NHE is a major mechanism for intracellular pH regulation in most cell types. Myocytes have ubiquitous NHE-1 subtype, which is a major contributor to ischemic and reperfusion injury since it is the primary regulator of intracellular pH. Therefore, NHE-1 inhibitors exert marked cardioprotective effects during ischemia, and may halt chronic maladaptive myocardial remodeling and the development of heart failure [99,100]. It appears that NHE-1 may even represent a common downstream mediator for various hypertropic factors such as angiotensin II, ET-1, and β_1-adrenergic receptor activation. Amiloride has NHE inhibitory properties. However, clinical trials program in ZONIPORIDE (CP-597396, Pfizer) and cariporide (Sanofi/Aventis), both new selective inhibitor of NHE-1, have reportedly been halted.

Oral phosphodiesterase (PDE3) inhibitors

Cyclic nucleotide phosphodiesterases such as PDE3 degrade cyclic nucleotides. They are therefore important in cyclic AMP (cAMP) and possibly cyclic GMP-mediated signaling in cardiac and vascular smooth muscle myocytes. Normally, cAMP phosphorylates various proteins (i.e. protein kinase A) that in turn phosphorylate proteins that modulate the entry of Ca^{2+} into the contractile apparatus. Drugs that inhibit phosphodiesterases raise cAMP levels, leading to enhanced inotropic and vasodilatory actions that have proven to be useful in the short-term treatment of heart failure and severe pulmonary hypertension. With long-term oral usage, however, oral PDE3 inhibitors increase mortality in patients with advanced heart failure (NYHA III–IV) – first in the PROMISE (Prospective Randomized Milrinone Survival Evaluation) trial for milrinone [101] and the PICO (Pimobendan in Congestive Heart Failure) trial for pimobendan (Vetmedin, Abbott) [102]. It is presumed that continuous stimulation of cAMP may be detrimental due to tachycardia, arrhythmias, and "overwork" of the inotropic state of myocardial cells. However, patients with mild to moderate heart failure treated with concomitant β-blockers and low-dose pimobendan therapy show improvement in morbidity and mortality [103]. Furthermore, therapy with pimobendan facilitated initiation of carvedilol in patients with severe heart failure [104]. Phase II studies with the PDE3 inhibitor toborinone (OPC-18790, Otsuka) are in progress.

Enoximone (MDL 17043, Myogen) is an orally active selective PDE3 inhibitor. Like milrinone, it enhances the inotropic state of the heart by increasing the levels of cAMP, thereby increasing phosphorylation of various proteins that regulate Ca^{2+} availability. Enoximone was widely studied in the 1980s along with its analog piroximone. Both drugs demonstrated markedly positive inotropic properties. However, they also raised heart rate, were arrhythmogenic, and are believed to increase the potential for excessive mortality when used long-term. However, enoximone is still used in some countries, particularly France. Interest in oral enoximone has been recently resurrected by the possibility that the concomitant use of a β-receptor antagonist and enoximone may offer theoretical advantages. The inotropic response to enoximone in patients receiving β-adrenergic blockade is preserved or even enhanced, unlike the mutually antagonistic effects of β-blockade and dobutamine. Beta-blockers and enoximone, when given concomitantly, may reduce the up-regulation of inhibitory $G_{\alpha i}$ protein. In theory, the favorable effects of enoximone and β-blockers are operationally additive. Additionally, enoximone might be used as a bridge to β-blocker initiation in patients who might otherwise be intolerant to β-blocker therapy because of advanced heart failure.

The Phase II results from EMOTE (A Phase II Randomized, Double-Blind, Placebo-Controlled Parallel Study of Oral Enoximone in Intravenous Inotrope-Dependent Subjects) has recently been presented. A total of 201 patients with advanced heart failure (NYHA III–IV, inotrope dependent, LVEF ($\leq$25%, LVEDD ($\geq$5.4 cm or 2.7 cm/m^2) were randomized to receive enoximone (25/50 mg 3 times per day) versus placebo. The primary endpoint of successful inotrope weaning at 30 days was achieved by 61% patients in the enoximone group and 51% in the placebo-treated group (not statistically significant). However, there was a benefit of lower rates of death or re-initiation of IV inotrope therapy at 60- and 90-day periods favoring enoximone [105]. The safety and efficacy of low-dose oral enoximone has been tested in a Phase III program, which includes the ESSENTIAL (Studies of Oral Enoximone Therapy in

Advanced Heart Failure, including ESSENTIAL-I in North and South America, and ESSENTIAL-II in Europe), and EMPOWER (Enoximone Plus Extended-Release Metoprolol Succinate in Subjects with Advanced Chronic Heart Failure). The results of these trials have been announced, and oral enoximone did not improve long-term morbidity and mortality in patients with advanced heart failure [106, 107]. At present, there are no plans to continue further development of oral enoximone as heart failure therapy.

Novel drug classes with promising clinical development

Arginine vasopressin antagonists

Neurohormonal excesses are well known to contribute to the pathophysiology of heart failure. Plasma arginine vasopressin (AVP) levels are increased in patients with heart failure and likely contribute to progression of the syndrome through activation of V_{1a} and V_2 receptors [108]. Activation of the V_{1a} receptors causes vasoconstriction, platelet aggregation, and adrenocorticotrophic hormone (ACTH) stimulation. Activation of the V_2 receptors within the renal collecting duct promotes sodium and water retention. Experimental studies indicate that blockade of the V_{1a} or V_2 receptors, either alone or in combination, results in a beneficial hemodynamic profile and less ventricular remodeling following myocardial injury [109,110]. Based on these concepts, there has been a long-standing interest in the development of AVP receptor antagonists for the treatment of heart failure [111].

There are also AVP antagonists that combine V_{1a} and V_2 receptor blockade. The V_{1a} receptor blockade in a post-infarction model reduces myocardial remodeling. In the recent ACTIV CHF (Acute and Chronic Therapeutic Impact of a Vasopressin Antagonist in Congestive Heart Failure) study, 319 patients treated with tolvaptan (OPC-41061, Otsuka), a selective V2 vasopressin receptor antagonist, had significant weight reduction due to fluid loss compared with placebo [112]. Tolvaptan improved serum sodium levels, and did not cause electrolyte imbalance, affect hemodynamics, or worsen renal function. All-cause mortality was 5.4% in the tolvaptan groups, and 8.7% in the placebo group, a difference that did not reach statistical significance. Result from the larger Phase III trial,

EVEREST (Effects of Vasopressin Antagonists in Heart Failure: Outcome Study with Tolvaptan), will soon be announced. EVEREST hopes to demonstrate that low-dose (30 mg/day) oral tolvaptan can improve clinical outcomes in as well as symptoms in patients with AHFS treated with standard therapy. Meanwhile, hemodynamic effects of tolvaptan will be further clarified in the ongoing ECLIPSE (Multicenter, Randomized, Double-blind, Placebo-controlled Study to Evaluate the Effect of Single Oral Tolvaptan Tablets on Hemodynamic Parameters in Subjects with Heart Failure) trial. Another dual antagonist, lixivaptan (cardiokine) is currently undergoing Phase II evaluation for the same indication.

The benefits of selective V_2 antagonist such as conivaptan (Vaprisol or YM087, Yamanouchi Pharmaceuticals) has been best seen in the treatment of hyponatremia, and several Phase II studies have been completed but the results have not been published[113]. It is not clear whether conivaptan will be developed as a heart failure drug. Other selective V_2 receptor antagonists, SR-121463b (Sanofi-Synthelabo) and VPA-985 (Wyeth-Ayerst), are also being tested in Phase-II clinical trials for hyponatremia. It is a hope that these drugs will be useful in the treatment of fluid overloaded states by increasing free-water excretion, improving dilutional hyponatremia, promoting peripheral vasodilation, and improving cardiac performance. How they should be used in conjunction or instead of standard loop diuretics will remain a challenge if these drugs are approved for AHFS or chronic maintenance. Furthermore, the lack of an agreeable endpoint for clinical trials in AHFS has discouraged many of these compounds from pursuing clinical development [114].

Adenosine receptor blockers

Adenosine is an endogenous vasoactive substance whose action is mediated through at least four receptors [115]. The most prevalent receptors are type 1, which promote vasoconstriction, and type 2, comprised of two subtypes (2A and 2B), which promote vasodilation. In the kidney, type 1 receptors located on pre-glomerular afferent vessels and in the tubules, and are involved in the regulation of glomerular filtration. Whole-body fluid balance is strongly dependent on the ability of the kidney to maintain stable intraglomerular hydraulic pressure. Several selective adenosine type 1 receptor antagonists have been developed. These agents enhance fluid (diuresis) and sodium (natriuresis) excretion in animals and experimental models of fluid retention by increasing afferent arteriolar dilation and thus intraglomerular hydraulic pressure [116]. This is also observed in normal and edematous humans [117]. In both animals and humans, these effects are generally achieved without major changes in glomerular filtration. Animal studies have confirmed the location of adenosine type 1 (A_1) receptors in relevant tissue sites in the kidney. Clinical trial results with adenosine antagonists had mixed results. The early results with BG9719/CVT-124 (Adentri, Biogen) in heart failure suggested promise [118], whereas trials in hypertension and renal failure have been more equivocal.

Clinical trials with another second-generation adenosine A_1 receptor antagonist, BG-9928 (Biogen Idec/Medicines Company) are also underway. The AB-CHF (A Phase II Randomized, Double-Blind, Placebo-Controlled, Trial Comparing Adenosine Blockade with BG9928 with Placebo for the Prevention of Worsening Renal Function in Patients with Acute Decompensated Heart Failure) is designed to initiate this drug therapy at the Emergency Department, with the goal to demonstrate efficacy in lowering the incidence of worsening renal insufficiency. Another novel intravenous A_1 receptor antagonist, KW-3902 (NovaCardia), has shown diuretic properties via impressive increases in glomerular filtration rates (GFR) and renal plasma flow. This is particularly apparent in those that were less responsive to loop diuretics over time during AHFS, where over 50% increase in GFR was documented with the use of KW-3902. This drug currently is being tested in a multi-center Phase III trials program, PROTECT (A Placebo-Controlled Randomized Study of the Selective A_1 Adenosine Receptor Antagonist KW-3902 for Patients Hospitalized With Acute Heart Failure and Volume Overload to Assess Treatment Effect on Congestion and Renal Function) studies, as adjunctive therapy to diuretics in decompensated heart failure. A separate study looking at patients with diminishing responses to loop diuretics will also be conducted. However, cases of seizure have been reported at high infusion doses as blocking adenosine receptors may lower seizure threshold in vulnerable subjects, therefore safety of this drug class has to be established.

Renin inhibitors

Along the same lines of thought to counteract the "escape" phenomenon in the renin–angiotensin–aldosterone system (RAAS) system, there has been a long history of efforts to develop competitive receptor antagonists to block the downstream effects of angiotensin and/or aldosterone. In contrast, halting the detrimental effects of the RAAS at the most upstream point of the cascade may offer theoretical advantages for cardiovascular protection. With the success of β-adrenergic blockers (which are well-known inhibitors of renin production), the possibility adverse effects of a "built-up" of plasma renin activity from downstream RAAS blockade [6] is now realized. There have been many attempts to synthesize an oral selective renin inhibitor [119], and only recently a non-peptide inhibitor of renin, aliskiren, has been successfully developed. Aliskiren (SPP100, Novartis) has been shown to inhibit the production of angiotensin I and II in healthy volunteers, and is an effective anti-hypertensive agent in early clinical trials [120]. Aliskiren is currently being evaluated in a mechanistic multicenter study in stable patients with hypertensive heart failure, called the ALOFT (Aliskiren Observation of Heart Failure Treatment) trial, and Phase III studies are in the planning stages if the results from ALOFT are encouraging.

Novel drug classes with challenging clinical development

Calcium sensitizers

Levosimendan (Simdax, Abbott) is a novel calcium sensitizer developed in Europe that improves myocardial contractility without increasing myocardial oxygen demand [121–123]. Levosimendan binds to troponin-C in the myocyte, and is hypothesized to exert effects of calcium sensitization, thereby enhancing contractility without disturbing the energy balance of the heart [124]. It is associated with a modest increase in heart rate, a substantial increase in cardiac output, and a reduction in LV filling pressure. Both levosimendan and OR-1896 are phosphodiesterase inhibitors that promote vasodilation, although the inotropic effects thought to be independent of the type of PDE inhibited [125]. Whether the inotropic effects of levosimendan is due to PDE inhibition or calcium sensitization remains highly debated [126].

In patients with severe low-output heart failure syndrome, levosimendan is thought to be more efficacious than dobutamine. The pharmacokinetics and pharmacodynamics of levosimendan are also highly complex and not well understood. There is an active metabolite of levosimendan, OR-1896, that has active inotropic properties long after the discontinuation of the infusion [127]. The benefit of intravenous levosimendan in the LIDO (Levosimendan Infusion Versus Dobutamine in severe Low-Output Heart Failure, $n = 203$) study entailed a lower rate of worsening heart failure and a lower mortality than intravenous dobutamine (6.8% versus 17% at 31 days and 26% versus 38% at 6 months, respectively) [128]. In the setting of pulmonary edema within 5 days of an acute MI, short-term intravenous infusion of levosimendan was associated with a reduction of worsening heart failure without risk of hypotension and ischemia when compared to placebo in the post-MI LV failure study, RUSSLAN (Randomized Study on Safety and Effectiveness of Levosimendan in patients with Left Ventricular Failure After an Acute Myocardial Infarction study, $n = 504$) [129]. Levosimendan has been approved in Europe for the treatment of low-output heart failure, primarily based on data from the LIDO study. Recently, the CASINO (Calcium Sensitizer or Inotrope or None in Low-Output Heart Failure) study was prematurely halted as the results further suggested that levosimendan significantly improves 6-month survival when compared with placebo or dobutamine in patients with decompensated heart failure [130]. Six-month mortality in patients randomized to levosimendan was 15.3%, while the mortality rate in the placebo and dobutamine groups were 24.7% and 39.6%, respectively. Following the promising results of the REVIVE-1 (Randomized, Multicenter Evaluation of Intravenous Levosimendan Efficacy versus Placebo, $n = 100$) trial, two pivotal, Phase III randomized, placebo-controlled trials, REVIVE-2 in the United States and Australia ($n = 800$), and SURVIVE (Survival Of Patients With Acute Heart Failure In Need Of Intravenous Inotropic Support, $n = 700$) trial has been completed and announced but not published. Overall, patients treated with levosimendan had less self-reported dyspnea at day 5, but no differences in clinical event rates were found. These some-what disappointing results have dampened the enthusiasm of this compound, and provided challenges for levosimendan to be approved in the United States without further studies.

Calcium transient modulators

Other drugs that improve calcium homeostasis include the calcium handling modulator, caldaret (MCC-135, Mitsubushi/Takeda). The presumed mechanism of action of MCC-135 is to enhance calcium reuptake by the sarcoplasmic reticulum (SR) without any anti-adrenergic or PDE effects. However, the results were not as impressive in a multicenter Phase II study [131], and limited information have been announced regarding the future development of this compound in the heart failure arena.

Ranolazine (Ranexa, CV Therapeutics) was originally thought to shift myocardial energy metabolism away from free fatty acids toward glucose for the production of adenosine triphosphate (ATP), but now ranolazine is being considered as a late sodium current inhibitor that reduces calcium overload in the myocardium. Ranolazine has anti-ischemic effects without reducing blood pressure or heart rate, side effects commonly seen with the use of traditional anti-ischemic agents. However, prolonged QT intervals (likely due to its sodium channel effects) have worried regulatory agencies regarding the safety profile of this compound. Therefore, ranolazine has promise as a drug that could supplement existing therapy without added concerns about hypotensive or bradycardic side effects. Ranolazine has been shown to lessen the frequency of angina attacks and increase symptom-free exercise duration in the setting of chronic ischemic heart disease [132], and is in the process of seeking for regulatory approval for the indication for treating angina. A large, multicenter study using intravenous ranolazine MERLIN-TIMI 36 (Metabolic Efficiency with Ranolazine for Less Ischemia in Non-ST Elevation Acute Coronary Syndromes, $n = 5500$) is currently underway to study the effects of ranolazine in acute coronary syndromes. In the setting of cardiac dysfunction, preclinical data have confirmed that ranolazine reduces short- and long-term myocardial ischemic injury in various animal models [133-135]. In addition, early preclinical observations suggest positive effects of ranolazine in the management of congestive heart failure [136]. There is hope that these drugs may some day be developed as part of the heart failure regimen.

Immunomodulation therapy

There has been a recent shift from targeting specific cytokines and their receptors to a broad-spectrum anti-inflammatory strategy via the exploitation of the physiologic anti-inflammatory immune response to apoptotic cells. The basis of this novel technology is the concept that removal of apoptotic cells may trigger the immune system to modulate key inflammatory mediators. Immunomodulation uses a device technology to extract a small amount of patients' blood and expose cells to oxidative stress (a combination of heating to 108°F, ultraviolet light and ozone) to render them senescent. The senescent cells that are re-administered to the patient intramuscularly subsequently undergo apoptosis. Exposure to the apoptotic cells accelerates the natural process of cell turnover to induce an anti-inflammatory response by macrophages and lymphocytes. Preliminary results from a randomized, double-blind, Phase II study of 75 patients with advanced heart failure demonstrated significant reduction in morbidity and mortality following implementation of Celacade (VAS-991, Vasogen) [137]. Neutral results from a large pivotal, Phase III mortality and morbidity study of Celacade, ACCLAIM (Advanced Chronic Heart Failure Clinical Assessment of Immune Modulation Therapy, LVEF <30%, NYHA II–IV, $n = 2000$) have been announced, although there were some indication of mortality benefit in the NYHA class II patient subset.

Other non-specific immunomodulatory strategies including plasmapheresis and immunoglobulin infusions are also under active investigations.

Xanthine oxidase inhibition

Chronic heart failure is associated with hyperuricemia and elevations in circulating markers of inflammation which often translates to poor prognosis [138,139]. Activation of xanthine oxidase, through free radical release, causes leukocyte and endothelial cell activation. Oxypurinol, a xanthine oxidase inhibitor and the metabolic derivative of the gout drug, allopurinol, may act as hydroxyl radical scavengers, and help to restore endothelial and myocardial dysfunction [140]. Early proof-of-concept studies, EXOTIC (European Xanthine Oxidase Inhibitors Trial In Cardiac Disease) and EXOTIC-EF (Evaluation of Xanthine Oxidase Inhibition on Cardiac Ejection Fraction), demonstrated

improvement in cardiac function following administration of intravenous oxypurinol without significant safety concerns. Recent reports of the "La Plata" study on oral oxypurinol showed significant improvement in LV ejection fraction at 28 days of follow-up, but no significant differences in 6-min walk test results. The pivotal OPT-CHF (Oxypurinol Therapy for CHF) study is designed to demonstrate the efficacy and safety of oral oxypurinol vs. placebo in a randomized, double-blind, 24-week trial in 400 patients in up to 50 centers. The OPT-CHF trial has finished enrollment in December 2005, and the preliminary results did not show any survival benefit in advanced heart failure [141].

Novel targets of therapy

Modulation of fatty acid and glucose metabolism

Metabolic modulation has long been considered to be a potential strategy in heart failure therapy [142–144]. The primary substrate of the heart is long-chain fatty acids (about 70%), mainly in the form of oleate and palmitate. The key in vivo regulator is the arterial plasma free fatty acid concentrations: fatty acid uptake and oxidation increases in proportion to the arterial plasma concentration. High fatty acid levels in turn reduce myocardial efficiency by increasing myocardial oxygen requirements in the setting of ischemia and sympathetic overactivation [145]. Therefore, partial fatty acid oxidation (pFOX) inhibition serves as a promising target of therapy particularly in the setting of ischemic cardiomyopathy. The anti-anginal drug trimetazidine (Teveten, Solvay), which has been widely used outside the United States, is an inhibitor of the long-chain activity of 3-ketoacyl-CoA thiolase. Trimetazidine (20 mg 3 times a day) has been shown to improve long-term LV systolic and diastolic function, symptoms, glucose metabolism, and endothelial function when compared to placebo in patients with ischemic cardiomyopathy, with [143,146] or without diabetes [147,148].

Inhibitors of carnitine palmitoyl-transferase I (CPT I), the key enzyme for the transport of long-chain acyl-coenzyme A (acyl-CoA) compounds into mitochondria, have been developed as agents for treating type 2 diabetes mellitus [149]. Findings that the CPT I inhibitor, etomoxir, has positive inotropic effects on heart muscle, were unexpected and can be attributed to selective changes in the dysregulated gene expression of hypertrophied cardiac myocytes. The first clinical trial with etomoxir in patients with heart failure showed that etomoxir improved the clinical status and several parameters of heart function [150]. Putative molecular mechanisms likely involve an increased expression of SERCA2, the Ca^{2+} pump of SR and α-myosin heavy chain (α-MHC) of failing heart muscle [151]. Etomoxir could also act on peroxisome proliferator activated receptor alpha (PPAR-α), thus up-regulating the expression of various enzymes that participate in β-oxidation [136]. However, etomoxir research has been halted due to lack of efficacy in Phase II studies. Whether newer cholesteryl ester transfer protein (CETP) inhibitors such as torcetrapib (CP-529414, Pfizer) [152] will be tested in this population also remains in question.

Glucose is a more efficient fuel, particularly when oxygen supply is diminished. Glucagon-like peptide-1 (GLP-1) is a novel way to tackle the metabolic balance by enhancing myocardial and whole-body glucose metabolism. So-called incretins or "gut hormones," GLP-1 is naturally synthesized in intestinal endocrine cells in two principal major molecular forms, as GLP-1 (7–36) amide and GLP-1 (7–37) [153]. There has been several human studies showing potential benefits of GLP-1 infusions in improving functional capacity, enhancing endothelial function, as well as improving cardiac performance [154–156]. The PROCLAIM study (Effect of AC2592 Administered by Continuous Subcutaneous Infusion in Subjects With Advanced Chronic Congestive Heart Failure) is a proof-of-concept study in patients with advanced heart failure (NYHA III–IV) using a continuous subcutaneous infusion of AC2592 (Amylin Pharmaceuticals). Other potential strategies for enhancing GLP-1 actions including long-acting analogs such as albugon (Human Genome Science/GlaxoSmithKline), and blocking its breakdown by dipeptidyl peptidase (DPP-IV) via DPP-IV inhibitors such as NVP-DPP728 (Novartis), MK0431 (Merck), saxagliptin (Bristol-Myers Squibb), and others. However, many of these compounds, however, are still in early clinical trial phases for diabetic indications and are unlikely to be tested in the heart failure arena in the near future.

Advanced glycosylation end-products cross-link breakers

Glucose and other reducing sugars react non-enzymatically with proteins leading to the formation of advanced glycosylation end-products (AGEs) and AGE-derived protein cross-linking. Formation of AGEs is a normal physiologic process, which is accelerated under the hyperglycemic condition of diabetes. Under normal conditions, AGEs build up slowly and then accumulate over years. Numerous studies have indicated that AGEs contribute to the pathologic events leading to diabetic complications, including nephropathy, retinopathy, vasculopathy, and neuropathy. They may also be important in acute coronary syndromes. Potential therapeutic approaches to prevent these complications include pharmacologic inhibition of AGE formation and disruption of pre-formed AGE-protein cross-links [157]. Animal models and preliminary clinical trials have shown that the AGE-inhibitor, pimagedine (aminoguanidine HCl, Alteon) and the cross-link breaker, alagebrium (ALT-711, Alteon), are able to reduce the severity of the multiple end-results of advanced glycosylation [158]. These agents are potential treatments for glucose-derived complications of diabetes and ageing. Data from the DIAMOND (Distensibility Improvement and Remodeling in Diastolic Heart Failure) trial have been positive. Patients who received alagebrium for 16 weeks in the DIAMOND trial experienced a rapid remodeling of the heart, resulting in a statistically significant reduction in LV mass, as well as a marked improvement in LV diastolic filling. Positive results from several Phase II studies for alagebrium including the SAPPHIRE (Systolic and Pulse Pressure Hemodynamic Improvement by Restoring Elasticity), and the SILVER (Systolic Hypertension Interaction with Left Ventricular Remodeling) trials have also been reported [159]. Results from a parallel, open-label study on patients with systolic heart failure and diastolic dysfunction called PEDESTAL (Patients with Impaired Ejection Fraction and Diastolic Dysfunction: Efficacy and Safety Trial of Alagebrium) were presented at the recent American Heart Association scientific sessions, and showed trends consistent with DIAMOND. However, recent safety concerns have emerged regarding liver toxicity in male rats treated with alagebrium, and the clinical development of this drug class in hypertension and erectile dysfunction has been discontinued. Nevertheless if the benefits outweigh the risks, this novel approach will be highly promising.

Matrix Metalloproteinases Inhibitors

Collagen deposition leading to increased stiffness can result from alterations in the balance of promoters and inhibitors of matrix metallo proteinases (MMPs) [160]. However, this concept of inhibiting MMPs to reduce collagen deposition suffers from problem of using a therapeutic target that has widespread effects that extend beyond the failing myocardium. Recent results from the PREMIER (Prevention of MI Early Remodeling) study showed that the prototype MMP inhibitor, PG-116800 did not show significant benefits in preventing left ventricular remodeling over placebo following myocardial infarction [161]. This inhibitor has yet to be tested in the setting of diastolic heart failure. Several other drugs are also being considered to target MMP/TIMPs in this population; but until a more specific target can be identified, this strategy remains largely theoretical.

Copper chelating therapy

Another intriguing concept that has emerged over the past few years is the role of copper metabolism in the development of diabetic cardiomyopathy. Cooper and colleagues published several key articles illustrating the efficacy of trientine, a copper chelating agent for Wilson's disease, in reversing LV remodeling (predominantly regression of hypertrophy) without lowering blood sugar [162, 163]. It was also shown to substantially improve cardiomyocyte structure, and to reverse elevation in LV collagen and ß-1 integrin. These data are believed to implicate accumulation of elevated loosely bound copper in the mechanism of diabetic cardiomyopathy and to support the use of selective copper chelation in the treatment of this condition. This hypothesis is now being tested in a new formulation of trientine (under the name Laszarin™, Protemix Inc.). Early phase reports of oral treatment with trientine results in elevated copper excretion in humans with type 2 diabetes and, following 6 months of treatment, causes elevated LV mass to decline significantly toward normal [163]. To date, trientine has been well- tolerated by patients in clinical trials, and it has a long safety profile in the

treatment of Wilson's disease. A Phase IIb clinical trial of trientine administration in patients with diabetic heart failure with a quality of life (exercise tolerance) outcome is currently underway. Larger clinical trials are in the planning stages. Nevertheless, our understanding of why copper chelation may work is rudimentary; it is unclear whether it will work outside the setting of diabetes mellitus, and whether structural changes may directly translate into clinical benefits.

Nitric oxide modulation

Nitric oxide is synthesized in endothelial cells and has a wide range of functions that are vital for maintaining a healthy cardiovascular system. Reduced nitric oxide availability has been implicated in the initiation and progression of many cardiovascular diseases, including heart failure [164]. The administration of exogenous nitric oxide to help prevent disease progression is an attractive therapeutic option. Nitric oxide donor drugs represent a useful means of systemic nitric oxide delivery. Moreover, organic nitrates have been used for many years to provide effective symptomatic relief from angina pectoris. However, nitrates have limitations and a number of alternative nitric oxide donor classes have now emerged.

Nebivolol (Nebilet®, Bertek/Mylan) is a new, long-acting, lipophilic, cardioselective β_1-adrenergic receptor blocker that is used for treating hypertension in Europe. It lacks intrinsic sympathomimetic activity and does not significantly affect glucose or plasma lipid metabolism. It has mild vasodilating properties that are attributed to its interaction with the L-arginine/nitric oxide pathway, which results in enhanced release of endothelial nitric oxide [165]. Recent publication of the SENIORS (Study of the Effects of Nebivolol Intervention on Outcomes and Rehospitalisation in Seniors with Heart Failure) trial showed significant reduction in combined endpoint of death and hospitalization even though all-cause mortality did not reach statistically significant differences between nebivolol and placebo [144].

BiDil (Nitromed) is a new preparation of two old drugs, isosorbide dinitrate and hydralazine. In principle, it delivers nitric oxide from the nitrate moiety and therefore has the potential to improve endothelial function and myocardial performance. Hydralazine appears to retard nitrate tolerance, in addition to reducing systemic vascular resistance.

Retrospective data from the V-HeFT studies suggest that African-Americans with heart failure may preferentially respond better to the hydralazine–isosorbide dinitrate combination than to ACE inhibitors. These concepts have been the subject of a recent, randomized control trial (A-HeFT, or African-American Heart Failure Trial) that demonstrated marked reduced mortality and morbidity in African-American patients with advanced heart failure when treated with BiDil versus placebo on top of standard therapy including ACE inhibitors, β-adrenergic blockers and/or aldosterone antagonists [167]. However, there is still much debate regarding the confounding factors of blood pressure reduction versus true effects of improving nitric oxide bioavailability, and whether these observations can be generalized in the general heart failure population at large.

While increased availability of nitric oxide may be beneficial in chronic heart failure patients and profound endothelial dysfunction, excessive vasodilatory consequences may be detrimental. There is increasing recognition of a syndrome with frank circulatory collapse, either from large anterior MI, or a sepsis-like presentation, which is sometimes referred to as "cytokine storm." In this setting, vasodilatory therapy clearly is inappropriate, and vasopressor drugs such as norepinephrine and vasopressin are often required. Large MI, complicated by cardiogenic shock, may be accompanied by a severe inflammatory response. This in turn releases various mediators, including cytokines, leading to high levels of nitric oxide and peroxynitrite production with subsequent deleterious hemodynamic effects. Indeed, a recent small case series of 11 patients with cardiogenic shock reported marked improvements following infusion of a nitric oxide synthase inhibitor, N(G)-monomethyl-L-arginine (L-NMMA or tilarginine, Arginox) at 1 mg/kg bolus plus 1 mg/kg/h infusion for 5 h [168]. On the other hand, blocking nitric oxide synthases may lead to similar downstream effects of other vasoconstrictors in reducing end-organ tissue oxygenation at the microcirculatory level. The SHOCK-2 (Should we Emergently Revascularize Occluded Coronaries for Cardiogenic Shock) trial is a Phase II dose-ranging study of 79 patients with persistent cardiogenic shock randomized to tilarginine at different doses versus placebo, and found significant reduction in high-dose treatment groups (1.5 mg/kg bolus plus 1.5 mg/kg/h infusion over 5 h) compared to placebo even though the overall difference was not statistically significant [169]. This led to the approval of tilarginine as an orphan drug by the FDA in 2005. A multinational pivotal Phase III study, TRIUMPH (Tilarginine Acetate Injection in a Randomized International Study in Unstable AMI Patients with Cardiogenic Shock) has recently announced its termination based on lack of efficacy, which cause doubt for its broad use.

Hormone and enzyme replacement therapy

Anderson–Fabry disease is an X-linked inherited disorder of metabolism due to mutations in the gene encoding α-galactosidase A, a lysosomal enzyme [170]. The enzymatic defect leads to the organ accumulation of incompletely metabolized glycosphingolipids, including kidneys, cornea, peripheral nerves, and the heart. Severe pain in the extremities, hypohidrosis, and end-organ dysfunction are the leading symptoms in patients with Anderson–Fabry disease. Inability to prevent the progression of glycosphingolipid deposition causes significant morbidity, often associated with significant impact on quality of life and diminished lifespan from early onset strokes, heart attack, and progressive renal failure. The disease manifests primarily in hemizygous males. However, there is increasing recognition that heterozygous (carrier) females may also develop disease-related complications. It is now recognized that some patients with LV hypertrophy may in fact have Anderson–Fabry disease [171]. However, there is not a widely available blood test to verify the disease, and there are uncertainties about when treatment should be started or even the long-term benefits of this therapeutic strategy. Agalsidase beta (Fabrazyme®, Genzyme), have been tested in clinical studies [172,173] and have gained approval for clinical use. The challenge, however, is to identify patients who have Anderson–Fabry disease and those who may be eligible for and can afford this expensive therapy.

There has been a long-standing, historical interest in using thyroid hormone and its analogs in the treatment of patients with heart failure [174]. Thyroid hormone has many favorable effects on the failing cardiovascular system, including increased myocardial contractility and heart rate, cardiac output, and blood volume, in addition to reducing systemic vascular resistance. Thyroid hormones have shown to produce inotropic, lusitropic, and vasodilator effects in patients with acute heart failure [175]. Thyroid hormone also stimulates the secretion of erythropoietin. In contrast, hypothyroidism has long been associated with impaired cardiac function [176]. Based on these long-standing observations, a number of small observational studies have examined the potential use of thyroid hormone in the treatment of heart failure. Intravenous triiodothyronine has been used acutely to treat advanced heart failure [177], and is associated with hemodynamic improvement and resolution of symptoms. However, the long-term use of oral thyroid hormone in the treatment of heart failure is problematic, and it may be safer to use a thyroid hormone analog such as 3,5-diiodothyropropionic acid (DITPA, Titan Pharmaceuticals) [178,179]. Indeed, a Phase II study using DITPA in patients with advanced symptomatic heart failure and low-T3 syndrome is ongoing.

The past decade has also seen the development of growth hormone and its secretagogs, such as CP-424391 (Pfizer), as therapies for heart failure. The rationale behind their use is that growth hormone may stimulate the growth of myocardial cells and improve organ function. A small, preliminary study indicated that recombinant human growth hormone, given to patients with idiopathic dilated cardiomyopathy, increased myocardial mass and reduced the size of LV chamber, resulting in improvement in hemodynamics, myocardial energy metabolism, and clinical status [180]. Favorable effects have been noted in experimental heart failure using insulin growth factor-1 (IGF-1) [181]. However, a randomized, double-blind, placebo-controlled trial of human recombinant growth hormone in patient with chronic heart failure due to dilated cardiomyopathy failed to demonstrate short-term improvement in clinical status [182]. Its use in critically ill patients also did not improve outcome and even tended to increase mortality.

Potential beneficial effects of ghrelin, a novel growth hormone releasing peptide isolated from the stomach, have been observed. Ghrelin levels are elevated in cachetic patients with advanced heart failure [183]. In humans, infusion of ghrelin improves hemodynamics acutely [184]. Long-term administration reverses cardiac remodeling, improves exercise capacity, and attenuates the development of cardiac cachexia in patients with chronic heart failure [185,186]. It is likely that further human studies on ghrelin will be conducted. Various other analogs of endogenous hormones, such as adrenomedullin and urocortin-II, are also in the early stages of clinical trial programs.

Novel non-pacing devices

Ultrafiltration/Aquapheresis

Optimization of fluid balance and the restoration of desirable levels of preload and afterload via the mechanical removal of fluid by ultrafiltration (or aquapheresis) has been a longstanding target for nephrologists in managing patients with ESRD [187]. Slow continuous ultrafiltration and continuous refilling of the intravascular volume from the interstitium may stabilize circulating blood volume and preserve organ perfusion. A new simplified peripheral ultrafiltration system (Aquadex-100, CHF Solutions Inc.) has been developed to remove up to 0.5 L of fluid per hour without central arterial or venous access [188]. However, appropriate patient selection and clinical efficacy remains to be determined. Several completed studies, including RAPID-CHF (Relief for Acutely Fluid Overloaded Patients with Decompensated congestive heart failure), OFFLOAD (Observational unit treatment of Fluid Overload) and EUPHORIA (Early Ultrafiltration Therapy in Patients with Decompensated Heart Failure and Observed Resistance to Interventions with Diuretic Agents) trials, have demonstrated safety and efficacy of ultrafiltration systems in the urgent care setting. The ongoing multicenter UNLOAD (Ultrafiltration versus IV Diuretics for Patients Hospitalized for Acute Decompensated Congestive Heart Failure trial, patients with fluid overloaded AHFS treated with aquapheresis achieved more volume removal, weight loss, and clinical outcomes compared to those received conventional intravenous diuretics [44].

Targeted renal therapy via intra-renal infusion

Intra-renal (IR) infusion therapy has been limited to experimental animal and human mechanistic studies on renal perfusion and glomerular feedback mechanisms. With the increasing recognition of the "cardio-renal syndrome" as a poor prognostic factor particularly in patients admitted with decompensated heart failure on aggressive diuretic regimens, targeted renal therapy via direct cannulation of the renal arteries may provide potential salvage of renal function and reduce morbidity and mortality. Several trials using IR infusion of nesiritide have been initiated using a novel selective infusion catheter system for the renal arteries (Benephit™ Infusion System, FlowMedica) in patients with heart failure and cardio-renal syndrome. The premise is that targeted renal infusion of a vasoactive drug may provide direct renal effects without producing hemodynamic compromise.

Aortic flow augmentation device

A novel invasive approach for severely decompensated patients utilizes mechanical afterload reduction by a peripherally accessed, external rotary blood pump to enhance blood flow in the descending aorta. A multicenter pivotal study, MOMENTUM (Multicenter trial of the Orqis Medical CRS Enhanced Treatment of CHF, Unresponsive to Medical therapy), is currently in the planning stages to test the safety and efficacy for this aortic flow augmentation device, the Cancion Cardiac Recovery System (Orqis Medical) [189]. Preliminary animal and human studies on its hemodynamic efficacies have been promising, albeit very invasive [190–193]. As technology for ventricular assist device (VAD) therapy advances, it is likely that smaller and more efficient VADs will be designed specific for contractile support of the failing heart [194,195].

Novel mechanical assist devices

Mechanical assist devices have focused on improving forward flow by providing either pulsatile or non-pulsatile pumps as "replacements" of myocardial function. However, currently available mechanical devices are invasive and mainly focus on salvaging patients with end-stage systolic dysfunction. Most of these strategies are highly invasive, with potential complications that can be extensive and devastating, which has limited their indications. Better implantation techniques and smaller sizes with lower thrombotic and infectious complications will likely lead to broader adoption (see Chapter – regarding mechanical assist devices). Besides the ongoing clinical

development of ventricular assist devices that focuses on improving cardiac output (such as HeartMate II, Jarvik, and VentrAssist, some new devices are specifically targeting the diastolic recoil properties that may improve diastolic dysfunction. The ImCardia (CorAssist Cardiovascular Inc) is an elastic, self-expanding device with a special silicon lattice material that is attached to the external surface of the LV[196]. The ImCardia harnesses the heart's systolic energy during recoil from systole in order to reduce diastolic intra-cardiac pressure. The device operates without the need for external source of energy. Human feasibility trials are commencing in the near future.

Conclusions

The development of new pharmacologic therapy for the treatment of heart failure has undergone substantial growth in recent years, largely driven by the increase in prevalence of cases. Many of the novel drugs never progress beyond Phase I or II trials. The trials and potential drugs mentioned in this review is only a partial list of what is under evaluation. Because of the vast heterogeneity of the syndrome and the lack of a single recognizable lesion, drugs cannot be easily targeted toward a single mechanism or lesion. Although some recent clinical trials in heart failure have been disappointing, the process of developing drugs to treat heart failure is long and tortuous. There is currently a much greater appreciation of how to develop new drugs and test them in the clinical arena. Although a novel drug may alter surrogate markers and the progression of heart failure, unless there is a measurable improvement in clinical outcome, such as mortality and morbidity, it is unlikely to be approved. Currently, regulatory agencies do not accept improvement in surrogate markers as a sole measure for approval. The usual approval process requires that the "total package," including improvement in survival, morbidity, and surrogate markers, all moving in a positive direction. There must be an internal constituency of all the surrogate markers, and by far improvement in LV remodeling appears to be most tightly coupled to improvement in morbidity and mortality. In the future, it is possible that novel pharmacologic therapies will be required to retard or reverse the progression of LV remodeling in addition to demonstrating improvement in mortality and the need to for hospitalizations. Drug development for patient with acute decompensated heart failure and diastolic heart failure is a vexing problem. We do not know which "outcome" to measure, how to measure it, or when to measure it. Improvement in hemodynamic profile is necessary, but not sufficient. The availability of new devices and infusion systems is likely going pave the way for an interventional approach to this growing problem, particularly with the goal of renal preservation.

For now, there is a growing recognition that early pharmacologic intervention in patients at risk of developing heart failure may delay or even prevent the onset of heart failure. Thus from a public health standpoint, early pharmacologic intervention may provide a larger preventive benefit than a polypharmacy approach at end-stage heart failure [1]. This hypothesis is supported by several clinical trials on at-risk patients where a decreased incidence of heart failure was observed with the use of ACE inhibitors or angiotensin receptor blockers [197–201]. It is possible, albeit unproven, that the very early use of renin–angiotensin–aldosterone inhibitors and β-adrenergic blockers may markedly delay or prevent the development of heart failure if initiated in Stage A (patients with multiple risk factors for developing heart failure without any signs and symptoms or structural abnormalities) [202]. To date, there are no randomized, controlled trials that vigorously tested the prevention hypothesis in early heart failure, in part, due to our inability to easily screen and detect patients with asymptomatic heart disease. Undertaking a trial to test this hypothesis would also be a formidable task because the event rate is relatively low and the sample size would have to be huge. Along this line of thinking, there is an attempt to design a trial using biomarkers (in the case of cardiac dysfunction, plasma NT-proBNP levels) to add aliskiren to standard therapy to prevent the development of heart failure (TIMI 43, or "AVANT-GARDE"). Many experts now agree that the future of heart failure management resides in the preventive arena, and novel therapeutic approaches should consider in patients at earlier stages of heart failure.

References

1 Yusuf S, Pitt B. A lifetime of prevention: the case of heart failure. *Circulation* 2002; **106**: 2997–2998.

2 American Heart Association. *Heart and Stoke Statistics – 2006 Update*. American Heart Association, Dallas, Texas, 2005.

3 Lloyd-Jones DM, Larson MG, Leip EP *et al.* Lifetime risk for developing congestive heart failure: the Framingham Heart Study. *Circulation* 2002; **106**: 3068–3072.

4 Packer M. The impossible task of developing a new treatment for heart failure. *J Card Fail* 2002; **8**: 193–196.

5 Weber KT. Aldosterone in congestive heart failure. *N Engl J Med* 2001; **345**: 1689–1697.

6 Tang WH, Vagelos RH, Yee YG *et al.* Neurohormonal and clinical responses to high- versus low-dose enalapril therapy in chronic heart failure. *J Am Coll Cardiol* 2002; **39**: 70–78.

7 Pitt B, Zannad F, Remme WJ *et al.* The effect of spironolactone on morbidity and mortality in patients with severe heart failure. Randomized Aldactone Evaluation Study Investigators. *N Engl J Med* 1999; **341**: 709–717.

8 Tang WHW, Francis GS. Spironolactone in chronic heart failure: All's well that ends well. *J Am Coll Cardiol* 2002; **41**: 215–216.

9 Ziillich AJ, Carter BL. Eplerenone – a novel selective aldosterone blocker. *Ann Pharmacother* 2002; **36**: 1567–1576.

10 Krum H, Nolly H, Workman D *et al.* Efficacy of eplerenone added to renin–angiotensin blockade in hypertensive patients. *Hypertension* 2002; **40**: 117–123.

11 Weinberger MH, Roniker B, Krause SL, Weiss RJ. Eplerenone, a selective aldosterone blocker, in mild-to-moderate hypertension. *Am J Hypertens* 2002; **15**: 709–716.

12 Pitt B, Remme W, Zannad F *et al.* Eplerenone, a selective aldosterone blocker, in patients with left ventricular dysfunction after myocardial infarction. *N Engl J Med* 2003; **348**: 1309–1321.

13 Rocha R, Williams GH. Rationale for the use of aldosterone antagonists in congestive heart failure. *Drugs* 2002; **62**: 723–731.

14 Pitt B, Reichek N, Willenbrock R *et al.* Effects of eplerenone, enalapril, and eplerenone/enalapril in patients with essential hypertension and left ventricular hypertrophy: the 4E-left ventricular hypertrophy study. *Circulation* 2003; **108**: 1831–1838.

15 Cicoira M, Zanolla L, Rossi A *et al.* Long-term, dose-dependent effects of spironolactone on left ventricular function and exercise tolerance in patients with chronic heart failure. *J Am Coll Cardiol* 2002; **40**: 304–310.

16 Suzuki G, Morita H, Mishima T *et al.* Effects of long-term monotherapy with eplerenone, a novel aldosterone blocker, on progression of left ventricular dysfunction and remodeling in dogs with heart failure. *Circulation* 2002; **106**: 2967–2972.

17 Zannad F, Alla F, Dousset B, Perez A, Pitt B. Limitation of excessive extracellular matrix turnover may contribute to survival benefit of spironolactone therapy in patients with congestive heart failure: insights from the randomized

aldactone evaluation study (RALES). RALES Investigators. *Circulation* 2000; **102**: 2700–2706.

18 Grandi AM, Imperiale D, Santillo R *et al.* Aldosterone antagonist improve diastolic function in essential hypertension. *Hypertension* 2002; **40**: 647–652.

19 Mottram PM, Haluska B, Leano R, Cowley D, Stowasser M, Marwick TH. Effect of aldosterone antagonism on myocardial dysfunction in hypertensive patients with diastolic heart failure. *Circulation* 2004; **110**: 558–565.

20 Cowie MR, Mendez GF. BNP and congestive heart failure. *Prog Cardiovasc Dis* 2002; **44**: 293–321.

21 Maisel AS, Krishnaswamy P, Nowak RM *et al.* Rapid measurement of B-type natriuretic peptide in the emergency diagnosis of heart failure. *N Engl J Med* 2002; **347**: 161–167.

22 Mills RM, Hobbs RE, Young JB. BNP for heart failure: role of nesiritide in cardiovascular therapeutics. *Congest Heart Fail* 2002; **8**: 270–273.

23 Intravenous nesiritide vs nitroglycerin for treatment of decompensated congestive heart failure: a randomized controlled trial. Publication Committee of VMAC Investigators. *J Am Med Assoc* 2002; **287**: 1531–1540.

24 Burger AJ, Elkayam U, Neibaur MT. Comparison of the occurrence of ventricular arrhythmias in patients with acutely decompensated congestive heart failure receiving dobutamine versus nesiritide therapy. *Am J Cardiol* 2001; **88**: 35–39.

25 Sackner-Bernstein JD, Kowalski M, Fox M, Aaronson K. Short-term risk of death after treatment with nesiritide for decompensated heart failure: a pooled analysis of randomized controlled trials. *J Am Med Assoc* 2005; **293**: 1900–1905.

26 Sackner-Bernstein JD, Skopicki HA, Aaronson KD. Risk of worsening renal function with nesiritide in patients with acutely decompensated heart failure. *Circulation* 2005; **111**: 1487–1491.

27 Suwa M, Seino Y, Nomachi Y, Matsuki S, Funahashi K. Multicenter prospective investigation on efficacy and safety of carperitide for acute heart failure in the "real world" of therapy. *Circ J* 2005; **69**: 283–290.

28 Mitrovic V, Luss H, Nitsche K *et al.* Effects of the renal natriuretic peptide urodilatin (ularitide) in patients with decompensated chronic heart failure: a double-blind, placebo-controlled, ascending-dose trial. *Am Heart J* 2005; **150**: 1239.

29 Rademaker MT, Cameron VA, Charles CJ, Richards AM. Integrated hemodynamic, hormonal, and renal actions of urocortin 2 in normal and paced sheep: beneficial effects in heart failure. *Circulation* 2005; **112**: 3624–3632.

30 Schafer A, Fraccarollo D, Eigenthaler M *et al.* Rosuvastatin reduces platelet activation in heart failure: role of NO bioavailability. *Arterioscler Thromb Vasc Biol* 2005; **25**: 1071–1077.

31 Tousoulis D, Antoniades C, Bosinakou E *et al.* Effects of atorvastatin on reactive hyperemia and inflammatory process in patients with congestive heart failure. *Atherosclerosis* 2005; **178**: 359–363.

32 Yildirir A, Muderrisoglu H. Non-lipid effects of statins: emerging new indications. *Curr Vasc Pharmacol* 2004; **2**: 309–318.

33 Liao JK. Statin therapy for cardiac hypertrophy and heart failure. *J Investig Med* 2004; **52**: 248–253.

34 Pliquett RU, Cornish KG, Zucker IH. Statin therapy restores sympathovagal balance in experimental heart failure. *J Appl Physiol* 2003; **95**: 700–704.

35 von Haehling S, Anker SD. Statins for heart failure: at the crossroads between cholesterol reduction and pleiotropism? *Heart* 2005; **91**: 1–2.

36 Segal R, Pitt B, Pode-Wilson P, Sharma D, Bradstreet DC, Ikeda LS. Effects of HMG-COA reductase inhibitors (statins) in patients with heart failure. *Eur J Heart Fail* 2000; **(Suppl 2)**: 96 [abstract].

37 Mozaffarian D, Nye R, Levy WC. Statin therapy is associated with lower mortality among patients with severe heart failure. *Am J Cardiol* 2004; **93**: 1124–1129.

38 Ray JG, Gong Y, Sykora K, Tu JV. Statin use and survival outcomes in elderly patients with heart failure. *Arch Intern Med* 2005; **165**: 62–67.

39 Horwich TB, MacLellan WR, Fonarow GC. Statin therapy is associated with improved survival in ischemic and nonischemic heart failure. *J Am Coll Cardiol* 2004; **43**: 642–648.

40 Sola S, Mir MQ, Rajagopalan S, Helmy T, Tandon N, Khan BV. Statin therapy is associated with improved cardiovascular outcomes and levels of inflammatory markers in patients with heart failure. *J Card Fail* 2005; **11**: 607–612.

41 Anker SD, Clark AL, Winkler R *et al.* Statin use and survival in patients with chronic heart failure – results from two observational studies with 5200 patients. *Int J Cardiol* 2006. Available online July 17, 2006 at www.internationaljournal ofcardiology.com

42 Foody JM, Shah R, Galusha D, Masoudi FA, Havranek EP, Krumholz HM. Statins and mortality among elderly patients hospitalized with heart failure. *Circulation* 2006; **113**: 1086–1092.

43 Sola S, Mir MQ, Lerakis S, Tandon N, Khan BV. Atorvastatin improves left ventricular systolic function and serum markers of inflammation in nonischemic heart failure. *J Am Coll Cardiol* 2006; **47**: 332–337.

44 Cleland JG, Coletta AP, Nikitin NP, Clark AL. Clinical trials update from the American College of Cardiology: Darbepoetin alfa, ASTEROID, UNIVERSE, paediatric carvedilol, UNLOAD and ICELAND. *Eur J Heart Fail* 2006; **8**: 326–329.

45 Tavazzi L, Tognoni G, Franzosi MG *et al.* Rationale and design of the GISSI heart failure trial: a large trial to assess the effects of *n*-3 polyunsaturated fatty acids and rosuvastatin in symptomatic congestive heart failure. *Eur J Heart Fail* 2004; **6**: 635–641.

46 Silverberg DS, Wexler D, Iaina A. The importance of anemia and its correlation in the management of severe congestive heart failure. *Eur J Heart Fail* 2002; **4**: 681–686.

47 Anker SD, Sharma R, Francis DP, Pitt B, Poole-Wilson PA, Coats AJ. Haemoglobin predicts survival in patients with chronic heart failure with a U-shaped curve: a substudy of the ELITE-II trial, *XVIIth Congress of the European Society of Cardiology*, Berlin, Germany, 2002 [abstract #P2302].

48 Maggioni AP, Latini R, Anand I *et al.* Prevalence and prognostic role of anemia in patients with heart failure in the IN-CHF Registry and the Val-HeFT trial, *XVII Congress of the European Society of Cardiology*, Berlin, Germany, 2002 [abstract 1480].

49 Horwich TB, Fonarow GC, Hamilton MA, MacLellan WR, Borenstein J. Anemia is associated with worse symptoms, greater impairment in functional capacity and a significant increase in mortality in patients with advanced heart failure. *J Am Coll Cardiol* 2002; **39**: 1780–1786.

50 Corwin HL, Gettinger A, Pearl RG *et al.* Efficacy of recombinant human erythropoietin in critically ill patients: a randomized controlled trial. *J Am Med Assoc* 2002; **288**: 2827–2835.

51 Parsi A. Anaemia in heart failure: its diagnosis and management. *Eur J Heart Fail* 2003; **5**: 3–4.

52 Donne RL, Foley RN. Anaemia management and cardiomyopathy in renal failure. *Nephrol Dial Transplant* 2002; **17**: 37–40.

53 Silverberg DS, Wexler D, Blum M *et al.* The use of subcutaneous erythropoietin and intravenous iron for the treatment of the anemia of severe resistant congestive heart failure improves cardiac and renal functions and functional cardiac class, and markedly reduces hospitalizations. *J Am Coll Cardiol* 2000; **35**: 1737–1744.

54 Silverberg DS, Wexler D, Sheps D *et al.* The effect of correction of mild anemia in severe, resistant congestive heart failure using subcutaneous erythropoietin and intravenous iron: a randomized controlled study. *J Am Coll Cardiol* 2001; **37**: 1775–1780.

55 Cleland JG, Coletta AP, Clark AL, Velavan P, Ingle L. Clinical trials update from the European Society of Cardiology Heart Failure meeting and the American College of Cardiology: darbepoetin alfa study, ECHOS, and ASCOT-BPLA. *Eur J Heart Fail* 2005; **7**: 937–939.

56 Levin ER. Endothelins. *N Engl J Med* 1995; **333**: 356–363.

57 Miyauchi T, Masaki T. Pathophysiology of endothelin in the cardiovascular system. *Ann Rev Physiol* 1999; **61**: 391–415.

58 Rodeheffer RJ, Lerman A, Heublein DM, Burnett Jr. JC. Increased plasma concentrations of endothelin in congestive heart failure in humans. *Mayo Clin Proc* 1992; **67**: 719–724.

59 Yanagisawa M, Kurihara H, Kimura S *et al.* A novel potent vasoconstrictor peptide produced by vascular endothelial cells. *Nature* 1988; **332**: 411–415.

60 Cowburn PJ, Cleland JGF. Endothelin antagonists for chronic heart failure: do they have a role? *Eur Heart J* 2001; **22**: 1772–1784.

61 Masaki T, Miwa S, Sawamura T, Ninomiya H, Okamoto Y. Subcellular mechanisms of endothelin action in vascular system. *Eur J Pharmacol* 1999; **375**: 133–138.

62 Cowburn PJ, Cleland JGF, McArthur JD *et al.* Endothelin B receptors are functionally important in mediating vasoconstriction in the systemic circulation in patients with left ventricular systolic dysfunction. *J Am Coll Cardiol* 1999; **33**: 932–938.

63 Kiowski W, Sutsch G, Hunziker P *et al.* Evidence for endothelin-1-mediated vasoconstriction in severe chronic heart failure. *Lancet* 1995; **346**: 732–736.

64 Packer M, McMurray J, Massie BM *et al.* Clinical effects of endothelin receptor antagonism with bosentan in patients with severe chronic heart failure: results of a pilot study. *J Card Fail* 2005; **11**: 12–20.

65 Kalra PR, Moon JC, Coats AJ. Do results of the ENABLE (Endothelin Antagonist Bosentan for Lowering Cardiac Events in Heart Failure) study spell the end for nonselective endothelin antagonism in heart failure? *Int J Cardiol* 2002; **85**: 195–197.

66 Abraham WT. Enrasentan Cooperative Randomized Evaluation (ENCOR). *American College of Cardiology 50th Annual Scientific Session*. Atlanta, GA, 2001.

67 Anand I, McMurray J, Cohn JN *et al.* Long-term effects of darusentan on left-ventricular remodelling and clinical outcomes in the Endothelin A Receptor Antagonist Trial in Heart Failure (EARTH): randomised, double-blind, placebo-controlled trial. *Lancet* 2004; **364**: 347–354.

68 Kelland NF, Webb DJ. Clinical trials of endothelin antagonists in heart failure: a question of dose? *Exp Biol Med* (Maywood) 2006; **231**: 696-699.

69 Teerlink JR, McMurray JJ, Bourge RC *et al.* Tezosentan in patients with acute heart failure: design of the Value of Endothelin Receptor Inhibition with Tezosentan in Acute heart failure Study (VERITAS). *Am Heart J* 2005; **150**: 46–53.

70 McMurray JJ. Value of Endothelin Receptor Inhibition with Tezosentan in Acute Heart Failure Study (VERITAS), *American College of Cardiology 2005 Scientific Sessions*, Orlando, Florida, 2005.

71 Channick RN, Simonneau G, Sitbon O *et al.* Effects of the dual endothelin-receptor antagonist bosentan in patients with pulmonary hypertension: a randomized placebo-controlled study. *Lancet* 2001; **358**: 1119–1123.

72 Weber MA. Vasopeptidase inhibitors. *Lancet* 2001; **358**: 1525–1532.

73 Troughton RW, Rademaker MT, Powell JD *et al.* Beneficial renal and hemodynamic effects of omapatrilat in mild and severe heart failure. *Hypertension* 2000; **36**: 523–530.

74 McClean DR, Ikram H, Mehta S, *et al.* Vasopeptidase inhibition with omapatrilat in chronic heart failure: acute and

long-term hemodynamic and neurohumoral effects. *J Am Coll Cardiol* 2002; **39**: 2034–2041.

75 Rouleau JL, Pfeffer MA, Stewart DJ *et al.* Comparison of vasopeptidase inhibitor, omapatrilat, and lisinopril on exercise tolerance and morbidity in patients with heart failure: IMPRESS randomised trial. *Lancet* 2000; **356**: 615–620.

76 Packer M, Califf RM, Konstam MA *et al.* Comparison of omapatrilat and enalapril in patients with chronic heart failure: the Omapatrilat Versus Enalapril Randomized Trial of Utility in Reducing Events (OVERTURE). *Circulation* 2002; **106**: 920–926.

77 Kostis JB, Packer M, Black HR, Schmieder R, Henry D, Levy E. Omapatrilat and enalapril in patients with hypertension: the Omapatrilat Cardiovascular Treatment vs. Enalapril (OCTAVE) trial. *Am J Hypertens* 2004; **17**: 103–111.

78 Omapatrilat Cardiovascular Treatment Assessment Versus Enalapril (OCTAVE): to compare the efficacy and safety of omapatrilat against enalapril in the treatment of hypertension, *American College of Cardiology 51st Annual Scientific Session*, Atlanta, GA, 2002.

79 Kostis JB, Cobbe S, Johnston C. Design of the Omapatrilat in Persons with Enhanced Risk of Atherosclerotic events (OPERA) trial. *Am J Hypertens* 2002; **15**: 193–198.

80 Bralet J, Marie C, Gros C, Schwartz JC, Lecomte JM. Fasidotril: the first dual inhibitor of neprilysin and ACE. *Cardiovasc Drug Rev* 2000; **18**: 1–24.

81 Palkhiwala SA, Yu A, Frishman WH. Imidazoline receptor agonist drugs for treatment of systemic hypertension and congestive heart failure. *Heart Dis* 2000; **2**: 83–92.

82 Reid JL. Update on rilmenidine: clinical benefits. *Am J Hypertens* 2001; **14**: 322S–324S.

83 Coats AJ. Heart failure 99 – the MOXCON story. *Int J Cardiol* 1999; **71**: 109–111.

84 Cohn JN. The Effect of sustained-release moxonidine on morality and morbidity in patients with congestive heart failure: results of the MOXCON study, *XIV Congress of the European Society of Cardiology*, Vienna, Austria, 1999.

85 Doggrell SA. Moxonidine: some controversy. *Expert Opin Pharmacother* 2001; **2**: 337–350.

86 Swedberg K, Bristow MR, Cohn JN *et al.* Effects of sustained-release moxonidine, an imidazoline agonist, on plasma norepinephrine in patients with chronic heart failure. *Circulation* 2002; **105**: 1797–1803.

87 Rajfer SI, Davis FR. Role of dopamine receptors and the utility of dopamine agonists in heart failure. *Circulation* 1990; **82**: I-97–I-102.

88 Francis GS, Parks R, Cohn JN. The effects of bromocriptine in patients with congestive heart failure. *Am Heart J* 1983; **106**: 100–106.

89 Tjeerdsma G, Van Wijk LM, Molhoek GP, Boomsma F, Haaksma J, Van Veldhuisen DJ. Autonomic and hemodynamic effects of a new selective dopamine agonist,

CHF1035, in patients with chronic heart failure. *Cardiovasc Drugs Ther* 2001; **15**: 139–145.

90 Mann DL. Inflammatory mediators and the failing heart: past, present, and the foreseeable future. *Circ Res* 2002; **91**: 988–998.

91 Deswal A, Petersen NJ, Feldman AM *et al.* Cytokines and cytokine receptors in advanced heart failure: an analysis of the cytokine database from the *vasonarinone* trial (VEST). *Circulation* 2001; **103**: 2055–2059.

92 Torre-Amione G, Kapadia S, Benedict CR. Proinflammatory cytokine levels in patients with depressed left ventricular ejection fraction: a report from the Studies of Left Ventriular Dysfunction (SOLVD). *J Am Coll Cardiol* 1996; **27**: 1201–1206.

93 Coletta AP, Clark AL, Banarjee P, Cleland JG. Clinical trials update: RENEWAL (RENAISSANCE and RECOVER) and ATTACH. *Eur J Heart Fail* 2002; **4**: 559–561.

94 Krum H. Tumor necrosis factor-a blockade as a therapeutic strategy in heart failure (RENEWAL and ATTACH): unsuccessful, to be specific. *J Card Fail* 2002; **8**: 365–368.

95 Aukrust P, Yndestad A, Ueland T, Damas JK, Gullestad L. Anti-inflammatory trials in chronic heart failure. *Heart Fail Monit* 2006; **5**: 2–9.

96 Gullestad L, Ueland T, Fjeld JG *et al.* Effect of thalidomide on cardiac remodeling in chronic heart failure: results of a double-blind, placebo-controlled study. *Circulation* 2005; **112**: 3408–3414.

97 Batchelder K, Mayosi BM. Pentoxifylline for heart failure: a systematic review. *S Afr Med J* 2005; **95**: 171–175.

98 Morris K. Targeting the myocardial sodium–hydrogen exchange for treatment of heart failure. *Expert Opin Ther Targets* 2002; **6**: 291–298.

99 Chen L, Chen CX, Gan XT, Beier N, Scholz W, Karmazyn M. Inhibition and reversal of myocardial infarction-induced hypertrophy and heart failure by NHE-1 inhibition. *Am J Physiol Heart Circ Physiol* 2004; **286**: H381–H387.

100 Karmazyn M. Role of sodium–hydrogen exchange in cardiac hypertrophy and heart failure: a novel and promising therapeutic target. *Basic Res Cardiol* 2001; **96**: 325–328.

101 Packer M, Carver JR, Rodeheffer RJ *et al.* Effect of oral milrinone on mortality in severe chronic heart failure. *N Engl J Med* 1991; **325**: 1468–1475.

102 The Pimobendan in Congestive Heart Failure (PICO) investigators. Effects of pimobendan on exercise in patients with heart failure: main results from the PICO trial. *Heart Fail Rev* 1996; **76**: 223–231.

103 The EPOCH Study Group. Effects of pimobendan on adverse cardiac events and physical activities in patients with mild to moderate chronic heart failure. The Effects of Pimobendan on Chronic Heart Failure Study (EPOCH Study). *Circ J* 2002; **64**: 149–157.

104 Yoshikawa T, Baba A, Suzuki M *et al.* Effectiveness of carvedilol alone versus carvedilol + pimobendan for severe congestive heart failure. *Am J Cardiol* 2000; **85**: 1495–1497.

105 Feldman AM. Oral Enoximone in Intravenous Inotrope-Dependent Subjects (EMOTE). In: Heart Failure Society of America 2004 Annual Scientific Sessions; Toronto, Canada; 2004.

106 Cleland JG, Coletta AP, Lammiman M *et al.* Clinical trials update from the European Society of Cardiology meeting 2005: CARE-HF extension study, ESSENTIAL, CIBIS-III, S-ICD, ISSUE-2, STRIDE-2, SOFA, IMAGINE, PREAMI, SIRIUS-II and ACTIVE. *Eur J Heart Fail* 2005; **7**: 1070–1075.

107 Lowes BD, Shakar SF, Metra M *et al.* Rationale and design of the enoximone clinical trials program. *J Card Fail* 2005; **11**: 659–669.

108 Goldsmith SR. Congestive heart failure: potential role of arginine vasopressin antagonists in the therapy of heart failure. *Congest Heart Fail* 2002; **8**: 251–256.

109 Yatsu T, Tomura Y, Tahara A. Cardiovascular and renal effects of conivaptan hydrochloride (YM087), a vasopressin V_{1A} and V_2 receptor antagonist, in dogs with pacing-induced congestive heart failure. *Eur J Pharmacol* 1999; **376**: 239–246.

110 Naitoh M, Suzuki H, Murakami M. Effects of oral AVP receptor antagonists OPC21268 and OPC31260 on congestive heart failure in conscious dogs. *Am J Physiol* 1994; **267**: H2245–H2254.

111 Sanghi P, Uretsky BF, Schwarz ER. Vasopressin antagonism: a future treatment option in heart failure. *Eur Heart J* 2005; **26**: 538–543.

112 Gheorghiade M, Gattis WA, O'Connor CM *et al.* Effects of tolvaptan, a vasopressin antagonist, in patients hospitalized with worsening heart failure: a randomized controlled trial. *J Am Med Assoc* 2004; **291**: 1963–1971.

113 Russell SD, Selaru P, Pyne DA *et al.* Rationale for use of an exercise end point and design for the ADVANCE (A Dose evaluation of a Vasopressin ANtagonist in CHF patients undergoing Exercise) trial. *Am Heart J* 2003; **145**: 179–186.

114 Francis GS, Tang WH. Vasopressin receptor antagonists: will the "vaptans" fulfill their promise? *J Am Med Assoc* 2004; **291**: 2017–2018.

115 Gottlieb SS. Renal effects of adenosine A1-receptor antagonists in congestive heart failure. *Drugs* 2001; **61**: 1387–1393.

116 Lucas Jr. DG, Patterson T, Hendrick JW *et al.* Effects of adenosine receptor subtype A1 on ventricular and renal function. *J Cardiovasc Pharmacol* 2001; **38**: 618–624.

117 Gottlieb SS, Skettino SL, Wolff A *et al.* Effects of BG9719 (CVT-124), an A1-adenosine receptor antagonist, and furosemide on glomerular filtration rate and natriuresis in patients with congestive heart failure. *J Am Coll Cardiol* 2000; **35**: 56–59.

118 Gottlieb SS, Brater DC, Thomas I *et al.* BG9719 (CVT-124), an A1 adenosine receptor antagonist, protects against the decline in renal function observed with diuretic therapy. *Circulation* 2002; **105**: 1348–1353.

119 Stanton A. Therapeutic potential of renin inhibitors in the management of cardiovascular disorders. *Am J Cardiovasc Drugs* 2003; **3**: 389–394.

120 Gradman AH, Schmieder RE, Lins RL, Nussberger J, Chiang Y, Bedigian MP. Aliskiren, a novel orally effective renin inhibitor, provides dose-dependent antihypertensive efficacy and placebo-like tolerability in hypertensive patients. *Circulation* 2005; **111**: 1012–1018.

121 Figgitt DP, Gillies PS, Goa KL. Levosimendan. *Drugs* 2001; **61**: 613–627.

122 Cleland JG, McGowan J. Levosimendan: a new era for inodilator therapy for heart failure? *Curr Opin Cardiol* 2002; **17**: 257–265.

123 Kivikko M, Lehtonen L. Levosimendan: a new inodilatory drug for the treatment of decompensated heart failure. *Curr Pharm Des* 2005; **11**: 435–455.

124 Kaheinen P, Pollesello P, Levijoki J, Haikala H. Effects of levosimendan and milrinone on oxygen consumption in isolated guinea-pig heart. *J Cardiovasc Pharmacol* 2004; **43**: 555–561.

125 Szilagyi S, Pollesello P, Levijoki J *et al.* The effects of levosimendan and OR-1896 on isolated hearts, myocyte-sized preparations and phosphodiesterase enzymes of the guinea pig. *Eur J Pharmacol* 2004; **486**: 67–74.

126 Hasenfuss G, Pieske B, Castell M, Kretschmann B, Maier LS, Just H. Influence of the novel inotropic agent levosimendan on isometric tension and calcium cycling in failing human myocardium. *Circulation* 1998; **98**: 2141–2147.

127 Kivikko M, Lehtonen L, Colucci WS. Sustained hemodynamic effects of levosimendan. *Circulation* 2003; **107**: 81–86.

128 Follath F, Cleland JGF, Just H. Efficacy and safety of intravenous levosimendan, a novel calcium sensitiser, in severe low output failure. *Lancet* 2002; **360**: 196–202.

129 Moiseyev VS, Poder P, Andrejevs N *et al.* Randomized study on safety and effectiveness of levosimendan in patients with left ventricular heart failure after an acute myocardial infarction (the RUSSLAN study). *Eur Heart J* 2002; **23**: 1422–1432.

130 Zairis MN. Calcium Sensitizer or Inotrope or None in Low Output Heart Failure (CASINO), *American College of Cardiology 2004 Scientific Sessions*, New Orleans, Lousiana, 2004.

131 Zile M, Gaasch W, Little W *et al.* A phase II, double-blind, randomized, placebo-controlled, dose comparative study of the efficacy, tolerability, and safety of

MCC-135 in subjects with chronic heart failure, NYHA class II/III (MCC-135-GO1 study): rationale and design. *J Card Fail* 2004; **10**: 193–199.

132 Chaitman BR, Pepine CJ, Parker JO *et al.* Effects of ranolazine with atenolol, amlodipine, or diltiazem on exercise tolerance and angina frequency in patients with severe chronic angina: a randomized controlled trial. *J Am Med Assoc* 2004; **291**: 309–316.

133 Chandler MP, Stanley WC, Morita H *et al.* Short-term treatment with ranolazine improves mechanical efficiency in dogs with chronic heart failure. *Circ Res* 2002; **91**: 278–280.

134 Sabbah HN, Chandler MP, Mishima T *et al.* Ranolazine, a partial fatty acid oxidation (pFOX) inhibitor, improves left ventricular function in dogs with chronic heart failure. *J Card Fail* 2002; **8**: 416–422.

135 Sabbah HN, Imai M, Morita H, Stanley WC, Blackburn B. Long-term therapy with ranolazine prevents progressive left ventricular dysfunction and remodeling in dogs with chronic heart failure. *Circulation* 2004; **110**: 679–680.

136 Rupp H, Zarain-Herzberg A, Maisch B. The use of partial fatty acid oxidation inhibitors for metabolic therapy of angina pectoris and heart failure. *Herz* 2002; **27**: 621–636.

137 Torre-Amione G, Sestier F, Radovancevic B, Young J. Effects of a novel immune modulation therapy in patients with advanced chronic heart failure: results of a randomized, controlled, phase II trial. *J Am Coll Cardiol* 2004; **44**: 1181–1186.

138 Doehner W, Anker SD. Uric acid in chronic heart failure. *Semin Nephrol* 2005; **25**: 61–66.

139 Leyva F, Anker SD, Godsland IF *et al.* Uric acid in chronic heart failure: a marker of chronic inflammation. *Eur Heart J* 1998; **19**: 1814–1822.

140 Kogler H, Fraser H, McCune S, Altschuld R, Marban E. Disproportionate enhancement of myocardial contractility by the xanthine oxidase inhibitor oxypurinol in failing rat myocardium. *Cardiovasc Res* 2003; **59**: 582–592.

141 Freudenberger RS, Schwarz Jr. RP, Brown J *et al.* Rationale, design and organisation of an efficacy and safety study of oxypurinol added to standard therapy in patients with NYHA class III–IV congestive heart failure. *Expert Opin Investig Drugs* 2004; **13**: 1509–1516.

142 O'Meara E, McMurray JJ. Myocardial metabolic manipulation: a new therapeutic approach in heart failure? *Heart* 2005; **91**: 131–132.

143 Ferrari R, Cicchitelli G, Merli E, Andreadou I, Guardigli G. Metabolic modulation and optimization of energy consumption in heart failure. *Med Clin North Am* 2003; **87**: 493–507, xii–xiii.

144 Taegtmeyer H. Cardiac metabolism as a target for the treatment of heart failure. *Circulation* 2004; **110**: 894–896.

145 Simonsen S, Kjekshus JK. The effect of free fatty acids on myocardial oxygen consumption during atrial pacing and catecholamine infusion in man. *Circulation* 1978; **58**: 484–491.

146 Thrainsdottir IS, von Bibra H, Malmberg K, Ryden L. Effects of trimetazidine on left ventricular function in patients with type 2 diabetes and heart failure. *J Cardiovasc Pharmacol* 2004; **44**: 101–108.

147 Di Napoli P, Taccardi AA, Barsotti A. Long term cardioprotective action of trimetazidine and potential effect on the inflammatory process in patients with ischaemic dilated cardiomyopathy. *Heart* 2005; **91**: 161–165.

148 Vitale C, Wajngaten M, Sposato B *et al.* Trimetazidine improves left ventricular function and quality of life in elderly patients with coronary artery disease. *Eur Heart J* 2004; **25**: 1814–1821.

149 Bristow M. Etomoxir: a new approach to treatment of chronic heart failure. *Lancet* 2000; **356**: 1621–1622.

150 Schmidt-Schweda S, Holubarsch C. First clinical trial with etomoxir in patients with chronic congestive heart failure. *Clin Sci (Lond)* 2000; **99**: 27–35.

151 Rupp H, Jacob R. Metabolically-modulated growth and phenotype of the rat heart. *Eur Heart J* 1992; **13(Suppl D)**: 56–61.

152 Brousseau ME, Schaefer EJ, Wolfe ML *et al.* Effects of an inhibitor of cholesteryl ester transfer protein on HDL cholesterol. *N Engl J Med* 2004; **350**: 1505–1515.

153 Meier JJ, Nauck MA. Glucagon-like peptide 1(GLP-1) in biology and pathology. *Diabetes Metab Res Rev* 2005; **21**: 91–117.

154 Thrainsdottir I, Malmberg K, Olsson A, Gutniak M, Ryden L. Initial experience with GLP-1 treatment on metabolic control and myocardial function in patients with type 2 diabetes mellitus and heart failure. *Diabetes Vasc Dis Res* 2004; **1**: 40–43.

155 Nystrom T, Gutniak MK, Zhang Q *et al.* Effects of glucagon-like peptide-1 on endothelial function in type 2 diabetes patients with stable coronary artery disease. *Am J Physiol Endocrinol Metab* 2004; **287**: E1209–E1215.

156 Nikolaidis LA, Mankad S, Sokos GG *et al.* Effects of glucagon-like peptide-1 in patients with acute myocardial infarction and left ventricular dysfunction after successful reperfusion. *Circulation* 2004; **109**: 962–965.

157 Vasan S, Foiles PG, Founds HW. Therapeutic potential of AGE inhibitors and breakers of AGE protein crosslinks. *Expert Opin Investig Drugs* 2001; **10**: 1977–1987.

158 Kass DA, Sharprio EP, Kawaguchi M *et al.* Improved arterial compliance by a novel advanced glycation endproduct crosslink breaker. *Circulation* 2001; **104**: 1464–1470.

159 Bakris GL, Bank AJ, Kass DA, Neutel JM, Preston RA, Oparil S. Advanced glycation end-product cross-link breakers: a novel approach to cardiovascular pathologies

related to the aging process. *Am J Hypertens* 2004; **17**: 23S–30S.

160 Ahmed SH, Clark LL, Pennington WR *et al.* Matrix metalloproteinases/tissue inhibitors of metalloproteinases: relationship between changes in proteolytic determinants of matrix composition and structural, functional, and clinical manifestations of hypertensive heart disease. Circulation 2006; **113**: 2089–2096.

161 Cleland JG, Coletta AP, Freemantle N, Velavan P, Tin L, Clark AL. Clinical trials update from the American College of Cardiology meeting: CARE-HF and the remission of heart failure, Women's Health Study, TNT, COMPASS-HF, VERITAS, CANPAP, PEECH and PREMIER. *Eur J Heart Fail* 2005; **7**: 931–936.

162 Cooper GJ, Chan YK, Dissanayake AM *et al.* Demonstration of a hyperglycemia-driven pathogenic abnormality of copper homeostasis in diabetes and its reversibility by selective chelation: quantitative comparisons between the biology of copper and eight other nutritionally essential elements in normal and diabetic individuals. *Diabetes* 2005; **54**: 1468–1476.

163 Cooper GJ, Phillips AR, Choong SY *et al.* Regeneration of the heart in diabetes by selective copper chelation. *Diabetes* 2004; **53**: 2501–2508.

164 Paulus WJ. The role of nitric oxide in the failing heart. *Heart Fail Rev* 2001; **6**: 105–118.

165 McNeely W, Goa K. Nebivolol in the management of essential hypertension: a review. *Drugs* 1999; **57**: 633–651.

166 Flather MD, Shibata MC, Coats AJ *et al.* Randomized trial to determine the effect of nebivolol on mortality and cardiovascular hospital admission in elderly patients with heart failure (SENIORS). *Eur Heart J* 2005; **26**: 215–225.

167 Taylor AL, Ziesche S, Yancy C *et al.* Combination of isosorbide dinitrate and hydralazine in blacks with heart failure. *N Engl J Med* 2004; **351**: 2049–2057.

168 Cotter G, Kaluski E, Blatt A *et al.* L-NMMA (a nitric oxide synthase inhibitor) is effective in the treatment of cardiogenic shock. *Circulation* 2000; **101**: 1358–1361.

169 Dzavik V. Tilarginine for acute myocardial infarction complicated by cardiogenic shock, *American Heart Association 2004 Scientific Sessions*, New Orleans, Lousiana, 2004.

170 Perrot A, Osterziel KJ, Beck M, Dietz R, Kampmann C. Fabry disease: focus on cardiac manifestations and molecular mechanisms. *Herz* 2002; **27**: 699–702.

171 MacDermot KD, Holmes A, Miners AH. Anderson–Fabry disease: clinical manifestations and impact on disease in a cohort of 98 hemizygote males. *J Med Genet* 2001; **38**: 750–760.

172 Eng CM, Guffon N, Wilcox WR. Safety and efficacy of recombinant human alpha-galactosidase A-replacement therapy in Fabry's disease. *N Engl J Med* 2001; **345**: 9–16.

173 Schiffmann R, Kopp JB, Austin HA. Enzyme replacement therapy in Fabry disease: a randomized controlled trial. *J Am Med Assoc* 2001; **285**: 2743–2749.

174 Morkin E, Pennock GD, Spooner PH, Bahl JJ, Goldman S. Clinical and experimental studies on the use of 3,5-diiodothyropropionic acid, a thyroid hormone analogue, in heart failure. *Thyroid* 2002; **12**: 527–533.

175 Spooner PH, Morkin E, Goldman S. Thyroid hormone and thyroid hormone analogues in the treatment of heart failure. *Coron Artery Dis* 1999; **10**: 395–399.

176 Hamilton MA. Prevalence and clinical implications of abnormal thyroid hormone metabolism in advanced heart failure. *Ann Thorac Surg* 1993; **56**: S48–S52.

177 Hamilton MA, Stevenson LW, Foranow GC *et al.* Safety and hemodynamic effects of intravenous triiodothyronine in advanced congestive heart failure. *Am J Cardiol* 1998; **81**: 443–447.

178 Pennock GD, Rava TE, Bahl JJ, Goldman S, Morkin E. Combination treatment with captopril and the thyroid hormone analogue, 3,5-diiodothyropropionic acid: a new approach to improve left ventricular performance in heart failure. *Circ J* 1993; **88**: 1289–1298.

179 Morkin E, Pennock GD, Spooner PH, Bahl JJ, Underhill Fox K, Goldman S. Pilot studies on the use of 3,5-diiodothyropropionic acid, a thyroid hormone analog, in the treatment of congestive heart failure. *Cardiology* 2002; **97**: 218–225.

180 Fazio S, Sabatini D, Capaldo B *et al.* A preliminary study of growth hormone in the treatment of dilated cardiomyopathy. *N Engl J Med* 1996; **334**: 809–814.

181 Jenkins RC, Ross RJ. The growth hormone IGF-I axis in dilated cardiomyopathy. *Clin Endocrinol (Oxf)* 1999; **50**: 415–416.

182 Osterziel KJ, Strohm O, Schuler J *et al.* Randomised, double-blind, placebo-controlled trial of human recombinant growth hormone in patients with chronic heart failure due to dilated cardiomyopathy. *Lancet* 1998; **351**: 1233–1237.

183 Nagaya N, Uematsu M, Kojima M *et al.* Elevated circulating level of ghrelin in cachexia associated with chronic heart failure: relationships between ghrelin and anabolic/catabolic factors. *Circulation* 2001; **104**: 2034–2038.

184 Nagaya N, Miyatake K, Uematsu M *et al.* Hemodynamic, renal, and hormonal effects of ghrelin infusion in patients with chronic heart failure. *J Clin Endocrinol Metab* 2001; **86**: 5854–5859.

185 Nagaya N, Kangawa K. Ghrelin improves left ventricular dysfunction and cardiac cachexia in heart failure. *Curr Opin Pharmacol* 2003; **3**: 146–151.

186 Nagaya N, Moriya J, Yasumura Y *et al.* Effects of ghrelin administration on left ventricular function, exercise capacity, and muscle wasting in patients with chronic heart failure. *Circulation* 2004; **110**: 3674–3679.

187 Sheppard R, Panyon J, Pohwani AL *et al.* Intermittent outpatient ultrafiltration for the treatment of severe refractory congestive heart failure. *J Card Fail* 2004; **10**: 380–383.

188 Jaski BE, Ha J, Denys BG, Lamba S, Trupp RJ, Abraham WT. Peripherally inserted veno-venous ultrafiltration for rapid treatment of volume overloaded patients. *J Card Fail* 2003; **9**: 227–231.

188 Wasler A, Radovancevic B, Fruhwald F, Tripolt M, Klein W, Tscheliessnigg K. First use of the Cancion cardiac recovery system in a human. *ASAIO J* 2003; **49**: 136–138.

190 Tuzun E, Conger J, Gregoric ID *et al.* Evaluation of a new cardiac recovery system in a bovine model of volume overload heart failure. *ASAIO J* 2004; **50**: 557–562.

191 Czerska B, Oren RM, Bohm M *et al.* Orqis cancion cardiac recovery system: hemodynamic effects of a novel minimally invasive approach to cardio-renal support in severe acute heart failure, *Heart Failure Society of America 7th Annual Scientific Session*, Toronto, Canada, 2004.

192 Oren RM, Czerska B, Bohm M *et al.* Cancion cardiac recovery system: effects on renal, echocardiographic, and health status parameters during and following treatment with a novel, minimally invasive approach to cardio-renal support in severe acute heart failure, *Heart Failure Society of America 7th Annual Scientific Sessions*, Toronto, Canada, 2004.

193 Zile M. continuous aortic flow augmentation using orqis cancion cardiac recovery system in patients with severe heart failure: determinants of the hemodynamic response, *American College of Cardiology 2005 Scientific Session*, Oralando, Florida, 2005.

194 Pennington DG, Smedira NG, Samuels LE, Acker MA, Curtis JJ, Pagani FD. Mechanical circulatory support for acute heart failure. *Ann Thorac Surg* 2001; **71**: S56–S59; discussion S82–S85.

195 Entwistle III JW. Short- and long-term mechanical ventricular assistance towards myocardial recovery. *Surg Clin North Am* 2004; **84**: 201–221.

196 Feld Y, Dubi S, Reisner Y, Schwammenthal E, Elami A. Future strategies for the treatment of diastolic heart failure. *Acute Card Care* 2006; **8**: 13–20.

197 Yusuf S, Sleight P, Pogue J, Bosch J, Davies R, Dagenais G. Effects of an angiotensin-converting-enzyme inhibitor, ramipril, on cardiovascular events in high-risk patients. The Heart Outcomes Prevention Evaluation Study Investigators. *N Engl J Med* 2000; **342**: 145–153.

198 Effects of ramipril on cardiovascular and microvascular outcomes in people with diabetes mellitus: results of the HOPE study and MICRO-HOPE substudy. Heart Outcomes Prevention Evaluation Study Investigators. *Lancet* 2000; **355**: 253–259.

199 Dahlof B, Devereux RB, Kjeldsen SE *et al.* Cardiovascular morbidity and mortality in the Losartan Intervention For Endpoint reduction in hypertension study (LIFE): a randomised trial against atenolol. *Lancet* 2002; **359**: 995–1003.

200 Braunwald E, Domanski MJ, Fowler SE *et al.* Angiotensin-converting-enzyme inhibition in stable coronary artery disease. *N Engl J Med* 2004; **351**: 2058–2068.

201 Fox KM. Efficacy of perindopril in reduction of cardiovascular events among patients with stable coronary artery disease: randomised, double-blind, placebo-controlled, multicentre trial (the EUROPA study). *Lancet* 2003; **362**: 782–788.

202 Hunt SA, Abraham WT, Chin MH *et al.* ACC/AHA 2005, Guideline update for the Diagnosis and Management of Chronic Heart Failure in the Adult: a report of the American College of Cardiology/American Heart Association Task Force on Practice Guidelines (writing Committee to update the 2001 Guidelines for the Evaluation and Management of Heart Failure). *Circulation* 2005; **112**: 154–235.

CHAPTER 5

Implantable cardioverter defibrillators and biventricular pacemakers in congestive heart failure

Mandeep Bhargava & Bruce L. Wilkoff

The last few decades have seen major advancements in the management of patients with congestive heart failure (CHF). The myriad of newer therapies and the newer insights into older therapies have contributed significantly to the reduction in mortality and morbidity in patients with heart failure. This chapter will explore the clinical expression of ventricular arrhythmias in these patients and also discuss the role of implantable cardioverter defibrillators (ICD) and cardiac resynchronization therapy (CRT) in modifying the natural history of this growing epidemic.

Sudden cardiac death in heart failure

Sudden cardiac death (SCD) has changed in definition a long way since the original description of this term by Kuller *et al.* in 1966 [1]. Most definitions now would account for SCD as death from unexpected circulatory arrest, usually from a cardiac arrhythmia, occurring within 1 h of the onset of symptoms [2]. The importance of defining this syndrome was realized due to the need to compare the randomized therapies in large clinical trials. The definition has been changed variously in accordance with the need for evaluating the results in various trials and continues to have its limitations in differentiating arrhythmic and non-arrhythmic deaths. Hinkle and Thaler [3] tried to differentiate between the two, classifying arrhythmic deaths as those in

which the subject collapsed abruptly and the pulse ceased prior to circulatory collapse, whereas circulatory failure deaths were those in which peripheral circulation collapsed before the cessation of the pulse. Such a classification revealed that 58% of the deaths in heart failure were arrhythmic and the remaining were due to circulatory collapse. Most of the arrhythmic deaths are out of hospital deaths and most deaths due to circulatory collapse occur in hospital. Studies have reported the incidence of seemingly arrhythmic deaths as being between 23% and 49% [4–7].

The need for differentiating between arrhythmic and non-arrhythmic deaths became important in order to risk stratify patients for SCD and to scientifically apply the various pharmacological and non-pharmacological treatment modalities for patients with heart failure and left ventricular (LV) dysfunction. This led to the publication of a standardized reporting system for classification of deaths in ICD trials by the North American Society of Pacing and Electrophysiology (NASPE) Policy Conference in 1993 [8]. They classified deaths as either sudden cardiac, non-sudden cardiac, operative or non-cardiac. *SCDs* were those which were either a witnessed cardiac arrest, or within 1 h of the onset of acute symptoms or an unexpected unwitnessed death in a patient known to be well in the previous 24 h. *Non-SCDs* were those due to progressive CHF and/or a low output state preceding the ventricular arrhythmias, if any. *Operative deaths* were those within 30 days of attempted ICD implant or before hospital discharge or the direct result of an ICD implant-related complication. *Non-cardiac deaths* included the rest of the events.

Ventricular arrhythmias causing SCD in heart failure

A number of complex inter-relationships predispose to the occurrence of ventricular arrhythmias in patients with heart failure. Though the mechanisms, type and frequency of the arrhythmias may differ in patients with and without coronary artery disease, all patients with heart failure are at higher risk of developing ventricular arrhythmias. Many of these could be fatal and life threatening. The correct application of the different management strategies for these arrhythmias requires some insight into the pathogenesis of these electrical disturbances.

The mechanisms that trigger these arrhythmias could either be substrate specific to patients with coronary artery disease, dilated, restrictive or hypertrophic cardiomyopathy or could be due to common electrophysiological, environmental and drug-related issues in these patients. Cellular hypertrophy, myocardial stretch and interstitial fibrosis leading to prolongation of action potential duration, spatial heterogeneity, reduction of conduction velocity predispose to re-entry circuits, and the increase in triggered activity favors the development of ventricular tachyarrhythmias in these patients [9–13]. Abnormal neurohormonal responses like increased central sympathetic outflow, stimulation of the renin-angiotensin system and the persistent stimulation of the adrenergic system cause enhanced automaticity [14,15]. Other important triggers like hypokalemia and hypomagnessemia, especially common in the setting of chronic diuretic therapy may lead to *torsades de pointes*.

Coronary artery disease

There is strong evidence to suggest association between coronary artery disease and ventricular tachyarrhythmias causing SCD. It is believed to be responsible for 65% of sudden deaths in men and up to 40% in women [16]. Most of the patients with heart failure have coronary artery disease-related scars as the etiopathologic mechanism. Autopsy data have shown that even patients with dilated cardiomyopathy could have scars in up to 14% of patients [17]. The most probable mechanism that leads to SCD in these patients is an initial occurrence of sustained monomorphic ventricular tachycardia (VT), which would subsequently degenerate into ventricular fibrillation (VF). This patient population provides an extremely durable substrate for re-entry circuits due to scar-related zones of slow conduction intermingled with normal areas of viable myocardium [18–20]. The characteristic feature of such tachycardias is that they have a reproducible initiation and termination by critically timed extrastimuli and activation mapping demonstrates reentrant excitation [21]. Most of these circuits are probably due to intramural re-entry but many could have endocardial and epicardial extensions. The recurrence rate of these arrhythmias is more than 40% after the initial presentation, at a rate of 3–5% annually over 15 years. The inducibility in the electrophysiology (EP) laboratory exceeds 90% even up to 6 years after the index event [21,22]. Analysis of the data from the bipolar electrograms retrieved from such patients suggest that there may be more than one mechanism for the causation of episodic VT, but sustained episodes with uniform morphology and stable cycle length are due to fixed re-entry circuits in the region of inexcitable scar tissue [23].

Initial VF in patients with coronary artery disease is most often the result of either an acute ischemic episode resulting from a recent thrombotic occlusion of a coronary artery or due to the degeneration from a sustained VT in the setting of prior myocardial infarction (MI). The data in relation to the association with a recent thrombotic occlusion is conflicting and various studies show the incidence of such phenomenon from less than 20% to more than 95% in survivors of SCD [24–27]. In conclusion, the mechanism of VF is poorly understood. However, in the setting of ischemia, LV dysfunction does predispose to ventricular arrhythmias and in the setting of heart failure, ischemia does lead to the lowering of threshold for the development of fatal arrhythmic events. As mentioned earlier, the occurrence of VF is most often related to the degeneration of sustained monomorphic episodes of VT, which in turn may be related to ischemia or other factors as electrolyte imbalances or neurohormonal activation [28,29].

Polymorphic VT is less common in patients with LV dysfunction. It is mostly associated with episodes of long QT syndrome, electrolyte imbalances, drug exposures and toxicity or bradycardia related to sinus or atrioventricular (AV) node dysfunction. Such bradycardia could either be related to the degeneration associated with the underlying disease or the effect of drugs. In situations when polymorphic VT is associated with bradycardia, it is referred to as "*torsades de pointes*" and responds well to catecholamines and pacing. The significance of polymorphic VT is that it suggests a higher likelihood of recurrence and identifies patients who are unlikely to tolerate drugs like amiodarone and other QT prolonging drugs [21,30].

It is a controversial issue whether less complex ventricular arrhythmias like ventricular premature beats (VPBs) and non-sustained VTs are predictors of SCD. There are conflicting results on this aspect from two retrospective analyses [31,32]. The trials which addressed this issue partly were the Argentinian Study Group for the Prevention of Cardiac Insufficiency (GESICA-GEMA) Investigators [33]. The incidence of non-sustained arrhythmias in patients with heart failure was found to be 33.5% and the combination of the VPBs and non-sustained VT conferred a relative risk of 2.2 for total mortality and 5.5 for sudden death. This data had the limitation that most patients in this study had non-ischemic dilated cardiomyopathy including Chagas' disease. Another trial throwing some light on this issue was the Prospective Randomized Milrinone Survival Evaluation (PROMISE) trial, which showed that 48% of the deaths occurring in patients with an LV ejection fraction (LVEF) of less than 0.35 and New York Heart Association (NYHA) Class III–IV heart failure were sudden and the strongest predictor of mortality was the frequency of non-sustained episodes of VT [34].

In summary, it is clear that patients with ischemic cardiomyopathy provide a fertile base for the occurrence of all types of ventricular tachyarrhythmias, which in turn predispose to SCD. Most of the sustained VTs may originate by more than one mechanism, but their sustenance is guided by the provision of a reliable substrate of heterogenous myocardium through reentrant mechanisms. VF is frequent and is either a consequence of degeneration of sustained VT or due to acute deteriorating factors of which ischemia is probably the most common. VPBs and non-sustained VT may not be fatal in their individual capacity, but SCDs are seemingly closely related to their presence and frequency in patients with severe LV systolic dysfunction. They are however, not reliable predictors of sudden death in an individual patient.

Non-ischemic dilated cardiomyopathy

The pathophysiological basis for ventricular arrhythmias in patients with non-ischemic dilated cardiomyopathy has been less well understood. Endocardial plaques and myocardial scar are frequently observed in these patients. The ventricular myocardium is characterized by patchy areas of interstitial fibrosis. Most of the patients in this category have relatively normal electrograms and activation patterns from the endocardial surface, especially when compared with patients of ischemic cardiomyopathy. Hence, these patients are not as good of a substrate for scar-related re-entrant arrhythmias. However, patients who do present with sustained VT, have more of scar-related heterogeneity in conduction and easy inducibility and reproducibility of VT by programmed stimulation. Such patients have low amplitude, wide, and fractionated endocardial electrograms [35]. Using three-dimensional mapping, Hsia *et al.* have shown that in patients with sustained VT and non-ischemic cardiomyopathy referred for an ablation, the majority of the patients had only a modest area (<25%) of endocardial abnormality [36]. These low voltage abnormal areas were located near the ventricular base in the perivalvular regions and 88% of the mapped VTs originated from the ventricular base, corresponding to regions with abnormal endocardial electrograms. Delacretaz *et al.* [37] found that in patients with non-ischemic cardiomyopathy, 58% of patients showed the above characteristics suggesting scar-related re-entry as the pathophysiological basis. Another 20–40% of patients may have bundle branch re-entry tachycardia and these patients have the highest efficacy with catheter ablation with success rates close to 100%.

Frequent ventricular ectopy and non-sustained VT are relatively more common than sustained VT, in patients with non-ischemic cardiomyopathy. Such non-sustained arrhythmias may be present in up to 60–87% of patients. Unlike patients presenting with sustained monomorphic VT, the inducibility of sustained VT at EP study in patients presenting with a cardiac arrest or non-sustained ventricular arrhythmias is extremely low (75–100% versus 0–15%, respectively). In patients presenting with non-sustained VT or a cardiac arrest, even despite a negative EP study, there continues to be a high risk of VT/VF recurrence and sudden death. This persists despite drug suppression or slowing of any inducible arrhythmia. Hence, the predictive role of such arrhythmias and the utility of EP studies in determining long-term prognosis and guiding therapy in these patients has been fairly limited [38–41]. This also suggests that the genesis of non-sustained arrhythmias in this group of patients is more likely to be due to mechanisms of focal automaticity or triggered mechanisms, unlike sustained monomorphic VT, which seems to be related to scar-related re-entry phenomenon similar to that in patients with ischemic cardiomyopathy.

Risk stratification for SCD in heart failure

A large number of variables have been studied to predict the risk of SCD in patients with heart failure and especially so in the presence of coronary artery disease. The most potent predictor for long-term survival continues to be the LV function [42,43]. Other entities like 24 h holter monitoring, invasive electrophysiologic testing, signal averaged electrocardiogram (SAECG), baroreflex sensitivity and heart rate variability, either in isolation or in combination, have been unable to predict the high risk groups accurately or to guide anti-arrhythmic or ICD therapy [44–48].

As has become increasingly clear by the various secondary prevention trials for ICD therapy [49–51] and with the discussion above, there now seems to be little doubt that patients with sustained monomorphic VT and VF and those with polymorphic VT are a high risk group for recurrence of such arrhythmias and SCD. Hence, aggressive and expensive therapy in such groups is justified. For long, there has been debate regarding the role of invasive electrophysiologic testing in patients with non-sustained VT and frequent VPBs in the setting of LV dysfunction, more so in the presence of coronary artery disease. Invasive EP testing has been shown to be positive in 20–45% of patients with non-sustained VT in such situations and these are the patients who are capable of sustaining re-entry as the mechanism of recurrent arrhythmias [52–54]. It is not clear whether such testing would reliably identify the patients who have other mechanisms for sustained VT.

Wilber *et al.* [52] had shown that inducibility of sustained monomorphic VT by programmed electrical stimulation in patients with coronary artery disease and LV dysfunction was reliable in guiding subsequent anti-arrhythmic therapy. Their study revealed that inducible sustained monomorphic VT despite anti-arrhythmic drugs (AADs) in such settings would have a risk of SCD in up to 50% patients over the next 2 years. In patients who had suppression of the tachycardia with drugs, the risk was around 11% but even those patients in whom there was no inducible tachycardia there was a 2–6% risk of cardiac arrest and SCD. As mentioned before, the reliability of such testing is even lower in patients with idiopathic dilated cardiomyopathy because it is neither reliable in reproducing VT even in patients with sustained spontaneous VT or syncope nor is the absence of an inducible VT a marker of low risk for sudden death [36,55]. However, with the results of the Multicenter Automatic Defibrillator Implantation Trial (MADIT) II and the SCD in Heart Failure Trial (SCD-HeFT) as discussed later, all the above data is likely to require major reconsideration and the value of EP testing stands challenged once again.

Another strong clinical predictor of SCD in patients with heart failure and LV dysfunction is the history of syncope. Unexplained syncope in patients with heart failure has been associated with a history of sudden death in up to 45% of patients [57] and invasive testing frequently demonstrates an arrhythmic cause in most of these patients. Although most of them have been found to have sustained monomorphic VT, abnormalities of the sinus node, AV junction and supraventricular arrhythmias are not uncommon [58]. As discussed before, the role of invasive EP testing in patients of dilated cardiomyopathy with a history of syncope is much less reliable [59] as it fails to show a consistent arrhythmic cause, but these patients continue to remain at a very high risk for SCD.

Impact of drugs on SCD in heart failure

There have been major advancements in the knowledge of the role of drugs in the changing profile of morbidity and mortality in heart failure. One of the earliest drugs that was found to make a significant impact on the course of the disease were the angiotensin-converting enzyme (ACE) inhibitors. Most of the trials evaluating the role of ACE inhibitors in heart failure have shown a significant reduction or a trend towards lowering the mortality and morbidity in these patients [60–62]. More recently there have been reports of significant improvement in mortality in patients with aldo-sterone antagonists though the mechanism for the same is incompletely understood. The Randomized Aldactone Evaluation Study (RALES) trial [63] showed a 30% improvement in total mortality. There had been fears regarding the safety with the use of Digoxin in patients with heart failure, especially so in patients with coronary artery disease. However, the more recent prospective randomized study, the Digitalis Investigation Group (DIG) trial, showed the safety of the use of digoxin in patients with an LVEF of less than 45% [64]. These patients did not show any difference in the incidence of tachyarrhythmias between the digoxin and the placebo group. The inci-dence of bradyarrhythmias was slightly higher in the digoxin group but was not associated with any increase in mortality. There was a trend towards a reduction in the progression of symptoms and death due to heart failure in patients in the digoxin group and this was more so and statistically significant in patients with non-ischemic cardiomyopathy.

The role of the various AADs has also been widely studied. The Cardiac Arrhythmia Suppression Trials (CAST) [65,66] have well demonstrated that though the Class I drugs (flecainide, encainide, and mori-cizine) can effectively reduce the ectopy in patients with heart failure, there was a significant increase in the mortality in patients taking these drugs. Even propafenone has been shown to be associated with adverse results [51]. Most of the contribution of the poor results with these drugs has been mainly attri-buted to the increased risk of proarrhythmias asso-ciated with these drugs, especially so in patients with coronary artery disease and LV dysfunction.

The Class II agents, the beta-blockers, though not primarily used as anti-arrhythmics in heart failure, are another group of agents that have revolutionized the treatment of heart failure. It has now been increasingly realized that adrenergic stimulation con-tributes significantly to the pathophysiologic processes relating to the progression of heart failure. Beta-blockers have effectively controlled this phe-nomenon and the fears regarding their negative inotropy and chronotropy contributing to the wors-ening of heart failure have been put to rest. There is an increasing aggressiveness to their early use in heart failure and in the maximum tolerated doses. Both, the

selective and non-selective agents have been found to be equally useful [67–69], and those with additional alpha-blocking properties have shown more promis-ing results, likely due to an additional effect of reduc-ing the afterload in these patients. The trials have uniformly shown consistent reduction in death, from both, the progression to heart failure and SCDs due to arrhythmic events. The benefit has extended to all classes of heart failure and in patients with both ischemic and non-ischemic cardiomyopathies.

Sotalol has been tried in patients with MI and LV dysfunction but has not shown any promise. In fact, it has been associated with a higher risk of sudden death likely due to the increased risk of *torsades de pointes* in these patients [70]. It is predominantly a Class III agent and also has beta-blocking proper-ties. Dofetilide has been shown to be a promising anti-arrhythmic, but failed to contribute positively to the mortality benefit in patients with LV dysfunc-tion [71].

Despite the gamut of side effects that can be asso-ciated with this drug, the only AAD that has consis-tently shown to be fairly safe and effective in patients with heart failure has been Amiodarone. Initially developed as an antianginal agent, this drug gradu-ally became popular as a Class III anti-arrhythmic drug by virtue of its ability to block the outward potassium currents. It also has mild antiadrenergic and calcium channel blocking properties in addition to mild Class I anti-arrhythmic effects and is used in the management of almost all types of supraventric-ular and ventricular tachyarrhythmias.

A large number of trials have been carried out to study the role of Amiodarone in patients after MI [72–74] and CHF [75–77]. The patient selection has been either on the basis of frequent ventricular ectopy or on the basis of echocardiographic evi-dence of LV dysfunction. Hence, all of these trials have tried to study the role of Amiodarone as a pri-mary prophylactic agent in the subset of population at a higher risk of SCD. Most of the trials have shown that Amiodarone has shown a significant decrease in the overall mortality or at least a trend towards the same in comparison to the placebo group. There has been a significant decrease in the frequency of fatal ventricular arrhythmias and the incidence of sudden death, which has been the major contributor to the reduced overall mortality. The effect has been more prominent in patients with an increased heart rate and in patients with more severe ventricular dysfunction and heart failure. However, the recently published SCD-HeFT trial [78] suggests that Amiodarone, like all other AADs, needs to be used with extreme caution, especially in patients with more severe heart failure. It has been well tolerated in patients with severe ventricular dysfunction in doses less than 300–400 mg/day, though the incidence of side effects and discontinuation rates have been significant.

The role of Amiodarone as the lone secondary prophylactic agent against a placebo may be difficult to study in this era of implantable defibrillators. The only randomized secondary prevention trial of amiodarone comparing it with conventional antiarrhythmic therapy is The Cardiac Arrest in Seattle: Conventional Versus Amiodarone Drug Evaluation (CASCADE) Study [79]. This study enrolled patients who were out of hospital survivors of a VF arrest in the absence of an acute MI. Most of them had coronary artery disease and about a half of them had LV dysfunction. The mean LVEF was 35%. The patients were treated either with Amiodarone or with conventional AADs and were followed by serial electrophysiologic testing or Holter monitoring if the VT was not inducible. Amiodarone was found to significantly reduce the number of cardiac deaths, recurrences of the arrhythmia, the number of syncopal events, and the frequency of ICD shocks.

Amiodarone continues to be a popular drug for the management of arrhythmias in patients with heart failure. There is convincing, though indirect evidence to suggest that it is more effective and safer than other AADs for the prevention of recurrence of VT/VF, and probably in comparison to placebo too. A meta-analysis [80] of the primary prevention trials shows that there is a major trend towards the improvement in overall cardiac mortality (13–15%) and a significant reduction in the risk of arrhythmic deaths (29%). The role of the drug in comparison to the ICDs is discussed later in the chapter but the drug is well tolerated in the hemodynamics of CHF, is fairly effective and is safe if monitored carefully. The risk of proarrhythmia is low and although many authors [81] believe that hard evidence is lacking for justifying its use as a primary prophylactic therapy against SCD, it will continue to be the "poor man's defibrillator", at least for secondary prophylaxis and in developing countries, till a reasonable alternative is available. Once again, the results of the SCD-HeFT trial, do not show any mortality benefit in patients with heart failure when amiodarone was compared with placebo for primary prophylaxis for SCD. In fact, the results were more detrimental in patients with NYHA Class III heart failure. However, it would be difficult to make a final conclusion in this subgroup of patients from this trial alone, as patients with NYHA Class III constituted only 30% of patients in this trial.

ICDs in heart failure

The concept of defibrillation was not new to the management of ventricular tachyarrhythmias. However, the development of the ICD has had a remarkable impact on the prevention of SCD. Michael Mirowski, first pioneered the earliest models of the device in the 1960s, after he got frustrated seeing the death of his friend and mentor by recurrent ventricular arrhythmias. He finally innovated and implanted the first device [82] in human beings in 1980 and since then the "magic shock box" has evolved a long way from being a treatment in desperation to almost the gold standard of therapy, and now often a treatment of first choice in many patients. There has now been more than decade follow up in patients in many trials that have undergone an ICD implantation and the role of the device in the various disease states is expanding by the day.

There have been numerous trials to study the role of the ICD in patients with coronary artery disease and LV dysfunction as these patients form the largest base of the population to benefit from the device. The role of the ICD has been differently studied in patients who have either experienced or survived an episode of SCD or have shown a high risk for the likelihood of suffering from such an episode.

The ICD is not just an automatic "shock box", but is essentially a very intelligent and sophisticated device. It has two main components, including a pulse generator and the leads. The combination of these two components enables the device sense the electrical activity in the ventricle (or the atria as the case may be) beat by beat and to identify the abnormal rhythms by various programmed algorithms. They then are able to accumulate charge within a capacitor and deliver a high energy shock so as to revert these fatal arrhythmias into normal rhythm. The initial ICDs had capacitors that were bulky and the device needed to be implanted in the anterior wall of the abdomen. The energy was delivered through surgically placed pericardial patches. However, advancements in integrated circuit design and capacitor technology have produced an ICD small enough to be implanted in the pre-pectoral fossa and employ transvenous leads precisely like pacemakers. The devices provide rate-adaptive single or dual chamber anti-bradycardia pacemaker functionality, and store electrograms and diagnostic information which can be easily retrieved by telemetry. Now these devices can also deliver resynchronization therapy for heart failure.

ICD therapy: secondary prevention trials

There are four major multicenter international trials which have assessed the efficacy of the ICD in comparison with drugs in patients who have survived an episode of SCD or a life-threatening arrhythmia. The entry criteria for patients in each of these trials have been an episode of VT/VF, and understandably, most of these patients had coronary artery disease and LV dysfunction.

Anti-arrhythmics Versus Implantable Defibrillator trial (AVID)

This was the first and the largest of the secondary prevention trials [49]. The study included patients who had either sustained a VF arrest or a syncopal VT or a VT in the setting of an LVEF of less than 40% or symptoms of severe hemodynamic compromise

(near syncope, heart failure, or angina). A total of 1016 patients were randomized to receive either Class III anti-arrhythmic drug therapy or ICD therapy. The primary end point of the study was all cause mortality.

The patient profile was very similar in the two groups as regards the age, sex, and LVEF. More than 80% of the patients had coronary disease and the mean LVEF was 31% in the patients receiving AADs and 32% in the ICD group. Almost 60% of the patients had functional NYHA Class II–III while those with Class IV were excluded. Among the patients in the drug therapy group, 96% of them received amiodarone and the rest of them received sotalol. The patients were followed up for a period of 3 years. An interim analysis in April 1997 by the Data and Safety Monitoring Board recommended a premature termination of the trial because the difference in the all cause mortality between the two groups had crossed the statistical limits enforcing an early termination of the study (Figure 5.1). The ICD group had a significant mortality benefit by 29%. The 1 year mortality was 11% in the ICD group as compared to 18% in the drug therapy group. The mortality benefit in the ICD group was clearly due to the reduction in the sudden, arrhythmic deaths [83] and the maximum benefit was achieved in patients with an LVEF of less than 35% [84]. This benefit was sustained throughout the study period and was 27%

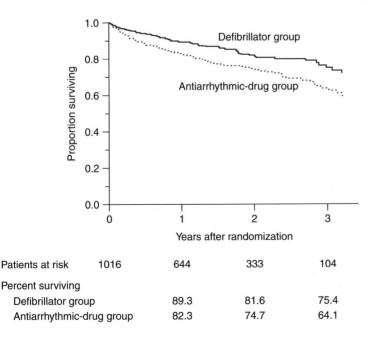

Patients at risk	1016	644	333	104
Percent surviving				
Defibrillator group		89.3	81.6	75.4
Antiarrhythmic-drug group		82.3	74.7	64.1

Figure 5.1 Overall survival (unadjusted for baseline characteristics) in the two groups treated with a defibrillator or with antiarrhythmic drugs in the AVID trial. Survival was better in the ICD group with a *P* value <0.02. (From the Antiarrhythmics Versus Implantable Defibrillators (AVID) Investigators, *N Engl J Med* 1997; **337**:1576–83. Reprinted with permission.) Copyright © 1997 Massachusetts Medical Society. All rights reserved.

at 2 years and 31% at 3 years. The average lifespan of a patient was found to be increased by about 2.7 months at the end of 3 years from the index event.

The Canadian Implantable Defibrillator Study (CIDS)

This multicenter trial [50] included 659 patients who were randomized to either receive an ICD or amiodarone. The entry criteria were similar to that in the Anti-arrhythmics Versus Implantable Defibrillator (AVID) trial except that the cut off point for the LVEF was 35% and it also included patients with a VT of more than 150 beats per minute or patients with inducible VT in individuals with unmonitored syncope. Initially it was decided that the primary endpoint was to study the arrhythmic deaths and the deaths occurring within 30 days from the initiation of therapy but this was subsequently changed to all cause mortality. The mean LVEF of the patients was 33% and 34% in the two groups, respectively, and patients in NYHA Class IV were also included. The results showed that there was a modest decrease in the all cause mortality (20%, $P = 0.14$) and in the incidence of arrhythmic deaths (30%, $P = 0.09$) at 5 years in patients receiving ICD therapy, but the difference was not statistically significant. The incidence of coronary artery disease and the mean LVEF was similar to that in the AVID trial but of note was the fact that there was a significant crossover rate at 5 years of follow up (30% from ICD to amiodarone and 16% from amiodarone to ICD). A *post hoc* subgroup analysis showed that the maximum benefit with the ICD was in patients with the highest risk of SCD, which composed of the older patients with an LVEF of less than 35% with NYHA Class III/IV heart failure [85].

The Cardiac Arrest Study Hamburg

The Cardiac Arrest Study Hamburg was a multicenter randomized study to compare ICD therapy against the efficacy of drugs [86]. The drugs used for comparison were propafenone, amiodarone and metoprolol and a 3:1 ratio of randomization assignment between the drug and ICD arms was used. A total of 349 patients who were survivors of cardiac arrest were enrolled in the study. As with all the other trials, almost three-fourths of the patients had coronary artery disease. However, the mean LVEF of the patients in this study was higher (46%) and about

10% of the patients had no structural heart disease. After 5 years of the start of the trial, in 1992, the propafenone arm had to be discontinued when an interim analysis [87] revealed that there was a higher mortality in the propafenone group (29% versus 11%). Almost all the excess mortality was due to an additional incidence of sudden deaths (11 in the propafenone group versus none in the ICD group). At the end of the study, which was at a mean follow up of 57 months, there was a 23% reduction in the all cause mortality with ICD therapy when compared with drugs (amiodarone and metoprolol). These results were borderline significant ($P = 0.08$) despite the fact that about three-fourths of the patient were in NYHA Class II, the mean LVEF and the incidence of patients with normal hearts were higher and more than half the patients received epicardial lead systems by thoracotomy, which in itself increased the perioperative mortality to some extent. The authors felt that all these factors could have led to the underestimation of the beneficial effects of the ICD.

The Dutch study

This was a small study [88] which enrolled 60 consecutive patients who were survivors of a VT/VF cardiac arrest, a greater than 4 week old MI and inducible VT with programmed electrical stimulation. The patients were randomized to either an ICD implantation ($n = 29$) or to conventional treatment ($n = 31$). The conventional treatment included an EP guided therapy with drugs and if this failed the patients underwent catheter/surgical ablation therapy. In the event of failure of ablation too (as guided by an EP study), the patients underwent an ICD implantation. Though the study was small, the protocol was quite aggressive in the management of patients not undergoing an ICD implantation. The mean LVEF of the patients in both groups was low (29% in the conventional group and 30% in the ICD group) and the Killip and NYHA Class distribution was similar. The results showed that there was a significant reduction in mortality in the ICD group (14% versus 35%) and this was predominantly due to the reduction in the sudden deaths.

ICD therapy: primary prevention trials

It is but natural that the impact of ICD therapy in the secondary prevention trials generated enthusiasm in trying to identify the high-risk population which was likely to sustain a cardiac arrest in the future. The importance of primary prevention stems from the fact that in most environments, not more than 5% of people can be resuscitated successfully after a cardiac arrest. The search for such clinical indicators to identify this high-risk population continues to make headway and is likely to have a significant impact on multiple aspects of therapy for heart disease, scientifically, ethically, and economically.

The issue of primary prevention of SCD and the role of the ICD in this context is importantly driven by the accurate assessment of the underlying disease and the accurate determination of the variables that can risk stratify and define the "high-risk population". This is important in the otherwise seemingly symptomless population, because ICD implantation is a surgical procedure not completely void of any risks, and its implantation has economic implications as well. Hence the knowledge from primary prevention trials is important in filtering out the eligible population which is likely to benefit from the implantation of an ICD. The major primary prevention trials to date and are discussed below.

Multicenter Automatic Defibrillator Implantation Trial (MADIT)

This was the first study that tried to compare the effect of prophylactic ICD therapy and anti-arrhythmic drug therapy among patients at a high risk of sudden death. Since non-sustained VT in patients with a prior MI and LV dysfunction is associated with 2-year mortality in the range of 30% [43,89] these parameters were used to select the high-risk population. The patients included in the study had a prior Q-wave MI, an LVEF of less than 35%, evidence of non-sustained VT and an inducible, non-suppressible, sustained, monomorphic VT on invasive electrophysiologic testing. The study included 196 patients, of which 101 patients received drug therapy and 95 patients received an ICD. The mean LVEF in the two groups of patients was not significantly different (25% and 27%, respectively). Almost two-thirds of the patients in either group were in NYHA Class II–III heart failure. The most commonly used drug was Amiodarone (in about 80% of the patients) but 9% of the patients were on no AADs at all.

The results of the trial [90] were so dramatic that the trial had to be prematurely terminated in 1996.

There was 39% mortality in the anti-arrhythmic group versus 12% mortality in the ICD group ($P = 0.009$). The arrhythmic deaths in the two groups were 13 and 3 respectively. In the ICD group, almost 60% of the patients had received a shock in the first 2 years after the implantation. *Post hoc* analysis [91] again showed that the greatest benefit was seen in patients with the worst ventricular function.

This was the first trial to show that ICD could improve survival in a symptomless high-risk population of coronary artery disease. There have been criticisms on the MADIT trial in relation to the fact that fewer patients in the conventional group were on beta-blockers. There were some issues of poor compliance with the drugs and the type of drug used, but nonetheless it was the first trial which conceptualized the importance of "risk stratification" and the role of invasive EP study in achieving this goal objectively.

The Coronary Artery Bypass Graft Patch trial (CABG-PATCH)

The CABG-patch trial enrolled patients undergoing coronary artery bypass graft (CABG) surgery if they had an LVEF of less than 36% and an abnormal SAECG. The patients were randomly assigned to receive either an ICD using epicardial lead systems at the time of surgery or to receive no other anti-arrhythmic therapy at all. By the design of the trial itself, all patients had coronary artery disease. The mean LVEF of the patients was 27%. About three-fourth of the patients had NYHA Class II–III heart failure. The study recruited 900 patients and they were followed up for a mean of 32 months prior to the termination of the study. The results showed that the total mortality was not different in the two groups [92]. The total mortality was 27% in the ICD group versus 24% in the control group. The study suggested that coronary revascularization may have decreased the trigger for arrhythmic events and that SAECG could not prove to be a reliable non-invasive alternative to invasive EP testing as an investigation for risk stratification for SCD.

Multicenter Unsustained Tachycardia Trial (MUSTT)

The Multicenter Unsustained Tachycardia Trial [93] was not initially designed to evaluate the efficacy of the ICD, but to study the role of an EP study guided approach to prevent SCD in patients with a prior

MI, an LVEF of less than 40% and evidence of non-sustained VT. A total of 2202 patients were enrolled and they underwent invasive EP study. Of these, 65% of the patients were non-inducible and they were followed up as a registry. From the remaining 35% of patients, 704 were randomized to either receive no specific treatment ($n = 353$) or to receive EP guided treatment ($n = 351$). EP guided drug testing was done to select the anti-arrhythmic drug, but in those patients who were non-suppressible, an ICD was implanted. Most of the patients in the drug therapy group were receiving Class IA agents. The mean LVEF was 30%. At 5 years of follow up it was found that the total mortality was 24% in the ICD group, 48% in the group receiving no therapy at all and 55% in the group of patients receiving AADs. The incidence of sudden death was 9% in the ICD group versus 37% in the non-ICD group; once again confirming that the major benefit of the ICD is by reducing the arrhythmic deaths. This study not only confirmed the superiority of the ICD in comparison of drugs, but also showed the alarming harmfulness of drugs (especially Class IA agents) in patients with coronary artery disease and LV dysfunction.

Multicenter Automatic Defibrillator Implantation Trial II (MADIT II)

One of the more recent trials that focused on the issue of primary prevention for SCD is the MADIT II Trial [56,94]. This trial directly addressed the issue whether LV function, the strongest known predictor of survival in coronary artery disease, could in itself be used for the risk stratification of patients for SCD in order to decide whether they are likely to benefit from ICD therapy. The trial began in July 1997 and the results became available in 2002. However, the results had far reaching implications and caused sensation for electrophysiologists all around the globe.

The trial enrolled all patients over the age of 21 years who had evidence of a prior MI more than 4 weeks old, a recent echocardiographic demonstration of severe LV dysfunction (as defined by an LVEF equal to or less than 30%) and they were randomized in a 3:2 ratio to either defibrillator therapy or conventional therapy. A total of 1232 patients were enrolled, of whom 742 received a defibrillator and 490 were allocated to receive conventional drug therapy. Those patients who had undergone a recent bypass surgery in the preceding 3 months, or had experienced a recent infarction in the preceding 1

month or who had NYHA Class IV heart failure were excluded from the study. The baseline clinical characteristics and adjuvant medical therapy were similar in the two groups at the start of the study.

The results showed that the survival curves ran close for the first 9 months but then began to diverge. During the average follow up of 20 months, the mortality rates in the conventional therapy group and the ICD group were 19.8% and 14.2%, respectively. There was a significant reduction in the all cause mortality in the ICD group and it was about 21% in the first year and 28% each in the second and third year, respectively (Figure 5.2). The hazard ratio of 0.69 of the two curves was indication of the fact that there was a 31% reduction in the risk of death at any interval among the patients in the defibrillator group as compared with patients in the group receiving conventional therapy. Although the subgroup analysis of patients when classified according to age, sex, LVEF, NYHA Class, hypertension, diabetes, and blood urea did not show any significant difference, it was notable that the difference in mortality was most prominent in patients who had a QRS duration of more than 120 ms. Interestingly, the hospitalizations were higher in the ICD group and it was hypothesized to be due to either longer survival in this group, ICD shocks-related admissions or worsening heart failure due to shock-related myocardial injury or backup ventricular pacing.

The trial added a new dimension for the risk stratification and management of patients with coronary artery disease and showed the possibility that invasive catheterization for this purpose may be on the verge of replacement by a simple non-invasive assessment of the LVEF. Although, it may still be argued whether the distribution of patients with an inducible ventricular arrhythmia was the same in the two groups and that the issue of the type of the anti-arrhythmic therapy used was not addressed, the results are here to stay for a while and would have a wide ranging economic implication based on the fact that this would make 400,000 new patients eligible for the device annually in addition to the 3–4 million who would already be on the waiting list in the United States alone.

Defibrillators In Acute MI Trial (DINAMIT)

The MADIT II trial made a significant impact on the practice and management of patients with coronary

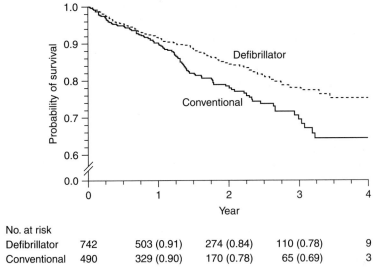

Figure 5.2 Kaplan Meier estimates of the probability of survival in the groups assigned to receive either a defibrillator or conventional medical therapy in the MADIT II trial. Survival was significantly better in the defibrillator group with a *P* value of 0.007. (From Moss AJ, Zareba W, Hall WJ, *et al. N Engl J Med* 2002; **346**: 877–883. Reprinted with permission.) Copyright © 2002 Massachusetts Medical Society. All rights reserved.

artery disease and severe LV dysfunction. The utility of defibrillators in improving long-term survival in these patients re-emphasized the role of the arrhythmic etiology of SCD in these patients. Most of the defibrillator trials excluded patients who had a recent revascularization or an acute MI. In fact, the CABG patch trial failed to show any benefit of ICDs in patients undergoing revascularization, the likely cause being that patients were enrolled too early for an ICD. The role of prophylactic defibrillators shortly after an acute MI was never really well defined and the Defibrillators In Acute MI Trial (DINAMIT) tried to answer this question objectively [95].

This open label trial randomized patients into two groups, to either receive ICD therapy (332 patients) or no ICD therapy (342 patients). The patients underwent randomization into either of these two groups if they had an acute MI within the last 6–40 days, had a LVEF of 35% or less and had impaired cardiac autonomic function (which was assessed by either a depressed heart rate variability or an elevated average 24-hour heart rate on Holter monitoring). During a mean follow up of 30 ± 13 months, there were 62 deaths in the group of patients who received an ICD and 58 deaths in patients who did not receive an ICD. There was no difference in the mortality between the two groups of patients, clearly showing that there was no beneficial role of an ICD in patients shortly after an acute MI.

Defibrillators In Non-Ischemic Cardiomyopathy Treatment Evaluation trial (DEFINITE)

The issue of the prophylactic use of defibrillators in patients with non-ischemic cardiomyopathy continued to be a debatable one for a long time. The use of electrophysiologic studies in these patients was never found to be rewarding and the information on the pathophysiology of ventricular arrhythmias in these patients was also less defined. Two small studies, the Cardiomyopathy Trial (CAT) and the Amiodarone versus ICD trial (AMIOVIRT) tried to answer the question whether prophylactic therapy with defibrillators in patients with non-ischemic cardiomyopathy was better than standard medical therapy or amiodarone, respectively [96,97]. Both trials had relatively small number of patients and short duration of follow up and were unable to show any evidence in favor of the ICDs.

The DEFibrillators In Non-Ischemic Cardiomyopathy Treatment Evaluation (DEFINITE) trial [98] was an investigator-initiated prospective trial which randomized 458 patients with non-ischemic cardiomyopathy, an LVEF of less than 36% and significant ventricular ectopy [defined in this trial as a mean premature ventricular contractions (PVC) count of more than 10 per hour or non-sustained VT of more than 120 bpm] into two groups. A total of 229 patients received standard medical therapy with ACE inhibitors and beta-blockers and the other 229 patients received an ICD in addition to standard medical therapy. The mean LVEF of the patients in the study was 21%. The patients were followed up for a mean of 29.0 ± 14.4 months and 68 deaths occurred during this time. Of these, 28 deaths occurred in the ICD group and 40 deaths in the group of patients treated with standard medical therapy ($P < 0.008$). It was notable that the number of arrhythmia-related episodes of SCD were significantly lower in patients with an ICD, with 3 in the ICD group and 14 in the non-ICD group ($P = 0.006$; hazard ratio 0.20). Although the difference in total mortality was not statistically significant, there was a demonstrable trend towards survival benefit in patients with an ICD and a significant reduction in the number of arrhythmic deaths. The authors believed that the study became underpowered due to the fact that the number of arrhythmic deaths was observed to be one-third of the total number of deaths, against an expected value of 50%. They thought that this might have contributed to the fact that the difference in the primary end point (in this case, total mortality) was not significant.

Sudden Cardiac Death in Heart Failure Trial (SCD-HeFT)

The SCD-HeFT trial [78] was a long awaited trial with the expectations to answer a lot of questions before major changes could be made to the policies governing ICD implantation in patients with heart failure. With the role of ICDs becoming unchallenged in the field of secondary prevention, most of the recent research has focused on better defining the role of ICDs in primary prevention of SCD. With the lack of predictability of non-invasive and invasive electrophysiologic studies, especially in patients with non-ischemic cardiomyopathy, the emphasis of patient selection has mainly been dependent on the LV function, which till today continues to be the best prognostic indicator of long-term survival in patients with heart failure.

The SCD-HeFT trial enrolled 2521 patients from September 1997 to July 2001 and these patients were randomly assigned in equal proportions to receive therapy with either placebo, amiodarone or a single chamber ICD, in addition to their usual heart failure management. All patients enrolled in the study were over 18 years of age, had an LVEF of 35% or less and had NYHA Class II or III chronic stable heart failure.

The trial was designed to include patients with both, ischemic and non-ischemic LV systolic dysfunction. All patients were followed till October 2003 for the primary end point of the trial, which was death from any cause.

After randomization, there were 847 patients in the placebo group, 845 patients in the amiodarone group and 829 patients in the ICD group. The median LVEF of the patients was 25%. The cause of heart failure was ischemic in 52% and non-ischemic in 48% of the patients. About 70% of the patients in were in functional NYHA Class II and 30% in NYHA Class III. The median follow up was for 45.5 months. The use of beta-blockers at last follow-up was a little lower in the Amiodarone group (72% versus 79% in the placebo group and 82% in the ICD group), but otherwise the three groups were very similar in their baseline characteristics. During the study period there were a total of 666 deaths (26%). This included 244 deaths in the placebo group (29%), 240 deaths in the amiodarone group (28%) and 182 deaths in the ICD group (22%). Hence, although amiodarone was no better than placebo reducing the risk of mortality, there was a 23% reduction in the risk of death in patients who received an ICD. There was an absolute reduction of 7.2% in the risk of mortality in these patients after 5 years (Figure 5.3). The results did not vary according to the ischemic or non-ischemic etiology of the patients.

There were a few other interesting observations in this trial which were not the predefined end points of the study but do leave room for thought. A total of 259 patients (31%) were known to receive a shock from their device from any cause. Of these, 177 patients (21% of the ICD cohort or 68% of those who received a shock) did so for a rapid VT or VF (appropriate shocks). Hence, during the 5 years of follow up, the average annual rate for any shock from the device was 7.5% and that for an appropriate shock was 5.1%. The reduction in the risk of death in the overall patient population was not dependent on the cause of CHF, but the patients with NYHA Class III CHF demonstrate a pattern which was typically different from that of the overall population or of the previous trials. This group showed no significant reduction in the risk of overall mortality in the ICD group when compared with placebo. On the other hand, Amiodarone was associated with a 44% increase in the risk of death in this

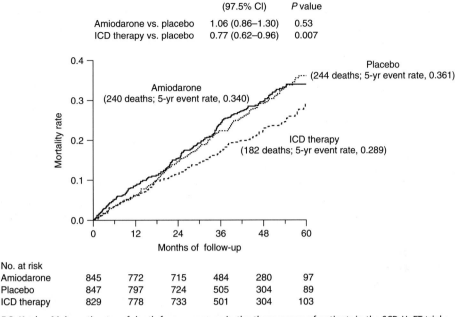

	Hazard ratio (97.5% CI)	P value
Amiodarone vs. placebo	1.06 (0.86–1.30)	0.53
ICD therapy vs. placebo	0.77 (0.62–0.96)	0.007

No. at risk

Amiodarone	845	772	715	484	280	97
Placebo	847	797	724	505	304	89
ICD therapy	829	778	733	501	304	103

Figure 5.3 Kaplan Meier estimates of death from any cause in the three group of patients in the SCD-HeFT trial. (From Bardy GH, Lee KL, Mark DB, *et al. N Engl J Med* 2005; **352**: 225–237. Reprinted with permission.) Copyright © 2005 Massachusetts Medical Society. All rights reserved.

group. In view of the trial design, the small number of patients in this group and conflicting results with previous ICD trials, it may be fair at this point of time to agree with the authors that these results may not be sufficient evidence to withhold ICD therapy in patients with NYHA Class III CHF, but it does merit the use of caution in prescribing Amiodarone in these patients without an ICD. The history of AADs in patients with CHF has never been exciting, and now even Amiodarone has been put to question.

ICD therapy: post-implant issues

There have been various post-implant issues with ICD therapy. The implantation of the device can be fraught with complications. Apart from the usual risks of hematomas and pneumothorax, there is a risk of device system infection of 1–2% which almost always requires extraction of the device and leads. There may be dislodgement of the atrial or the ventricular leads in 1–4% of patients. In distinction to lead dislodgement in pacemakers, the consequence of lead dislodgement or mechanical failure can cause inappropriate shocks or failure of the device to convert VF. Late complications related to insulation breaks, conductor fractures, and lead dysfunction are not rare and were particularly a

problem with the early transvenous leads. There can also be problems related to thrombosis and occlusion of the veins. Many of these causes can lead to the need for extraction of the leads and removal of the device, and this in itself is fraught with the risk of major complications in up to 2% of patients.

The ICDs can have a significant impact on the quality of life (QOL). With the increasing survival in these patients from protection by malignant arrhythmias, they are more likely to have progression and worsening of their heart failure. In patients with ICDs, there may be problems related to psychological or even cosmetic distress that may need reassurance and appropriate attention. Some countries may prohibit such patients from driving public vehicles; or even their own, for the safety of others. In situations where patients present with recurrent syncopal events from their arrhythmias, this is of special concern.

ICDs could also have potential interactions with drugs which the general practitioners need to be aware of. The drugs could alter the sensing and detection of the events by diminishing the slew rate and the rate of the tachycardia. They could lead to an increase in the pacing and the defibrillation thresholds. This is potentially important with Lidocaine and Amiodarone. Magnetic resonance and radiotherapy could cause problems to the device and need appropriate precautions. The surgical cautery could trigger the device and hence the ICD therapy needs to be switched off during such procedures.

Recurrent shocks from the device could be a potential problem, especially so if the shocks are inappropriate. This is usually the case in either patients with atrial fibrillation or in patients with recurrent episodes of non-sustained VT. Atrial fibrillation is most often the cause of inappropriate shocks. Most of the times, troubleshooting can be done by a simple reprogramming of the device in accordance with the patient's needs or by the addition of the appropriate pharmacotherapy to treat the underlying rhythm disturbance.

ICD therapy: conclusions

It is now increasingly clear, that patients with CHF from LV systolic dysfunction form a subgroup that is at a high risk of SCD. Most of these patients have coronary artery disease but a fair number have a non-ischemic dilated cardiomyopathy. In either case, the long-term survival is predominantly dependent on the left ventricular function.

Patients with ischemic cardiomyopathy are especially predisposed to re-entrant ventricular arrhythmias due to provision of a fertile substrate around scars within areas of normal myocardium, and such mechanisms are more easily identifiable by an invasive electrophysiologic testing. Such patients have a very high incidence of recurrence of a VT/VF episode if they are lucky to survive the first episode. Hence, as a mode of secondary prevention of SCD in such patients, ICD therapy is the first line treatment. However, ICD therapy may have a still larger role to play in the primary prevention of sudden death in these patients as evidenced by the recent trials. An inducible VT in these patients does seem to help in selecting patients who are likely to benefit from the ICD, but lately it seems that the non-invasive assessment of the LVEF may be all that is required.

Patients with non-ischemic cardiomyopathy are also predisposed to the occurrence of ventricular arrhythmias. As of the current data available, it seems logical to suggest that ICD therapy should be the chosen mode of therapy for secondary prevention. The role of the ICD in primary prevention is less clear in view of the poorer sensitivity and specificity

of the EP study in these patients, but patients who have non-sustained VT and a positive EP study are likely to do better with an ICD as per the little information available from the trials. Patients with a bundle branch re-entrant tachycardia would do well with a catheter ablation in view of its high rate of success. The current data does not define the role of the ICD in this subgroup of patients if the EP study is negative, but there is data to suggest that the patients who present with syncope would do better with an ICD even if the test does not show any inducible tachycardia [59,99].

With the availability of the results of the MADIT II and the SCD-HeFT trial and the more recent Medicare guidelines, for patients with LVEF of less than or equal to 35%, it is likely that the implantation of a defibrillator would soon become the standard of care for all patients for primary prophylaxis of SCD. It is important to remember that patients are unlikely to benefit if they are within 3 months of a revascularization procedure, within a month of their MI or if the primary myocardial disease is less than 3 months of duration. This is the minimum amount of time after which their LV function should be reassessed before the decision for implanting an ICD is taken. For patients who have had syncope of unknown origin or have sustained a VF arrest or sustained monomorphic VT in the presence of an LVEF of 40% or less, ICD therapy would definitely be the standard of care. The current guidelines [100] also emphasize on the role of ICD therapy in patients with and inducible VT/VF in the setting of LV dysfunction, but the guidelines would be expecting major revisions and the role of electrophysiologic studies to guide ICD therapy is likely to get limited to patients with an LVEF between 35% and 40% or for patients who have frequent non-sustained VT in the immediate post-MI or post-revascularization period.

There has also been a controversy regarding the role of defibrillators in patients with functional NYHA Class IV as these patients have a relatively high incidence of progressive worsening of heart failure and death from the same. Hence, the proportion of benefit by reducing the incidence of SCDs by an ICD may not be that impressive. However, as has been discussed later in the chapter, patients in this category may be fair candidates for an ICD if they were to receive a device anyway, for example, for reasons of intraventricular conduction needing biventricular pacing or for sinus or AV node dysfunction needing a pacemaker.

Biventricular pacing in CHF

Concept of dyssynchrony and pacing in heart failure

The importance of the concept of pacing in heart failure was first realized when it was reported that patients could benefit from dual chamber pacing by the manipulation of the AV delay. It was first reported by Hochleitner and colleagues that physiologic dual chamber pacing programmed to a short AV delay could help in the early withdrawal of inotropic support in patients with heart failure [101] and that these patients had symptomatic improvement on follow up. Other researchers [102,103] found that dual chamber pacing with optimization of the AV delay could help patients with heart failure in reducing their symptoms, improving cardiac output and oxygen consumption, reducing diastolic mitral regurgitation and also improve exercise capacity. However, long-term follow up of controlled randomized trials [104,105] showed that this benefit was restricted to patients with evidence of prolonged AV conduction time and pre-systolic mitral regurgitation, which resulted in reduced diastolic filling times. Patients with NYHA Class III and IV heart failure did not show any significant improvement. Hence, although the evidence may suggest that dual chamber pacing may help in CHF, it was realized that the benefit of this therapy is inconsistent and restricted to patients who may show acute hemodynamic benefit. The mode of benefit was predominantly due to the optimization of the AV delay and both shorter and longer than the optimum AV delays had deleterious effects [102,106]. In fact, as suggested by the Dual Chamber And VVI Implantable Defibrillator (DAVID) trial [107], dual chamber pacing in patients with LV systolic dysfunction is associated with worsening of heart failure and increased mortality.

Scientific data has shown that the failing heart not only exhibits depression of cardiac contractility, but there is also significant alteration of the conduction pathways in these patients. This is not just an electrocardiographic aberration, but there is emerging data to show that it has wide ranging clinical implications that cannot be ignored. Almost 30% of patients with CHF can have a wide QRS complex suggestive of intraventricular conduction delay

[108,109]. The onset of the QRS complex is followed by a delay in the onset of the ejection of blood into the aorta. This interval, termed the pre-ejection interval is prolonged in patients with intraventricular conduction defects and a resultant wide QRS complex. This causes a delay in the early diastolic filling of the ventricle in the subsequent cardiac cycle, which then impinges on to the atrial systole. Hence this electromechanical delay causes a prolongation of the LV contraction and relaxation intervals, worsening of mitral regurgitation and a shortening of the diastolic filling time [110–113]. This has a direct effect on the stroke volume and cardiac output, as it is well known that the efficiency of the failing heart is fairly dependent on the diastolic filling in accordance with the Frank–Starling law.

Adding more support to the adverse effects of intraventricular conduction delay in these patients is the evidence that it is associated with clinical instability and increased risk of death in heart failure [114–116]. In fact, Baldasseroni et al. [117] have reported a recent study of 5517 patients of heart failure of which 45.6% had ischemic heart disease, 36% had dilated cardiomyopathy, and 12.6% had hypertensive heart disease. A total of 25.2% of these patients had left bundle branch block (LBBB), 6.1% of patients had right bundle branch block (RBBB) and 6.1% had another form of intraventricular delay. It was interesting to note that patients with LBBB had more severe heart failure (higher proportion of patients with NYHA Class III and IV), reduced systolic blood pressure, increased incidence of third heart sound and more abnormal cardiothoracic ratios. The proportion of patients with an LVEF of less than 30% was also higher in the LBBB group and they also had a significantly higher mortality in comparison to patients without LBBB or any other intraventricular conduction defect (16.1% versus 11.9%; hazard ratio 1.7). LBBB was found to be an independent predictor of mortality and this negative effect was not influenced by age, heart failure severity or of drug prescriptions. Even the recent MADIT II trial has shown that the major advantage of the benefit of mortality in patients with an LVEF of 30% or less was most apparent in patients with a wide QRS complex [94]. LBBB results in dyssynchrony and abnormal septal motion even in patients with normal LV function [118] and it is possible that even these patients may have a higher incidence of progression to cardiomyopathy [119].

Role of cardiac resynchronization

The concept of biventricular pacing or what is now commonly called Cardiac Resynchronization Therapy (CRT) emerged in the late 1980s and the early 1990s. In the initial animal studies, Burkhoff et al. [120] showed that there was a linear relationship that exists between the decrease in the LV pressures and an increase in the width of the QRS complex. Following this, Lattuca and his colleagues [121] showed that simultaneous pacing of the left ventricle (LV) and the right ventricle (RV) could result in the narrowing of the QRS complex and a reduction in the intraventricular dyssynchrony, both electrically and mechanically. After the initial reports in the early 80s in four patients [122], it was in 1996 that Cazeau et al. [123] first showed the beneficial effects of biventricular pacing through a systematic analysis. In 1998, Leclerq et al. [124] studied the acute hemodynamic effects of biventricular pacing in patients with severely symptomatic heart failure and intraventricular conduction defects. They showed improvement in cardiac index and the pulmonary capillary wedge pressures. In 1999, Kass et al. [125] suggested the concept that LV pacing alone could probably compete or even better the results of biventricular pacing and that RV pacing was not only of no benefit, but could be harmful. However, most of these initial studies were acute hemodynamic studies and provided no information on the long-term effects of LV or biventricular pacing.

In a nutshell, the prime targets of pacing therapy and cardiac resynchronization have been either a correction of the faulty AV synchrony as discussed earlier, or more commonly and more importantly, to correct the abnormal intraventricular dyssynchrony caused by the latency of conduction through the ventricles themselves. Under normal circumstances, the LV contracts in a synchronous manner within all its segments, such that there is a variability of only about 40 ms in the electro-mechanical activation of its various segments. This produces the most optimal and efficient ejection. However, when one of the segments is prematurely activated and the others delayed (as in patients with intraventricular conduction delay), it leads to regions of early and delayed mechanical activity as well [126–128]. Both of these segments, the premature and the delayed segments could represent areas of wasted contraction and effort, as the former would contribute to an isovolumic contraction without any effective ejection of blood, whereas the delayed segments would be contracting at times when there would be either a higher stress in the areas which have already been activated or a paradoxical stretch in them if they are already in the phase of repolarization [129]. This leads to a reduction in the cardiac output, delayed relaxation and an increase in the end-systolic wall stress, which in effect would increase the myocardial oxygen consumption [130–133]. Studies have also shown that this could lead to triggering of calcium release which could lead on to the pro-arrhythmic effects of dyssynchrony [134].

Biventricular pacing: rationale, technique, and limitations

The previous discussion well illustrates the problems that intraventricular conduction delay can have adverse effects on the myocardial contractility and efficiency. It is with this background that researchers tried to evaluate the role of LV and biventricular pacing in this subset of patients.

The initial clinical studies focused on the optimization of the AV delay but as previously discussed, the applicability of this approach was restricted to a select few patients with AV conduction problems and not to all patients with intraventricular conduction defects. In fact it was then believed that RV apical pacing might be adding to the discoordination of the segments and further worsening the LV function. Even RV outflow tract pacing was tried [135], but without success. Hence, the focus was changed to try methods to seek an early activation of the left free wall instead. The result was the inception of biventricular and LV pacing. The aim of biventricular pacing was not only to correct the AV synchrony but also to ensure a uniformity of the ventricular activation, contraction and relaxation sequences. Since then, biventricular pacing has been shown to markedly improve cardiac output, increase systolic pressure, lower pulmonary capillary wedge pressures [136,137], enhance ventricular systolic function and pressure–volume loops [125] and improve the magnitude and synchrony of wall contraction [138,139]. Another interesting phenomenon that these initial studies showed was that the stimulation of the LV alone at a single site also had equivalent results as those of biventricular pacing [125,136,140]. The reason of this phenomenon was not very clear and in long-term studies the emphasis continued to remain on biventricular pacing.

There have also been reports of reduced mitral regurgitation with biventricular pacing. The preliminary presentation of the *Multicenter InSync Randomized Clinical Evaluation* (MIRACLE) Study [141] showed reduction in the systolic mitral regurgitation from 7 to 4 cm². One possible explanation for this is that the patients with heart failure have functional systolic mitral regurgitation and this is usually worse with the normal pattern of activation which causes contraction from the apex towards the base. With biventricular pacing, the sequence of activation is reversed and so occurs from the base to the apex [142]. This reversal leads to a premature activation of the base of the heart and is hypothesized to cause a squeezing effect on the annulus which may be leading to the reduction in the mitral regurgitation.

Another important mechanism that has been proposed is that patients with left bundle branch block may have a delayed onset of the diastole in the LV in comparison to the RV. This may cause an earlier filling of the RV which would decrease the potential space available for the LV filling. Biventricular pacing may reverse this problem and hence the LV may enter diastole earlier and this may improve the diastolic filling of the LV [143].

The standard procedure for the implantation of the biventricular pacemaker initially involves placing the atrial and RV leads in the usual manner. The RV lead is usually placed at the apex as the approach is to try and have the maximum separation between the RV and the LV leads. The LV lead was initially placed surgically, but this procedure is more invasive and involves a thoracotomy or thoracoscopy under general anesthesia. At our institution, this approach is limited only to patients where either the patient is undergoing an open heart surgery for other causes or there is a failure in placing the transvenous lead with an existing indication for a biventricular pacing.

The epicardial approach was gradually replaced by the transvenous approach which involved the canulation of the coronary sinus with an open lumen catheter. This paves the way for a balloon catheter, which is used to perform an occlusion venography and to identify the posterior and lateral branches of the coronary sinus. The lead is then directed in these branches so as to try and achieve a stable position in one of the posterolateral branches so as to have a maximum separation from the RV apical lead and to also avoid pacing the diaphragm. The sheath is then peeled away over the lead (or removed using a slitter in some models as required) and then secured in the pectoral pocket. The initial success rates with this approach were lower, but with improved operator experience and hardware, the success rates have been over 90%. The clinical benefits with placement of the coronary sinus lead in the posterior or lateral portions of the heart far outweigh the benefits offered by placing the lead in the anterior interventricular branches. At our institute, in case there is failure to place the lead transvenously in an optimum branch, it is preferable to implant the lead surgically on the epicardial surface directly.

Clinical trials on resynchronization therapy

The final status of any interventional therapy is best judged by its comparison with the existing therapies in randomized controlled clinical trials. The impact of biventricular pacing has been under very close and keen observation but it has finally made its place secure in the armamentarium against congestive heart failure (CHF). There is now large amount of data from well designed clinical trials over the last few years which has shown that the benefits of biventricular pacing are objective, quantifiable, difficult to ignore, additive to conventional therapy and more than just a placebo effect.

The *Pacing Therapies for CHF (PATH-CHF) trial* was a multicenter randomized trial that evaluated the benefits of LV and biventricular pacing in patients with moderate to severe CHF and intraventricular conduction defects [140]. Patients were randomly assigned to either biventricular pacing or to an atrio-univentricular pacing mode (the mode was chosen as LV or RV on the basis of an acute hemodynamic study during implantation) and were paced in this manner for 4 weeks. Subsequently pacing was switched off for the second 4 weeks and the pacing mode was crossed over to the other mode in the third 4 weeks. At the end of 12 weeks, the patients were followed for 1 year after being placed in the best chronic pacing mode as was obtainable on the basis of the first 12 weeks. Both, the acute and long-term results showed favorable results in the hemodynamics with improvement in the 6 min walking distance, QOL, LVEF and the heart rate variability, with both LV and biventricular pacing without any significant superiority of one over the other.

The *VIGOR-CHF Trial* was the first trial in the United States on CRT where an epicardial LV lead was used in 18 patients and the effect of the therapy was studied in these patients who were in NYHA Class III or IV, had a mean LVEF of 27 ± 6% and a QRS duration of 167 ± 29 s [144]. The investigators evaluated the Myocardial Performance Index (MPI) which was defined as the ratio of isovolumetric contraction and relaxation time relative to the ejection time. An improvement in the MPI was observed in 14 out of the 18 patients and it decreased from 0.77 ± 0.30 before implantation to 0.61 ± 0.19 with biventricular pacing.

The *Medtronic InSync Study* was a multicenter European and Canadian Trial which examined the safety and efficacy of a multisite pacing in refractory heart failure [145]. A total of 68 patients with NYHA Class III or IV, drug refractory heart failure, with an LVEF of 35% or less, a QRS duration of greater than 150 ms and LV End-Diastolic Diameter (LVEDD) of 60 mm or more underwent implantation of a biventricular pacemaker. The patients showed significant improvement in their NYHA functional Class, 6 min walking distance and QOL indices and this correlated well with their reduction in QRS duration and the increase in their LVEF.

In another small study by *Alonso et al.* [146], 26 patients with drug refractory CHF of NYHA Class III or IV, an LVEF of 35% or less, an LVEDD of 60 mm or more and a QRS width of more than 120 ms were enrolled. The patients received biventricular dual chamber pacemakers and were then classified as responders or non-responders as per the symptomatic benefit that they reported from the pacemaker in terms of the NYHA Class and the exercise tolerance. The mean LVEF of the patients was 23 ± 8%, the mean LVEDD was 5 ± 9 mm and the mean QRS duration was 178 ± 24 ms. There were 19 responders and 7 non-responders. The patients classified as responders showed an average improvement of 1.3 in their NYHA Class status and an increase in the oxygen consumption by a mean of about 50%. It was interesting that the only difference in the variables of the two groups on follow-up was the post-pacing QRS duration which was significantly lower in the responders (a mean of 154 versus

177 ms, respectively) and the authors postulated that this variable was possibly a good parameter to assess the efficacy of biventricular pacing.

The *Multisite Stimulation in Cardiomyopathy (MUSTIC) Trial* results represent the first published randomized data with biventricular pacing [147]. This was a single blind randomized crossover trial in which patients received a biventricular pacemaker and were then randomized to a period of 3 months of active atrial-biventricular pacing or to an inactive mode where they were kept at a backup VVI pacing rate of 40 beats per minute. These patients were then crossed over after 3 months to the opposite mode for the next 3 months. Of the 67 patients chosen, 48 were successfully randomized to follow up. The results showed a 22% improvement in the exercise tolerance as assessed by the 6 min walk test, a 32% improvement in the QOL indices, an 8% increase in the peak oxygen consumption and a two-thirds reduction in the frequency of admission from heart failure in patients with active pacing. In addition to this, 85% of the patients preferred the active biventricular pacing mode and only 4% of the patients favored the inactive mode. The other patients had no preference for either.

The same group followed up patients in a similar study design for a longer period of time [148]. A total of 42 such patients in sinus rhythm and 33 in atrial fibrillation were successfully followed up for 12 months and they reported sustained improvement in not only these parameters but also in the LVEF (increase by 4–5%) and the mitral regurgitation (decrease by 45–50%). It was interesting to note such a high percentage of patients in atrial fibrillation and the fact that the benefit of biventricular pacing appeared to be equivalent in patients with atrial fibrillation also.

One of the largest initial experiences in a randomized double blind long-term follow-up of patients with biventricular pacing has been reported by the *MIRACLE Trial* Study Group [149]. This clinical trial included 453 patients with moderate to severe symptoms of heart failure associated with an LVEF of 35% or less, an LVEDD of 55 mm or more and with a QRS interval of 130 ms or more. Of these, 228 patients were randomly assigned to the resynchronization group and the other 225 patients remained as the control group. Optimal conventional therapy for CHF was continued in both the groups and the patients were followed up to see the improvement in their NYHA functional Class, the QOL indices, and the distance walked in 6 min as the primary end points. The patients were also evaluated for changes in the LVEF and the time on the treadmill during exercise testing.

The baseline characteristics were similar in the both groups in terms of the age and sex distribution, the symptomatic and echocardiographic variables, the hemodynamic parameters and the drugs that they were receiving. About 90–93% of patients was receiving ACE-I or angiotensin receptor blockers (ARBs) and about 55–62% of the patients were on beta-blockers. The mean QRS duration was 165 ± 20 ms in the control group and 167 ± 21 ms in the cardiac-resynchronization group. The results showed a significant benefit for the patients with CRT and that the differences were apparent as early as 1 month after the treatment and were sustained without any attenuation throughout the study period of 6 months. The patients with resynchronization therapy showed a higher increase in the 6 min walking distance ($+39$ m versus $+10$ m; $P < 0.005$), more significant improvement in the QOL index (-18.0 versus -9.0 points; $P = 0.001$), more improvement in the LVEF ($+4.6\%$ versus -0.2%; $P < 0.001$) and

a larger increase in the time on treadmill exercise testing ($+81$ s versus $+19$ s; $P = 0.001$). There was a nearly 50% reduction in the requirement of intravenous medication and need for hospitalization. In addition, there was also improvement in the peak oxygen consumption, the end-diastolic dimension, the mitral regurgitant jet and the duration of the QRS interval. At 6 months, the risk of death or hospitalization was 40% lower in the resynchronization group (Figure 5.4).

However, there were certain areas of concern. The median duration of the procedure was 2.7 h and even up to 7 h in a few patients. The fluoroscopy time was not reported but is likely to have been significantly higher than the other procedures. There were two procedure related deaths in the 571 patients. The incidence of coronary sinus dissection was 4% and another 2% had coronary sinus perforation, though most of these patients recovered without any sequelae. The incidence of infection was 1.5% and there was a failure to implant the device in eight patients. Moreover, only 67% of the patients in the resynchronization group showed symptom benefit and there was no survival advantage that could be documented.

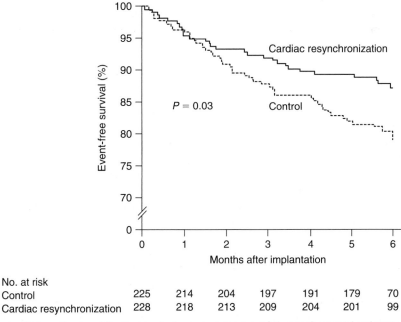

No. at risk

Control	225	214	204	197	191	179	70
Cardiac resynchronization	228	218	213	209	204	201	99

Figure 5.4 Kaplan Meier estimates of the time to death or worsening heart failure in the control and resynchronization groups in the MIRACLE trial. The risk of an event was 40% lower in the CRT group; *P* value 0.03. (From Abraham WT, Fisher WG, Smith AL, *et al. N Engl J Med* 2002; **346**: 1845–1853. Reprinted with permission.) Copyright © 2002 Massachusetts Medical Society. All rights reserved.

Another well-designed trial, which compared the effects of either CRT alone or in combination with defibrillator capabilities, is the *Comparison of Medical Therapy, Pacing and Defibrillation in Heart Failure (COMPANION) trial.* This trial [150] was designed to see if resynchronization therapy with or without defibrillators would reduce the risk of death and hospitalization among patients with advanced heart failure with accompanying delay in their intraventricular conduction. Among 1520 patients who were included in this trial, randomization was done in a 1:2:2 design such that 308 patients received optimal pharmacological therapy alone, 617 patients received optimal medical therapy with biventricular pacemakers (CRT group) and 595 patients received optimal medical therapy with biventricular pacemaker-defibrillators (CRT-D group). The criteria at enrollment included an LVEF of 35% or less, NYHA Class III or IV heart failure from ischemic or non-ischemic cardiomyopathy, a QRS interval of more than 120 ms and a PR interval of more than 150 ms, sinus rhythm, absence of absolute indications for a pacemaker or a defibrillator, and a hospitalization for the treatment of heart failure or equivalent in the preceding 12 months. The primary end point was the combined risk of death or hospitalization from any cause and the secondary end point was death from any cause.

The results showed that there was no significant difference in the baseline characteristics between the three groups. The implantation was successful in 87% of patients in the CRT group and 91% of patients in the CRT-D group with a median procedure time of 164 min and 176 min in the two groups, respectively. The median duration of follow-up for the primary end point in the three groups was 11.9 months, 16.2 months and 15.7 months, respectively and that for the secondary end point was 14.8 months, 16.5 months and 16.0 months, respectively. The 12-month rate of the primary composite end point of death from any cause or hospitalization from any cause was 68% in the pharmacologic therapy group as compared with 56% in the CRT group and 56% in the CRT-D group. Thus, either group with resynchronization therapy, either with or without defibrillators, showed a 20% risk reduction in the primary end point. The secondary end point of death from any cause was reduced by 24% in the CRT group when compared with pharmacologic therapy alone ($P = 0.06$) and by 36% in the CRT-D

group; the latter being statistically significant ($P = 0.003$). As with any other heart failure trial, the risk of death or hospitalization from heart failure was also measured and this was found to be lower by 25% in the CRT group ($P = 0.002$) and 28% lower in the CRT-D group ($P < 0.001$).

Despite the extremely complex nature of the analysis and results of the trial, it was clear that there was significant reduction in the risk of a composite of death and severe symptomatic states from the use of resynchronization therapy in patients with CHF. The magnitude of the benefit becomes more noteworthy when it is realized that this is in addition to the best medical therapy that patients were already receiving. The benefit was maximized when resynchronization therapy was combined with defibrillation capabilities and was progressively more with the increasing duration of the QRS interval. The benefit of this treatment extended to patients with both, ischemic and non-ischemic cardiomyopathy.

A major recent breakthrough has been the impact of resynchronization therapy alone on the survival in patients with heart failure. This has been elegantly demonstrated in the *Cardiac Resynchronization – Heart Failure (CARE-HF) Trial* [151]. This was an international, multicenter, randomized trial which compared the effect of standard pharmacotherapy alone with that of the combination of standard pharmacotherapy with CRT (without a defibrillator) on the risk of death and unplanned hospitalization for major cardiac events in patients with LV systolic dysfunction and cardiac dyssynchrony. The enrollment of the trial was done from January 2001 to March 2003 at 82 European centers. The primary end point was death from any cause or an unplanned hospitalization for a major cardiovascular event. The principal secondary end point was death from any cause.

A total of 813 patients were enrolled for the trial and were followed up for a mean of 29.4 months. The patients were 18 years or older, had heart failure for at least 6 weeks, had NYHA Class III or IV functional status despite standard pharmacologic therapy, an LVEF of 35% or less and a QRS interval of more than 120 ms. For patients with a QRS interval between 120 and 149 ms, two of the three criteria for dyssynchrony had to be met for inclusion in the trial. These criteria included an aortic pre-ejection delay of more than 140 ms, an interventricular mechanical delay of more than 40 ms or delayed activation of the posterolateral wall [152–154]. After randomization, 404 patients received medical therapy alone and 409 patients received medical therapy with cardiac resynchronization. During follow-up, the primary end point of death from any cause or hospitalization for a major cardiac event was reached in 224/404 patients in the group on medical therapy alone (55%) versus 159/409 patients in the group which received CRT in addition (39%). This amounted to a significant reduction of death or hospitalization from resynchronization therapy alone in the absence of a backup defibrillator (hazard ratio 0.63; $P < 0.001$) (Figure 5.5a). There was also a significant reduction in the secondary end point of death from any cause. In comparison to 120 deaths from any cause in the patients on medical therapy alone (30%), there were only 82 deaths (20%) in the patients treated with cardiac resynchronization in addition ($P < 0.002$) (Figure 5.5b).

The COMPANION Trial did show a survival benefit from all cause mortality in patients who received resynchronization therapy with defibrillator capabilities. Previous meta-analysis has also shown [155,156] that CRT can have a survival benefit. However, this is the first trial to show independently that CRT alone can improve survival in patients with heart failure. In fact, 29 patients (7%) in the resynchronization therapy group died of sudden death, signifying the potential additive effect that defibrillator capabilities could have further had on the mortality benefit in this group. As per the author's calculations from the current trial, one death and three hospitalizations were prevented for every nine devices that were implanted in the CARE-HF trial. Other end points were also analyzed in the study. There was a significant improvement in the LVEF, the end-systolic volume index, the area of mitral regurgitation, the interventricular mechanical delay, the NYHA functional Class, the levels of N-terminal probrain natriuretic peptide, the systolic blood pressure on follow up, among the other things that were monitored during the trial. It was interesting to note though, that the incidence of atrial arrhythmias or ectopy was higher in the cardiac-resynchronization group.

The biventricular pacemaker-defibrillator

We have already seen that the incidence of SCD is high in patients with heart failure and a large proportion of them are due to ventricular arrhythmias.

Although a few studies have shown that biventricular pacing may diminish the need for ICD therapy in terms of the number of shocks delivered by the device [157], it does not necessarily obviate the need for an ICD. Till the recently published CARE-HF trial, there was insufficient data to show that resynchronization therapy alone leads to any survival advantage or any reduction in the incidence of SCD. Up to 35% of patients with cardiomyopathy and a potential indication for a biventricular pacing have been shown to have inducible ventricular arrhythmia [158]. The MADIT II and SCD-HeFT trials mentioned above, have shown that ICDs should form part of the therapy for patients with severe LV systolic dysfunction. All this data would suggest that most of the patients who require biventricular pacing for systolic dysfunction would also be candidates for an implantable defibrillator as these patients often have an LVEF of 35% or less. Hence, it is recognized that these patients may be candidates for an additional device with defibrillator capabilities.

With these indications, it is likely that biventricular defibrillators would almost totally replace the biventricular pacemakers for managing patients with heart failure. However, cost considerations are still likely to help the biventricular pacemakers to survive, at least in the developing world. It is also important to individualize patient therapy with or without ICDs as all patients may not find repeated shocks from an ICD as their preference, especially, if they are interested only in the improvement in the QOL rather than the quantity of life.

The safety and efficacy of biventricular defibrillators has been studied in the *MIRACLE-ICD Trial* [159] in patients with NYHA Class III and IV heart failure. The patients were randomized into two groups after receiving a biventricular pacemaker-defibrillator. All patients had the defibrillator functions of the device activated but were randomly assigned to two groups to have the CRT function turned "off" or turned "on". At 6 months of follow-up, the patients with resynchronization therapy activated, had improved QOL, improved functional status and better exercise capacity. There was no increased risk of pro-arrhythmia or compromised ICD function, and these findings were especially important in light of the findings of the inadvertent effects of pacing in the DAVID trial. The *MIRACLE-ICD II Trial* also showed that the benefits of biventricular pacing with

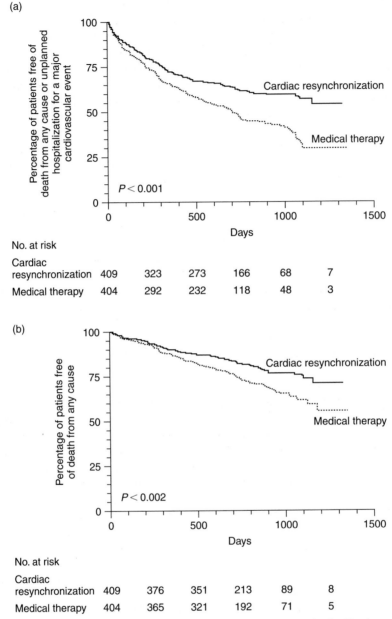

Figure 5.5 Figure 5a and 5b are Kaplan Meier estimates of the time for the primary end point (death or unplanned hospitalization; *P* value < 0.001) or the secondary end point (all cause mortality; *P* value < 0.002), respectively, in the CARE-HF trial. This was the first trial to show a significant reduction in all cause mortality from cardiac resynchronization even without a defibrillator. (From Cleland JGF, Daubert JC, Erdmann E, *et al. N Engl J Med* 2005; **352**: 1539–1549. Reprinted with permission.) Copyright © 2005 Massachusetts Medical Society. All rights reserved.

such devices extended to improvement in cardiac structure and function in terms of improvement in the LV diastolic and systolic volumes and the LVEF [160]. Other studies have shown that the benefits of such devices may even extend to patients with NYHA Class II symptoms [161]. The *VENTAK-CHF/ CONTAK-CD Trial* randomized 490 patients with CHF and wide QRS to receive either pacing or no pacing from a biventricular-defibrillator system. The results are still under review in relation to the effect on mortality but the initial report suggests symptomatic benefit in heart failure [144].

It is likely that even antitachycardia pacing may be affected by the site of stimulation as this may guide the ability of a stimulated impulse to enter a re-entry circuit and with two stimulation sites being used by the biventricular pacemaker, this may make it more effective than RV-ATP alone. One of the major concerns with the biventricular devices has been the issue of double counting and this occurs because two different electrograms obtained from the right and the left ventricle are fed into a single amplifier. Double counting can be a source of inappropriate therapy in up to 14% of patients and is most often due to sinus tachycardia or could be due to VT also [162–164]. However, the newer devices use only the RV lead for sensing and bypass the problem.

Biventricular pacing: future perspectives and unanswered questions

The field of biventricular pacing is new and rapidly evolving, both for the medical specialists and the industry. The more answers that come, pave way for more questions and quest for improvement. There are still a lot of ongoing trials that are likely to throw light on the important aspects related to the clinical application of the device.

Many of the initial problems with the device have paved way for advancements in understanding and technology. The initial devices sensed both the RV and the LV and hence gave problems with inappropriate shocks due to double counting. The newer devices have RV only sensing to overcome this problem. There is also a capability to separately program the LV and RV pacing outputs to better pace the two leads with varying output and help in battery conservation. There is also evolution of over the wire leads and bipolar leads with various programmability options. This can help to achieve lower thresholds and avoid phrenic nerve capture and even help leads to function from relatively suboptimal positions during difficult placement. The *VENTAK-CHF Trial* is assessing the safety and efficacy of biventricular antitachycardia pacing and defibrillation in this subset of patients. The value of biventricular pacing in atrial fibrillation is being assessed in the *LV-Based Cardiac Stimulation Post-AV Node Ablation Evaluation (PAVE) Trial*. It is interesting because patients are given a standard dual chamber pacemaker after AV node ablation and the RV and the LV leads are connected

to the ventricular and the atrial channels respectively and LV dysfunction is not an essential criterion for inclusion in the study. In addition, this trial and the Bi versus Left Ventricular Pacing: an International Pilot Evaluation on Heart Failure Patients with Ventricular Arrhythmias (*BELIEVE*) and the Optimal Pacing Site Study (*OPSITE*) *Trials* are also trying to assess the difference if any between single site LV pacing and biventricular pacing. Other studies trying to assess the mortality benefit if any of biventricular pacing include the Pacing for Cardiomyopathies (*PACMAN*), Pacing Therapies in Congestive Heart Failure (*PATH-CHF II*), *and* Ventricular Resynchronization Therapy Randomized Trial (*VECTOR*) *Trials*. There are also studies evaluating the role of V–V timing programmability through these devices.

There have also been parallel and significant strides in the development of hardware and techniques to widen the applicability of biventricular pacing. There is an availability of more trackable over the wire leads which also have a lower profile and can help in patients with an unfavorable coronary sinus anatomy. Steerable sheaths are available to increase the chances of successful cannulation of the coronary sinus. Several alternative approaches as the trans-septal and the pericardial approaches have been tried but the risk of strokes and tamponade preclude the use of these techniques as of now.

But despite all these issues, many questions remain unanswered in relation to the role of biventricular pacing. The sustenance of benefit and the effect on survival has already been discussed. It still remains important to differentiate which patients will and which will not respond to biventricular pacing. Multiple techniques using echocardiography and magnetic resonance imaging (MRI) have been used but they have as yet to come with firm conclusions. There has however, been an increased realization of the fact that electrical dyssynchrony perhaps represents only a tip of the iceberg in terms of the patients who need cardiac resynchronization. Many techniques which measure the intraventricular dyssynchrony using septal to posterior or lateral wall motion delays, time to peak velocities in the various myocardial segments, tissue strain analysis, tissue doppler analyses, pre-ejection intervals, etc., have shown that the real patients who benefit from CRT are likely those who have mechanical dyssynchrony in the various myocardial segments. As a corollary to this fact, it is not surprising that a large number of patients who have a narrow QRS (less than 120 ms) have been noted to have mechanical dyssynchrony. The role of biventricular pacing is being studied in these patients and the initial results seem encouraging. If such patients were to improve from cardiac resynchronization, it would not only open a new channel of therapy for a lot of patients, it would open doors for research on a number of questions relating to the possible mechanisms of heart failure and the reasons of benefit from resynchronization. The role of LV pacing alone and the role of resynchronization in patients with atrial fibrillation is being assessed. It remains important to assess the role in patients with NYHA Class II and in patients with normal systolic function with intraventricular conduction defects. Various mechanisms of benefit have been proposed, but the exact mechanisms still remain unclear and it remains to be determined whether the benefit would be extendable for patients with RBBB and atrial fibrillation. There is still uncertainty about the best site of pacing in both the LV and the RV and the relationship of the benefit with the post-pacing QRS duration. As per the current information it appears that the anterior branches of the coronary sinus are definitely inferior choices in comparison to the LV free wall. It will also be interesting to see whether LV pacing alone may be as effective as biventricular pacing and if so, why?

Biventricular pacing (cardiac resynchronization): conclusions

There is evidence to suggest that conduction defects are coupled with mechanical dyssynchrony and have a significant association with the deterioration of the failing heart, if not as an etiological role. The correction of this dyssynchrony leads to acute and possibly long-term hemodynamic and symptomatic clinical benefit. Biventricular pacing is an innovative advancement in the field of correcting this dyssynchrony and emerges as a powerful armamentarium in the evolving therapies for the failing heart. There is enough data to show that biventricular pacing benefits a large number of patients with symptom reduction and improved hemodynamics. Most patients who are candidates for biventricular pacing are also at significant risk of SCD. Therefore, within economic constraints, biventricular defibrillators are likely to become the rule for such patients. It is also important to realize that not all patients benefit from CRT.

About one-third of the patients with delayed electrical activation on the ECG may not benefit from the device. It remains elusive how to identify these patients pre-operatively. Echocardiography and MRI are being investigated to try and identify patients who are likely to be responders or non-responders. It may also be important to study these tools to try and identify patients who may be having evidence of dyssynchronous segmental contraction but still have evidence of a narrow QRS morphology on the ECG. It would be interesting to investigate how such patients would benefit from CRT or Multisite Pacing.

Currently, the ideal candidate for a biventricular device seems to be a patient with NYHA Class III or IV heart failure despite medical therapy if he/she has a left bundle branch block pattern, a QRS of ≥ 150 ms and a left ventricular end diastolic dimension of more than 55 mm. Patients with a QRS of 120–149 ms have also shown to have benefit, more so if they have associated evidence of mechanical dyssynchrony. Patients with conduction abnormalities other than left bundle branch block are also considered for therapy if they have a wide QRS pattern but have been less well represented in the trials and hence, lesser information is available about the response in these patients. The information on the benefit in patients with NYHA Class II symptoms and with a narrow QRS should be available soon.

References

1 Kuller LH, Lilienfeld A, Fisher R. Epidemiological study of sudden and unexpected deaths due to arteriosclerotic heart disease. *Circulation* 1966; **34**: 1056–1068.

2 Poole JE, Bardy GH. Sudden Cardiac Death. In: Zipes D & Jalife J, eds. *Cardiac Electrophysiology: From cell to bedside*, WB Saunders Co, Philadelphia, PA, 2000: 615–640.

3 Hinkle Jr LE, Thaler HT. Clinical classification of cardiac deaths. *Circulation* 1982; **65**: 457–464.

4 SOLVD Investigators. Effect of enalapril on mortality and the development of heart failure in asymptomatic patients with reduced left ventricular ejection fractions. *N Engl J Med* 1992; **327**: 685–691.

5 Cohn JN, Archibald DG, Ziesche S *et al.* Effect of vasodilator therapy on mortality in chronic congestive heart failure. Results of a veterans administration cooperative study. *N Engl J Med* 1986; **314**: 1547–1552.

6 Cohn JN, Johnson G, Ziesche S *et al.* A comparison of enalapril with hydralazine-isosorbide dinitrate in the treatment of chronic congestive heart failure's. *N Engl J Med* 1991; **325**: 303–310.

7 Singh SN, Fletcher RD, Fisher SG *et al.*, for the survival trial of antiarrhythmic therapy in congestive heart failure. Amiodarone among patients with congestive heart failure and asymptomatic ventricular arrhythmias. *N Engl J Med* 1995; **333**: 77–82.

8 Kim SG, Fogoros RN, Furman S *et al.* Standardized reporting of ICD patient outcome: *The report of a North American Society of Pacing and Electrophysiology Policy Conference*, February 9–10, PACE 1993; **16**: 1358–1362.

9 Cameron JS, Myerburg RJ, Wong SS. Electrophysiological consequences of chronic experimentally induced left ventricular pressure overload. *J Am Coll Cardiol* 1983; **2**: 481–487.

10 Tomaselli GF, Beuckelmann DJ, Calkins HJ *et al.* Sudden cardiac death in heart failure. The role of abnormal repolarization. *Circulation* 1994; **90**: 2534–2539.

11 Vermeulen JT, McGuire MA, Opthof T *et al.* Triggered activity and automaticity in ventricular trabeculae of failing human and rabbit hearts. *Cardiovasc Res* 1994; **28**: 1547–1554.

12 Aronson RS. Mechanisms of arrhythmias in ventricular hypertrophy. *J Cardiovasc Electrophysiol* 1991; **2**: 249–261.

13 Franz MR, Cima R, Wang D. Electrophysiological effects of myocardial stretch and mechanical determinants for stretch-activated arrhythmias. *Circulation* 1992; **86**: 968–978.

14 Schreir RW, Abraham WT. Mechanisms of disease: Hormones and hemodynamics in heart failure. *N Engl J Med* 1999; **341**: 577–585.

15 Abraham WT, Port JD, Bristow MR. Neurohormonal receptors in the failing heart. In: Poole-Wilson PA, Colucci WS, Massie BM, Chatterjee K & Coates AJS, eds. *Heart Failure*, Churchill Livingstone, NY, 1997: 127–141.

16 Thomas A, Knapman P, Krikler D *et al.* Community study of the causes of "natural" sudden death. *Brit Med J* 1988; **297**: 1453–1456.

17 Roberts WC, Siegel RJ, McManus BM. Idiopathic dilated cardiomyopathy: analysis of 152 necropsy cases. *Am J Cardiol* 1987; **60**: 1304–1355.

18 Josephson ME, Almendral JM, Buxton AE *et al.* Mechanisms of ventricular tachycardia. *Circulation* 1987; **75**: 41–47.

19 deBakker JMT, van Capelle FJL, Janse MJ *et al.* Macroreentry in the infarcted human heart: Mechanism of ventricular tachycardia among patients with chronic ischemic heart disease: Electrophysiologic and anatomic correlation. *Circulation* 1988; **77**: 589–606.

20 deBakker JMT, van Capelle FJL, Janse MJ *et al.* Slow conduction in the infarcted human heart: "Zigzag" course of activation. *Circulation* 1993; **88**: 915–926.

21 Josephson ME. *Clinical Cardiac Electrophysiology: Techniques and Interpretations.* 2nd edn. Philadelphia/London, Lea and Feiberger, 1993.

22 Brembilla-Perrot B, Houriez P, Claudon O *et al.* Long term reproducibility of ventricular tachycardia induction with electrophysiological testing in patients with coronary heart disease and depressed left ventricular ejection fraction. *PACE* 2000; **23**: 47–53.

23 Sweeney MO, Guy ML, McGovern B *et al.* Natural history of spontaneous sustained monomorphic ventricular tachycardia in coronary disease revealed by local bipolar electrograms retrieved from implantable cardioverter-defibrillators. *Circulation* 1996; **94(Suppl 1)**: I–568 [Abstract].

24 Liberthson RR, Nagel EL, Hischman JC *et al.* Prehospital ventricular fibrillation: Prognosis and follow up course. *N Engl J Med* 1974; **291**: 317–321.

25 Schaffer WA, Cobb LA. Recurrent ventricular fibrillation and modes of death in survivors of out-of-hospital ventricular fibrillation. *N Engl J Med* 1975; **293**: 259–262.

26 Baroldi G, Falzi G, Mariani F. Sudden coronary death: a postmortem study in 208 selected cases compared with 97 "control" subjects. *Am Heart J* 1970; **98**: 20–31.

27 Stevenson W, Weiner I, Yeatman L *et al.* Complicated atherosclerotic lesions: A potential cause of ischemic ventricular arrhythmias in cardiac arrest survivors who do not have inducible ventricular tachycardia. *Am Heart J* 1988; **116**: 1–6.

28 Nikolic G, Bishop RL, Singh JB. Sudden death during Holter monitoring. *Circulation* 1982; **66**: 218–225.

29 Pratt CM, Francis MJ, Luck JC *et al.* Analysis of ambulatory electrocardiograms in 15 patients during spontaneous ventricular fibrillation with special reference to preceding arrhythmic events. *J Am Coll Cardiol* 1982; **2**: 789–797.

30 Middlekauff HR, Stevenson WG, Saxon LA *et al.* Amiodarone and torsades de pointes in patients with advanced heart failure. *Am J Cardiol* 1995; **76**: 499–501.

31 Meinertz T, Hofman T, Kasper W *et al.* Significance of ventricular arrhythmias in idiopathic dilated cardiomyopathy. *Am J Cardiol* 1984; **53**: 902–907.

32 Huang SK, Messer JV, Denes P. Significance of ventricular tachycardia in idiopathic dilated cardiomyopathy. *Am J Cardiol* 1983; **51**: 507–512.

33 Doval HC, Nul DR, Grancelli HO *et al.*, for the GESICA-GEMA Investigators. Nonsustained ventricular tachycardia in severe heart failure: Independent marker of increased mortality due to sudden cardiac death. *Circulation* 1996; **94**: 3198–3203.

34 Teerlink JR, Jalaluddin M, Anderson S *et al.*, on behalf of the PROMISE (Prospective Randomized Milrinone Survival Evaluation) Investigators. Ambulatory ventricular arrhythmias among patients with heart failure do not specifically predict an increased risk of sudden death. *Circulation* 2000; **101**: 40–46.

35 Cassidy DM, Vassallo JA, Miller JM *et al.* Endocardial catheter mapping in humans with sinus rhythm: Relationship to underlying heart disease and ventricular arrhythmias. *Circulation* 1986; **73**: 645–652.

36 Hsia HH, Callans DJ, Marchlinski FE. Characterization of endocardial electrophysiological substrate in patients

with nonischemic cardiomyopathy and monomorphic ventricular tachycardia. *Circulation* 2003; **108**: 704–710.

37 Delacretaz E, Stevenson WG, Ellison KE *et al*. Mapping and radiofrequency catheter ablation of the three types of sustained monomorphic ventricular tachycardia in nonischemic heart disease. *J Cardiovasc Electrophysiol* 2000; **11**: 11–17.

38 Das S, Morady F, DiCarlo L *et al*. Prognostic usefulness of programmed ventricular stimulation in idiopathic dilated cardiomyopathy without symptomatic ventricular arrhythmias. *Am J Cardiol* 1986; **59**: 998–1000.

39 Kron J, Hart M, Schual-Berke S, Niles N *et al*. Idiopathic dilated cardiomyopathy: role of programmed electrical stimulation and holter monitoring in predicting those at risk of sudden death. *Chest* 1988; **93**: 85–90.

40 Meinertz T, Treese N, Kasper W *et al*. Determinants of prognosis in idiopathic dilated cardiomyopathy as determined by programmed electrical stimulation. *Am J Cardiol* 1985; **56**: 337–341.

41 Brachman J, Hilbel T, Grunig E *et al*. Ventricular arrhythmias in dilated cardiomyopathy. *PACE* 1997; **20**: 2714–2718.

42 Mukharji J, Rude RE, Poole WK *et al*. The MILIS study group: Risk factors for sudden death after acute myocardial infarction: Two year study follow up. *Am J Cardiol* 1984; **54**: 31–36.

43 Bigger JT, Fleiss JL, Kleiger R *et al*. The multicenter post infarction program: The relationship between ventricular arrhythmias, left ventricular dysfunction and mortality in the years after myocardial infarction. *Circulation* 1984; **69**: 250–258.

44 Moss AJ, Davis HT, DeCamilla J *et al*. Ventricular ectopic beats and their relation to sudden and non-sudden cardiac death after myocardial infarction. *Circulation* 1979; **60**: 998–1003.

45 Marchlinski FE, Buxton AE, Waxman HL *et al*. Identifying patients at risk of sudden death after myocardial infarction: Value of the response of programmed stimulation, degree of ventricular ectopic activity and the severity of left ventricular dysfunction. *Am J Cardiol* 1993; **12**: 1190–1196.

46 Gomes JA, Winters SL, Stewart D *et al*. The prognostic significance of quantitative signal-averaged variables relative to clinical variables, site of myocardial infarction, ejection fraction and ventricular premature beats: A prospective study. *J Am Coll Cardiol* 1988; **1**: 377–384.

47 LaRovere MT, Specchia G, Mortara A *et al*. Baroreflex sensitivity, clinical correlates and cardiovascular mortality among patients with a first myocardial infarction: A prospective study. *Circulation* 1988; **78**: 816–824.

48 Kleiger RE, Miller JP, Bigger Jr JT *et al*. Heart rate variability: A variable predicting mortality following acute myocardial infarction. *Am J Cardiol* 1988; **59**: 541–548.

49 The antiarrhythmic versus implantable defibrillator (AVID) investigators. A comparison of antiarrhythmic-drug therapy with implantable defibrillators in patients resuscitated from near-fatal ventricular arrhythmias. *N Engl J Med* 1997; **337**: 1576–1583.

50 Connolly SJ, Gent M, Roberts RS *et al*., for the CIDS Investigators. Canadian Implantable Defibrillator Study: A randomized trial of the implantable cardioverter defibrillator against amiodarone. *Circulation* 2000; **101**: 1297–1302.

51 Ferguson JJ. Meeting highlights: 47th Annual Scientific Sessions of the American College of Cardiology. *Circulation* 1998; **97**: 2377–2381.

52 Wilber J, Olshansky B, Moran JF *et al*. Electrophysiological testing and nonsustained ventricular tachycardia: Use and limitations among patients with coronary artery disease and impaired ventricular function. *Circulation* 1990; **82**: 350–358.

53 Buxton AE, Lee KL, Fisher JD *et al*., for the Multicenter Unsustained Tachycardia Trial Investigators. A randomized study for the prevention of sudden death among patients with coronary artery disease. *N Engl J Med* 1999; **341**: 1882–1890.

54 Klein RC, Machell C. Use of electrophysiological testing among patients with a nonsustained ventricular tachycardia: Prognostic and therapeutic implications. *J Am Coll Cardiol* 1989; **14**: 155–161.

55 Kadish A, Schnaltz S, Calkins H *et al*. Management of nonsustained ventricular tachycardia guided by electrophysiologic testing. *PACE* 1993; **16**: 1037–1050.

56 Coats AJ. MADIT II, the Multi-center Automatic Defibrillator Implantation Trial II stopped early for mortality reduction, has ICD therapy earned its evidence-based credentials? *Int J Cardiol* 2002; **82**: 1–5.

57 Middlekauff HR, Stevenson WG, Stevenson LW *et al*. Syncope in advanced heart failure: High sudden death risk in advanced heart failure: High sudden death risk regardless of syncope etiology. *J Am Coll Cardiol* 1993; **21**: 110–116.

58 Mittal S, Iwai S, Stein KM *et al*. Long-term outcome of patients with unexplained syncope treated with an electrophysiologic-guided approach in the implantable cardioverter-defibrillator era. *J Am Coll Cardiol* 1999; **34**: 1082–1089.

59 Knight BP, Goyal R, Pelosi F *et al*. Outcome of patients with nonischemic dilated cardiomyopathy and unexplained syncope treated with an implantable defibrillator. *J Am Coll Cardiol* 1999; **33**: 1964–1970.

60 SOLVD Investigators. Effect of enalapril on mortality and the development of heart failure in asymptomatic patients with reduced left ventricular ejection fractions. *N Engl J Med* 1992; **327**: 685–691.

61 CONSENSUS Trial Study Group. Effects of enalapril on mortality in severe congestive heart failure. *N Engl J Med* 1987; **316**: 1429–1435.

62 Pfeffer MA, Braunwald E, Moye LA *et al*. Effect of captopril on mortality and morbidity among patients with left ventricular dysfunction after myocardial infarction.

Results of the survival and ventricular enlargement trial. *N Engl J Med* 1992; **327**: 669–677.

63 Pitt B, Zannad F, Remme WJ *et al.*, for the randomized aldactone evaluation study investigators. The effect of spironolactone on morbidity and mortality among patients with severe heart failure. *N Engl J Med* 1999; **341**: 709–717.

64 Garg R, Gorlin R, Smith T *et al.*, for the Digitalis Investigation Group. The effect of digoxin on mortality and morbidity in patients with heart failure. *N Engl J Med* 1997; **336**: 525–533.

65 The Cardiac Arrhythmia Suppression Trial (CAST) Investigators. Effect of encainide and flecainide on mortality in a randomized trial of arrhythmia suppression after myocardial infarction. *N Engl J Med* 1989; **321**: 406–412.

66 The Cardiac Arrhythmia Suppression Trial II Investigators. Effect of the antiarrhythmic agent moricizine on survival after myocardial infarction. *N Engl J Med* 1992; **327**: 227–233.

67 MERIT-HF Study Group. Effect of metoprolol CR/XL in chronic heart failure: Metoprolol CR/XL randomized intervention trial in congestive heart failure (MERIT-HF). *Lancet* 1999; **353**: 2001–2007.

68 CIBIS II Investigators. The cardiac insufficiency bisoprolol study II: A randomized trial. *Lancet* 1999; **353**: 9–13.

69 Packer M, Bristow MR, Cohn JN *et al.*, for the U.S. Carvedilol Heart Failure Study Group. The effect of carvedilol on morbidity and mortality among patients with chronic heart failure. *N Engl J Med* 1996; **334**: 1349–1355.

70 Pratt CM, Camm AJ, deRuyter H *et al.* Effect of d-sotalol on mortality in patients with left ventricular dysfunction after recent and remote myocardial infarction. *Lancet* 1996; **348**: 7–12.

71 Torp-Pedersen CT, Moller M, Bloch-Thomsen PE *et al.* Dofetilide among patients with congestive heart failure and left ventricular dysfunction. *N Engl J Med* 1999; **341**: 857–865.

72 Burkart F, Pfisterer M, Kiowski W *et al.* Effect of antiarrhythmic therapy on mortality in survivors of myocardial infarction with asymptomatic complex ventricular arrhythmias: Basel Antiarrhythmic Study of Infarct Survival (BASIS). *J Am Coll Cardiol* 1990; **16**: 1711–1718.

73 Cairns JA, Connolly SJ, Roberts RS *et al.*, for the CAMIAT Investigators. Randomized trial of outcome after myocardial infarction in patients with frequent or repetitive ventricular premature depolarizations: CAMIAT. *Lancet* 1997; **349**: 675–682.

74 Julian DG, Camm AJ, Frangin G, Janse MJ, Munoz A, Schwartz PJ, Simon P, for the EMIAT Investigators. Randomized trial of effect of amiodarone on mortality in patients with left ventricular dysfunction after recent myocardial infraction: EMIAT. *Lancet* 1997; **349**: 667–674.

75 Doval HC, Nul DR, Grancelli HO *et al.*, for Grupo de Estudio de la Sobrevida en la Insuficiencia Cardiaca en Argentina (GESICA). Randomized trial of low-dose amiodarone in severe congestive heart failure. *Lancet* 1994; **344**: 493–498.

76 Singh SN, Fletcher RD, Fisher SG *et al.*, for the Survival Trial of Antiarrhythmic Therapy in Congestive Heart Failure (STAT-CHF): Amiodarone in patients with congestive heart failure and asymptomatic ventricular arrhythmia. *N Engl J Med* 1995; **333**: 77–82.

77 Garguichevich JJ, Ramos JL, Gambarte A *et al.* Effect of amiodarone therapy on mortality in patients with left ventricular dysfunction and asymptomatic complex ventricular arrhythmias: Argentine Pilot Study for Sudden Death (EPAMSA). *Am Heart J* 1995; **130**: 494–500.

78 Bardy GH, Lee KL, Mark DB *et al.*, for the Sudden Cardiac Death in Heart Failure Trial (SCD-HeFT) Investigators. Amiodarone or an implantable cardioverter-defibrillator for congestive heart failure. *N Engl J Med* 2005; **352**: 225–237.

79 Greene HL. The CASCADE Study: Randomized antiarrhythmic drug therapy in survivors of the cardiac arrest in Seattle. CASCADE Investigators. *Am J Cardiol* 1993; **72**: 70F–74F.

80 Amiodarone Trials Meta-Analysis Investigators. Effect of prophylactic amiodarone on mortality after acute myocardial infarction and in congestive heart failure: meta-analysis of individual data from 6500 patients in randomized trials. *Lancet* 1997; **350**: 1417–1424.

81 Connolly SJ. Evidence-based analysis of amiodarone efficacy and safety. *Circulation* 1999; **100**: 2025–2034.

82 Mirowski M, Reid PR, Mower MM *et al.* Termination of malignant ventricular arrhythmias with an implanted automatic defibrillator in human beings. *N Engl J Med* 1980; **303**: 322–324.

83 The AVID Investigators. Causes of death in the antirhythmics versus implantable defibrillator (AVID) trial. *J Am Coll Cardiol* 1999; **34**: 1552–1559.

84 Domanski MJ, Saksena S, Epstein AE *et al.* Relative effectiveness of the implantable cardioverter-defibrillator and antiarrhythmic drugs in patients with varying degrees of left ventricular dysfunction who have survived malignant ventricular arrhythmias. AVID Investigators – Antiarrhythmic versus Implantable Defibrillators. *J Am Coll Cardiol* 1999; **34**: 1090–1095.

85 Sheldon R, Connolly S, Krahn A *et al.* Identification of patients most likely to benefit from implantable cardioverter-defibrillator therapy: the Canadian Implantable Defibrillator Study. *Circulation* 2000; **101**: 1660–1664.

86 Siebels J, Cappato R, Ruppel R *et al.* Preliminary results of the Cardiac Arrest Study Hamburg. *Am J Cardiol* 1993; **72**: 109F–113F.

87 Kuck KH, Cappato R, Siebels J *et al.* Randomized comparison of antiarrhythmic drug therapy with implantable defibrillators in patients resuscitated from cardiac arrest-the

Cardiac Arrest Study Hamburg. *Circulation* 2000; **102**: 748–754.

88 Wever EFD, Hauer RNW, van Capelle FJI *et al.* Randomized study of implantable defibrillator as first choice therapy versus conventional strategy in the postinfarct sudden death survivors. *Circulation* 1995; **91**: 2195–2203.

89 Buxton AE, Marchlinski FE, Waxman HL, Flores BT, Cassidy DM, Josephson ME. Prognostic factors in nonsustained ventricular tachycardia. *Am J Cardiol* 1984; **53**: 1275–1279.

90 Moss AJ, Hall WJ, Cannom DS *et al.* Improved survival with an implanted defibrillator in patients with coronary artery disease at high risk for ventricular arrhythmia: the Multicenter Automatic Defibrillator Implant Trial Investigators. *N Engl J Med* 1996; **335**: 1933–1940.

91 Moss AJ, Fadl Y, Zareba W *et al.* Survival benefit with an implantable defibrillator in relation to mortality risk in chronic coronary heart disease. *Am J Cardiol* 2001; **88**: 516–520.

92 Bigger JT, for the Coronary Artery Bypass Graft (CABG) Patch Trial Investigators. Prophylactic use of implanted cardiac defibrillators in patients at high risk for ventricular arrhythmias after coronary-artery bypass graft surgery. *N Engl J Med* 1997; **337**: 1569–1575.

93 Buxton AE, Lee KL, Fisher JD *et al.* A randomized study of the prevention of sudden death in patients with coronary artery disease: Multicenter unsustained tachycardia trial investigators. *N Engl J Med* 1999; **341**: 1882–1890.

94 Moss AJ, Zareba W, Hall WJ *et al.* Prophylactic implantation of a defibrillator in patients with myocardial infarction and reduced ejection fraction. *N Engl J Med* 2002; **346**: 877–883.

95 Hohnloser SH, Kuck KH, Dorian P *et al.*, on behalf of the Defibrillator in Acute Myocardial Infarction Trial (DINAMIT) Investigators. Prophylactic use of an implantable cardioverter-defibrillator after acute myocardial infarction. *N Engl J Med* 2004; **351**: 2481–2488.

96 Bansch D, Antz M, Boczor S *et al.* Primary prevention of sudden cardiac death in idiopathic dilated cardiomyopathy: the cardiomyopathy trial (CAT). *Circulation* 2002; **105**: 1453–1458.

97 Strickberger A, Hummel JD, Bartlett TG *et al.* Amiodarone versus implantable cardioverter-defibrillator: randomized trial in patients with nonischemic cardiomyopathy and asymptomatic nonsustained ventricular tachycardia – AMIOVIRT. *J Am Coll Cardiol* 2003; **41**: 1707–1712.

98 Kadish A, Dyer A, Daubert J *et al.*, for the Defibrillators in Non-Ischemic Cardiomyopathy Treatment Evaluation (DEFINITE) Investigators. Prophylactic defibrillator implantation in patients with nonischemic dilated cardiomyopathy. *N Engl J Med* 2004; **350**: 2151–2158.

99 Grimm W, Hoffman JJ, Muller HH *et al.* Implantable defibrillator event rates in patients with idiopathic dilated cardiomyopathy, nonsustained ventricular tachycardia on Holter and a left ventricular ejection fraction of less than 30%. *J Am Coll Cardiol* 2002; **39**: 788–789.

100 ACC/AHA/NASPE 2002 Guideline update for implantation of cardiac pacemakers and antiarrhythmia devices: summary article. A report of the American College of Cardiology/American Heart Association Task Force on practice guidelines. *Circulation* 2002; **106**: 2145–2161.

101 Hochleitner M, Hortnagl H, Freidrich L *et al.* Long term efficacy of physiologic dual chamber pacing in the treatment of end stage idiopathic dilated cardiomyopathy. *Am J Cardiol* 1992; **70**: 1320–1325.

102 Brecker SJD, Ziao HB, Sparrow J *et al.* Effects of dual chamber pacing with short atrioventricular delay in dilated cardiomyopathy. *Lancet* 1992; **340**: 1308–1312.

103 Nishimura RA, Hayes DL, Holmes DR *et al.* Mechanism of hemodynamic improvement by dual chamber pacing for severe left ventricular dysfunction: an acute Doppler and catheterization hemodynamic study. *J Am Coll Cardiol* 1995; **25**: 281–288.

104 Linde C, Gadler F, Edner M *et al.* Results of atrioventricular synchronous pacing with optimized delay in patients with severe congestive heart failure. *Am J Cardiol* 1995; **75**: 919–923.

105 Gold MR, Feliciano Z, Gottlieb SS *et al.* Dual chamber pacing with a short atrioventricular delay in congestive heart failure: a randomized study. *J Am Coll Cardiol* 1995; **26**: 967–973.

106 David D, Michelson EL, Naito M *et al.* Diastolic "locking" of the mitral valve: the importance of atrial systole and intraventricular volume. *Circulation* 1983; **67**: 640–645.

107 Wilkoff BL, Cook JR, Epstein AE *et al.* Dual-chamber pacing or ventricular backup pacing in patients with an implantable defibrillator: the Dual Chamber and VVI Implantable Defibrillator (DAVID) Trial. *J Am Med Assoc* 2002; **288**: 3115–3123.

108 Farwell D, Patel NR, Hall A, Ralph S, Sulke AN. How many people with heart failure are appropriate for biventricular resynchronization? *Eur Heart J* 2000; **21**: 1246–1250.

109 Aaronson KD, Schwartz JS, Chen TM, Wong KL, Goin JE, Mancini DM. Development and prospective validation of a clinical index to predict survival in ambulatory patients referred for cardiac transplant evaluation. *Circulation* 1997; **95**: 2660–2667.

110 Xiao HB, Brecker SJ, Gibson DG. Effects of abnormal activation on the time course of the left ventricular pressure pulse in dilated cardiomyopathy. *Brit Heart J* 1992; **68**: 403–407.

111 Littmann L, Symanski JD. Hemodynamic implications of left bundle branch block. *J Electrocardiol* 2000; **33(Suppl)**: 115–121.

112 Saxon LA, Kerwin WF, Cahalan MK *et al.* Acute effects of intraoperative multisite ventricular pacing on left ventricular function and activation/contraction sequence in: a

report from the Italian Network on Congestive Heart Failure. *Am Heart J* 2002; **143**: 398–405.

113 Kerwin WF, Botvinick EH, O'Connell JW *et al.* Ventricular contraction abnormalities in dilated cardiomyopathy: effect of biventricular pacing to correct interventricular dyssynchrony. *J Am Coll Cardiol* 2000; **35**: 1221–1227.

114 Xiao HB, Roy C, Fujimoto S, Gibson DG. Natural history of abnormal conduction and its relation to prognosis in patients with dilated cardiomyopathy. *Int J Cardiol* 1996; **53**: 163–170.

115 Unverferth DV, Magorien RD, Moeschberger ML, Baker PB, Fetters JK, Leier CV. Factors influencing the one-year mortality of dilated cardiomyopathy. *Am J Cardiol* 1984; **54**: 147–152.

116 Shamim W, Francis DP, Yousufuddin M *et al.* Intraventricular conduction delay: a prognostic marker in chronic heart failure. *Int J Cardiol* 1999; **70**: 171–178.

117 Baldasseroni S, Opasich C, Gorini M *et al.* Left bundle branch block (LBBB) is associated with increased 1-year sudden and total rate in 5517 outpatients with congestive heart failure: a report from the Italian Network on Congestive Heart Failure. *Am Heart J* 2002; **143**: 398–405.

118 Ozdemir K, Altunkeser BB, Danis G *et al.* Effect of the isolated left bundle branch block on systolic and diastolic functions of left ventricle. *J Am Soc Echocardiog* 2001; **14**: 1075–1079.

119 Hayashi T, Sakai Y, Kobayashi S *et al.* Correlation between interventricular septal motion and left ventricular systolic-diastolic function in patients with left bundle branch block. *J Cardiol* 2000; **35**: 181–187.

120 Burkhoff D, Oikawa RY, Sagawa K. Influence of pacing site on canine left ventricular contraction. *Am J Physiol* 1986; **251**: H428–H435.

121 Lattuca JJ, Cohen TJ, Mower MM. Biventricular pacing to improve cardiac hemodynamics. *Clin Rev* 1990; **38**: 882A.

122 De Teresa PA, Chamoro JL. An even more physiologic pacing: changing the sequence of ventricular activation. *Proceedings, VIIth World Symposium on Cardiac Pacing*, Vienna, Austria 1983: 95–100.

123 Cazeau S, Ritter P, Lazarus A *et al.* Multisite pacing for end stage heart failure: early experience. *PACE* 1996; **19**: 1748–1757.

124 Leclerq C, Cazeau S, Le Breton H *et al.* Acute hemodynamic effects of biventricular DDD pacing in patients with end-stage heart failure. *J Am Coll Cardiol* 1998; **32**: 1825–1831.

125 Kass DA, Chen CH, Curry C *et al.* Improved left ventricular mechanics from acute VDD pacing in patients with dilated cardiomyopathy and ventricular conduction delay. *Circulation* 1999; **99**: 1567–1573.

126 Prinzen FW, Augustijn CH, Arts T *et al.* Redistribution of myocardial fiber strain and blood flow by asynchronous activation. *Am J Physiol* 1990; **259**: H300–H308.

127 Prinzen FW, Hunter WC, Wyman BT *et al.* Mapping of regional myocardial strain and work during ventricular pacing: experimental study using magnetic resonance tagging. *J Am Coll Cardiol* 1999; **33**: 1735–1742.

128 Wyman BT, Hunter WC, Prinzen FW *et al.* Mapping propagation of mechanical activation in the paced heart with MRI tagging. *Am J Physiol* 1999; **276**: H881–H891.

129 Curry CC, Nelson GS, Wyman BT *et al.* Mechanical dyssynchrony in dilated cardiomyopathy with intraventricular conduction delay as depicted by 3-D tagged magnetic resonance imaging. *Circulation* 2000; **101**: e2.

130 Park RC, Little WC, O'Rourke RA. Effect of alteration of left ventricular activation sequence on the left ventricular end-systolic pressure-volume relation in closed-chest dogs. *Circ Res* 1985; **57**: 706–717.

131 Heyndrickx GR, Vantrimpont PJ, Rousseau MF *et al.* Effects of asynchrony on myocardial relaxation at rest and during exercise in conscious dogs. *Am J Physiol* 1988; **254**: H817–H822.

132 Baller D, Wolpers HG, Zipfel J *et al.* Comparison of the effects of right atrial, right ventricular apex and atrioventricular sequential pacing on myocardial oxygen consumption and cardiac efficiency: a laboratory investigation. *PACE* 1988; **11**: 394–403.

133 Owen CH, Esposito DJ, Davis JW *et al.* The effects of ventricular pacing on the left ventricular geometry, function, myocardial oxygen consumption, and efficiency of contraction in conscious dogs. *PACE* 1998; **21**: 1417–1429.

134 Sarubbi B, Ducceschi V, Santangelo L *et al.* Arrhythmias in patients with mechanical ventricular dysfunction and myocardial stretch: role of mechano-electric feedback. *Can J Cardiol* 1998; **14**: 245–252.

135 Victor F, Leclerq C, Mabo P *et al.* Optimal right ventricular pacing site in chronically implanted patients: a prospective randomized crossover comparison of apical and outflow tract pacing. *J Am Coll Cardiol* 1999; **33**: 311–316.

136 Blanc JJ, Etienne Y, Gilard M *et al.* Evaluation of different ventricular pacing sites in patients with severe congestive heart failure: results of an acute hemodynamic study. *Circulation* 1997; **96**: 3272–3277.

137 Mansourati J, Etienne Y, Gilard M *et al.* Left ventricular based pacing in patients with chronic heart failure: comparison of acute hemodynamic benefits according to underlying heart disease. *Eur J Heart Fail* 2000; **2**: 195–199.

138 Saxon LA, Kerwin WF, Cahalan MK *et al.* Acute effects of intraoperative multisite ventricular pacing on left ventricular function and activation/contraction sequence in patients with depressed ventricular function. *J Cardiovasc Electrophysiol* 1998; **9**: 13–21.

139 Kerwin WF, Botvinick EH, O'Connell JW *et al.* Ventricular contraction abnormalities in dilated cardiomyopathy: effect of biventricular pacing to correct interventricular dyssynchrony. *J Am Coll Cardiol* 2000; **35**: 1221–1227.

140 Auricchio A, Stellbrink C, Block M *et al*. Effect of pacing chamber and atrioventricular delay on acute systolic function of paced patients with congestive heart failure: The Pacing Therapies for Congestive Heart Failure Study Group. The Guidant Congestive Heart Failure Study Group. *Circulation* 1999; **99**: 2993–3001.

141 Abraham W. MIRACLE trial data. Presented at the *North American Society of Pacing and Electrophysiology Meeting*, Boston, 2001.

142 Toussaint JF, Lavergne T, Ollitraut J *et al*. Biventricular pacing in severe heart failure patients reverses electromechanical dyssynchronization from apex to base. *PACE* 2000; **23**: 1731–1734.

143 Morris-Thurgood JA, Turner MS, Nightingale AK *et al*. Pacing in heart failure: improved ventricular interaction in diastole rather than systolic resynchronization. *Europace* 2000; **2**: 271–275.

144 Saxon LA, Boehmer JP, Hummels H *et al*., for the VIGOR CHF and the VENTAK CHF Investigators. Biventricular pacing in patients with congestive heart failure: Two prospective randomized trials. *Am J Cardiol* 1999; **83**: 130D–135D.

145 Gras D, Mabo P, Tang T *et al*. Multisite pacing as a supplemental treatment of congestive heart failure: Preliminary results of the Medtronic Inc. InSync Study. *PACE* 1998; **21**: 2249–2255.

146 Alonso C, Leclercq C, Victor F *et al*. Electrocardiographic predictive factors of long-term clinical improvement with multisite biventricular pacing in advanced heart failure. *Am J Cardiol* 1999; **84**: 1417–1421.

147 Cazeau S, Leclercq C, Lavergne T *et al*. Effects of multisite biventricular pacing in patients with heart failure and intraventricular conduction delay: Multisite Stimulation in Cardiomyopathies (MUSTIC) Study Investigators. *N Engl J Med* 2001; **344**: 873–880.

148 Linde C, Leclercq C, Rex S *et al*. Long-term benefits of biventricular pacing in congestive heart failure: results from the Multisite Stimulation in Cardiomyopathy (MUSTIC) study. *J Am Coll Cardiol* 2002; **40**: 111–118.

149 Abraham WT, Fisher WG, Smith AL *et al*., for The Multicenter InSync Randomized Clinical Evaluation (MIRACLE) Study Group. Cardiac resynchronization in chronic heart failure. *N Engl J Med* 2002; **346(24)**: 1845–1853.

150 Bristow MR, Saxon LA, Boehmer J *et al*., for the Comparison of Medical Therapy, Pacing, and Defibrillation in Heart Failure (COMPANION) Investigators. Cardiac-Resynchronization Therapy with or without an implantable defibrillator in advanced chronic heart failure. *N Engl J Med* 2004; **350**: 2140–2150.

151 Cleland JGF, Daubert JC, Erdmann E *et al*., for the Cardiac Resynchronization – Heart Failure (CARE-HF) Study Investigators. The effect of cardiac resynchronization on morbidity and mortality in heart failure. *N Engl J Med* 2005; **352**: 1539–1549.

152 Cleland JGF, Daubert JC, Erdmann E *et al*. The CARE-HF study (Cardiac Resynchronization in Heart Failure study): rationale, design and end points. *Eur J Heart Fail* 2001; **3**: 481–489.

153 Calvert MJ, Freemantle N, Cleland JGF. The impact of heart failure on health-related quality of life data acquired in the baseline phase of the CARE-HF study. *Eur J Heart Fail* 2005; **7**: 243–251.

154 Cleland JGF, Daubert JC, Erdmann E *et al*. Baseline characteristics of patients recruited to the CARE-HF study. *Eur J Heart Fail* 2005; **7**: 205–214.

155 Bradley DJ, Bradley EA, Baughman KL *et al*. Cardiac resynchronization and death from progressive heart failure: a meta-analysis of randomized controlled trials. *J Am Med Assoc* 2003; **289**: 730–740.

156 Salukhe TV, Dimopoulos K, Francis D. Cardiac resynchronization may reduce all-cause mortality: meta-analysis of preliminary COMPANION data with CONTAK-CD, InSync ICD, MIRACLE and MUSTIC. *Int J Cardiol* 2004; **93**: 101–103.

157 Higgins SL, Yong P, Sheck D *et al*. Biventricular pacing diminishes the need for implantable cardioverter defibrillator therapy. Ventak CHF Investigators. *J Am Coll Cardiol* 2000; **36**: 828–831

158 Lam C, Rose M, Jaeger F *et al*., Wide QRS duration predicts inducibility of sustained ventricular arrhythmia. *Circulation* 2000; **102(Suppl 2):** II–675 [abstract].

159 Young JB, Abraham WT, Smith AL *et al*., for the Multicenter InSync ICD Randomized Clinical Evaluation (MIRACLE ICD) Trial Investigators. Combined cardiac resynchronization and implantable cardioversion defibrillation in advanced chronic heart failure. *J Am Med Assoc* 2003; **289**: 2685–2694.

160 Abraham WT, Young JB, Leon AR *et al*., on behalf of the Multicenter InSync ICD II Study Group. Effects of cardiac resynchronization on disease progression in patients with left ventricular systolic dysfunction, an indication for an implantable cardioverter-defibrillator, and mildly symptomatic chronic heart failure. *Circulation* 2004; **110**: 2864–2868.

161 Kuhlkamp V, for the InSync 772 ICD World Wide Investigators. Initial experience with an implantable cardioverter-defibrillator incorporating cardiac resynchronization therapy. *J Am Coll Cardiol* 2002; **39**: 790–797.

162 Wilkoff BL, Kuhlkamp V, Volosin K *et al*. Critical analysis of dual-chamber implantable cardioverter-defibrillator arrhythmia detection: results and technical considerations. *Circulation* 2001; **103**: 381–386.

163 Gaita F, Bocchiardo M, Porciani MC *et al*. Should stimulation therapy for congestive heart failure be combined with defibrillation backup? *Am J Cardiol* 2000; **86**: 165K–168K.

164 Bocchiardo M, Achtelik M, Gaita F *et al*. Efficacy of biventricular sensing and treatment of ventricular arrhythmias. *PACE* 2000; **23**: 1989–1991.

CHAPTER 6

Managing a heart failure clinic

Nancy M. Albert

Introduction

Chronic left ventricular systolic dysfunction or heart failure (HF) is a common disabling condition affecting about 2.2% of the US population [1,2]. Today, about 5 million people are living with HF and about 550,000 new cases are diagnosed each year [2]. Some patients with HF lead an independent and full life, especially when ventricular remodeling is mild and hormones producing vasodilation, diuresis and natriuresis counterbalance the vasoconstricting forces. However, moderate to marked limitations that interfere with employment or usual activities of daily living and result in emotional, economic and social distress, and costs burdens many patients.

In the last decade, there have been remarkable advances on many fronts related to understanding of the pathophysiology of HF, the natural history of the syndrome, as well as important advances in pharmacologic, surgical, device, and medical therapeutics. One such advance has been the move from treating HF symptoms to treating the multi-faceted HF condition. Through research, it is known that HF can progress even when the patient remains asymptomatic. Core drug therapies that promote regression of ventricular remodeling or prevent its progression benefit patients by prolonging survival, decreasing debilitating symptoms and improving morbidity. Based on the belief that patients will benefit from comprehensive treatment of the condition rather than just treating symptoms, a disease management approach has been advocated. One aspect of disease management is the use of a "HF clinic". A HF clinic program can aid in the verification of diagnosis, ensure full care planning, facilitate optimization of drug therapies, promote changes in lifestyle and self-management, increase patient and family understanding of their condition and treatment options and guide patients toward supportive resources to promote adherence of the plan of care and wellness.

Specifically, an HF clinic refers to a nurse-run and coordinated, algorithm-driven, physician supervised, interdisciplinary outpatient model. This chapter will provide support for the use of an HF clinic in the continuum of care. It will focus on components inherent in successful start-up and operation. Then, attention will be given to issues and barriers impacting clinical success and current limitations in knowledge of HF clinics.

Why an HF clinic?

There is much evidence to support the use of a HF clinic in outpatient management. The current state of HF care, which is epitomized by a cycle of acute care hospitalizations and acute episodic outpatient care by a primary or emergency care provider, has not led to a great improvement in patient quality of life or prognosis. When patients with decompensated HF were followed after discharge from an emergency department of a community hospital, 61% returned to the emergency department or were admitted to the hospital within 3 months and the median time to failure was 30 days [3]. In a Department of Veterans Affairs study of patterns of hospital and clinic use and risk-adjusted death in 1996, the cohort of 31,429 patients had a total of 34,907 hospital discharges. The average patient had 14 inpatient days, 6–7 visits with a primary care physician, 15 other visits for consultations or tests, and 1–2 emergent care visits during a 12-month period. The overall adjusted risk adjusted mortality at 5 years was 64% [4].

To assess whether survival had improved over time in a general population of patients with HF admitted to a Scottish hospital with an HF diagnosis, crude case fatality rates in 1986 were compared to those from 1987 to 1995. For the entire cohort, fatality rates were 19.9% at 30 days, 44.5% at 1 year, 76.5% at 5 years and 87.6% at 10 years [5]. In this group of 66,547 patients, the median age of males and females was 72 and 78 years, respectively and age had the most powerful effect on survival. Thus within 30 days and after 30 days post-hospitalization median survival rates improved in both men and women from 1987 to 1995 when compared to 1986, but only modestly (i.e., median 30 day mortality in 1995 declined to 18.6% and 1-year mortality declined to 42.4%).

Using the same Scottish database, Stewart and colleagues assessed 16,224 men and 14,842 women after their first hospitalization for HF in 1991 and compared their 5-year survival to patients being admitted for the first time with myocardial infarction and the four most common types of cancer for each sex. With the exception of lung cancer, those hospitalized for HF had the poorest survival (approximately 25% for both sexes) [6]. By comparison, large, multi-center clinical trial research conducted in recent years in the United States and Europe has yielded encouraging short-term survival benefit and improved quality of life [7]. While HF prognosis remains grim despite advances in pharmacologic therapies, there is hope that team management as recommended by the Cardiovascular Nursing Council of the American Heart Association (AHA) [8] will improve survival and enhance functional capacity and quality of life. A HF clinic that delivers care by practitioners with HF expertise and uses an integrated approach to manage the syndrome based on the current AHA and American College of Cardiology (ACC) guidelines [7] can potentially impact prognosis and also decrease the rate of hospital recidivism.

The current state of recommended HF care is complex. Proven pharmacologic therapies must be administered to the right patients and at the right dosage levels. The healthcare provider must juggle multiple medications and pay close attention to potential side effects, drug interactions, contraindications due to comorbidities, drug impact on serum electrolyte levels, and serum drug levels that might prove harmful. Many patient factors add to the complexity, such as level of depression, patient understanding of the effects and side effects of drugs, financial constraints, access to a pharmacy, willingness to use therapy when traveling from home, ability to read labels and follow administration directions, and ability to open drug containers. In addition, healthcare providers must keep pace with advancements that may impact patient subgroups (minorities, women) or influence polypharmacy drug interaction. The average community-based primary care physician may not be able to keep pace with the latest research findings.

Edep and colleagues characterized physician practices by survey to learn if there was a difference in HF management by specialty and how physicians related to guideline recommendations [9]. Researchers found significant differences between physician groups (general practitioners, internists and cardiologists) in each of the major guideline recommendations (evaluation of left ventricular function, angiotensin converting enzyme (ACE) inhibitor use, and ACE inhibitor dosages). Cardiologists reported practices that were more in conformity with published guidelines than the other physician groups. These differences were large and statistically significant [9]. One rationale for not using specialty physicians is that inpatient costs would increase. Harjai et al. compared caregiver specialty during patient hospitalization for HF to assess hospital costs, length of stay and in-hospital mortality. In 614 consecutive patients admitted to a large teaching center, researchers found no difference in any of the outcome endpoints and concluded that specialty care was not more expensive than that provided by generalists [10].

In an outpatient setting, many HF specialty programs, conducted by cardiologists, nurses and other healthcare providers who specialize in the care of patients with HF and cardiac transplantation, have reported favorable morbidity outcomes (subsequent hospitalizations, length of hospital stay, quality of life, and exercise tolerance) after as little as 3 months of program implementation. The first published report of an HF clinic program was in 1983 [11]. Subsequently, reports of programs that offered different combinations of care strategies followed. While program features differed in each report, two things were common HF clinic elements: adjustments in medical therapy consistent with guideline recommendations and patient support (that was evidenced in many ways: medication, exercise, nutrition and lifestyle education classes; written education materials; vigilance monitoring for adherence to the plan of care; home care; and telephonic support initiated by the patient) [12–24]. In a meta-analyses of comprehensive or multidisciplinary strategies of support for older patients with chronic HF [25] and a systematic review of multidisciplinary strategies for patients at high risk for hospital re-admission [26], pooled data reflected improvements in mortality, hospitalization, cost of care and other clinical outcomes [25–27]. Specialized HF clinic personnel are more likely to keep abreast of research-based advancements and are more likely to follow AHA/ACC drug recommendations since they are constantly practicing the art and science of HF management and develop a greater repertoire of actions when dealing with the complexities of management. Ultimately, patients benefit since modulation of the progression of HF and enhanced quality of life are associated with drug and medical therapy optimization.

Nurses usually carry out detailed patient education of the complex aspects of HF pathophysiology and management. Nurses who specialize in the care of patients with HF have a stronger knowledge base about important education topics as compared to nurses with a critical care or medical–surgical background [28]. This knowledge base may translate into educational messages that lead to improved patient outcomes. In a randomized trial of post-hospitalization education and support provided by knowledgeable cardiac nurses, not only did 1-year readmission rates decrease by 39% in the intervention group (and not in the control group), but the combination of 1-year hospitalization or death also decreased significantly (risk reduction: 31%, $P = 0.01$) [29].

Numerous reports have provided evidence of oversights in promoting non-pharmacologic strategies that might prevent hospitalization. Many hospitalizations may be avoided if healthcare providers frequently reassess variables known to precipitate decompensation and also promote patient adherence in self-care, self-management (including symptom monitoring), and preventive recommendations. Issues to be addressed are a failed social support

system; diet, fluid and exercise non-adherence; premature hospital discharge; inadequate discharge planning and/or follow-up; failure to seek prompt medical attention when symptoms emerge or worsen; lack of understanding of the HF syndrome, therapy benefits, and actions that can improve outcomes; and lack of understanding of actions that cause detriment [30–34]. In a randomized, controlled study of 98 patients with advanced HF receiving optimal medical care by HF specialty cardiologists, patients were assigned to routine or multidisciplinary care. Those assigned to multidisciplinary care by a nurse specialist and dietician had decreased rehospitalization or death 3 months post-intervention [35]. A HF clinic that uses specialized nurses is poised to meet the non-pharmacologic issues inherent in a chronic, progressive condition like HF, especially when a multidisciplinary approach is used, the program includes some aspect of vigilance monitoring, and encourages patients to communicate freely and at any time of the day [36].

Why an HF clinic? Specialized HF care physicians, nurses and other healthcare providers can close the gap between the state of knowledge concerning HF, optimized treatments, and delivery of care. Deficiencies that exist in the traditional care system can be recognized and overcome through a coordinated approach of prevention, education, and research-based disease management strategies.

Getting started

Financial and patient outcome successes attributed to care provided in an HF clinic are based on factors that must be recognized and attended to in the planning phase. Questions to think about are listed in Table 6.1 and include structural, process of care and reimbursement issues [37,38]. It is important to know your market (are you the only HF specialty team in town with expertise?), know what other care providers offer, understand the level of care coordination across care settings (are patients transferred to the appropriate care setting or team as their HF condition worsens?), and learn the local barriers that prevent patients from receiving optimized care.

Once preliminary questions are answered and there is insight in the level of support available, a multidisciplinary planning team should be brought

Table 6.1 Questions to ask in the early planning phase and impact of knowledge.

Questions	Impact of knowledge gained
Who is requesting that a HF clinic program be developed? Who wants it to succeed? • Community primary care providers • Large (general) cardiology practice group • An advanced practice nurse • Hospital administrator(s) • Nursing administrator • Managed care organization • HF specialty physicians • Cardiac rehabilitation specialists • Pharmacist	Those requesting a HF clinic will have overt and hidden agendas that may impact the focus and goals of the program and these may be different than the goals of those who want the program to succeed (if not one in the same). For example, a hospital administrator may want to decrease HF related hospitalizations to improve finances, but may only want the clinic practitioners to focus on discharge planning, not comprehensive HF care.
What does recent patient data of quality indicators of HF care reflect? • Is left ventricular ejection fraction assessed in every patient? • Are ACE-inhibitors and beta-blockers prescribed to most patients and at high enough doses? • Is there written evidence of preventive therapies (i.e., smoking cessation)? • Is there written evidence of patient understanding in diet, exercise, weight monitoring, medications and when to notify the healthcare team of worsening condition? • What are the 7 and 30 day re-hospitalization rates of the local hospital? • What is the in-hospital and 30 day mortality rates of the local hospital? • How do hospitalization and mortality rates compare with other local HF care providers?	Putting together a HF clinic takes time, effort, and funding. Prior to initiating a plan of action, it is important to learn what the current status quo is so that you can build on specific needs. If recent quality indicators of HF care reflect optimized patient data, the clinic may not succeed financially, especially if the stakeholders are relying on patient referrals.
How will patients be transferred or referred into the HF clinic? • Are you depending on primary care referrals? Cardiology referrals? Referrals prior to hospital discharge? • Do the current practitioners have enough HF volume to offset the cost associated with adding healthcare providers to meet the needs of the program?	If relying on outsiders to provide you with the required patient volume to break-even financially, you must be very sure that providers will actually make referrals to your HF clinic. This requires discussion and collaboration by the two (or more) parties prior to program planning. If primary care providers only plan to refer patients that are transplant candidates, then your program may need to have a different focus (i.e., include advanced HF research protocols) than a program with a broader patient base.
Describe your local HF patient population: • Elderly? Obese? Smokers? More hypertension and diastolic dysfunction than systolic dysfunction? Comorbidities? • Education level? Literacy level? Insurance coverage? • Are there general economic issues (high unemployment rates; lack of income)? • Are there general barriers to care (unsafe neighborhood, lack of local pharmacy, lack of support services-cab or wheels on meals)?	Knowing your local patient population will prevent development of actions that patients will not benefit from (i.e., reading level in patient education materials must meet the abilities of most patients; if your property manager charges a parking fee or parking is not readily available near the facility, patients may cancel appointments).

(Continued)

Table 6.1 (*Continued*)

Questions	Impact of knowledge gained

Does the infrastructure support a program that promotes services across the continuum of care?
    Care settings: home care, emergency care, acute care, critical care, palliative care, subacute care.
    • Are AHA/ACC guidelines followed in all care settings?
    • Is there coordination across care settings if a patient must be transferred?
Is there clinical expertise in HF across care settings?
	If programs are not available across the continuum of care, it is prudent to create *more than* an outpatient program when planning the HF clinic to ensure optimized care when acute care or special services are required.

Does the infrastructure support a program that treats patients with any level of HF (functional class I–IV) or only moderately to severely symptomatic patients? How much attention should be paid to preventive strategies; population-based education materials; telephonic monitoring programs?	Symptom management, psychosocial needs, education, support services and resources can be developed specifically for the level of severity of HF that the program is expecting to treat.
Do the partnering physicians follow the AHA/ACC evidence-based guidelines? Do the partnering physicians believe that algorithm or guideline-based care practices can meet many patient care needs? Can consensus be reached on pharmacologic treatment for diastolic dysfunction since evidence-based guidelines are not available?	Potential process of care issues should be discussed and agreed upon before implementation. If specific team members feel the guidelines are too aggressive or rigid or non-specific, they may not refer patients to the specialized HF clinic.
Will patients be mainly Medicare fee-for-service only? Have secondary insurance? Be in a managed care program? Is the health insurance market stable in your local environment?	Medicare fee-for-service does not include cardiac rehabilitation (in patients without coronary artery disease), education self-care techniques, nutrition counseling, telemonitoring, or home care unless home bound.
	In a volatile health reimbursement market, patients may change healthcare providers to meet reimbursement policies. All of the above can impact optimization of care.
What is the number of hospital discharges per year in DRG 127? What is the number of ambulatory care visits per year in your hospital or clinic for ICD-9 code 428.0? How many patients were treated last year in the hospital and ambulatory setting?	Is the HF volume in your center (hospital, office or clinic) large enough to support at least one full-time clinical nurse specialist or nurse practitioner with prescription privileges? Hiring a part-time employee(s) may interrupt services, especially on-going nurse–patient communication. This may decrease program benefits.

DRG: discharge related group; ICD: international classification of diseases.

together to shape the program. While a large group might be unwieldy, it is important that program users define the program's scope and overcome issues and barriers learned from answers to questions posed in Table 6.1. Then, much of the process work can be completed through electronic mail or small work groups. The planning process may take over a year if all elements are being generated by the team without the benefit of communicating and collaborating with groups experienced in developing, implementing and

evaluating a specific multidisciplinary program that is similar in goals to the proposed model. No matter if the planning team consults other organizations to learn from their trials and errors, expect to take a considerable amount of time in discussion with key stakeholders and potential users of the program.

It is important to determine who is most likely to benefit from HF clinic interventions [39]. Identifying patients most likely to benefit from the program might be difficult since potential benefits are derived from medical interventions that the program advocates, the patient population in need, patient health plans and available HF resources in the continuum of care that are beyond the scope of a HF clinic. Riegel *et al.* conducted a study to learn which patients would respond best to a HF disease management program. Patients were matched on age, comorbidity and preadmission functional class, then half were given a disease management intervention and the other half received usual care. In the investigators primary analysis, there were no differences between groups in overall or HF hospitalization rates and total costs at 6 months. However, they found that preadmission patients in functional class II used less acute care, leading to a reduction in total costs by 68% compared to patients in the usual care group. Patients in functional class I preadmission had a 288% increase in total costs and a 14-fold increase in HF costs [40].

Another factor to consider is the scope of clinic services. Will the HF clinic focus on patients with systolic dysfunction alone or include patients with HF and preserved left ventricular function due to hypertension, post-myocardial infarction, or other factors? Since restrictive and hypertrophic cardiomyopathy are less common, planning should include deciding whether these patients are best served in a formalized HF clinic program or require individualized physician care. It must be determined whether the program should focus on treating common comorbidities associated with HF, such as diabetes, atrial fibrillation, hypercholesterolemia, and depression. Finally, the scope regarding routine laboratory monitoring and treatment of serum anti-coagulation level in patients on warfarin therapy should be considered.

There are important considerations that are critical for a successful program, both in start-up and long-term operation. The single most important key element to success revolves around personnel: (1) choosing the right physician champion, (2) employing specialized, knowledgeable HF nurse(s) who effectively collaborate with physicians, and (3) utilizing the skills of a clinical nurse specialist to initiate and maintain protocols (algorithms) and actions related to new technology that are consistent with the ever-changing recommended guidelines and aid in the optimization of cost-effective care. Table 6.2 lists qualities and roles of each personnel type that can benefit a program. For all 3 groups of

personnel, it is important that they are effective communicators with administrators, physicians, multidisciplinary team members, and patients and have a background of working closely with patients so that they understand factors that impact medical care.

Physicians aligned with the HF clinic must be supportive of the benefits of using an advance practice nurse caregiver to aid in meeting program goals. Nurses are integral to the process of care since they are challenged with providing coordinated and integrative services as part of any clinical role. In a HF clinic, their background and education allows for systems thinking in the context of incorporating a patient's values, environment, family, illness experiences and view of health and wellness into the plan of care [41]. When nurses recommend interdisciplinary services, they coordinate activities around the needs of the patient and family and are available by phone to adjust the plan of care when the focus changes from primary prevention to secondary prevention to tertiary care planning and end-of-life.

A second element of success centers on the use of evidence-based guidelines, algorithms and nomograms developed specifically for the HF clinic. These must be accurate, provide enough detail to be safely and effectively used by all healthcare providers as appropriate, include cut-off points or values that set the limits of independent practice by the nurse caregiver, and also be simple and easy to use so that they are not perceived as a burden to caregivers or do not cause untold complications. Ultimately, an algorithm-driven program should provide enough heterogeneity to meet the complexities of patients with chronic HF, but be specific enough to provide "best practice", cost-effective, productive, accountable care and prevent concerns among physicians related to medical liability of nurse caregiver actions. Guidelines should reflect consensus among caregivers, since they are unlikely to be used when the content is threatening or opinions vary from the written plan of care.

A third element to successful clinic start-up and an important aspect of gaining consensus in the use of algorithms is education. This can be carried out by providing all personnel with comprehensive materials in a three-ring binder and pocket-sized laminated cards that provide the same content in a reduced size. Education is also carried out at

Table 6.2 Personnel qualities and roles in an HF clinic.

Qualities/qualifications	Roles
Physician champion	
Leader in HF management	Approves algorithms and guidelines developed for program; assures validity of content; keeps pace with advances in HF pharmacotherapeutics
Advocate to change other physicians practices	Physician education; consultant to other disease management programs associated with this clinic
Belief that recommended guidelines are appropriate and advocates usage	Collaborates with other caregivers to ensure guidelines are followed; overcomes barriers to guideline use among team members
Awareness of benefits of HF nurse caregiver as team member; understands HF nurse caregiver capabilities	Provides support, encouragement; acts as consultant; communicates benefits of nursing role; promotes autonomous actions as appropriate to nursing degree/license, background, certification(s)
Litigator; motivator; quality leader; builds consensus	Lead quality assurance or performance improvement initiatives; provide feedback at annual performance appraisal; mitigate conflicts, discuss problems or questions; provide feedback to team members
HF clinic nurse caregiver	
Advance practice nurse (nurse practitioner or clinical nurse specialist) with prescription privileges; able to coordinate and integrate discontinuous care	Provide direct billable care that includes primary/secondary atherosclerosis prevention strategies; medication changes that promote therapeutic dosing; diagnostic testing and interpretation; routine follow-up care and emergent care when symptoms worsen
Strong background in managing patients with HF	Consults with primary care physician; facilitates consultation/referrals with specialists, admitting physician, other multidisciplinary care providers; keeps current in literature, especially medical care knowledge
Experience with computer documentation and information software programs	Enter data into database for quality initiatives and outcomes analysis; assists in measuring program and patient outcomes
Patient advocate	Assessment of patient psychosocial status and placement in appropriate programs to meet needs; patient education; vigilance monitoring for adherence to the plan of care
Clinical nurse specialist (masters prepared nurse with HF specialty)	
Project development	Program planning: task force point person; learn costs associated with current care; works within administrative rules; develops care management algorithms based on current guidelines; develops budget, data collection variables for outcomes analysis, nurse caregiver key job roles, paperwork to facilitate day-to-day operations
Educator	Educate nurse caregiver(s) in program plan and algorithm/guidelines; ongoing education for self and nurse caregiver(s) by article review, in-services, formal education
Consultant	Coordinates and participates in site visits, telephone consultation (patient and organization), and education workshops for outside organizations; develops, initiates, manages or oversees continuum of care programs
Program maintenance	Revise algorithms and guidelines to keep pace with recommended guidelines; develop new guidelines as needed; assess program quality; promote effective operations
Research	Use database to answer questions related to program effectiveness; develop prospective research questions and protocols; facilitate new technology or systems that promote time efficiencies and optimal patient outcomes

monthly meetings with staff, nurses and other key personnel. At meetings, key components of the program can be reinforced, new additions or changes can be reviewed and individuals can provide feedback on process or quality issues.

It is important to understand that organizational systems that are directly associated with the HF clinic may be inadequate to support the processes needed. During the development phase of the HF clinic, processes might require revision to facilitate the new plans of care. For example, a program-specific order sheet or care pathway that encourages patient transfer directly from the HF clinic to another setting when emergent, acute, subacute or palliative care is recommended must be associated with transfer procedures and forms devised to assist patients in recording daily weight and sodium and fluid intake for self-assessment must be associated with the education plan. The HF clinic may benefit from the purchase of new equipment; such as a waiting room TV with videotape machine, a computer with Internet access for HF education programs, point of care serum B-type natriuretic peptide testing equipment or a biothoracic impedance hemodynamic monitor that can be used in patient assessment.

A fifth element to success revolves around the notion that the HF clinic is one program in the continuum of HF care and should not be developed in isolation from other HF services or care areas. Systemization of processes among care teams and departments improves quality of care and leads to better long-term outcomes. When patients require emergent care, if is beneficial to utilize a facility in which emergency physicians treat the HF syndrome using protocols developed specifically to optimize HF diagnosis and treatment and not just manage the symptoms of decompensation. An aggressive emergency department short-stay unit program decreased early hospital recidivism in patients who were discharged from the short-stay unit to home [42]. Formalized home-based HF programs have not only decreased the frequency of unplanned hospitalizations and out-of-hospital mortality within 6 months of discharge but benefits persisted over a 4-year period, thus, decreasing costs [43,44]. The development of an inpatient management program led one group to demonstrate improvements in core HF drug use, daily weight compliance, left ventricular function assessment,

hospital costs and hospital length of stay [45]. Some continuum of care programs are depicted in Figure 6.1. When utilized to meet individual patient and general program needs, they promote close follow-up, timely interventions and aggressive effective care. While hospital or site-specific personnel can develop these HF programs independently, a well-conceived program requires HF expertise and collaboration.

Additionally, the collaborative effort between the team implementing the program and the HF specialty team must be maintained over time to ensure on-going proven efficacious therapies, since it is not expected that generalists in acute, palliative, subacute, home, emergency or other care settings will keep abreast of complex HF therapies. It is possible to have one advanced practice nurse to carry out a dual role of HF clinic nurse caregiver and disease management programs coordinator; however, nurturing and maintaining multiple programs require intermittent but regular visibility; regular review of protocols, algorithms and patient educational materials; staff educational inservices and quality improvement consultation. Separating the roles and duties will not only increase nurse visibility in the HF clinic, thereby augmenting revenue, but will also increase visibility and extend communication among other teams that provide HF services.

Before implementation: what's next?

Prior to start-up of HF clinic operations, resources and protocols must be established to track specific patient and clinical outcomes, support patient self-management, facilitate adherence to the plan of care, streamline the process of vigilance monitoring, and promote multidisciplinary services. The development of the aforementioned systems might take time and be expensive depending on the complexity and resources chosen to carry out the plan.

Data collection and analysis of patient variables over time is important if there is a need to justify program expenses, ensure the program meets pre-set clinical goals, grow the market (through advertising or promotion), or show evidence of specific quality patient outcomes. While it is a noble idea to collect data on demographics, personal and family history, diagnostic tests, quality of life measures, symptoms, functional class, pharmacotherapeutics,

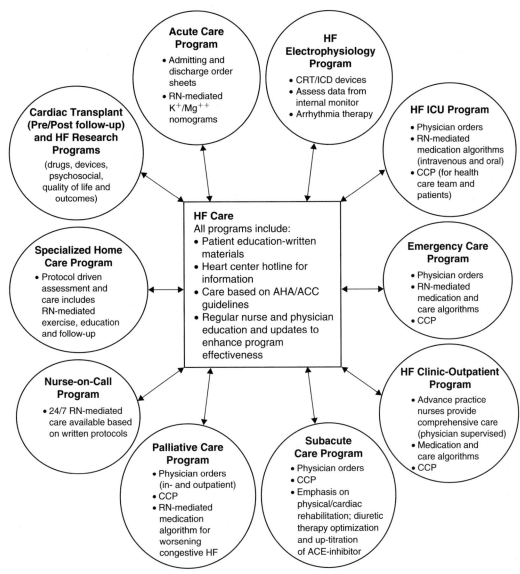

Figure 6.1 Continuum of care programs.
CCP: coordinated care pathway; CRT: cardiac resynchronization therapy; ICD: implantable cardioverter/defibrillator; RN: registered nurse.

hospitalization, office and emergency care visits, etc. over time; collection of data elements (and entry into a computer database) distances the nurse caregiver from patients, thereby decreasing patient access to the program and potential revenue. In addition, there may be data management costs and institutional review board paperwork associated with creating a useable database that can support analysis of data at many levels as well as data cleaning prior to analysis. A statistician may need to be employed every time questions are generated. In an effort to maintain a high level of clinical availability for the nurse caregiver, it is important to carefully determine exactly what variables are important to collect, simplify the data collection process (especially in regard to surveys that address psychosocial variables and quality of life) and then determine if current computer billing or medical record documentation systems can support much of (or all of) the program's data collection needs.

Prior to implementation, self-management directives need to be agreed upon by the team and then resources must be created to guide and motivate the patient and family toward behavior change. Decisions might include determining whether to have a standard or individualized response to weight gain (when to notify the team, taking extra diuretics, using fluid restriction or limiting the diet restrictions to a greater degree) or developing systems to enhance a patient's self-efficacy for carrying out specific behaviors. Plans to promote self-management may be relatively inexpensive to prepare (i.e., education materials) while others take longer to plan and implement and utilize more resources (i.e., home care, telephonic or web communication or support/education group). Ultimately, the best plans are those that have a high patient participation level and in which the ratio of cost to benefit is maximized. Again, if implementation and/or program evaluation plans involve using the nurse caregiver's time, then HF clinic activities will be compromised and program revenue will decline.

Facilitating adherence to the plan of care is no easy task since a 'one size fits all' approach will not work. Adherence is impacted by physical, economic, social, cultural, and psychological support. In addition, adherence can be strengthened or hindered by a patient's or family's self-confidence in carrying out desired behaviors, self-esteem and understanding of education that specifies the importance of carrying out specific behaviors and actions. In order for the nurse to advocate on the patient's behalf, the clinic visit must be long enough to allow time for communication. A 1-h initial visit and 30-min subsequent visits are needed to carry out usual clinic activities of physical exam and subjective patient assessment, assessment of effectiveness of current therapies, implementation of the plan of care, and provision of education. During the visit period, the nurse must also make time to re-assess patient education needs, learn about strengths and weaknesses in the patient's support system and then use interdisciplinary resources to promote or improve adherence.

Repetition in communicating education information is important and patients must understand the impact of their actions on outcome. In a study

to learn the factors that influenced knowledge and adherence of self-care in patients with HF, researchers conducted a needs assessment survey in 113 patients. While two-thirds of patients reported receiving information about self-care, only 14% of survey responders said they knew "a lot" and 37% said they knew "little to nothing". In addition, 40% of responders did not recognize the importance of limiting salt or weighing themselves [46]. Interestingly, longer duration of HF did not lead to a higher knowledge score. Patients had higher knowledge if they were hospitalized in the last year or if they received both information and advice about self-care from a doctor and a nurse [46]. These results are a reminder that knowledge does not equal adherence! In addition, the results might reflect that patients who perceive their HF condition to be "serious" (i.e., due to hospitalization) may be more open to receiving knowledge and carrying our self-care. Future research is needed to learn if there is a link between perceived seriousness of the HF condition and adherence to the plan of care.

Vigilance monitoring is used in many outpatient programs and comes in many forms. Frequent nurse-initiated telephone contact, computer communication and other means are available to assist or push patients toward carrying out appropriate behaviors. Constant two-way communication that reflects on-going support, especially in patients who are socially isolated due to age or physical disability, promotes desired outcomes. Unfortunately, the "best" form of vigilance monitoring is unknown since published reports use a variety of monitoring systems and monitoring is usually one of many interventions in a study. It is known however, that trials employing telephone contact to improve coordination of primary care services failed to find beneficial effects [47]. It is unknown if studies conducted with HF specialty teams would lead to the same results.

As discussed with data collection, on-going program development, self-management directives and vigilance monitoring are time intensive, especially if nurse-initiated or nurse-mediated. In addition, the patient becomes reliant on the nurse's advice and request for information and may not internalize behaviors without on-going support. One way to provide monitoring but *not* impact the nurses' clinic schedule to a great degree is to have a 1-800 telephone contact number for patients to call in their issues, questions, requests for advice or requests for a change in the plan of care. In this way, the patient learns to recognize important symptoms or changes reflecting worsening of condition and actively intervenes, hopefully in the early stage. Future research is needed to learn what systems work best or if any system is good as long as patient contact is regular and meaningful.

Finally, multidisciplinary services can be incorporated into the program in a direct or indirect manner. When social work, nutrition, palliative care, pharmacy, cardiac rehabilitation or other service providers offer a formalized training program, a request should be made to use their services on a regular basis in the HF clinic. Having a multidisciplinary presence in the clinic on a regular basis not only provides valuable resources for patients but also acts as a great clinical opportunity for the person in training. For HF clinics that cannot support on-site multidisciplinary personnel, services are more likely to be utilized by patients when mechanisms are put in place to facilitate timely patient assessment and intervention without requiring patients to travel a long distance or be inconvenienced to a great degree. Keeping a list of department contact people and phone numbers at close hand may assist in the consultation process. In addition, on-going communication with task force members maintains program enthusiasm and diminishes inefficiencies in daily operations.

Barriers impacting HF clinic success

A HF clinic will be viable over a long period of time only if the healthcare community supports it. There are many reasons why the phrase "if you build it, patients will come" does not hold true when implementing a HF clinic program. Table 6.3 lists specific post-implementation issues and perceived barriers that impact physician acceptance [48,49].

While the perceived barriers to sending patients for care in a HF clinic listed in Table 6.3 are false (with the exception of potential lack of survival benefit), perceptions of healthcare providers are often difficult to change. Healthcare team members must be willing to be educated and to make changes in standard processes of care. Even when physicians

verbalize benefits of sending patients to a HF clinic; such as, limited time for patient education and monitoring, little confidence in their knowledge about the complexities of HF management and lack of financial incentive to start their own HF clinic program, the physician champion and other physician supporters must provide formal education in the following areas to achieve external success: (a) current quality data that reflects specific problems with traditional care system, (b) how the HF clinic works, and (c) how the HF clinic will benefit both patients and physicians who use the service. This is a daunting task since physicians may not have the time to provide or attend more than a few educational programs and may have even less time to meet individually with the HF clinic team to receive firsthand experiences of issues and barriers that limit success.

Overcoming barriers

As already mentioned, it is difficult to change ingrained perceptions without spending time, effort and cost in on-going education, mentoring, and consultation services. Another option in gaining patient volume is to directly target patients and their families. This can be achieved through direct marketing by offering a seminar and lunch program on HF to the public. To advertise for the program, an announcement can be placed in a local newspaper or a brochure can be mailed to homes of people who are known in the community to be on a certain drug regime (i.e., beta-blockers + ACE inhibitors + diuretic). Another option is to have large posters made that can be placed on an easel or hung in a prominent place in the hallway, lobby, elevator of the local hospital(s), medical office, etc., associated with the program. In addition, one-page handouts, wallet cards or refrigerator magnets can be placed in central meeting areas of local hospital(s) (i.e., individual floor waiting rooms, cafeteria) that contain key contact information.

"Continuum of care" programs offer another avenue of referrals to a HF clinic. Case managers, social workers and other multidisciplinary service personnel can recommend the program when they consult with patients. In addition, it is possible to proactively gain patient volume by incorporating HF clinic personnel services in a continuum of care

Table 6.3 Issues and barriers to success once implemented.

Slow to gain acceptance due to	Perceived barriers
Use of algorithms, guidelines and pathways	Not all cardiologists and internal medicine practitioners are true believers in a systematized process: • Decreased ability to risk stratify patients (cookbook medicine) • Resistance to standardization of care • Oversimplification of protocols in patients with complex comorbidities • Doubt the benefit of this approach; especially if research trial patient demographics vary significantly from patient population being served
Use of nurses	• Physicians do not understand the capabilities or know the training of an advance practice nurse • Physicians do not want to give up care to a nurse • Physicians enjoy hands on practice and/or want to control decision-making • Supervising physician has a fear of miscommunication or believes there will be a lack of communication and consultation regarding patient care issues • Patient satisfaction will decrease • Fear of legal liability
Lack of provider understanding of which HF patients to refer, when to refer patients and why to refer patients to the program	• Physicians think that HF specialty referrals (and therefore a HF clinic) are for patients with an advanced condition requiring transplant evaluation or research protocols • Physicians believe that it is not the right time to refer if asymptomatic or only mild symptoms, if elderly or if patient/family does not make a request for new or aggressive therapeutic options • Patients with HF have a primary diagnosis when entering the healthcare system that is not decompensated HF (i.e., new onset atrial fibrillation or pneumonia) • Physicians believe they are optimizing care and do not need to utilize a specialty program
Political/Financial constraints	• After consultation in a HF clinic, the patient will be lost to internal medicine or general cardiology follow-up • Lack of documented patient care updates to facilitate coordination of care between teams • Fear that patient will be angry when billed for physician services but not treated by a physician • Fear that cost of care will increase and simultaneously, the patient will not see immediate benefits, causing unease in the physician–patient relationship • Insurance carrier will not pay for specialty services or more aggressive therapies • Fear of increased admissions (especially in a managed care market)
Patient and physician beliefs	• Patients believe HF comes and goes (with symptoms) and cannot understand necessity for expensive polypharmacy and lifestyle changes • Patients do not understand the seriousness of HF and do not request a second opinion or specialty services

(Continued)

Table 6.3 (*Continued*)

Slow to gain acceptance due to	Perceived barriers
	• Physicians believe a patient who is non-compliant will not benefit from program
	• Physicians may have ingrained beliefs about specific therapies and do not want to use "proven therapies" (i.e., promoting rest instead of exercise, not initiating beta-blocker therapy in functional class I or IV patients or continued use of non-steroidal anti-inflammatory agents when a patient became fluid overloaded after initiating)
	• Physicians do not see survival benefits (and therefore do not place value on the service)

program. For example, whenever a patient arrives at the local Emergency Department and does not have a primary physician who is associated with that hospital, an automatic referral can be made to a HF specialist to meet and consult on that patient's care. Before discharge from the Emergency Department, it would be expected that the physician–patient evaluation would take place. This evaluation gives continuity of follow-up care; ensures that patients who are candidates for cardiac arrhythmia and dyssynchrony devices, cardiac transplantation, or research protocols have the opportunity to receive services; and promotes optimization of medication therapies while the patient is still in the hospital [50].

Report card

Many reports of HF management models have led the Cardiovascular Roundtable, a subgroup of the Advisory Board Company members (administrators in approximately 2000 hospitals and healthcare settings in the United States), to focus on gathering data and publishing studies on progressive HF management and clinical practices. After an intensive review of specific nurse-led, cardiologist-led and case manager programs, they graded nurse-led clinic programs a B+ (effective) and cardiologist-led programs an A (very effective) on a A–C grading scale, based on the criteria listed in Table 6.4 [51,52]. Many cardiologist-led programs use nurses and other multidisciplinary team caregivers to provide expert clinical management, structured follow-up and intensive education (similar to what has been described in this chapter); thus, a cardiologist-led

management model can augment care services beyond the traditional care approach and effectively achieve improved outcomes.

Limitations

There are limitations in HF clinic program research that might impact the beneficial outcomes seen in many studies. Programs have not been powered to study mortality as an endpoint [53]. Many programs use a non-randomized, pre–post-intervention design and even when patients were randomly assigned to traditional care or disease management, some researchers had carefully selected criteria for inclusion, thereby limiting the intervention to those most likely to benefit [54]. When the patient is entered after hospitalization (no matter the assigned group), the reduction in hospitalizations and cost data post-intervention may be inflated. A better approach would be to develop a research protocol that allows post-hospitalization *and* ambulatory patients to receive the care provided in a HF clinic, then study all-comers. Many of the trials had a small sample size and selection bias (most caregivers were cardiologists, not internal medicine practitioners; patients generally had advanced HF; and minorities and women were not well represented), and only reported finding after the first 3- or 6-month post-intervention. Results from reports in the literature are confined to patients who had multiple visits and generally chose to partake and follow the plan of care. Many patients choose not to adhere to scheduled follow-up or to medication and lifestyle recommendations in a program that is not a structured clinical trial. In addition, it is still unknown if a HF clinic,

Table 6.4 Cardiovascular roundtable grading matrix for nurse-led HF programs.

Criteria	Grade	
	Nurse-led	Cardiologist-led
1 Optimizes medical care	A−	A+
2 Reduces emergency department and hospital utilization	A	A+
3 Attracts physician buy-in and referrals	B−	A+
4 Promotes patient self-management	A	A
5 Creates hospital revenue opportunities	B	B+
6 Impacts payer bottom line	C	C+
Overall grade	B+	A

Note: Grades developed after interviews with programs and dissemination of data provided from program sites. Grading score: A, very effective; B, effective; C, somewhat effective.

led by HF nurse specialists but supervised by general internists or primary care physicians would have the same impact as the programs supervised by HF specialty cardiologists.

A HF clinic as described in this chapter is reliant on a specially trained HF nurse who not only understands how to medically manage the HF condition based on AHA/ACC management guidelines, educate patients at their level of understanding and collaborate with others to optimize patient functioning, but is also able to independently carry out actions that reflect the above. The nurse must be comfortable with decision-making and take responsibility for making changes in the plan of care. An assertive approach, especially when the supervising physician does not show interest in following the recommended management guidelines, requires an open, honest physician–nurse relationship with healthy discussions and negotiations in care planning and actions. Most HF clinic research reports did not adequately describe the nurse's background except that they worked for a cardiologist service. The results of these studies may not be generalizable to different HF programs, especially when nurse suggestions for optimized care based on current evidence are abandoned by their cardiologist preceptor. Examples would be choosing to withhold ACE-inhibitor therapy in the elderly or in those with a baseline serum creatinine greater than 1.8 mg/dL but under 2.5 mg/dL, or choosing to administer intravenous outpatient inotropic or vasodilator infusions in patients whose oral therapies are not optimized.

In summary, most studies have concluded that HF clinics were effective in achieving endpoints under study, especially when the focus was multidisciplinary and utilized evidence-based practices. If programs can continuously attain recommended treatment goals and maintain patient changes over a long time period, the burden of poor prognosis and quality of life might be diminished. In addition, by attending to traditional risk factors for cardiovascular disease (sedentary lifestyle, smoking, obesity, hyperlipidemia, hypertension), HF clinic programs might reduce cardiovascular mortality, improve functional capacity and reduce the risk of myocardial ischemia and infarction.

References

1 Davis RC, Hobbs FD, Kenkre JE *et al.* Prevalence of left ventricular systolic dysfunction and heart failure in high risk patients: community based epidemiological study. *Brit Med J* 2002; **325**: 1156–1160.

2 American Heart Association. *Heart Disease and Stroke Statistics – 2004 Update.* American Heart Association, Dallas, Tex, 2003.

3 Rame JE, Sheffield MA, Dries DL *et al.* Outcomes after emergency department discharge with a primary diagnosis of heart failure. *Am Heart J* 2001; **142**: 714–719.

4 Ashton CM, Peterson NJ, Souchek J *et al.* Rates of health services utilization and survival in patients with heart failure in the Department of Veterans Affairs Medical Care System. *Am J Med Qual* 1999; **14**: 55–63.

5 MacIntyre K, Capewell S, Stewart S *et al.* Evidence of improving prognosis in heart failure. Trends in case fatality in 66,547 patients hospitalized between 1986 and 1995. *Circulation* 2000; **102**: 1126–1131.

6 Stewart S, MacIntyre K, Hole DJ *et al.* More "malignant" than cancer? Five-year survival following a first admission for heart failure. *Eur J Heart Fail* 2001; **3**: 315–322.

7 Hunt SA, Abraham WT, Chin MH *et al.* ACC/AHA 2005, guideline update for the diagnosis and management of chronic heart failure in the adult article: a report of the American College of Cardiology/American Heart Association Task Force on Practical Guidelines (Writing committee to update the 2001 Guideline for the Evaluation and Management of Heart failure). [American College of Cardiology website]. Available: http://www.acc.org/clinical/guidelines/failure/index.pdf.

8 Grady KL, Dracup K, Kennedy G *et al.* Team management of patients with heart failure. A statement for healthcare professionals from the Cardiovascular Nursing Council of the American Heart Association. *Circulation* 2000; **102**: 2443–2456.

9 Edep ME, Shah NB, Tateo IM *et al.* Differences between primary care physicians and cardiologists in management of congestive heart failure: relation to practice guidelines. *J Am Coll Cardiol* 1997; **30**: 518–526.

10 Harjai KJ, Boulos LM, Smart FW *et al.* Effects of caregiver specialty on cost and clinical outcomes following hospitalization for heart failure. *Am J Cardiol* 1998; **82**: 82–85.

11 Cintron G, Bigas C, Linares E *et al.* Nurse practitioner role in a congestive heart failure clinic: in-hospital time, costs and patient satisfaction. *Heart Lung* 1983; **12**: 237–240.

12 Block L, Fredericks LA, Moore B *et al.* The design and implementation of a disease management program for congestive heart failure at a community hospital. *Congest Heart Fail* 1997; **3(4)**: 22–28, 36–37.

13 Chapman DB, Torpy J. Development of a heart failure center: A medical center and cardiology practice join forces to improve care and reduce costs. *Am J Manag Care* 1997; **3**: 431–437.

14 Fonarow GC, Stevenson LW, Walden JA *et al.* Impact of a comprehensive heart failure management program on hospital readmission and functional status of patients with advanced heart failure. *J Am Coll Cardiol* 1997; **30**: 725–732.

15 Hanumanthu S, Butler J, Chomsky D *et al.* Effect of a heart failure program on hospitalization frequency and exercise tolerance. *Circulation* 1997; **96**: 2842–2848.

16 Hershberger RE, Ni H, Nauman DJ *et al.* Prospective evaluation of an outpatient heart failure management program. *J Card Fail* 2001; **7**: 64–74.

17 O'Connell AM, Crawford MH, Abrams J. Heart failure disease management in an indigent population. *Am Heart J* 2001; **141**: 254–258.

18 Rich MW, Beckham V, Wittenberg C *et al.* A multidisciplinary intervention to prevent the readmission of elderly patients with congestive heart failure. *N Engl J Med* 1995; **333**: 1190–1195.

19 Riegel B, Thomason T, Carlson B *et al.* Implementation of a multidisciplinary disease management program for heart failure patients. *Congest Heart Fail* 1999; **5**: 164–170.

20 Roglieri JL, Futterman R, McDonough KL *et al.* Disease management interventions to improve outcomes in congestive heart failure. *Am J Manag Care* 1997; **3**: 1831–1839.

21 Schulman KA, Mark DB, Califf RM. Outcomes and costs within a disease management program for advanced congestive heart failure. *Am Heart J* 1998; **135**: S285–S292.

22 Smith LE, Fabbri SA, Pai R *et al.* Symptomatic improvement and reduced hospitalization for patients attending a cardiomyopathy clinic. *Clin Cardiol* 1997; **20**: 949–954.

23 West JA, Miller NH, Parker KM *et al.* A comprehensive management system for heart failure improves clinical outcomes and reduces medical resource utilization. *Am J Cardiol* 1997; **79**: 58–63.

24 Whellan DJ, Gaulden L, Gattis WA *et al.* The benefit of implementing a heart failure disease management program. *Arch Intern Med* 2001; **161**: 2223–2228.

25 Phillips CO, Wright SM, Kern DE *et al.* Comprehensive discharge planning with postdischarge support for older patients with congestive heart failure. *J Am Med Assoc* 2004; **219**: 1358–1367.

26 McAlister F, Stewart S, Ferrua S, McMurray JJ. Multidisciplinary strategies for the management of heart failure patients at high risk for admission. A systematic review of randomized trials. *J Am Coll Cardiol* 2004; **44**: 810–819.

27 Galbreath AD, Krasuski RA, smith B *et al.* Long-term healthcare and cost outcomes of disease management in a large, randomized, community-based population with heart failure. *Circulation* 2004; **110**: 3518–3526.

28 Albert NM, Collier S, Sumodi V *et al.* Nurses' knowledge of heart failure education principles. *Heart Lung* 2002; **31**: 102–112.

29 Krumholz HM, Amatruda J, Smith GL *et al.* randomized trial of an education and support intervention to prevent readmission of patients with heart failure. *J Am Coll Cardiol* 2002; **39**: 83–89.

30 Bennett SJ, Hustler GA, Baker SL *et al.* Characterization of the precipitants of hospitalization for heart failure decompensation. *Am J Crit Care* 1998; **7**: 168–174.

31 Butler J, Hanumanthu S, Chomsky D *et al.* Frequency of low-risk hospital admissions for heart failure. *Am J Cardiol* 1998; **81**: 41–44.

32 Friedman MM. Older adults' symptoms and their duration before hospitalization for heart failure. *Heart Lung* 1997; **26**: 169–176.

33 Jaarsma T, Halfens RJG, Saad HH. Readmission of older heart failure patients. *Progress Cardiovasc Nurs* 1996; **11(1)**: 15–20, 48.

34 Vinson JM, Rich MW, Sperry JC *et al.* Early readmission of elderly patients with congestive heart failure. *J Am Geriatr Soc* 1990; **38**: 1290–1295.

35 McDonald K, Ledwidge M, Cahill J *et al.* Heart failure management: multidisciplinary care has intrinsic benefit above the optimization of medical care. *J Card Fail* 2002; **8**: 142–148.

36 Albert NM, Young JB. Heart failure disease management: a team approach. *Clev Clin J Med* 2001; **68**: 53–62.

37 Linder AP. *Improving Quality of Care for Californians with Heart Failure.* California Healthcare Foundation, Oakland, CA, 2002.

38 Paul S. Ask the experts. *Crit Care Nurse* 2000; **20**: 81–82.

39 Rector TS, Venus PA. Judging the value of population-based disease management. *Inquiry* 1999; **36**: 122–126.

40 Riegel B, Carlson B, Glaser D *et al.* Which patients with heart failure respond best to multidisciplinary disease management? *J Card Fail* 2000; **6**: 290–299.

41 Kerfoot KM. Bridging the knowledge-treatment gap with nurse-managed care. *Prev Med Manag Care* 2000; **1**: 91–93.

42 Peacock WF, Remer EE, Aponte J *et al.* Effective observation unit treatment of decompensated heart failure. *Congest Heart Fail* 2002; **8**: 68–73.

43 Stewart S, Pearson S, Horowitz JD. Effects of a home-based intervention among patients with congestive heart failure discharged from acute hospital care. *Arch Intern Med* 1998; **158**: 1067–1072.

44 Stewart S, Horowitz JD. Home-based intervention in congestive heart failure. Long-term implications on readmission and survival. *Circulation* 2002; **105**: 2861–2866.

45 Cooper GS, Armitage KB, Ashar B *et al.* Design and implementation of an outpatient disease management program. *Am J Manag Care* 2000; **6**: 793–801.

46 Ni H, Nauman D, Burgess D *et al.* Factors influencing knowledge of and adherence to self-care among patients with heart failure. *Arch Intern Med* 1999; **159**: 1613–1619.

47 McAlister FA, Lawson FME, Teo KK *et al.* A systematic review of randomized trials of disease management programs in heart failure. *Am J Med* 2001; **110**: 378–384.

48 Knox D, Mischke L. Implementing a congestive heart failure disease management program to decrease length of stay and cost. *J Cardiovasc Nurs* 1999; **14**: 55–74.

49 Moser D. Heart failure management: optimal health care delivery programs. In: Fitzpatrick JF & Goeppinger J, eds. *Annual Review of Nursing Research, Vol. 18. Focus: Chronic Illness.* Springer Publishing Co, New York, NY, 2000: 91–126.

50 Peacock WF, Albert NM. Observation unit management of heart failure. *Emerg Med Clin N Am* 2001; **19**: 209–232.

51 Cardiovascular Roundtable of the Advisory Board Company. CHF Management Models. Model #2. Nurse-led programs. http://www.advisory.com/members/default.asp?collectionid=188&program=2

52 Cardiovascular Roundtable of the Advisory Board Company. CHF Management Models. Model #3. Cardiologist-led programs. http://www.advisory.com/members/default.asp?collectionid=188&program=2

53 Dahlstrom U. Heart failure clinics: organization, development and experiences. *Curr Opin Cardiol* 2001; **16**: 174–179.

54 Rich MW. Heart failure disease management: a critical review. *J Card Fail* 1999; **5**: 64–75.

CHAPTER 7

Novel imaging technologies for heart failure patients

Richard D. White

Introduction

With the growing epidemic of heart failure within the aging population of the western world, cardiovascular physicians will be contending more and more with generally increasingly complex problems in generally older patients. In the future, advanced cardiac imaging modalities should offer support to heart failure specialists in their efforts to fully understand the nature and extent of disease causing heart failure, to optimize and monitor effects of their medical treatment for it, and judiciously apply cardiac catheter-based or surgical interventions when most appropriate in their patients.

MRI and MDCT scanning: attributes and limitations

Magnetic resonance imaging
Attributes
Use of magnetic resonance imaging (MRI) for assessing the cardiovascular system has gradually become more widespread over the past two decades [1]. For imaging the heart, MRI has several well-recognized advantages over other imaging modalities. Unlike other imaging modalities, including cardiac multidetector computed tomography (MDCT), MRI carries with it no risk to the patient related to exposure to either ionizing radiation or iodinated contrast materials. In addition, MRI has well-established dynamic imaging capabilities for the assessment of global chamber function, tissue perfusion, regional myocardial mechanics, and blood flow [1–5]. Capabilities for myocardial characterization were greatly improved with the introduction of the delayed-enhancement

MRI (DE-MRI) technique, requiring injection of a non-iodine-based contrast agent (e.g. Gadolinium-DTPA) [6]. With DE-MRI, acute myocardial necrosis or remote myocardial scarring is clearly depicted as high intensity (bright appearing) and, consequently, is easily distinguishable from both normal and viable-ischemic areas (dark appearing) [7].

When static "dark-blood" imaging and dynamic "bright-blood" (cine) imaging (for overall morphologic, systolic and diastolic assessment, ventricular volumetric analysis, evaluation of regional ventricular wall thickening, and detection and grading of valve dysfunction), first-pass perfusion imaging with bolus administration of MRI contrast agents (for differentiation between preserved versus delayed versus negligible myocardial perfusion), dynamic myocardial grid-tag imaging (for assessment of left ventricle (LV) myocardial mechanics), velocity phase mapping (for measurement of forward bulk flow from versus reverse bulk flow into the ventricles over the cardiac cycle) and DE-MRI (for evaluation of the regional pattern and extent of myocardial necrosis or scarring) are combined into a single examination, a comprehensive assessment of peri-cardiac and cardiac anatomy, cardiac function, and myocardial viability can be performed with or without physiologically or pharmacologically induced stress [1,8–10].

Limitations
The application of cardiovascular MRI remains limited primarily by well-recognized contraindications that are commonly found in patients with heart failure; these include implanted active permanent pacemakers or defibrillators or retained components of either, due to their potential to

become dysfunctional and/or unwanted conductors (e.g. induction of ectopy or heating capable of burning) with the rapidly changing magnetic and radio-frequency environments during the imaging process [1,11]. In addition, the presence of ventricular assist devices precludes the performance of cardiac MRI for various reasons, including the risk of magnetic attraction. Due to similar MRI safety concerns, limitations of basic life-support and physiologic-monitoring equipment in the region of the MRI scanner are considerable. Although frequently encountered, patient claustrophobia can almost always be effectively relieved with anxiolytic therapy [1].

MDCT scanning

Attributes

Widespread utilization of computed tomography (CT) for cardiac imaging had in the past been limited by the need for specialized equipment, in particular electron-beam CT [12]. With the advent of MDCT technology [13], however, true 3-dimensional sub-second electrocardiographically (ECG) gated imaging of the heart became feasible [14]. As a result, motion (cardiac and respiratory) free imaging of the cardiac chambers, valves, coronary vessels, and surrounding tissues (e.g. pericardium) over an extended range could be accomplished with helical ECG-gated MDCT within a breath-hold period. While the primary expression of ECG-gated MDCT has been static 2-dimensional or 3-dimensional displays for morphologic assessment [14,15], multi-phasic reconstructions of the same data for cine imaging (e.g. for ventricular volumetric analysis) is now possible [16,17].

Initial clinical experience at large cardiac centers indicates that for morphologic assessment of cardiac disease, contrast-enhanced ECG-gated MDCT is comparable-to-superior to MRI from the standpoint of information supplied, especially pertaining to coronary artery abnormalities [18–20]; it is clearly superior from the standpoint of ease and expedience of performance. Of course, application of ECG-gated MDCT does not suffer from the aforementioned contra-indications commonly confronting MRI in routine clinical cardiac imaging.

Limitations

Unlike MRI, contrast-enhanced ECG-gated MDCT requires the patient to be exposed to the risks from X-rays (e.g. ionizing effects of radiation) and usually from iodinated contrast materials (e.g. possible allergic reaction or renal insufficiency). Nevertheless, with proper screening (e.g. denial of contrast for creatinine levels >1.5 g/dL or substitution of Gadolinium-DTPA) [21] or pre-treatment (e.g. steroid therapy for known allergy), almost all complications from contrast administration can be avoided.

MRI and MDCT scanning: applications to heart failure

Non-ischemic heart disease

Causes of primarily diastolic heart failure

Factors extrinsic to the myocardium (e.g. pericardial disease) or intrinsic to the myocardium (e.g. infiltrative disease) may lead to the development of heart failure characterized by diastolic dysfunction [22]. The differentiation between primarily diastolic heart failure and primarily systolic heart failure, moreover the distinction between causes of diastolic dysfunction, cannot reliably accomplished based on physical examination [23]. Consequently, patients with suspected diastolic heart failure can benefit greatly from the use of MRI and/or ECG-gated MDCT, with enhanced decisions regarding their medical versus surgical management, and if surgery is warranted, regarding the procedure needed (e.g. pericardiectomy for constrictive pericarditis or cardiac transplantation for end-stage restrictive disease). Both imaging modalities can overcome the limitations of trans-thoracic echocardiography (TTE) and trans-esophageal echocardiography (TEE) in directly visualizing the entire pericardium in patients with constrictive pericarditis as the cause of diastolic heart failure. The characteristic conical/tubular deformation of the LV and right ventricle (RV) due to the surrounding abnormally constricting pericardium, along with the associated bilateral atrial dilation and venous distention (vena cavae and pulmonary veins), can be easily detected using MRI and/or ECG-gated MDCT for reliable diagnosis of constrictive pericarditis [1,24,25]. ECG-gated MDCT has the advantage over MRI of clearly defining the extent of pericardial calcification [26–29].

Dynamic MRI facilitates the important assessment of ventricular filling patterns and pericardial surface interactions. Cine imaging can reveal the late-diastolic abrupt limitation to ventricular filling due to the surrounding abnormal pericardium in constrictive pericarditis and a diastolic septal "bounce" due to the rapid equalization of ventricular pressures [1,25,29,30]. Dynamic grid-tag imaging can demonstrate tethering of the visceral pericardium on the epicardial surface with the parietal pericardium due to adhesive components which may cause impaired systolic function of the RV and/or LV, mimicking restrictive cardiomyopathy [1].

Accordingly, MRI and/or ECG-gated MDCT can be used to exclude the presence of hemodynamically significant pericardial disease in patients presenting with heart failure primarily due to diastolic dysfunction [22,23]. Characteristic findings of restrictive cardiomyopathy, such as abnormally thickened ventricular myocardium, atrial dilation, venous distention, and/or fluid collections (ascites, pleural effusions) can be easily detected using either imaging modality [1,24,25,31,32]. Again, dynamic MRI permits the appreciation of abnormally prolonged (earlier phase) or rapid but abruptly terminated (later phase) patterns of ventricular filling due to stages of restrictive pathophysiology [1,22,23]. MRI has the added advantage over ECG-gated MDCT of being capable of detecting other associated functional abnormalities (e.g. systolic dysfunction, atrioventricular valve regurgitation) [1,25], and is more comprehensive in aiding the identification of the cause of restrictive disease (e.g. hypertropic obstructive cardiomyopathy, infiltrative disease) [31,32].

When used in combination with TTE or TEE assessment of intra-cardiac hemodynamics, MRI and/or ECG-gated MDCT provide valuable morphologic or functional information leading to more optimal identification of patients with constrictive pericarditis, their differentiation from patients with restrictive cardiomyopathy, and selection and planning of surgical approaches (i.e. global pericardial involvement versus primarily affecting one pericardial region for selecting anterior versus lateral pericardiectomy approach). Consequently, the preoperative evaluation may remain entirely non-invasive, precluding the need for right-heart catheterization.

Causes of primarily systolic heart failure
While TTE and TEE are important in evaluating patients with primary systolic heart failure, even

3-dimensional forms of echocardiography may be unable to fully evaluate a markedly dilated LV chamber, including all portions of its cavity and wall. Consequently, the extent of cavity dilation or abnormal wall morphology (e.g. thinning or adherent mural thrombus) may not be appreciated. The role of TTE and TEE may then be relegated to the evaluation or the mitral and aortic valve and to basic assessments of global ventricular function.

MRI and ECG-gated MDCT can image the heart with large fields of view, unlimited by acoustic windows. Therefore, both provide the basis for complete 3-dimensional quantitative assessments of the LV for volumes and function without the need for geometric assumptions [1,33]. MRI remains the more established of the two imaging modalities in this pursuit, with proven high reproducibility [1,34–36].

Cine MRI, in particular, has been shown to be useful in the evaluation of patients with dilated cardiomyopathy. This technique has been validated for the quantification of cavity volumes and ejection fractions of the LV and RV, LV mass, LV wall stress, and associated atrioventricular valve regurgitation [1,2,35,37–39]. It has been shown using cine MRI that, despite increase in LV mass due to eccentric hypertrophy, peak and end-systolic wall stress are significantly increased in patients with dilated cardiomyopathy [2,38]. Due to these capabilities, cine MRI has been used to monitor positive responses of LV volumes, ejection fraction, and wall stress to medical therapy [40].

Regional systolic function in dilated cardiomyopathy has been assessed using dynamic MRI. Loss in the normal increasing gradient of wall thickening from base to apex has been demonstrated using short-axis cine MRI [2]. On the other hand, the normal inverse relationship between regional ejection fraction and end-systolic wall stress from base to apex was shown to be maintained in dilated cardiomyopathy, although end-systolic wall stress was found to be higher than normal at all levels [41]. Dynamic myocardial grid-tag imaging has been used to estimate the extent of fiber and cross-fiber shortening in the LV in patients with dilated cardiomyopathy compared to normals; although the normal transition in fiber orientation and dependence on cross-fiber shortening in the endocardium was found to be maintained in dilated cardiomyopathy, fiber shortening was found to be markedly reduced [42].

In patients with dilated cardiomyopathy and studied with dynamic MRI before and following partial left ventriculectomy, the beneficial effects on clinical outcome of the presence of baseline septal stretching (positive strain) followed by post-surgical contraction (negative strain) on myocardial grid-tag imaging, suggesting a "contractile reserve", was demonstrated [43]. Again using dynamic myocardial grid-tag imaging, further reduction in the already impaired baseline LV twist after partial left ventriculectomy was shown, indicating that improved LV function was not reflective of improvement in this measure of myocardial mechanics [44].

On dynamic myocardial grid-tag imaging, baseline abnormal regional myocardial strains (e.g. reduced circumferential shortening and abnormally directed increased short-axis lengthening) in severe mitral regurgitation without evidence of dilated cardiomyopathy (e.g. normal LV ejection fraction) have been shown to persist after mitral valve repair [45].

Recently, the ability of DE-MRI to identify patterns of myocardial scarring characteristic of non-ischemic causes (e.g. myocarditis) of dilated cardiomyopathy has been recognized [46,47].

Ischemic heart disease
Cardiac consequences of myocardial infarction

As with non-ischemic heart disease, LV volumes and ejection fraction can be accurately measured in the setting of ischemic heart disease using MRI and/or ECG-gated MDCT, with the aforementioned relative advantages and disadvantages; this becomes particularly useful in patients with heart failure due to chronic ischemic heart disease (CIHD) [1,10,48–50]. Both global and regional LV wall thinning and dysfunction due to CIHD can be assessed using these imaging modalities [1,16,17, 51,52]. As well as dimensions, the characteristic location and configuration of a post-myocardial infarction (MI) aneurysm (typically antero-apical and broad based) [1,10,49] or pseudo-aneurysm (typically inferior and narrow necked) [1,53,54] of the LV can be easily delineated using either MRI and/or ECG-gated MDCT. Both complications predispose to intracavitary LV thrombus formation which can be detected by either imaging modality [1,10,53–56].

Mitral regurgitation due to ischemic changes affecting the LV can be semi-quantitatively assessed in a manner similar to that of TTE and TEE based on jet appearance [1,10,57] or quantitated volumetrically based on cine series and velocity phase maps [1,10,58].

Improved regional function following post-MI LV antero-apical aneurysmectomy has been demonstrated (Figure 7.1). Lengthening strain (representing ability of LV to thicken) increased significantly in the base and middle portions of the LV, especially in the inferior wall, while shortening strain (representing ability of LV to circumferentially shorten) did not change 6 weeks after linear repair with septal exclusion surgery [59].

Myocardial revascularization

Contrast-enhanced ECG-gated MDCT is the basis for coronary CT angiography (CTA). The sensitivity and specificity of coronary CTA for the detection of luminal stenosis >50% in comparison to selective coronary angiography have both continued to increase with improvements in technology [60–64]. However, although coronary CTA is currently limited in its ability to provide accurate measures of degree stenosis, it can differentiate between sub-total/total occlusion and normal/insignificantly narrowed conditions. Therefore, it can be used in a complementary diagnostic role to assess the status of a major epicardial coronary arterial segment beyond a high-grade lesion being considered to receive improved flow by either an interventional procedure or surgical bypass grafting. In addition, contrast-enhanced ECG-gated MDCT data sets simultaneously provide information about other cardiac structures, such as the myocardium of the LV, thereby offering insights into the direct relationship between the status of the coronary artery and the condition of the dependent myocardial region not offered by conventional angiography/ventriculography.

Exciting evidence of the ability of coronary CTA to identify and characterize early changes of atherosclerosis, prior to the onset of flow-limiting stenosis, is also emerging [65]. Coronary CTA has been shown to be able to detect and characterize non-calcified atherosclerotic plaques [20,66–69]. When compared to coronary intravascular ultrasound for the differentiation between atherosclerotic coronary

(a) (b)

(c) (d)

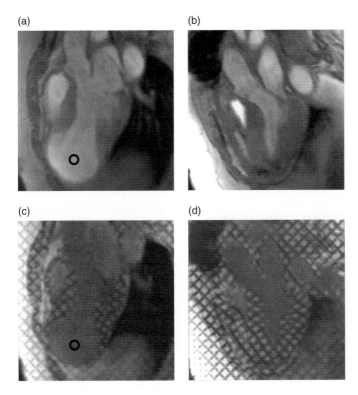

Figure 7.1 Improved LV function with successful antero-apical LV aneurysmectomy. Dynamic "bright-blood" and dynamic myocardial grid-tag MRI before (a, c) and after (b, d) LV aneurysmectomy shows improved LV morphology from obliteration of the aneurysm (circles), along with increased overall function.

plaque components it has demonstrated sufficiently different attenuation levels between them to permit their identification on coronary CTA. In addition, positive coronary arterial remodeling in the absence of stenosis-producing plaque, a combination associated with the development of acute coronary syndromes [70,71], can be successfully evaluated using coronary CTA.

The determination of the extent of LV myocardial necrosis and related dysfunction is important in managing patients with CIHD with heart failure. Even if only small amounts of residual viable myocardium are present, revascularization can be beneficial, with improvement in LV function or survival [72]. Current methods for evaluating viability include dobutamine stress echocardiography, single photon emission CT, and positron emission tomography; each has different accuracies in different clinical scenarios [73]. The major limitation with these modalities relates to their inability to directly detect and quantitate non-transmural myocardial necrosis or scarring. Consequently, the fact that an ischemic region is slightly scarred and potentially less responsive to revascularization or the fact

that a thinned and dysfunctional region with significant scarring contains some residual viable myocardium might go unappreciated with these modalities. This important insight can now be provided by MRI, especially when the DE-MRI technique is utilized to delineate myocardial necrosis or scarring [7,10]. An inverse correlation between the amount of myocardial scarring on non-stress DE-MRI and the probability of improved resting function after revascularization for both relatively intact LV function [74] and significant LV dysfunction [75] has been shown; in both settings, >50% scarring per segment indicated a very low likelihood of functional improvement of the segment with revascularizaration. Using cine MRI alone, LV end-diastolic wall thickness thresholds for high likelihood (65% of segments at >15 mm) and low likelihood (4% of segments at <6 mm) of functional improvement after revascularization have been reported [76].

With MRI myocardial-viability maps combining several imaging techniques, the relationship between the pattern and extent of LV myocardial scarring (by DE-MRI), LV end-diastolic wall thickness and

(a)   (b)

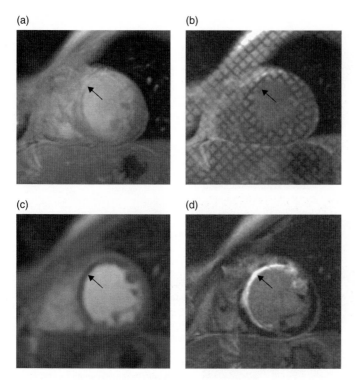

(c)   (d)

Figure 7.2 MRI myocardial-viability map. The MRI myocardial-viability map demonstrates abnormalities in LV end-diastolic wall thickness and regional wall thickening by dynamic "bright-blood" MRI (a), systolic mechanics of the LV myocardium by dynamic myocardial grid-tag MRI (b), LV myocardial perfusion by ultrafast first-pass perfusion MRI (c), and myocardial histology by DE-MRI (d) at rest in a CIHD patient. In this case, evidence of transmural MI (arrows) in the distribution of the left anterior descending coronary artery is shown.

regional wall thickening (by cine MRI), LV myocardial perfusion (by ultrafast first-pass perfusion MRI), and systolic mechanics of the LV myocardium (by dynamic myocardial grid-tag MRI), at rest or with induced stress, can be directly assessed in a CIHD patient during the planning of revascularization (Figure 7.2) [1,10]. The combination of results from the different MRI techniques provides more accurate identifiers of viable versus scarred myocardium and predictors of functional improvement with intervention or surgery [77–79].

Integrated imaging, using MDCT-derived coronary CTA and MRI-derived myocardial-viability maps, can non-invasively provide information about the morphologic and physiologic significance of obstructive and non-obstructive atherosclerotic coronary artery lesions. Lesion characteristics (e.g. severity of stenosis, plaque composition, and remodeling) and the condition of the coronary artery distal to the lesion (e.g. presence or absence of collaterals beyond an occlusive lesion) can be assessed in relation to the size and distribution of the resulting myocardial damage [10,80].

By visual cross-referencing of coronary CTA images and the corresponding myocardial-viability map in a coronary artery disease/CIHD patient, transmural MI in the distribution of an occluded and non-collateral-reconstituted epicardial coronary artery can be easily distinguished from a non-transmural MI in the distribution of an occluded but collateral-reconstituted epicardial artery (Figure 7.3) [10,80]. Thus, the situation where no revascularization is warranted (i.e. totally scarred myocardium) despite the satisfactory status of the distal coronary segment (i.e. patent distally) can be distinguished from the situation where revascularization is justified (i.e. residual viable myocardium and patent distal artery) [10,80]. In addition, diffuse reversible myocardial changes (e.g. hibernation) in a dilated LV may be attributed to coronary artery disease by visualized diffuse vascular disease of the coronary arteries and differentiated from non-ischemic dilated cardiomyopathy by absence of evidence of significant coronary atherosclerosis.

In an effort to link myocardial segments to known coronary arterial topography as defined by coronary angiography, the American Heart Association introduced a 17-segment model of the LV for standardized description applicable to all cardiac imaging modalities, including CT and MRI [81]; by this

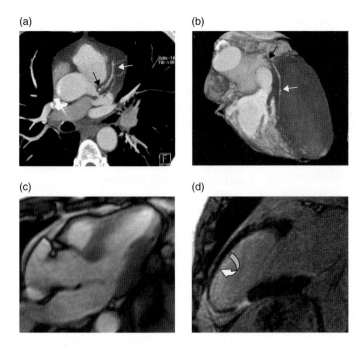

Figure 7.3 Integrated use of coronary CTA and myocardial-viability map. Non-transmural MI (curved arrow) beyond a proximally occluded (black arrows) but collateral-reconstituted (white arrows) left anterior descending coronary artery is shown on coronary CTA (a, b), dynamic "bright-blood" (c), and DE (d) MRI.

model, each myocardial segment is assigned to one of the three major coronary arteries. However, the assignment of coronary artery supply to LV regions remains empiric, based on population studies of patterns, and may not pertain to individual patients [80]. Therefore, the diagnostic evaluation and/or treatment planning in patients with coronary artery disease/CIHD has continued to rely on the following: (1) imaging assessments of myocardial viability by contrast-enhanced X-ray or nuclear ventriculography, TTE or TEE, nuclear myocardial tomography, contrast-enhanced CT, or MRI; (2) assessment of coronary artery anatomy by selective coronary angiography; and (3) mental fusion of information from (1) and (2), often by a non-imager planning revascularization [80]. However, high-spatial-resolution, static 3-dimensional or dynamic 2-dimensional co-registered displays of coronary CTA and myocardial-viability data are now possible. Such co-registered displays permit establishment of the direct spatial relationship between a specific coronary artery system anatomy and specific myocardial regions of the LV under consideration for treatment in an individual patient [82]. Consequently, additional insights about the appropriateness of and/or approach to revascularization of specific myocardial regions can be provided to the interventional cardiologist or to the cardiac surgeon.

Following interventional or surgical procedures to improve myocardial perfusion, both coronary MRI (including angiographic forms) and MDCT-based coronary CTA can be used for the non-invasive assessment of bypass grafts. For both imaging modalities, patency or occlusion of grafts can be established by the presence or absence of contrast enhancement, respectively [1,83–86]; because of their relatively larger size compared to internal mammary artery grafts, venous aortocoronary grafts can also be evaluated for degree of stenosis. MRI has the advantage of allowing measurements of flow velocity within a coronary artery bypass graft.

While the metallic mesh of coronary artery stents may limit confident grading of in-stent restenosis with MRI- or MDCT-derived CTA, determination of stent patency, and occlusion is usually possible [87–90].

Conclusion

MRI and ECG-gated MDCT are uniquely well suited to evolve into "front line" diagnostic tools for the assessment of the wide range of issues that confront cardiovascular physicians in their caring for patients suffering from heart failure.

Acknowledgment

The author wishes to express appreciation to his advanced imaging colleagues of the Cleveland Clinic Foundation (Drs. A. Stillman, R. Setser, S. Halliburton, P. Schoenhagen) and of Siemens Medical Solutions [MR Division (Chicago, IL and Malvern, PA): Drs. O. Simonetti, J. Bundy; Corporate Research (Princeton, NJ): Dr. T. O'Donnell; CT Division (Forchheim, Germany): Drs. B. Ohnesorge, T. Flohr] for their scientific support.

References

1 Schvartzman PR, White RD. Magnetic resonance imaging. In: Topol EJ, ed. *Textbook of Cardiovascular Medicine*, 2nd edn. Lippincott-Williams and Wilkins, Philadelphia, PA, 2002: 1213–1256.

2 Wagner S, Auffermann W, Buser P et al. Functional description of the left ventricle in patients with volume overload, pressure overload, and myocardial disease using cine magnetic resonance imaging. *Am J Cardiac Imag* 1991; **5**: 87–97.

3 Wilke N, Jerosch-Herold M, Zenovich A et al. Magnetic resonance first-pass myocardial perfusion imaging: clinical validation and future applications. *J Magn Reson Imag* 1999; **10**: 676–685.

4 Reichek N. MRI myocardial tagging. *J Magn Reson Imag* 1999; **10**: 609–616.

5 Lotz J, Meier C, Leppert A et al. Cardiovascular flow measurement with phase-contrast MR imaging: basic facts and implementation. *Radiographics* 2002; **22**: 651–671.

6 Simonetti OP, Kim RJ, Fieno DS et al. An improved MR imaging technique for the visualization of myocardial infarction. *Radiology* 2001; **218**: 215–223.

7 Kim RJ, Fieno DS, Parrish TB et al. Relationship of MRI delayed contrast enhancement to irreversible injury, infarct age, and contractile function. *Circulation* 1999; **100**: 1992–2002.

8 Reeder SB, Du YP, Lima JAC et al. Advanced cardiac MR imaging of ischemic heart disease. *Radiographics* 2001; **21**: 1047–1074.

9 Warren WP, Lima JAC. Cardiac MRI: where are we? *ACC Curr J Rev* 2001; September/October Issue: 35–41.

10 White RD. MR and CT assessment for ischemic cardiac disease. *J Magn Reson Imag* 2004; **19**: 659–675.

11 Shellock FG. *Reference Manual for Magnetic Resonance Safety, Implants, and Devices*, 2005 edn. Biomedical Research Publishing Group, Los Angeles, CA, 2004.

12 Lipton MJ, Higgins CB, Farmer D et al. Cardiac imaging with a high speed cine-CT scanner: preliminary results. *Radiology* 1984; **152**: 579–582.

13 Klingenbeck-Regn K, Schaller S, Flohr T et al. Subsecond multi-slice computed tomography: basics and applications. *Eur J Radiol* 1999; **31**: 110–124.

14 Klingenbeck-Regn K, Flohr T, Ohnesorge B et al. Strategies for cardiac CT imaging. *Int J Cardiovasc Imag* 2002; **18**: 143–151.

15 Cline H, Coulam C, Yavuz M et al. Coronary artery angiography using multislice computed tomography images. *Circulation* 2000; **102**: 1589–1590.

16 Hundt W, Siebert K, Wintersperger BJ et al. Assessment of global left ventricular function: comparison of cardiac multidetector-row computed tomography with angiography. *J Comput Assist Tomo* 2005; **29**: 373–381.

17 Koyama Y, Mochizuki T, Higaki J. Computed tomography assessment of myocardial perfusion, viability, and function. *J Magn Reson Imag* 2004; **19**: 800–815.

18 Kopp AF, Schroeder S, Kuettner A et al. Coronary arteries: retrospectively ECG-gated multi-detector row CT angiography with selective optimization of the image reconstruction window. *Radiology* 2001; **221**: 683–688.

19 Nieman K, Cademartiri F, Lemos PA et al. Reliable non-invasive coronary angiography with fast submillimeter multislice spiral computed tomography. *Circulation* 2002; **106**: 2051–2054.

20 Schoenhagen P, Halliburton SS, Stillman AE et al. Noninvasive imaging of coronary arteries: current and future role of multi-detector row CT. *Radiology* 2004; **232**: 7–17.

21 Remy-Jardin M, Dequiedt P, Ertzbischoff O et al. Safety and effectiveness of gadolinium-enhanced multi-detector row spiral CT angiography of the chest: preliminary results in 37 patients with contra-indications to iodinated contrast agents. *Radiology* 2005; **235**: 819–826.

22 Zile MR, Brutsaert DL. New concepts in diastolic dysfunction and diastolic heart failure: Part I. *Circulation* 2002; **105**: 1387–1393.

23 Zile MR, Brutsaert DL. New concepts in diastolic dysfunction and diastolic heart failure: Part II. *Circulation* 2002; **105**: 1503–1508.

24 Masui T, Finck S, Higgins CB. Constrictive pericarditis and restrictive cardiomyopathy: evaluation with MR imaging. *Radiology* 1992; **182**: 369–373.

25 Frank H, Globits S. Magnetic resonance imaging evaluation of myocardial and pericardial disease. *J Magn Reson Imag* 1999; **10**: 617–626.

26 Suchet IB, Horwitz TA. CT tuberculous constrictive pericarditis. *J Comput Assist Tomo* 1992; **16**: 391–400.

27 Olson MC, Posniak HV, McDonald V et al. Computed tomography and magnetic resonance imaging of the pericardium. *Radiographics* 1989; **9**: 633–649.

28 Breen JF. Imaging of the pericardium. *J Thorac Imag* 2001; **16**: 47–54.

29 Wang ZJ, Reddy GP, Gotway MB *et al.* CT and MR imaging of pericardial disease. *Radiographics* 2003; **23**: S167–S180.

30 Francone M, Dymarkowski S, Kalantzi M *et al.* Real-time cine MRI of ventricular septal motion: a novel approach to assess ventricular coupling. *J Magn Reson Imag* 2005; **21**: 305–309.

31 Soler R, Rodriguez E, Remuinan C *et al.* Magnetic resonance imaging of primary cardiomyopathies. *J Comput Assist Tomo* 2003; **27**: 724–734.

32 Schulz-Menger J, Friedrich MG. Magnetic resonance imaging in patients with cardiomyopathies: when and why. *Herz* 2000; **25**: 384–391.

33 Dulce MC, Mostbeck GH, Friese KK *et al.* Quantitation of the left ventricular volumes and function with cine MRI: comparison of geometric models and three-dimensional data. *Radiology* 1993; **188**: 371–376.

34 Semelka RC, Tomei E, Wagner S *et al.* Normal left ventricular dimensions and function: interstudy reproducibility of measurements with cine MR imaging. *Radiology* 1990; **174**: 763–768.

35 Semelka RC, Tomei E, Wagner S *et al.* Interstudy reproducibility of dimensional and functional measurements between cine magnetic resonance studies in the morphologically abnormal left ventricle. *Am Heart J* 1990; **119**: 1367–1373.

36 Pattynama PMT, Lamb HJ, van der Velde EO *et al.* Left ventricular measurements with cine and spin-echo MRI imaging: a study of reproducibility with variance component analysis. *Radiology* 1993; **187**: 261–268.

37 Strohm O, Schulz-Menger J, Pilz B *et al.* Measurement of left ventricular dimensions and function in patients with dilated cardiomyopathy. *J Magn Reson Imag* 2001; **13**: 367–371.

38 Auffermann W, Wagner S, Holt WW *et al.* Noninvasive determination of left ventricular output and wall stress in volume overload and in myocardial disease by cine magnetic resonance imaging. *Am Heart J* 1991; **121**: 1750–1758.

39 Prasad SK, Kotwinski P, Assomul R. The role of cardiovascular magnetic resonance in the evaluation of patients with heart failure. *Expert Rev Cardiovasc Ther* 2004; **2**: 53–59.

40 Doherty NE, Seelos KC, Suzuki JI *et al.* Application of cine NMR imaging for sequential evaluation of response to angiotensin-converting enzyme inhibitor therapy in dilated cardiomyopathy. *J Am Coll Cardiol* 1992; **19**: 1294–1302.

41 Fujita N, Duerinckx AJ, Higgins CB. Variation in left ventricular regional wall stress with cine magnetic resonance imaging: normal subjects versus dilated cardiomyopathy. *Am Heart J* 1993; **125**: 1337–1345.

42 McGowan GA, Shapiro EP, Azhari H *et al.* Non-invasive measurement of shortening in the fibre and cross fibre directions in the normal human left ventricle and idiopathic dilated cardiomyopathy. *Circulation* 1997; **96**: 535–541.

43 Setser RM, White RD, McCarthy PM *et al.* Noninvasive assessment of cardiac mechanics and clinical outcome after partial ventriculectomy. *Ann Thorac Surg* 2003; **76**: 1576–1585.

44 Setser RM, Kasper JM, Lieber M *et al.* Persistent abnormal left ventricular systolic torsion in dilated cardiomyopathy after partial left ventriculectomy. *J Thorac Cardiovasc Surg* 2003; **126**: 48–55.

45 Mankad R, McCreery CJ, Rogers Jr WJ *et al.* Regional myocardial strain before and after mitral valve repair for sever mitral regurgitation. *J Cardiovasc Magn Reson* 2001; **3**: 257–266.

46 Hunold P, Schlosser T, Vogt FM *et al.* Myocardial late enhancement in contrast-enhanced cardiac MRI: distinction between infarction scar and non-infarction-related disease. *Am J Roentgenol* 2005; **184**: 1420–1426.

47 Dill T, Ekinci O, Hansel J *et al.* Delayed contrast-enhanced magnetic resonance imaging for the detection of autoimmune myocarditis and long-term follow-up. *J Cardiovasc Magn Reson* 2005; **7**: 521–523.

48 Halliburton SS, Petersilka M, Schvartzman PR *et al.* Evaluation of left ventricular dysfunction using multiphasic reconstructions of coronary multi-slice computed tomography data in patients with chronic ischemic heart disease: validation against cine magnetic resonance imaging. *Int J Cardiovasc Imaging* 2003; **19**: 73–83.

49 Buck T, Hunold P, Wentz KU *et al.* Tomographic three-dimensional echocardiographic determination of chamber size and systolic function in patients with left ventricular aneurysm: comparison to magnetic resonance imaging, cine ventriculography, and two-dimensional echocardiography. *Circulation* 1997; **96**: 4286–4297.

50 Konermann M, Sanner BM, Horstmann E *et al.* Changes of the left ventricle after myocardial infarction: estimation with cine magnetic resonance imaging during the first six months. *Clin Cardiol* 1997; **20**: 201–212.

51 Pflugfelder PW, Sechtem UP, White RD *et al.* Quantification of regional myocardial function by rapid cine MR imaging. *Am J Roentgenol* 1988; **150**: 523–529.

52 Baer FM, Smolarz K, Jungehulsing M *et al.* Chronic myocardial infarction: assessment of morphology, function, and perfusion by gradient-echo magnetic resonance imaging and 99mTc-methoxyisobutyl-isonitrile-SPECT. *Am Heart J* 1992; **123**: 636–645.

53 Duvernoy O, Wikstrom G, Mannting F *et al.* Pre- and post-operative CT and MR in pseudoaneurysms of the heart. *J Comp Assist Tomo* 1992; **16**: 401–409.

54 Kahn J, Fisher MR. MRI of cardiac pseudoaneurysm and other complications of myocardial infarction. *Magn Reson Imag* 1991; **9**: 159–164.

55 Sechtem U, Theissen P, Heindel W *et al.* Diagnosis of left ventricular thrombi by magnetic resonance imaging and comparison with angiocardiography, computed tomography, and echocardiography. *Am J Cardiol* 1989; **64**: 1195–1199.

56 Selvanayagam JB, Spyrou N, Francis JM *et al.* Resolution of ventricular thrombus identified by contrast enhanced cardiac MRI. *Int J Cardiovasc Imaging* 2004; **20**: 369–370.

57 van der Wall EE, de Roos A, van Voorthuisen AE *et al.* Magnetic resonance imaging: a new approach for evaluating coronary artery disease. *Am Heart J* 1991; **121**: 1203–1220.

58 Sechtem U, Pflugfelder PW, Cassidy MM *et al.* Mitral or aortic regurgitation: quantification of regurgitant volumes with cine MR imaging. *Radiology* 1988; **167**: 425–430.

59 Kramer CM, Magovern JA, Rogers WJ *et al.* Reverse remodeling and improved regional function after repair of left ventricular aneurysm. *J Thorac Cardiovasc Surg* 2002; **124**: 700–706.

60 Hoffmann U, Moselewski F, Cury RC *et al.* Predictive value of 16-slice multidetector spiral computed tomography to detect significant obstructive coronary artery disease in patients at high risk for coronary artery disease: patient- versus segment-based analysis. *Circulation* 2004; **110**: 2638–2643.

61 Moon JY, Chung N, Choi BW *et al.* The utility of multidetector row spiral CT for detection of coronary artery stenoses. *Yonsei Med J* 2005; **46**: 86–94.

62 Dorgelo J, Willems TP, Geluk CA *et al.* Multidetector computed tomography-guided treatment strategy in patients with non-ST elevation acute coronary syndromes: a pilot study. *Eur Radiol* 2005; **15**: 708–713.

63 Dirksen MS, Jukema JW, Bax JJ *et al.* Cardiac multidetector-row computed in patients with unstable angina. *Am J Cardiol* 2005; **95**: 457–461.

64 Kuettner A, Beck T, Drosch T *et al.* Diagnostic accuracy of noninvasive coronary imaging using 16-detector slice spiral computed tomography with 188 ms temporal resolution. *J Am Coll Cardiol* 2005; **45**: 123–127.

65 Libby P. Current concepts of the pathogenesis of the acute coronary syndromes. *Circulation* 2001; **104**: 365–372.

66 Becker CR, Knez A, Ohnesorge B *et al.* Imaging of noncalcified coronary plaques using helical CT with retrospective EKG gating. *Am J Roentgenol* 2000; **175**: 423–424.

67 Schroeder S, Kopp AF, Baumbach A *et al.* Non-invasive detection and evaluation of atherosclerotic plaque with multi-slice computed tomography. *J Am Coll Cardiol* 2001; **37**: 1430–1435.

68 Schroeder S, Kopp A, Baumbach A *et al.* Non-invasive characterization of coronary lesion morphology by multi-slice computed tomography: a promising new technology for risk stratification of patients with coronary artery disease. *Heart* 2001; **85**: 576–577.

69 Fayad ZA, Fuster V, Nikolaou K *et al.* Computed tomography and magnetic resonance imaging for noninvasive coronary angiography and plaque imaging: current and potential future concepts. *Circulation* 2002; **106**: 2026– 2034.

70 Schoenhagen P, Tuzcu EM, Stillman AE *et al.* Noninvasive assessment of plaque morphology and remodeling in mildly stenotic coronary segments: comparison of 16-slice computed tomography and intravascular ultrasound. *Coronary Artery Dis* 2003; **14**: 459–462.

71 Achenbach S, Moselewski F, Ropers D *et al.* Detection of calcified and noncalcified coronary atherosclerotic plaque by contrast-enhanced, submillimeter multidetector spiral computed tomography: a segment-based comparison with intravascular ultrasound. *Circulation* 2004; **109**: 14–17.

72 Alderman EL, Fisher LD, Litwin P *et al.* Results of coronary artery surgery in patients with poor left ventricular function (CASS). *Circulation* 1983; **68**: 785–795.

73 Bonow RO. Identification of viable myocardium. *Circulation* 1996; **94**: 2674–2680.

74 Kim RJ, Wu E, Rafael A *et al.* The use of contrast-enhanced magnetic resonance imaging to identify reversible myocardial dysfunction. *N Engl J Med* 2000; **343**: 1445–1453.

75 Schvartzman PR, Srichai MB, Grimm RA *et al.* Nonstress delayed-enhancement magnetic resonance imaging of the myocardium predicts improvement of function after revascularization for chronic ischemic heart disease with left ventricular dysfunction. *Am Heart J* 2003; **146**: 535–541.

76 Klow NE, Smith HJ, Gullestad L *et al.* Outcome of bypass surgery in patients with chronic ischemic left ventricular dysfunction: predictive value of MR imaging. *Acta Radiol* 1997; **38**: 76–82.

77 Wintersperger BJ, Penzkofer HV, Knez A *et al.* Multislice MR perfusion imaging and regional myocardial function analysis: complimentary findings in chronic myocardial ischemia. *Int J Cardiac Imag* 1999; **15**: 425–434.

78 Lauerma K, Niemi P, Hanninen H *et al.* Multimodality MR imaging assessment of myocardial viability: combination of first-pass and late contrast enhancement to wall motion dynamics and comparison with FDG PET – Initial experience. *Radiology* 2000; **217**: 729–736.

79 Sensky PR, Jivan A, Hudson NM *et al.* Coronary artery disease: combined stress MR imaging protocol: one-stop evaluation of myocardial perfusion and function. *Radiology* 2000; **215**: 608–614.

80 White RD, Setser RM. Integrated approach to evaluating coronary artery disease and ischemic heart disease. *Am J Cardiol* 2002; **90**: 49L–55L.

81 Cerqueira MD, Weissman NJ, Dilsizian V *et al.* Standardized myocardial segmentation and nomenclature for

tomographic imaging of the heart: a statement for health-care professionals from the Cardiac Imaging Committee of the Council on Clinical Cardiology of the American Heart Association. *Circulation* 2002; **105**: 539–542.

82 Setser RM, O'Donnell TP, Smedira NG *et al.* Co-registered MRI myocardial viability maps and MDCT coronary angiogram displays and surgical revascularization planning: initial experience. *Radiology* 2005 (in press).

83 Bunce NH, Lorenz CH, John AS *et al.* Coronary artery bypass graft patency: assessment with true fast imaging with steady-state precession versus gadolinium-enhanced MR angiography. *Radiology* 2003; **227**: 440–446.

84 Stauder NI, Schuele AM, Hahn U *et al.* Perioperative monitoring of flow and patency in native and grafted internal mammary arteries using combined MR protocol. *Br J Radiol* 2005; **78**: 292–298.

85 Schlosser T, Konorza T, Hunold P *et al.* Noninvasive visualization of coronary artery bypass grafts using 16-detector row computed tomography. *J Am Coll Cardiol* 2004; **44**: 1238–1240.

86 Gurevitch J, Gasper T, Orlov B *et al.* Noninvasive evaluation of arterial grafts with newly released multidetector computed tomography. *Ann Thorac Surg* 2003; **76**: 1523–1527.

87 Sardanelli F, Zandrino F, Molinari G *et al.* MR evaluation of coronary stents with navigator echo and breath-hold cine gradient echo techniques. *Eur Radiol* 2002; **12**: 193–200.

88 Amano Y, Ishihara M, Hayashi H *et al.* Metallic artifacts of coronary and iliac arteries stents in MR angiography and contrast-enhanced CT. *Clin Imag* 1999; **23**: 85–89.

89 Gillard M, Cornily JC, Rioufol G *et al.* Noninvasive assessment of left main coronary stent patency with 16-slice computed tomography. *Am J Cardiol* 2005; **95**: 110–112.

90 Hong C, Chrysant GS, Woodard PK *et al.* Coronary artery stent patency assessed with in-stent contrast enhancement measured at multi-detector row CT angiography: initial experience. *Radiology* 2004; **233**: 286–291.

CHAPTER 8

Assessment of myocardial viability in ischemic cardiomyopathy

Raymond Q. Migrino

Coronary artery disease (CAD) remains the leading cause of mortality in the USA, and mortality rates are higher in patients with severely depressed left ventricular function [1,2]. Following acute myocardial infarction (MI), left ventricular enlargement is one of the strongest predictors of short-term and long-term mortality (Figure 8.1) [3]. Left ventricular dysfunction may be regional or global. It is important to distinguish whether myocardial segments that appear non-contractile or severely dysfunctional are viable (hibernating or stunned myocardium) or non-viable (scar or infarct). Revascularization may restore function in the former but not in the latter. The prevalence of viable myocardium in the setting of CAD is not well-established. In MI patients, up to 50% may have hibernating tissue mixed with scar tissue. Functional recovery of dysfunctional myocardial segments following surgical revascularization varies from 24% to 82% [4–6]. Assessing myocardial viability is important in identifying patients and coronary territories amenable to revascularization.

The spectrum of viable myocardium in CAD includes normal, ischemic or hibernating myocardium. The absence of viable myocardium, on the other hand, indicates scar or infarct. Normal myocardium has normal function at rest with augmentation following stress, as well as normal resting coronary flow and flow reserve. Ischemic myocardium may have normal or mildly decreased function at rest but function decreases with stress. The corresponding coronary flow may be normal or mildly diminished at rest, but coronary flow reserve is impaired. Hibernating myocardium is

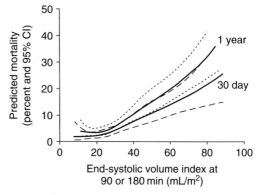

Figure 8.1 A model of the relationship between end-systolic volume index and 30-day and 1-year mortality in acute MI patients undergoing thrombolytic therapy. Reprinted from [3] with permission.

functionally impaired, but viability is evidenced by presence of contractile reserve, metabolic or electrical activity, and improvement in function following revascularization.

The surgical practice of revascularizing all stenotic arteries that are amenable to coronary bypass regardless of the contractile state of the myocardium led to interesting observations in the 1970s and 1980s that previously dysfunctional myocardium improves after bypass surgery [4,7–9]. Diamond *et al.* [10] and Rahimtoola [11] framed this phenomenon using the concept of "hibernating myocardium" which was originally defined as chronic, reversible left ventricular dysfunction due to CAD. Hibernating myocardium implies a state in which myocyte viability is present despite evidence of diminished function as manifested by absence or severe diminution of contractile function. The viability of myocytes is demonstrated by improvement or return of function after revascularization. The features that are consistent with hibernating myocardium are perfusion–contraction matching, recovery of myocardial substrate and energy metabolism during periods of ischemia, persistent inotropic reserve, and lack of necrosis [12].

With diminished coronary perfusion, a protective downregulation of myocyte function occurs to reduce oxygen demand and preserve viability for a prolonged period of time [13]. This model of chronic hypoperfusion, however, is being challenged by findings from positron emission tomography (PET) imaging studies of human subjects, which demonstrate that myocardial dysfunction is disproportionate to the degree of flow reduction [14]. In a majority of patients, flow to hibernating myocardium was 70–80% of baseline blood flow [15,16]. An alternate view of viable myocardium that is consistent with this finding is cumulative and repetitive stunning may occur despite absence or mild reduction of resting blood flow [17]. Intermittent ischemia arising from increased demand in the setting of impaired coronary flow reserve may account for the hypocontractile yet viable state of the myocyte. The distinction between a chronic low flow and near normal flow state as a cause of the dysfunctional yet viable myocardium is further clouded by the inability of PET imaging to resolve subendocardial from transmural myocardial flow. This may lead to an overestimation of blood flow [12]. It is quite possible that hibernating myocardium may exist in either a chronic low flow milieu, or one that is near-normal at rest but with impaired flow reserve.

In hibernating myocardium, the downregulation of contractile function leads to reduced energy demand and restoration of the myocardial energetic state. There is close matching of myocardial function and oxygen consumption as an adaptive response to ischemia. Metabolic changes include increased glucose uptake and reduced Kreb's cycle activity. During recruitment of inotropic reserve, there is a further increase in glucose uptake and lactate production [12].

Morphologic changes have been observed in hibernating myocytes (Table 8.1). Both degeneration and dedifferentiation have been described. There may be myofilament, contractile protein, and

Table 8.1 Morphologic changes associated with hibernating myocardium.

A. Myocyte changes
  Cardiomyocyte loss
  Myofilament and contractile protein loss
  Cytoskeletal degeneration
  Small mitochondria
  Glycogen deposits
  Heterochromatin distribution over nucleoplasm
  Apoptosis

B. Interstitial changes
  Cellular debris
  Increased macrophages
  Increased fibroblasts
  Increased collagen

sarcoplasmic reticulum loss. There is cytoskeletal disorganization, small mitochondria, glycogen deposits, heterochromatin distribution over the nucleoplasm, and apoptosis. Interstitial changes include presence of cellular debris, increased macrophages and fibroblasts, and increased collagen [12]. If blood flow is not restored, the process may lead to necrosis.

Clinical significance of myocardial viability

In patients with CAD and left ventricular dysfunction, surgical revascularization has been shown to confer survival benefits compared to medical therapy [9]. Surgical treatment is an independent prognostic factor for improved long-term survival in patients with multivessel disease and moderate to severe left ventricular dysfunction [18]. Revascularization is also associated with improved functional class and reduction of symptoms. However, patients with moderate to severe left ventricular dysfunction may have high operative mortality rates, ranging from 5% to 30%, depending on the degree of dysfunction and associated co-morbidities [19]. The potential long-term benefit of revascularization therefore needs to be tempered because of this high "upfront cost". As a result, efforts were undertaken to selectively identify patients who would benefit from revascularization. The assessment of myocardial viability aims to determine whether revascularization would confer clinical benefit. Clinical benefit has

Table 8.2 The mechanisms underlying the techniques used to assess myocardial viability.

Mechanism	Technique/s
Blood flow	Th-201, Tc-99m, Rb-82, C-11 acetate, first-pass Gd MRI, myocardial contrast echo
Cell membrane integrity	Th-201, Tc-99m, Rb-82, Gd contrast MRI
Energy dependent cell processes	Tc-99m, BMIPP
Metabolic utilization	F-18 FDG, C-11 acetate, C-11 palmitate, N-13 glutamate
Electromechanical activity	Electromechanical mapping (EMM)
Wall thickness	Echo, MRI
Contractile reserve	Dobutamine echo/MRI/gated SPECT, post extra-systolic potentiation

been evaluated in two general areas: recovery of segmental or global left ventricular function and more importantly, improvement in symptoms or survival.

A pooled review of studies employing the most commonly used techniques revealed equivalent high sensitivity in predicting functional recovery after revascularization using Tl-201 rest-redistribution, Tl-201 reinjection, Tc-99m sestamibi single photon emission computed tomography (SPECT) imaging, F-18 fluorodeoxyglucose positron emission tomography (F-18 FDG PET), and low-dose dobutamine stress echocardiography (DSE) (weighted average 90%, 86%, 81%, 88%, and 84%, respectively) (Table 8.2). Specificity was lower with Tl-201 rest-redistribution (54%), reinjection (47%), and Tc-99m (60%). F-18 FDG PET had intermediate specificity (73%) and DSE had the highest specificity (81%) [6]. The comparison of the different techniques, however, is limited by the lack of randomized data, the number of patients studied, definition of viability used, and differences in patient characteristics. Furthermore, the length of follow-up is frequently 3 months following revascularization. Full recovery, though detectable immediately post-procedure [20], may not be expected to occur until 6–12 months following revascularization [21]. Despite these limitations, the above techniques have shown robustness in identifying dysfunctional myocardium that would recover function following revascularization. Low-dose dobutamine echocardiography has the highest specificity, probably because it assesses contractile reserve (which implies recruitment of significant number of viable myocytes to be visually perceptible) rather than merely detecting metabolically or functionally intact myocytes that might benefit from revascularization but whose aggregate

number may be insufficient to result in functional improvement. A study of 70 patients with severe ischemic cardiomyopathy who underwent revascularization showed that the amount of scar is a stronger predictor of functional recovery (i.e. less scar predicts functional recovery) than FDG PET mismatch; other predictors include increasing age and presence of diabetes [22].

The more relevant issue is whether functional recovery translates to improvement in symptoms, reduction of ischemic events, and prolonged survival. The extent of myocardial viability has been shown to predict improvement in heart failure symptoms and exercise capacity following revascularization [23,24]. A meta-analysis of myocardial viability studies involving 3088 patients assessed clinical outcomes following revascularization [25]. The average left ventricular ejection fraction was 32% and average follow-up was 25 months. Patients underwent myocardial viability evaluation by thallium-201, F-18 FDG PET or dobutamine echocardiography. The three techniques were equivalent in predicting revascularization benefit (Figure 8.2). Patients with viability who underwent revascularization had the best survival and patients with viability who were medically treated had the worst survival (annual mortality rate 3.2% versus 16%, respectively) (Figure 8.3). Patients without viability had intermediate survival rates with a tendency towards increased mortality in revascularized as compared to medically treated patients (annual mortality rate 7.7% versus 6.2%, respectively). Furthermore, the improvement in survival with revascularization in patients with viable myocardium is more pronounced with greater degrees of left ventricular dysfunction. The meta-analysis presents important aggregation of data, but suffers important limitations

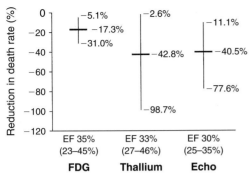

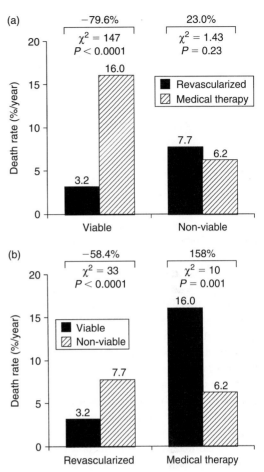

Figure 8.2. Decrease in mortality with revascularization of viable myocardium for each testing technique shown as mean value with 95% confidence limits. Note wide confidence limits, especially for thallium and echocardiography. No measurable differences in test performance were observed. EF = ejection fraction; FDG = F-18 fluorodeoxyglucose [25]. (Reprinted with permission from the American College of Cardiology Foundation. *Journal of the American College of Cardiology* 2002; **39**: 1156.)

Figure 8.3 (a) Death rates for patients with and without myocardial viability treated by revascularization or medical therapy. There is a 79.6% reduction in mortality for patients with viability treated by revascularization ($P < 0.0001$). In patients without myocardial viability, there was no significant difference in mortality with revascularization versus medical therapy. (b) Same data as (a) with comparisons based on treatment strategy in patients with and without viability. Annual mortality was lower in revascularized patients when viability was present versus absent (3.2% versus 7.7%, $P < 0.0001$). Annual mortality was significantly higher in medically treated patients when viability was present versus absent (16% versus 6.2%, $P = 0.001$). Revasc = revascularization [25]. (Reprinted with permission from the American College of Cardiology Foundation. *Journal of the American College of Cardiology* 2002; **39**: 1155.)

that should temper the interpretation and generalizability of its results. The studies used in the meta-analysis were non-randomized, observational studies. As such, the decisions for revascularization were not based solely on viability assessment but also on important co-morbidities and technical factors that were not adjusted for adequately in the studies. Furthermore, the quality of medical therapy in the studies was not uniform and may not be reflective of current advances. The study does point strongly to the fact that patients with viability who are candidates for revascularization do well after the procedure while those who are not do poorly. In patients without evidence of viability, revascularization does not appear to confer a survival advantage, although the same limitation cited above applies to this generalization.

To definitely establish that myocardial viability and revascularization therapy are independently predictive of clinical outcomes in CAD patients with left ventricular dysfunction would require a prospective, randomized controlled trial. This is probably not practical at this point. The next best thing would be to have clinical studies with provisions for adjusting for differences in clinical characteristics that may also affect clinical outcome and confound the results. No study adequately adjusts for baseline clinical variables that are relevant, such

as factors that affect the decision on whether revascularization or medical therapy would be undertaken (e.g. tiny or non-revascularizable arteries, significant co-morbidities, etc.). Furthermore, the

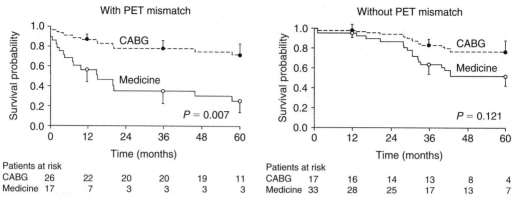

Figure 8.4 Plot shows adjusted Kaplan–Meier estimated survival probabilities for patients with left ventricular dysfunction treated medically and with coronary artery bypass graft (CABG) by presence or absence of PET mismatch, reflecting hibernating myocardium. (Reprinted with permission from Elsevier Science. Di Carli MF, Maddahi J, Rokhsar S, *et al*. Long-term survival of patients with CAD and left ventricular dysfunction: implications for the role of myocardial viability assessment in management decisions. *Journal of Thoracic and Cardiovascular Surgery* 1998; **116**: 997–1004.)

few studies that did adjust for independent clinical variables had a limited number of patients.

Despite these limitations, few studies did attempt to assess whether the presence of myocardial viability and/or the use of revascularization are independently predictive of clinical outcomes. Di Carli *et al.* [26] studied 93 patients with left ventricular dysfunction who had F-18 FDG PET assessment for viability. Coronary bypass surgery was performed in 43 patients and follow-up was done for 4 years. Using Cox proportional hazards model, viability assessed by PET mismatch was the strongest independent predictor of death; the other variables were heart failure class and prior MI. Adjusted for clinical variables, patients who underwent surgical revascularization had improved survival compared with medical therapy. In patients with PET mismatch, there was significant survival advantage in the bypass group as compared to the medically treated group. In the absence of PET mismatch, however, there was no difference in survival between surgical and medical management (Figure 8.4). Cuocolo *et al.* [27] studied 76 ischemic cardiomyopathy patients who had thallium-201 rest-redistribution testing. They found that the variables independently predictive of cardiac death are age, number of viable segments, and absence of revascularization procedure. On the other hand, Lee *et al.* [28] studied 129 patients with left ventricular dysfunction who had FDG-PET viability evaluation treated either medically or with bypass surgery. On Cox proportional hazards analysis, only

age and left ventricular ejection fraction but not myocardial viability and revascularization were independent predictors of survival. The presence of viability and absence of revascularization, however, were found to be independent predictors of ischemic events, defined as unstable angina or MI.

In a purely surgically revascularized group, 70 ischemic cardiomyopathy patients with thallium-201 viability assessment prior to coronary bypass surgery were studied. After adjusting for clinical variables, myocardial viability was found to be independently predictive of improved survival free from cardiac death or heart transplant [29]. On the other hand, in analyses of ischemic cardiomyopathy patients who were only treated medically, viable or ischemic myocardium detected by dobutamine echocardiography and thallium rest-redistribution were found to be independent predictors of death or ischemic events [30,31].

Although limited by the lack of randomized trials, these studies strongly support the use of myocardial viability assessment in the prognostic evaluation of CAD patients with left ventricular dysfunction and in guidance of therapy.

The mechanisms by which revascularization leads to improved survival have not been well defined. Improvement in left ventricular function certainly plays a role, but resting left ventricular function may not change following revascularization in severe ischemic cardiomyopathy [32] despite clear survival benefits in this patient group [22,33].

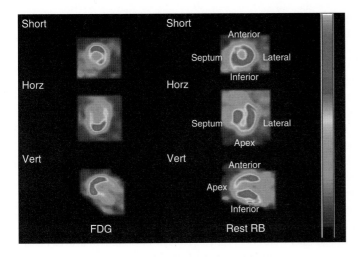

Figure 8.5 Myocardial viability from F-18 FDG PET. Resting Rb-82 perfusion scan is represented in the right column and FDG scan is in the left column with both scans shown in short axis, horizontal long axis, and vertical long axis slices. Perfusion scan shows anterior and apical perfusion defects. There is increased FDG uptake in these corresponding areas, indicating viability. (Images courtesy of Wael Jaber, M.D. and the Cleveland Clinic Nuclear Cardiology laboratory.)

Improved coronary flow in ischemic territories, reduced arrhythmogenesis, and attenuation of ventricular remodeling are possible additional mechanisms underlying the clinical benefit of revascularization.

Techniques to evaluate myocardial viability

The assessment of myocardial viability relies on techniques that evaluate different aspects of "living" myocytes (Table 8.2). They include tests that assess cell membrane function, energy dependent cell processes, metabolic utilization, electromechanical activity, and contractile reserve. Other techniques are indirect correlates, such as myocardial wall thickness and evaluation of blood flow.

PET

PET relies on the use of radionuclides that decay by positron emission. The positrons travel a few millimeters in tissues before annihilating and producing two 511-keV gamma rays that are 180 degrees apart. It confers several advantages over ordinary SPECT imaging. There is higher spatial resolution because of coincident imaging of higher energy gamma rays, attenuation is less of an issue because of the standard use of transmission scans for attenuation correction, and quantitative analyses of blood flow and metabolic rates can be done.

F-18 FDG

Myocytes under normal conditions utilize free fatty acids and glucose as the major sources of energy. With relative tissue hypoxia from ischemia, oxidative metabolism of free fatty acids is reduced and glucose metabolism becomes the preferred substrate. Energy production comes mainly from anaerobic glycolysis [34]. This change in bioenergetics has been utilized in myocardial viability assessment. F-18 FDG is a glucose analog that is actively transported via glucose transporters into the myocyte. It is phosphorylated by hexokinase in the cytoplasm but does not undergo further metabolism and remains trapped in the myocardium. Myocardial FDG uptake can be evaluated subjectively or can be compared to the uptake of a normal myocardial segment semiquantitatively. Uptake of FDG that is at least 50% of the uptake in normal reference myocardial segment is considered viable. Imaging with FDG is usually paired with perfusion imaging such as nitrogen-13 ammonia or rubidium-82 chloride using PET or with SPECT techniques using Tc-99m sestamibi or tetrofosmin. Segmental defects seen in perfusion imaging that show FDG uptake (flow–metabolism mismatch) signify viability whereas concordant segmental defects in both perfusion and FDG imaging (flow–metabolism match) signify non-viability (scar or infarct) (Figure 8.5). Normal myocardium may appear to have relatively reduced FDG uptake compared to ischemic segments because of preferential utilization of fatty acids [35].

There is heterogeneity in FDG uptake depending on the fasting state, glucose, and insulin levels. To reduce this heterogeneity, techniques such as oral glucose loading or intravenous administration of insulin have been utilized. Insulin clamp comprising a constant infusion of glucose, insulin, and potassium has also been utilized to maintain a steady state glucose and insulin in the circulation [35].

Although PET is more commonly used for FDG imaging, SPECT imaging on a gamma camera and ultra-high energy collimators is being used. The advantage of this approach is the wider availability of gamma cameras. The disadvantage is the lower resolution of SPECT compared to PET, although the images are usually adequate for clinical interpretation [35–38].

In a pooled evaluation of 12 small studies using FDG PET for assessment of prediction of improvement of regional contractile function, the average sensitivity of 88% was comparable to thallium-201, technetium-99m, and DSE techniques. The average specificity of 73% was higher than thallium-201 and technetium-99m but lower than DSE [6] (Table 8.2).

C-11 acetate, C-11 palmitate, and N-13 glutamate

Viable myocytes maintain oxidative metabolism. C-11 acetate has been used to assess both oxidative metabolism and to measure regional blood flow. Unlike FDG, the uptake of C-11 acetate does not depend on substrate utilization [39]. In post-MI patients undergoing revascularization, oxidative metabolic rates were reduced only in irreversibly injured segments. Segments with reversible dysfunction had baseline blood flow of 0.73 ± 0.18 mL/min/g, significantly higher than the flow in irreversibly dysfunctional segments, 0.43 ± 0.18 mL/min/g [40]. C-11 palmitate has also been used to assess oxidative metabolism. Another agent that is not widely used is N-13 glutamate labeled amino acid, which is increased in ischemic and viable myocardium and decreased in areas of myocardial necrosis [41].

SPECT imaging
Thallium-201

Thallium is a potassium analog that is used to assess both flow and viability. The uptake of thallium-201 early after injection represents regional myocardial blood flow but delayed redistribution occurs later reflecting gradual uptake by cells with membrane integrity. In normal myocytes, initial uptake is high but falls rapidly within hours. On the other hand, hibernating myocardium initially has low uptake which then increases. A segmental defect on initial resting thallium injection image that fills in 4 h later during redistribution signifies viable myocardium (Figure 8.6). This rest- and delayed-redistribution image protocol has been shown to have diagnostic accuracy for regional recovery [42]. In clinical practice, the typical stress and 4-h rest-redistribution imaging protocol with thallium has been shown to underestimate viable myocardium. Improved detection has been reported with reinjection of thallium after rest-redistribution imaging, identifying up to half of presumed irreversible defects [42–45]. An uptake of 50% relative to the uptake in a normal segment is the best predictor of functional recovery after revascularization [4,46].

In a pooled analysis of seven studies using thallium-201 stress-redistribution–reinjection protocol, the sensitivity in predicting regional functional recovery was high (weighted average 86%) but with low specificity (weighted average 47%). For rest-redistribution imaging, pooled analysis of 8 studies showed sensitivity of 90% and low specificity of 54% [6] (Table 8.2).

Technetium-99m

Technetium-99m sestamibi and tetrofosmin are two commonly used agents to assess myocardial perfusion. Extraction by myocytes occurs in proportion to coronary blood flow and is dependent on cell membrane integrity and mitochondrial function and thus myocardial viability. There is no uptake in necrotic myocardium. Unlike thallium-201, they have minimal redistribution [6,47–50]. Studies comparing Tc-99m sestamibi imaging with thallium-201 rest-redistribution or reinjection and F-18 FDG PET showed consistent findings that Tc-99m sestamibi is less accurate in detecting myocardial viability. Although the sensitivity in evaluating improvement in regional functional outcome is high (weighted mean 81%), the specificity was variable (35–86%, weighted mean 60%) [6,51–57]. The addition of nitrates before the administration of Tc-99m sestamibi has been reported to improve

(a)

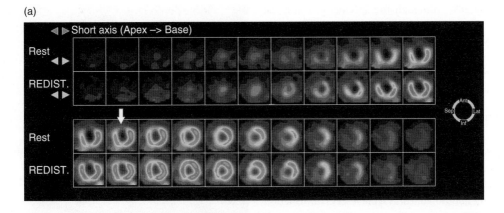

(b)

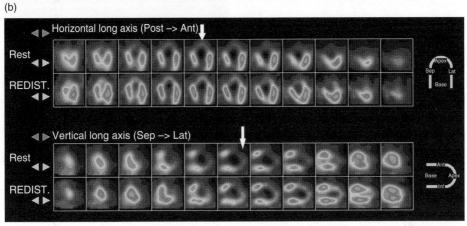

Figure 8.6 Thallium-201 rest and 3 hour redistribution image in a patient with prior MI. There is severe reduction in tracer activity in the anterior wall and apical regions (white arrows), which partially normalizes during redistribution signifying residual myocardial viability in the region.

sensitivity (weighted mean 91%) as well as specificity (weighted mean 88%) [6,58–60] (Table 8.2).

BMIPP

Iodine-123 15-(*p*-iodophenyl)-3-R,S-methylpentadecanoic acid (BMIPP) is a branched fatty acid analog that is taken up by myocytes and retained in the mitochondria. Studies have shown its utility in differentiating viable from non-viable myocardium and in predicting functional improvement after MI. A mismatch pattern with decreased BMIPP uptake relative to perfusion tracers such as technetium-99m sestamibi or thallium-201 is associated with myocardial viability. A matched diminution of BMIPP and perfusion tracer uptake is associated with scar [42,61]. In a study of 56 post-MI patients, BMIPP and thallium-201 perfusion mismatch within 30 days of the infarct was associated with

functional recovery and further improvement in the mismatch 2–3 months after percutaneous revascularization [62]. Using quantitative methods in 18 MI patients who underwent revascularization, a pattern of mismatch with technetium-99m sestamibi uptake <70% and BMIPP uptake at least 10% lower was found to be optimal in predicting global functional recovery [61].

Echocardiography
Wall thickness

In clinical practice, a thinned, akinetic myocardial segment usually portends scar and absence of viability. This has been confirmed by several studies. In 28 ischemic cardiomyopathy patients undergoing surgical revascularization, segmental diastolic wall thickness of ≥5 mm predicted functional recovery at 1 year with a sensitivity of 100% but a specificity of only 28%. Although the specificity is low, the negative predictive value was 100%. This simple test was not improved with the addition of DSE or thallium-201. Thus, diastolic wall thickness of <5 mm was deemed the best single and simple predictor of non-recovery of left ventricular function [63]. Similarly, a study of 45 patients with left ventricular dysfunction undergoing surgical coronary revascularization showed that an end-diastolic wall thickness of >6 mm had a high sensitivity for predicting functional recovery of 94% with similar low specificity of 48% [64]. Unlike the first study, however, the addition of contractile reserve information from DSE improved the specificity of the test to 77% without a significant loss of sensitivity. The role of diastolic wall thickness in the accuracy of prediction of viability by DSE was studied in 53 patients undergoing revascularization. The accuracy and sensitivity of DSE in predicting functional recovery was decreased in segments with thinned end-diastolic thickness [65].

DSE

Myocardial viability assessment by DSE is based on the recruitment of contractile reserve in viable myocytes. Dobutamine is administered at low (5–10 μg/kg/min) and higher (20–50 μg/kg/min) doses, with or without the addition of atropine. Dobutamine stimulates primarily β1-adrenoreceptors with minimal β2 and α1 effects. Low-dose infusion causes primarily inotropic stimulation and evokes contractile reserve of viable myocardium, causing segmental thickening. Higher doses cause inotropic and chronotropic stimulation, leading to increased myocardial oxygen demand in the setting of impaired coronary perfusion. This leads to an ischemic response, depletion of energy stores, and diminution or absence of contractility [66,67].

Two patterns of response were found to be predictive of viability. A biphasic pattern with improvement in segmental function at low doses and subsequent deterioration at higher doses is highly predictive of recovery of function following revascularization. The observed improvement at low dose probably represents recruitment of contractile reserve. A second pattern is progressive worsening of wall motion beginning at low doses. This has been attributed to severely diminished perfusion that even a low dose of dobutamine incites an ischemic response. A third

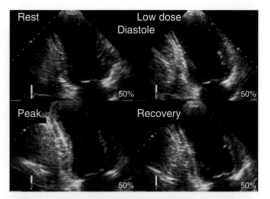

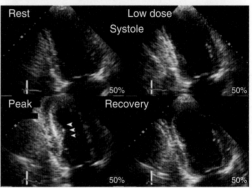

Figure 8.7 Myocardial viability assessed by DSE. Apical two-chamber view showing anterior and inferior walls in a 56-year-old male with moderate left ventricular dysfunction from CAD. The top panel shows end-diastolic frames and lower panel shows end-systolic frames during rest, low- and peak-dose dobutamine infusion and recovery. There is resting inferior akinesia that did not improve with low-dose dobutamine. However, with peak-dose dobutamine, there was improved thickening in the mid and distal inferior wall (white arrowheads). During recovery, the segmental abnormality returned. The presence of contractile reserve is consistent with viability in the inferior wall. Compared to biphasic response (improvement at low dose and deterioration of function at high dose), this pattern of response is not as predictive of functional improvement following revascularization. (Images courtesy of Michael Picard, MD and the Massachusetts General Hospital echocardiography laboratory.)

response, progressive improvement of function, had a low predictive value for recovery of function [66] (Figure 8.7).

In a pooled study of 16 studies utilizing low-dose DSE, the average sensitivity in predicting improvement of regional contractile function was 84% with specificity of 81% [6] (Table 8.2). The sensitivity of DSE is comparable to SPECT or PET based techniques, but its specificity is higher. Other advantages of DSE include availability, ease of use, and absence of radiation. The disadvantages include technical limitations in imaging patients with poor acoustic windows such as obese patients or patients with chronic lung disease and the subjective nature of the evaluation. The use of harmonic imaging and ultrasound contrast agents has greatly improved endocardial border detection and image interpretation [67]. In patients where surface transthoracic echocardiography does not provide adequate image quality, transesophageal echocardiography (TEE) can be employed. In a study of 52 patients who underwent successful revascularization, dobutamine-TEE was compared to dobutamine magnetic resonance imaging (MRI) in predicting functional recovery and the positive predictive values (85% versus 92%, respectively) and negative predictive values (80% versus 85%, respectively) of the two techniques were comparable [68]. Due to its invasive nature, dobutamine-TEE is not as widely utilized, however.

Myocardial contrast echocardiography

Myocardial contrast echocardiography (MCE) utilizes echogenic microbubbles approximating the size of red blood cells that opacifies the myocardium and provides information on myocardial perfusion from antegrade or collateral circulation. The underlying basis by which MCE assesses myocardial viability is that an intact microcirculation is needed for continued viability [69]. In MI, loss of myocytes is accompanied by loss of microvasculature [70]. Intravenous MCE is now being used to assess myocardial blood flow. A high-energy impulse is applied that causes bubble destruction and when new microbubbles enter the imaging field, the rate of increase and the peak plateau signal reflect myocardial blood flow velocity and cross-sectional volume of the microcirculation [71].

In patients with recent or remote MI, functional segmental recovery correlated well with degree of myocardial perfusion as assessed using intracoronary MCE [72–74]. In a study of 23 ischemic heart disease patients who had DSE and intracoronary MCE prior to revascularization, both techniques were equivalent in predicting functional recovery of hypokinetic segments. For akinetic segments, DSE and MCE had similar sensitivities (89% versus 94%, respectively), negative predictive values (93%

versus 97%, respectively) but MCE had poorer specificity (92% versus 67%) and positive predictive value (85% versus 55%). Using intracoronary MCE, thallium-201 and DSE in stable ischemic cardiomyopathy patients, Nagueh et al., [75] found comparable sensitivities for all three (93%, 100%, and 82%, respectively), but lower specificities for MCE and thallium-201 as compared to the biphasic response in DSE (45%, 36%, and 82%, respectively). In another study, intravenous MCE was performed together with Tc-99m sestamibi and dipyridamole–dobutamine stress echo in 17 MI patients and functional recovery following percutaneous revascularization was evaluated. The sensitivity of MCE compared to Tc-99m sestamibi and dipyridamole–dobutamine echo was high (96%, 77%, and 79%, respectively) and the specificity was low (58%, 93%, and 87%, respectively) [76]. The poorer specificity of MCE in these studies may be because myocardial perfusion is preserved in islands of viable myocytes surrounded by extensive fibrosis and revascularization fails to augment functional activity [77]. This is supported by the finding that with intravenous infusion of echo contrast, peak myocardial contrast intensity closely correlated with microvascular density and capillary area from endomyocardial biopsy, but a significant overlap in microvascular density was seen between segments with and without functional recovery [69].

MRI

MRI provides superior spatial resolution and the capability of tissue characterization, advantages over other techniques that enhance its potential to identify viable myocardium. Myocardial viability is evaluated by MRI through several parameters, including diastolic wall thickness, contractile reserve, tissue characteristics as well as gadolinium contrast first-pass effect, and delayed enhancement in myocardium. Other potential applications include use of MR spectroscopy for chemical composition characterization.

Diastolic wall thickness and contractile reserve

The high spatial resolution of MRI allows accurate measurement of wall thickness. Similar to previously discussed echocardiographic studies, a non-viable or scarred myocardial segment is associated with thinning and akinesia. Baer et al. [78] reported in

Table 8.3 Sensitivity and specificity for detection of regional contractile functional recovery in patients with CAD and left ventricular dysfunction following revascularization

Technique	Number of studies	Number of patients	Sensitivity[a]	Specificity[a]
F-18 FDG PET [6]	12	332	71–100 (88)	38–91 (73)
Tl-201 rest-redistribution [6]	8	145	44–100 (90)	22–92 (54)
Tl-201 reinjection [6]	7	209	80–100 (86)	38–80 (47)
Tc-99m sestamibi [6]	7	152	73–100 (81)	35–86 (60)
Tc-99m sestamibi + nitrate [6]	3	55	88–95 (91)	88–89 (88)
DSE [6]	16	448	71–97 (84)	69–96 (81)
Echo end-diastolic wall thickness [63,64]	2	73	94–100	28–48
Myocardial contrast echo [75–77,108]	4	109	84–98	19–58
MRI end-diastolic wall thickness [78]	1	43	92	56
Dobutamine MRI [78–81]	4	116	50–89	70–94
MRI lack of early hypoenhancement [82]	1	20	19	89
MRI lack of CDE [82,88]	2	32	82–98	64–76

a: range (weighted mean).

43 patients that short axis diastolic wall thickness of 5.5 mm or greater is indicative of viability in an infarct region based on functional recovery 4–6 months following revascularization with a sensitivity of 92% and specificity of 56%.

In the same study, contractile reserve was also studied. It was found that low-dose dobutamine-induced systolic wall thickening of 2 mm or greater was a better predictor of functional recovery as compared to diastolic wall thickness with sensitivity of 89% and specificity of 94%. There was a significant increase in left ventricular function in patients with contractile reserve as compared to those without [78].

The relationship between myocardial viability and contractile reserve (measured by low-dose dobutamine-induced systolic wall thickening) has also been reported in other studies. Gunning et al., [79] showed that dobutamine MRI was an insensitive (50%) but specific (81%) test in 23 patients. In a study of 25 patients, Trent et al. [80] used semiautomated edge detection methods to analyze thickening and motion in viability assessment with dobutamine, and found a sensitivity of 71% and specificity of 70%. Dobutamine MRI was also useful in predicting global functional recovery of akinetic myocardial segments after revascularization in 25 patients, with sensitivity of 76% and specificity of 100% [81] (Table 8.2). The robustness of this technique remains to be seen in larger series of patients.

Contrast-enhanced MRI

Myocardial viability can be assessed with cardiac MRI using relaxation contrast agents such as gadolinium chelates. Gadolinium, a large molecule contrast agent that is distributed in the extracellular space and is excluded from myocardial cells with intact membranes, decreases T1 and T2 relaxation of surrounding tissues. Two patterns have been observed to characterize patients with MI. First-pass images obtained immediately following contrast injection demonstrate hypoenhancement in the area of the infarct corresponding to reduced blood flow and microvascular obstruction. The second pattern is seen during delayed imaging (10–20 min after contrast administration) with signal hyperenhancement that corresponds to myocardial necrosis. In ischemically injured or infarcted tissue, the volume of distribution of the gadolinium in the myocardium is increased by interstitial edema but more significantly by loss of cellular membrane integrity allowing entrance of the contrast agent and by fibrosis. The exit of the agent is also delayed in areas of irreversibly damaged myocardium [67,82–86]. It is well-established in the animal model that the areas of contrast delayed enhancement (CDE) following gadolinium administration correspond to areas of infarct by triphenyl tetrazolim chloride staining at every stage of healing following MI [87] (Table 8.3).

The lack of CDE has been found to be more accurate in predicting viability and functional recovery as compared to lack of early hypoenhancement [82]. Other studies have corroborated the usefulness of lack of CDE as a marker of viability. In 12 patients with ischemic left ventricular dysfunction followed up to 3 months following revascularization, lack of CDE was associated with functional improvement with sensitivity of 98% and specificity of 76% [88] (Table 8.2). Kim *et al.* [89] demonstrated in 50 patients that the presence and transmural extent of CDE is related to functional recovery following revascularization (Figure 8.8). In myocardial segments without CDE, 78% had improved contractility as compared to 1.7% of segments with CDE in more than 75% of tissue. Segments with intermediate levels of CDE had functional improvement inversely proportional to the transmural extent of hyperenhancement. Several small series have supported this inverse relationship between segmental functional recovery and CDE in patients with acute MI treated either medically or with additional revascularization therapy [82,90–92]. Global left ventricular function improvement was found to be best predicted by the extent of myocardial segments with dysfunction but either did not have CDE or had transmural extent <25% of the left ventricular wall thickness [92]. It is of interest that in segments with transmural distribution of CDE, 5–15% still show functional improvement [91,92].

The advantages of CDE MRI in the evaluation of viability as compared to other modalities such as PET, SPECT or echocardiography include high spatial resolution that allows delineation of subendocardial or varying degrees of transmural involvement, and the ability to image all myocardial segments even in obese patients. Disadvantages include inability to image patients with pacemakers and defibrillators, an increasingly substantial segment of the ischemic cardiomyopathy population, as well lack of widespread availability. CDE MRI, although promising, still awaits validation at this time as an independent prognostic marker for survival in ischemic cardiomyopathy patients. Two preliminary trial results presented at a national meeting demonstrate the potential of CDE for risk prognostication. In 257 CAD patients followed up for an average of 13.8 months, patients with no CDE had better freedom from major adverse cardiac events (death, infarction, unstable angina, decompensated heart failure, and revascularization) as compared with those with CDE [93]. The presence of CDE was the variable with the highest hazard ratio (5.75, CI 2.8–11.5) as compared to other risk factors such as age, left ventricular function, prior MI, hypertension, diabetes, and abnormal electrocardiogram. The presence of CDE in >15% of the left ventricular mass was also shown to be independently associated with worse survival in a study of 100 CAD patients (average follow-up 25 months) on routine cardiac care, as compared with those with no CDE or CDE <15% of the myocardium [94]. Among several variables tested, only the presence of CDE and reduced left ventricular ejection fraction were found to be independent predictors of all-cause mortality.

MR spectroscopy

MR spectroscopy allows interrogation of the chemical composition and metabolism of myocardial tissue. Although clinical utility has not been established, preliminary data show promising results. The focus has been on assessing myocardial energetics. Using phosphorus-31 magnetic spectroscopy, Beer *et al.* [95] demonstrated in a study of eight patients that 6 months following revascularization, the phosphocreatine/ATP ratios of myocardial segments with functional recovery were comparable to normal controls. The segments that showed no functional recovery had reduced phosphocreatine/ATP ratios. Similarly, Yabe *et al.* [96] studied myocardial high-energy phosphate levels in 41 CAD patients. Phosphocreatine was significantly reduced in CAD patients with both fixed and reversible thallium defects, but ATP was reduced only in patients with fixed defects. Using hydrogen instead of phosphorus MR spectroscopy in 10 CAD patients, Bottomley and Weiss [97] reported that total creatine was lower in infarct regions compared to non-infarcted myocardium. These studies demonstrate that MR spectroscopy has the potential for spatially localized non-invasive determination of myocardial metabolic state. The main disadvantage with MR spectroscopy involves the need to use large voxel sampling size (10 to >20 mL) to compensate for its low intrinsic sensitivity and low metabolite concentrations, thus compromising spatial resolution. The technique is also technically demanding.

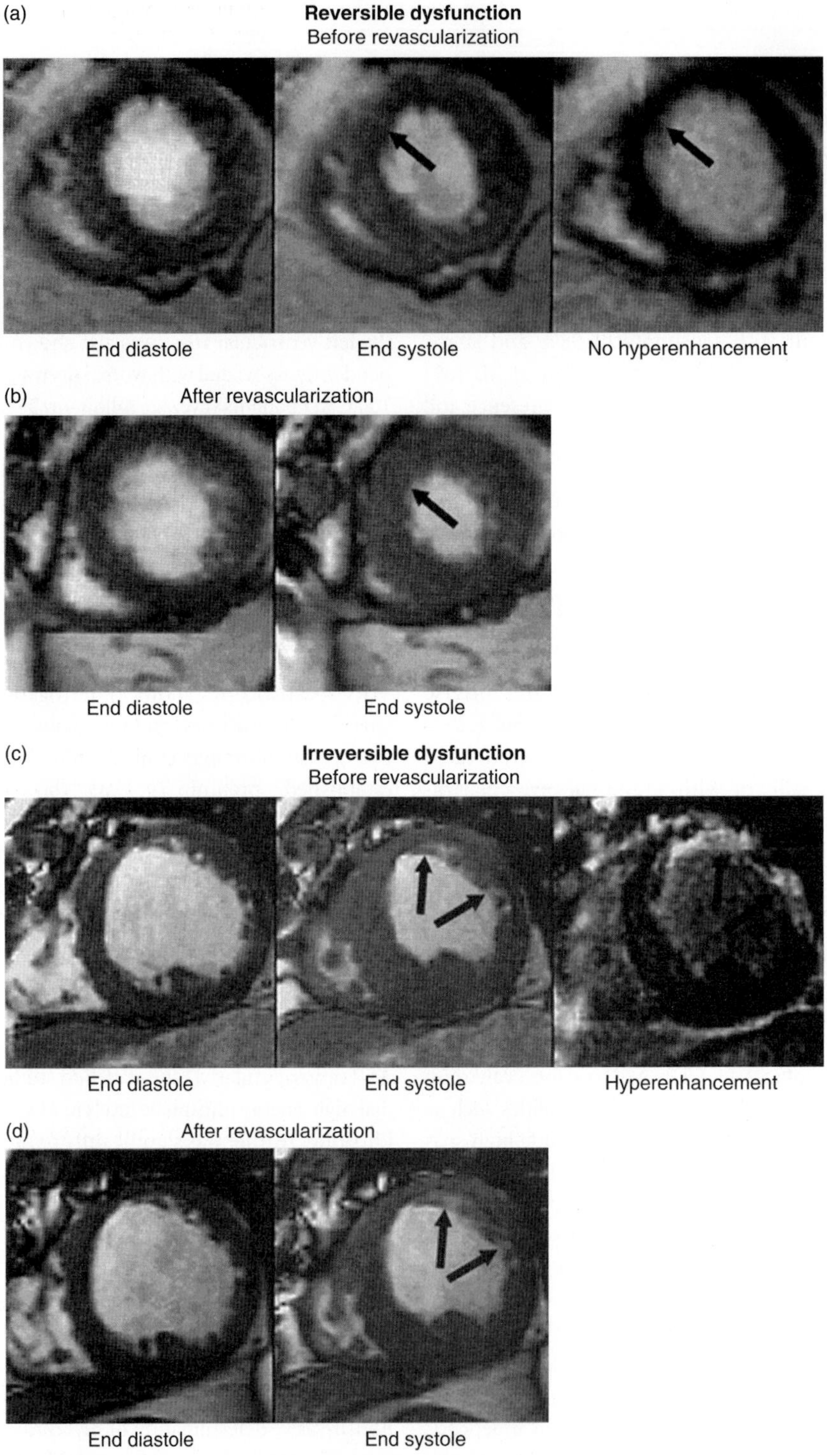

Figure 8.8 Representative cine images and contrast-enhanced images obtained by MRI in one patient with reversible ventricular dysfunction (Panels a and b) and one with irreversible ventricular dysfunction (Panels c and d). The patient with reversible dysfunction had severe hypokinesia of the anteroseptal wall (arrows) and this area was not hyperenhanced before revascularization. The contractility of the wall improved after revascularization. The patient with irreversible dysfunction had akinesia of the anterolateral wall (arrows), and this area was hyperenhanced before revascularization. The contractility of the wall did not improve after revascularization [89]. (Copyright © 2000 Massachusetts Medical Society. All rights reserved.)

Invasive methods of viability assessment

Electromechanical mapping

Electromechanical mapping (EMM) involves the measurement of endocardial unipolar voltages (UPV) and local shortening (LS) using ultra-low electromagnetic field energy and a tip-deflecting sensor catheter. Mostly performed without fluoroscopy, real-time three-dimensional maps can be created from both the electrical activity (UPV) and regional contractility data (LS) of the left ventricular endocardium. It has been shown in animal experiments that myocardial ischemia and MI were associated with reduced voltage potentials [98,99]. In a pig model of myocardial hibernation, there is preserved electrical activity in myocardial segments with reduced coronary perfusion and function [100].

EMM has been compared to more established imaging modalities for viability. It was found that regional UPV and LS values were proportional to thallium uptake score at rest and with redistribution in 61 patients with CAD [101]. In 51 CAD patients, the highest UPV and LS were found in normally perfused myocardial segments. There were intermediate values for viable myocardium, defined by fixed perfusion defect by technetium-99m tetrofosmin SPECT but with normal or limited FDG uptake, and lowest values in scar tissue [102]. Using lack of delayed enhancement contrast MRI as a gold standard for viability, Perin et al. [103] found significantly lower UPV in myocardial segments with subendocardial scar and even lower values in transmural scar segments as compared to normal myocardium. The threshold values for UPV and LS that would distinguish normal from viable and scarred myocardium are not clearly established. Perin et al. [103] suggested a threshold value of 7.9 mV (sensitivity and specificity 80%) and 6.9 mV (sensitivity 93% and specificity 88%) to distinguish normal from subendocardial and transmural scar, respectively. With FDG PET data, Keck et al. [102] found UPV of 4.5 mV as a threshold distinguishing viable from non-viable functionally impaired myocardial segments (sensitivity 65% and specificity 90%). Fuchs et al. [101] suggested UPV of 7.4 mV (sensitivity 78% and specificity 68%) and LS of 5% (sensitivity 65% and specificity 67%) as cutoff points to distinguish viable from non-viable myocardium using thallium data for comparison.

The disadvantage of EMM over other techniques involves the invasive nature of the technique. Its advantage involves the ability to detect ischemic and viable myocardial zones to guide local delivery of therapy that may be available in the future, such as gene therapy or myoblast transfer. No study is available yet that establishes the ability of EMM to predict functional recovery or clinical outcomes.

Cardiac catheterization

The use of left ventriculography to assess myocardial viability is currently of historical rather than clinical importance in light of the available non-invasive means of detection. However, left ventriculography done as part of routine coronary angiography procedure may provide important information regarding myocardial viability. Contractile reserve as a marker of myocardial viability was first established with angiography. Popio et al. [104] showed that improvement in regional contractility following premature ventricular contractions was associated with functional recovery following surgical revascularization in a study involving 31 patients. In another study, post extra-systolic potentiation was also used to detect residual myocardial function [105]. Contractile reserve as a means to assess viability was also examined using nitrates and catecholamines infusion [4,106,107].

Summary

The identification of viable myocardium has important functional and prognostic significance in the treatment of CAD with left ventricular dysfunction. Revascularization of viable myocardial segments is associated with improved survival, but benefit has not been established in revascularization of non-viable myocardium. There are several techniques being used to identify and quantify myocardial viability. The most established techniques include thallium-201 SPECT, F-18 FDG PET, and DSE. These techniques have comparable efficacy in predicting clinical outcomes and sensitivity in predicting regional functional recovery. DSE has higher specificity in predicting regional functional recovery compared to the other two techniques. Increasingly, MRI techniques, including dobutamine MRI and gadolinium CDE are being used in the assessment of myocardial viability. Other promising techniques are at early stages of evaluation, but should contribute to the enhancement of viability assessment.

References

1 The American Heart Association *1999 Heart and Stroke Statistical Update*. American Heart Association, Dallas, 1999.

2 Emond M, Mock MB, Davis KB, Fisher LD, Holmes Jr. DR, Chaitman BR *et al.* Long-term survival of medically treated patients in the Coronary Artery Surgery Study (CASS) Registry. *Circulation* 1994; **90(6)**: 2645–2657.

3 Migrino RQ, Young JB, Ellis SG, White HD, Lundergan CF, Miller DP *et al.* End-systolic volume index at 90 to 180 minutes into reperfusion therapy for acute myocardial infarction is a strong predictor of early and late mortality. The Global Utilization of Streptokinase and t-PA for Occluded Coronary Arteries (GUSTO)-I Angiographic Investigators. *Circulation* 1997; **96(1)**: 116–121.

4 Wijns W, Vatner SF, Camici PG. Hibernating myocardium. *N Engl J Med* 1998; **339(3)**: 173–181.

5 Brunken R, Tillisch J, Schwaiger M, Child JS, Marshall R, Mandelkern M *et al.* Regional perfusion, glucose metabolism, and wall motion in patients with chronic electrocardiographic Q wave infarctions: evidence for persistence of viable tissue in some infarct regions by positron emission tomography. *Circulation* 1986; **73(5)**: 951–963.

6 Bax JJ, Wijns W, Cornel JH, Visser FC, Boersma E, Fioretti PM. Accuracy of currently available techniques for prediction of functional recovery after revascularization in patients with left ventricular dysfunction due to chronic coronary artery disease: comparison of pooled data. *J Am Coll Cardiol* 1997; **30(6)**: 1451–1460.

7 Rees G, Bristow JD, Kremkau EL, Green GS, Herr RH, Griswold HE *et al.* Influence of aortocoronary bypass surgery on left ventricular performance. *N Engl J Med* 1971; **284(20)**: 1116–1120.

8 Chatterjee K, Swan HJ, Parmley WW, Sustaita H, Marcus HS, Matloff J. Influence of direct myocardial revascularization on left ventricular asynergy and function in patients with coronary heart disease. With and without previous myocardial infarction. *Circulation* 1973; **47(2)**: 276–286.

9 Alderman EL, Fisher LD, Litwin P, Kaiser GC, Myers WO, Maynard C *et al.* Results of coronary artery surgery in patients with poor left ventricular function (CASS). *Circulation* 1983; **68(4)**: 785–795.

10 Diamond GA, Forrester JS, deLuz PL, Wyatt HL, Swan HJ. Post-extrasystolic potentiation of ischemic myocardium by atrial stimulation. *Am Heart J* 1978; **95(2)**: 204–209.

11 Rahimtoola SH. A perspective on the three large multi-center randomized clinical trials of coronary bypass surgery for chronic stable angina. *Circulation* 1985; **72(6 Pt 2)**: V123–V135.

12 Heusch G, Schulz R. The biology of myocardial hibernation. *Trends Cardiovasc Med* 2000; **10(3)**: 108–114.

13 Dispersyn GD, Borgers M, Flameng W. Apoptosis in chronic hibernating myocardium: sleeping to death? *Cardiovasc Res* 2000; **45(3)**: 696–703.

14 Vanoverschelde JL, Wijns W, Depre C, Essamri B, Heyndrickx GR, Borgers M *et al.* Mechanisms of chronic regional postischemic dysfunction in humans. New insights from the study of noninfarcted collateral-dependent myocardium. *Circulation* 1993; **87(5)**: 1513–1523.

15 Maes A, Flameng W, Nuyts J, Borgers M, Shivalkar B, Ausma J *et al.* Histological alterations in chronically hypoperfused myocardium. Correlation with PET findings. *Circulation* 1994; **90(2)**: 735–745.

16 Heusch G. Hibernating myocardium. *Physiol Rev* 1998; **78(4)**: 1055–1085.

17 Bolli R. Myocardial 'stunning' in man. *Circulation* 1992; **86(6)**: 1671–1691.

18 Pigott JD, Kouchoukos NT, Oberman A, Cutter GR. Late results of surgical and medical therapy for patients with coronary artery disease and depressed left ventricular function. *J Am Coll Cardiol* 1985; **5(5)**: 1036–1045.

19 Baker DW, Jones R, Hodges J, Massie BM, Konstam MA, Rose EA. Management of heart failure. III. The role of revascularization in the treatment of patients with moderate or severe left ventricular systolic dysfunction. *J Am Med Assoc* 1994; **272(19)**: 1528–1534.

20 Topol EJ, Weiss JL, Guzman PA, Dorsey-Lima S, Blanck TJ, Humphrey LS *et al.* Immediate improvement of dysfunctional myocardial segments after coronary revascularization: detection by intraoperative transesophageal echocardiography. *J Am Coll Cardiol* 1984; **4(6)**: 1123–1134.

21 Vanoverschelde J-L, Melin JA, Depre C, Borgers M, Dion R, Wijns W. Time-course of functional recovery of hibernating myocardium after coronary revascularization (abstract). *Circulation* 1994; **90(Suppl I)**: I-378.

22 Beanlands RS, Ruddy TD, deKemp RA, Iwanochko RM, Coates G, Burns RJ *et al.* Positron emission tomography and recovery following revascularization (PARR-1): the importance of scar and the development of a prediction rule for the degree of recovery of left ventricular function. *J Am Coll Cardiol* 2002; **40(10)**: 1735–1743.

23 Di Carli MF, Asgarzadie F, Schelbert HR, Brunken RC, Laks H, Phelps ME *et al.* Quantitative relation between myocardial viability and improvement in heart failure symptoms after revascularization in patients with ischemic cardiomyopathy. *Circulation* 1995; **92(12)**: 3436–3444.

24 Marwick TH, Zuchowski C, Lauer MS, Secknus MA, Williams J, Lytle BW. Functional status and quality of life

in patients with heart failure undergoing coronary bypass surgery after assessment of myocardial viability. *J Am Coll Cardiol* 1999; **33(3)**: 750–758.

25 Allman KC, Shaw LJ, Hachamovitch R, Udelson JE. Myocardial viability testing and impact of revascularization on prognosis in patients with coronary artery disease and left ventricular dysfunction: a meta-analysis. *J Am Coll Cardiol* 2002; **39(7)**: 1151–1158.

26 Di Carli MF, Maddahi J, Rokhsar S, Schelbert HR, Bianco-Batlles D, Brunken RC *et al.* Long-term survival of patients with coronary artery disease and left ventricular dysfunction: implications for the role of myocardial viability assessment in management decisions. *J Thorac Cardiovasc Surg* 1998; **116(6)**: 997–1004.

27 Cuocolo A, Petretta M, Nicolai E, Pace L, Bonaduce D, Salvatore M *et al.* Successful coronary revascularization improves prognosis in patients with previous myocardial infarction and evidence of viable myocardium at thallium-201 imaging. *Eur J Nucl Med* 1998; **25(1)**: 60–68.

28 Lee KS, Marwick TH, Cook SA, Go RT, Fix JS, James KB *et al.* Prognosis of patients with left ventricular dysfunction, with and without viable myocardium after myocardial infarction. Relative efficacy of medical therapy and revascularization. *Circulation* 1994; **90(6)**: 2687–2694.

29 Pagley PR, Beller GA, Watson DD, Gimple LW, Ragosta M. Improved outcome after coronary bypass surgery in patients with ischemic cardiomyopathy and residual myocardial viability. *Circulation* 1997; **96(3)**: 793–800.

30 Williams MJ, Odabashian J, Lauer MS, Thomas JD, Marwick TH. Prognostic value of dobutamine echocardiography in patients with left ventricular dysfunction. *J Am Coll Cardiol* 1996; **27(1)**: 132–139.

31 Gioia G, Milan E, Giubbini R, DePace N, Heo J, Iskandrian AS. Prognostic value of tomographic rest-redistribution thallium 201 imaging in medically treated patients with coronary artery disease and left ventricular dysfunction. *J Nucl Cardiol* 1996; **3(2)**: 150–156.

32 Freeman AP, Walsh WF, Giles RW, Choy D, Newman DC, Horton DA *et al.* Early and long-term results of coronary artery bypass grafting with severely depressed left ventricular performance. *Am J Cardiol* 1984; **54(7)**: 749–754.

33 Di Carli MF, Hachamovitch R, Berman DS. The art and science of predicting postrevascularization improvement in left ventricular (LV) function in patients with severely depressed LV function. *J Am Coll Cardiol* 2002; **40(10)**: 1744–1747.

34 Visser FC. Imaging of cardiac metabolism using radiolabelled glucose, fatty acids and acetate. *Coronary Artery Dis* 2001; **12(Suppl 1)**: S12–S18.

35 Segall G. Assessment of myocardial viability by positron emission tomography. *Nucl Med Commun* 2002; **23(4)**: 323–330.

36 Fukuchi K, Sago M, Nitta K, Fukushima K, Toba M, Hayashida K *et al.* Attenuation correction for cardiac dual-head gamma camera coincidence imaging using segmented myocardial perfusion SPECT. *J Nucl Med* 2000; **41(5)**: 919–925.

37 Fukuchi K, Katafuchi T, Fukushima K, Shimotsu Y, Toba M, Hayashida K *et al.* Estimation of myocardial perfusion and viability using simultaneous 99mTc-tetrofosmin-FDG collimated SPECT. *J Nucl Med* 2000; **41(8)**: 1318–1323.

38 Delbeke D, Videlefsky S, Patton JA, Campbell MG, Martin WH, Ohana I *et al.* Rest myocardial perfusion/metabolism imaging using simultaneous dual-isotope acquisition SPECT with technetium-99m-MIBI/fluorine-18-FDG. *J Nucl Med* 1995; **36(11)**: 2110–2119.

39 Iskandrian AE, Verani MS. *Nuclear Cardiac Imaging: Principles and Applications*, 2nd edn. F.A. Davis Company, Philadelphia, 1996.

40 Wolpers HG, Burchert W, van den Hoff J, Weinhardt R, Meyer GJ, Lichtlen PR. Assessment of myocardial viability by use of 11C-acetate and positron emission tomography. Threshold criteria of reversible dysfunction. *Circulation* 1997; **95(6)**: 1417–1424.

41 Zimmermann R, Tillmanns H, Knapp WH, Helus F, Georgi P, Rauch B *et al.* Regional myocardial nitrogen-13 glutamate uptake in patients with coronary artery disease: inverse post-stress relation to thallium-201 uptake in ischemia. *J Am Coll Cardiol* 1988; **11(3)**: 549–556.

42 Al-Khouri F, Narula J. Radionuclide imaging for the assessment of myocardial viability in chronic LV dysfunction. *Echocardiography* 2000; **17(6 Pt 1)**: 605–612.

43 Dilsizian V, Rocco TP, Freedman NM, Leon MB, Bonow RO. Enhanced detection of ischemic but viable myocardium by the reinjection of thallium after stress-redistribution imaging. *N Engl J Med* 1990; **323(3)**: 141–146.

44 Tamaki N, Ohtani H, Yonekura Y, Nohara R, Kambara H, Kawai C *et al.* Significance of fill-in after thallium-201 reinjection following delayed imaging: comparison with regional wall motion and angiographic findings. *J Nucl Med* 1990; **31(10)**: 1617–1623.

45 Ohtani H, Tamaki N, Yonekura Y, Mohiuddin IH, Hirata K, Ban T *et al.* Value of thallium-201 reinjection after delayed SPECT imaging for predicting reversible ischemia after coronary artery bypass grafting. *Am J Cardiol* 1990; **66(4)**: 394–399.

46 Ragosta M, Beller GA, Watson DD, Kaul S, Gimple LW. Quantitative planar rest-redistribution 201Tl imaging in detection of myocardial viability and prediction of improvement in left ventricular function after coronary bypass surgery in patients with severely depressed left ventricular function. *Circulation* 1993; **87(5)**: 1630–1641.

47 Beanlands RS, Dawood F, Wen WH, McLaughlin PR, Butany J, D'Amati G *et al.* Are the kinetics of technetium-99m methoxyisobutyl isonitrile affected by cell

metabolism and viability? *Circulation* 1990; **82(5)**: 1802–1814.

48 Piwnica-Worms D, Kronauge JF, Chiu ML. Uptake and retention of hexakis (2-methoxyisobutyl isonitrile) technetium(I) in cultured chick myocardial cells. Mitochondrial and plasma membrane potential dependence. *Circulation* 1990; **82(5)**: 1826–1838.

49 Freeman I, Grunwald AM, Hoory S, Bodenheimer MM. Effect of coronary occlusion and myocardial viability on myocardial activity of technetium-99m-sestamibi. *J Nucl Med* 1991; **32(2)**: 292–298.

50 De Coster PM, Wijns W, Cauwe F, Robert A, Beckers C, Melin JA. Area-at-risk determination by technetium-99m-hexakis-2-methoxyisobutyl isonitrile in experimental reperfused myocardial infarction. *Circulation* 1990; **82(6)**: 2152–2162.

51 Marzullo P, Sambuceti G, Parodi O, Gimelli A, Picano E, Giorgetti A *et al*. Regional concordance and discordance between rest thallium 201 and sestamibi imaging for assessing tissue viability: comparison with postrevascularization functional recovery. *J Nucl Cardiol* 1995; **2(4)**: 309–316.

52 Marzullo P, Parodi O, Reisenhofer B, Sambuceti G, Picano E, Distante A *et al*. Value of rest thallium-201/technetium-99m sestamibi scans and dobutamine echocardiography for detecting myocardial viability. *Am J Cardiol* 1993; **71(2)**: 166–172.

53 Gonzalez P, Massardo T, Munoz A, Jofre J, Rivera A, Yovanovich J *et al*. Is the addition of ECG gating to technetium-99m sestamibi SPET of value in the assessment of myocardial viability? An evaluation based on two-dimensional echocardiography following revascularization. *Eur J Nucl Med* 1996; **23(10)**: 1315–1322.

54 Marzullo P, Sambuceti G, Parodi O. The role of sestamibi scintigraphy in the radioisotopic assessment of myocardial viability. *J Nucl Med* 1992; **33(11)**: 1925–1930.

55 Maes AF, Borgers M, Flameng W, Nuyts JL, van de Werf F, Ausma JJ *et al*. Assessment of myocardial viability in chronic coronary artery disease using technetium-99m sestamibi SPECT. Correlation with histologic and positron emission tomographic studies and functional follow-up. *J Am Coll Cardiol* 1997; **29(1)**: 62–68.

56 Udelson JE, Coleman PS, Metherall J, Pandian NG, Gomez AR, Griffith JL *et al*. Predicting recovery of severe regional ventricular dysfunction. Comparison of resting scintigraphy with 201Tl and 99mTc-sestamibi. *Circulation* 1994; **89(6)**: 2552–2561.

57 Maublant JC, Citron B, Lipiecki J, Mestas D, Bailly P, Veyre A *et al*. Rest technetium 99m-sestamibi tomoscintigraphy in hibernating myocardium. *Am Heart J* 1995; **129(2)**: 306–314.

58 Maurea S, Cuocolo A, Soricelli A, Castelli L, Nappi A, Squame F *et al*. Enhanced detection of viable myocardium by technetium-99m-MIBI imaging after nitrate administration in chronic coronary artery disease. *J Nucl Med* 1995; **36(11)**: 1945–1952.

59 Bisi G, Sciagra R, Santoro GM, Fazzini PF. Rest technetium-99m sestamibi tomography in combination with short-term administration of nitrates: feasibility and reliability for prediction of postrevascularization outcome of asynergic territories. *J Am Coll Cardiol* 1994; **24(5)**: 1282–1289.

60 Bisi G, Sciagra R, Santoro GM, Rossi V, Fazzini PF. Technetium-99m-sestamibi imaging with nitrate infusion to detect viable hibernating myocardium and predict postrevascularization recovery. *J Nucl Med* 1995; **36(11)**: 1994–2000.

61 Hambye AS, Vervaet A, Dobbeleir A, Dendale P, Franken P. Prediction of functional outcome by quantification of sestamibi and BMIPP after acute myocardial infarction. *Eur J Nucl Med* 2000; **27(10)**: 1494–1500.

62 Hashimoto A, Nakata T, Tsuchihashi K, Tanaka S, Fujimori K, Iimura O. Postischemic functional recovery and BMIPP uptake after primary percutaneous transluminal coronary angioplasty in acute myocardial infarction. *Am J Cardiol* 1996; **77(1)**: 25–30.

63 La Canna G, Rahimtoola SH, Visioli O, Giubbini R, Alfieri O, Zognio M *et al*. Sensitivity, specificity, and predictive accuracies of non-invasive tests, singly and in combination, for diagnosis of hibernating myocardium. *Eur Heart J* 2000; **21(16)**: 1358–1367.

64 Cwajg JM, Cwajg E, Nagueh SF, He ZX, Qureshi U, Olmos LI *et al*. End-diastolic wall thickness as a predictor of recovery of function in myocardial hibernation: relation to rest-redistribution T1-201 tomography and dobutamine stress echocardiography. *J Am Coll Cardiol* 2000; **35(5)**: 1152–1161.

65 Furukawa T, Haque T, Takahashi M, Kinoshita M. An assessment of dobutamine echocardiography and end-diastolic wall thickness for predicting post-revascularization functional recovery in patients with chronic coronary artery disease. *Eur Heart J* 1997; **18(5)**: 798–806.

66 Afridi I, Kleiman NS, Raizner AE, Zoghbi WA. Dobutamine echocardiography in myocardial hibernation. Optimal dose and accuracy in predicting recovery of ventricular function after coronary angioplasty. *Circulation* 1995; **91(3)**: 663–670.

67 Cho S, McConnell MV. Echocardiographic and magnetic resonance methods for diagnosing hibernating myocardium. *Nucl Med Commun* 2002; **23(4)**: 331–339.

68 Baer FM, Theissen P, Crnac J, Schmidt M, Deutsch HJ, Sechtem U *et al*. Head to head comparison of dobutamine-transoesophageal echocardiography and dobutamine-magnetic resonance imaging for the prediction of left ventricular functional recovery in patients with chronic coronary artery disease. *Eur Heart J* 2000; **21(12)**: 981–991.

69 Shimoni S, Frangogiannis NG, Aggeli CJ, Shan K, Quinones MA, Espada R *et al*. Microvascular structural correlates of myocardial contrast echocardiography in patients with coronary artery disease and left ventricular dysfunction: implications for the assessment of myocardial hibernation. *Circulation* 2002; **106(8)**: 950–956.

70 Kloner RA, Rude RE, Carlson N, Maroko PR, DeBoer LW, Braunwald E. Ultrastructural evidence of microvascular damage and myocardial cell injury after coronary artery occlusion: which comes first? *Circulation* 1980; **62(5)**: 945–952.

71 Lafitte S, Higashiyama A, Masugata H, Peters B, Strachan M, Kwan OL *et al*. Contrast echocardiography can assess risk area and infarct size during coronary occlusion and reperfusion: experimental validation. *J Am Coll Cardiol* 2002; **39(9)**: 1546–1554.

72 Camarano G, Ragosta M, Gimple LW, Powers ER, Kaul S. Identification of viable myocardium with contrast echocardiography in patients with poor left ventricular systolic function caused by recent or remote myocardial infarction. *Am J Cardiol* 1995; **75(4)**: 215–219.

73 Ragosta M, Camarano G, Kaul S, Powers ER, Sarembock IJ, Gimple LW. Microvascular integrity indicates myocellular viability in patients with recent myocardial infarction. New insights using myocardial contrast echocardiography. *Circulation* 1994; **89(6)**: 2562–2569.

74 Sabia PJ, Powers ER, Ragosta M, Sarembock IJ, Burwell LR, Kaul S. An association between collateral blood flow and myocardial viability in patients with recent myocardial infarction. *N Engl J Med* 1992; **327(26)**: 1825–1831.

75 Nagueh SF, Vaduganathan P, Ali N, Blaustein A, Verani MS, Winters Jr. WL *et al*. Identification of hibernating myocardium: comparative accuracy of myocardial contrast echocardiography, rest-redistribution thallium-201 tomography and dobutamine echocardiography. *J Am Coll Cardiol* 1997; **29(5)**: 985–993.

76 Borges AC, Richter WS, Witzel C, Witzel M, Grohmann A, Reibis RK *et al*. Myocardial contrast echocardiography for predicting functional recovery after acute myocardial infarction. *Int J Cardiovasc Imag* 2002; **18(4)**: 257–268.

77 deFilippi CR, Willett DL, Irani WN, Eichhorn EJ, Velasco CE, Grayburn PA. Comparison of myocardial contrast echocardiography and low-dose dobutamine stress echocardiography in predicting recovery of left ventricular function after coronary revascularization in chronic ischemic heart disease. *Circulation* 1995; **92(10)**: 2863–2868.

78 Baer FM, Theissen P, Schneider CA, Voth E, Sechtem U, Schicha H *et al*. Dobutamine magnetic resonance imaging predicts contractile recovery of chronically dysfunctional myocardium after successful revascularization. *J Am Coll Cardiol* 1998; **31(5)**: 1040–1048.

79 Gunning MG, Anagnostopoulos C, Knight CJ, Pepper J, Burman ED, Davies G *et al*. Comparison of 201Tl,

99mTc-tetrofosmin, and dobutamine magnetic resonance imaging for identifying hibernating myocardium. *Circulation* 1998; **98(18)**: 1869–1874.

80 Trent RJ, Waiter GD, Hillis GS, McKiddie FI, Redpath TW, Walton S. Dobutamine magnetic resonance imaging as a predictor of myocardial functional recovery after revascularisation. *Heart* 2000; **83(1)**: 40–46.

81 Sandstede JJ, Bertsch G, Beer M, Kenn W, Werner E, Pabst T *et al*. Detection of myocardial viability by low-dose dobutamine cine MR imaging. *Magn Reson Imag* 1999; **17(10)**: 1437–1443.

82 Gerber BL, Garot J, Bluemke DA, Wu KC, Lima JA. Accuracy of contrast-enhanced magnetic resonance imaging in predicting improvement of regional myocardial function in patients after acute myocardial infarction. *Circulation* 2002; **106(9)**: 1083–1089.

83 Higgins CB. Prediction of myocardial viability by MRI. *Circulation* 1999; **99(6)**: 727–729.

84 Lima JA, Judd RM, Bazille A, Schulman SP, Atalar E, Zerhouni EA. Regional heterogeneity of human myocardial infarcts demonstrated by contrast-enhanced MRI. Potential mechanisms. *Circulation* 1995; **92(5)**: 1117–1125.

85 Rochitte CE, Lima JA, Bluemke DA, Reeder SB, McVeigh ER, Furuta T *et al*. Magnitude and time course of microvascular obstruction and tissue injury after acute myocardial infarction. *Circulation* 1998; **98(10)**: 1006–1014.

86 Beller GA. Noninvasive assessment of myocardial viability. *N Engl J Med* 2000; **343(20)**: 1488–1490.

87 Fieno DS, Kim RJ, Chen EL, Lomasney JW, Klocke FJ, Judd RM. Contrast-enhanced magnetic resonance imaging of myocardium at risk: distinction between reversible and irreversible injury throughout infarct healing. *J Am Coll Cardiol* 2000; **36(6)**: 1985–1991.

88 Sandstede JJ, Lipke C, Beer M, Harre K, Pabst T, Kenn W *et al*. Analysis of first-pass and delayed contrast-enhancement patterns of dysfunctional myocardium on MR imaging: use in the prediction of myocardial viability. *Am J Roentgenol* 2000; **174(6)**: 1737–1740.

89 Kim RJ, Wu E, Rafael A, Chen EL, Parker MA, Simonetti O *et al*. The use of contrast-enhanced magnetic resonance imaging to identify reversible myocardial dysfunction. *N Engl J Med* 2000; **343(20)**: 1445–1453.

90 Bello D, Shah DJ, Farah GM, Di Luzio S, Parker M, Johnson MR *et al*. Gadolinium cardiovascular magnetic resonance predicts reversible myocardial dysfunction and remodeling in patients with heart failure undergoing beta-blocker therapy. *Circulation* 2003; **108(16)**: 1945–1953.

91 Beek AM, Kuhl HP, Bondarenko O, Twisk JW, Hofman MB, van Dockum WG *et al*. Delayed contrast-enhanced magnetic resonance imaging for the prediction of regional functional improvement after acute myocardial infarction. *J Am Coll Cardiol* 2003; **42(5)**: 895–901.

92 Choi KM, Kim RJ, Gubernikoff G, Vargas JD, Parker M, Judd RM. Transmural extent of acute myocardial infarction predicts long-term improvement in contractile function. *Circulation* 2001; **104(10)**: 1101–1107.

93 Chan CW, Yucel K, Reynolds G. Prediction of event-free survival by contrast enhanced cardiac magnetic resonance imaging in patients with symptoms of coronary artery disease. *J Cardiovasc Magn Reson* 2005; **7(1)**: 14–15 [abstract].

94 Kaushal R, Fieno D, Radin M, Shaoulian E, Narula J, Goldberger J et al. Infarct size is an independent predictor of mortality in patients with coronary artery disease. *J Cardiovasc Magn Reson* 2005; **7(1)**: 39–40 [abstract].

95 Beer M, Buchner S, Sandstede J, Viehrig M, Lipke C, Krug A et al. (31)P-MR Spectroscopy for the evaluation of energy metabolism in intact residual myocardium after acute myocardial infarction in humans. *Magma* 2001; **13(2)**: 70–75.

96 Yabe T, Mitsunami K, Inubushi T, Kinoshita M. Quantitative measurements of cardiac phosphorus metabolites in coronary artery disease by 31P magnetic resonance spectroscopy. *Circulation* 1995; **92(1)**: 15–23.

97 Bottomley PA, Weiss RG. Non-invasive magnetic-resonance detection of creatine depletion in non-viable infarcted myocardium. *Lancet* 1998; **351(9104)**: 714–718.

98 Kornowski R, Hong MK, Shiran A, Fuchs S, Pierre A, Collins SD et al. Electromechanical characterization of acute experimental myocardial infarction. *J Invasive Cardiol* 1999; **11(6)**: 329–336.

99 Kornowski R, Hong MK, Gepstein L, Goldstein S, Ellahham S, Ben-Haim SA et al. Preliminary animal and clinical experiences using an electromechanical endocardial mapping procedure to distinguish infarcted from healthy myocardium. *Circulation* 1998; **98(11)**: 1116–1124.

100 Fuchs S, Kornowski R, Shiran A, Pierre A, Ellahham S, Leon MB. Electromechanical characterization of myocardial hibernation in a pig model. *Coronary Artery Dis* 1999; **10(3)**: 195–198.

101 Fuchs S, Hendel RC, Baim DS, Moses JW, Pierre A, Laham RJ et al. Comparison of endocardial electromechanical mapping with radionuclide perfusion imaging to assess myocardial viability and severity of myocardial ischemia in angina pectoris. *Am J Cardiol* 2001; **87(7)**: 874–880.

102 Keck A, Hertting K, Schwartz Y, Kitzing R, Weber M, Leisner B et al. Electromechanical mapping for determination of myocardial contractility and viability. A comparison with echocardiography, myocardial single-photon emission computed tomography, and positron emission tomography. *J Am Coll Cardiol* 2002; **40(6)**: 1067–1074; discussion 1075–1078.

103 Perin EC, Silva GV, Sarmento-Leite R, Sousa AL, Howell M, Muthupillai R et al. Assessing myocardial viability and infarct transmurality with left ventricular electromechanical mapping in patients with stable coronary artery disease: validation by delayed-enhancement magnetic resonance imaging. *Circulation* 2002; **106(8)**: 957–961.

104 Popio KA, Gorlin R, Bechtel D, Levine JA. Postextrasystolic potentiation as a predictor of potential myocardial viability: preoperative analyses compared with studies after coronary bypass surgery. *Am J Cardiol* 1977; **39(7)**: 944–953.

105 Dyke SH, Cohn PF, Gorlin R, Sonnenblick EH. Detection of residual myocardial function in coronary artery disease using post-extra systolic potentiation. *Circulation* 1974; **50(4)**: 694–699.

106 Horn HR, Teichholz LE, Cohn PF, Herman MV, Gorlin R. Augmentation of left ventricular contraction pattern in coronary artery disease by an inotropic catecholamine. The epinephrine ventriculogram. *Circulation* 1974; **49(6)**: 1063–1071.

107 Helfant RH, Pine R, Meister SG, Feldman MS, Trout RG, Banka VS. Nitroglycerin to unmask reversible asynergy. Correlation with post coronary bypass ventriculography. *Circulation* 1974; **50(1)**: 108–113.

108 Meza MF, Ramee S, Collins T, Stapleton D, Milani RV, Murgo JP et al. Knowledge of perfusion and contractile reserve improves the predictive value of recovery of regional myocardial function postrevascularization: a study using the combination of myocardial contrast echocardiography and dobutamine echocardiography. *Circulation* 1997; **96(10)**: 3459–3465.

CHAPTER 9

Bypass surgery in the treatment of ischemic cardiomyopathy

Bruce W. Lytle

The most common operation performed for patients with congestive heart failure (CHF) is coronary bypass surgery. In the United States, the majority of patients with heart failure have a cardiomyopathy, that is, at least in part, ischemic in origin: coronary artery disease has contributed to their myocardial dysfunction. It has been long known that coronary bypass surgery improves or relieves angina and substantial evidence exists that bypass surgery prolongs the life expectancy of patients with ischemic cardiomyopathy. Recent series have also shown and quantified the improvement of symptoms of CHF following bypass surgery. In addition to advances in the safety and effectiveness of bypass surgery there have also been improvements in imaging techniques that allow identification of patient subsets particularly likely to benefit from revascularization.

Early in the bypass surgery era, randomized and comparative observational trials were undertaken to identify the impact of bypass surgery on long-term survival. The results of these trials indicated that patients with abnormal left ventricular (LV) function experienced an improved survival rate with prompt bypass surgery compared with the strategy of initial medical management with surgery being recommended later on if symptoms worsened (cross-over to surgery). The Veteran's Affairs (VA) Cooperative Study of coronary artery bypass surgery was the first such trial undertaken and began in 1972 [1]. Very early in the trial it was clear that patients with left main coronary artery diseased benefitted from bypass surgery and left main disease was an exclusion criteria for subsequent enrollment. With time, it was also clear that patients classified as "high-risk" angiographic group, defined as the combination of triple-vessel disease and impaired LV function, received survival benefit from surgery (Figure 9.1). It has been pointed out that by 15 years after operation

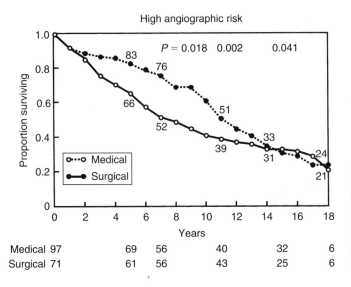

Figure 9.1 The initial randomized trial of surgery versus medical treatment, the VA study of stable angina showed a survival advantage for patients with triple-vessel disease and abnormal left ventricular function who underwent bypass surgery (reprinted with permission from [1]).

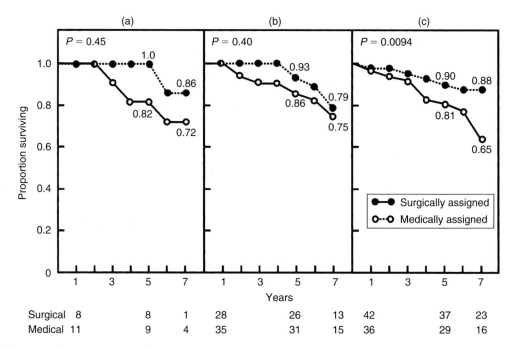

Figure 9.2 In the CASS randomized trial, there were trends toward improved survival rates for surgically treated patients with (a) single-, (b) double-, or (c) triple-vessel disease that achieved statistical significance (reprinted with permission from [2]).

the highly significant survival difference between the medical and surgical groups had disappeared. However, it is also important to note that only 30% of patients were still alive at that point and that by 18 years 62% of the patients originally randomized to receive medical treatment had "crossed-over" to receive bypass surgery, thus receiving whatever survival benefit bypass surgery provided. Furthermore, the VA trial was conducted in a primitive era of bypass surgery prior to internal thoracic artery (ITA) grafts and effective myocardial protection.

The Coronary Artery Surgery Study (CASS) was undertaken in the latter years of the 1970s and involved a randomized arm of patients with mild or moderate angina and a registry arm of patients who either did not qualify for randomization or who did qualify but were not randomized. In the randomized arm of the trial the patients with an ejection fraction (EF) of <50% were found to have an improved survival rate at 10 years after randomization whether or not they had symptoms prior to operation (Figure 9.2) [2]. Again, none of those patients had severe angina, and cross-over to surgical treatment was frequent as 38% of medically treated

patients had undergone surgery by 10 post-operative years [3].

In CASS, many more patients were included in the non-randomized registry than in the randomized arm, and registry analyses documented some important observations. For patients with mild angina and moderate impairment of LV function survival rates were improved according to a non-EF based LV scoring method [4]. Few patients with severe LV function were included in this registry study. For patients with severe angina there was a major difference in survival for patients with triple-vessel disease as 82% of the surgical group survived to 5 years, as opposed to 52% of the group initially treated medically (Figure 9.3) [5].

Another important study from the CASS registry involved the impact of bypass surgery on the risk of sudden death [6]. Sudden cardiac death (death within 1 h of the onset of symptoms) was the mode of death in 26% of the deaths that occurred during a 4.6-year follow-up. Surgery decreased the overall risk of sudden death in most patient subsets that were examined but was particularly effective in decreasing the rate of sudden death for patients

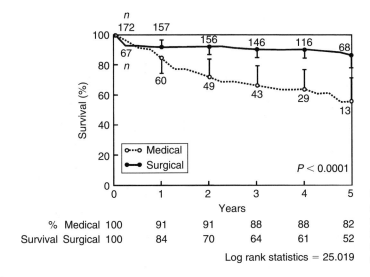

Figure 9.3 Non-randomized CASS patients with severe angina and triple-vessel disease experienced a marked improvement in survival rate with operation (reprinted with permission from [3]).

%	Medical	100	91	91	88	88	82
Survival	Surgical	100	84	70	64	61	52

Log rank statistics = 25.019

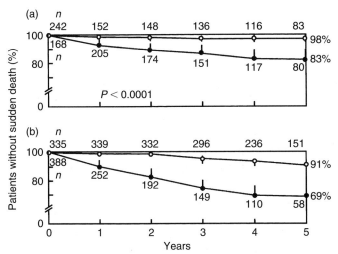

Figure 9.4 (a) Double-vessel disease. (b) Triple-vessel disease. In the non-randomized CASS registry, bypass surgery decreased the risk of sudden death for patients with a history of CHF and either two or triple-vessel disease (reprinted with permission from [6]).

with multi-vessel disease and a history of CHF. For example, for patients with triple-vessel disease with a history of CHF, by 5 years 31% of medically treated patients had suffered sudden death compared to 9% of those surgically treated (Figure 9.4) [6].

Data from the CASS registry also addressed the importance of the extent of revascularization on the survival rate of patients after bypass surgery. Bell and colleagues separated the surgically treated patients into subgroups based on the number of grafts performed as an indicator of complete versus incomplete revascularization. They found that the number of grafts relative to the number of vessels diseased did not impact on patients with normal ventricular function but that complete revascularization

significantly improved the survival rate of those with ischemic cardiomyopathy [7].

A second VA Trial involved patients with unstable angina. This trial also showed a survival benefit for patients with abnormal LV function and triple-vessel disease who underwent bypass surgery compared with those treated with initial medical management [8].

All of these trials were begun within the first decade of the bypass surgery era when intra- and postoperative strategies were relatively primitive. Since that time conceptual and technical improvements have lowered the short-term risks and improved the long-term outcomes associated with bypass surgery. Perioperative risks have diminished due to improvements in intraoperative myocardial protection, increased surgeon experience, and more consistent postoperative care strategies. The use of platelet inhibitors has been shown to improve vein graft patency rates and may diminish perioperative ischemic events [9], and the use of 3-hydroxy-3-methylglutaryl (HMG) co-enzyme A inhibitors decreases angiographic progression of atherosclerosis in bypass grafts and native coronary arteries, and decreases the risk of cardiac events within the first 3 years after bypass surgery [10,11]. ITA grafts were not used to any significant degree in any of the randomized trials. We now know that ITA grafts have superior early and late patency rates to vein grafts and that even to 20 years after operation the likelihood of late ITA graft failure is quite low. These improved patency rates are also clinically important and the use of the "left internal thoracic artery to left anterior descending coronary artery" (LITA-LAD) graft has been shown to prolong long-term survival rate and reduce the incidence of late cardiac events [12]. Also, observational data is now accumulating that the use of two ITA grafts may improve long-term survival rates and decrease the risk of reoperation when compared with the single ITA graft strategy [13].

The results of the randomized and observational trials of the 1970s were reasonably consistent, observational studies since that time have also seemed to indicate favorable outcomes for patients with abnormal LV function and surgical outcomes have improved dramatically since the trials were completed. These considerations have established bypass surgery as the treatment of choice for prolonging patient survival for patients with ischemic cardiomyopathy. Reviews by consensus panels have further established the principal that abnormal LV function combined with left main or multi-vessel coronary artery disease represents an indication for bypass surgery regardless of the severity of symptoms [14,15].

Non-operative therapies for patients with ischemic cardiomyopathy have also improved. Pharmacologic treatments including the use of angiotensin converting enzyme inhibitors, beta-blockers, and diuretics, often improve the symptoms of CHF and some randomized trials have also noted that pharmacologic therapies may decrease the mortality rate during short follow-up periods [16]. The availability of multiple anti-arrhythmic agents have decreased symptoms induced by arrhythmias but an influence on survival rate has been hard to show. Implantable defibrillators, however, have appeared to decrease the risk of death based on arrhythmia for some high-risk patient subgroups [17]. In view of these advances in non-operative therapy, it has been suggested that revascularization may not still be needed to improve the survival rate of patients with ischemic cardiomyopathy, and that more current randomized trials comparing modern bypass surgery with modern non-operative treatment are needed to re-establish the indications for revascularization.

My own view is different. Patients with ischemic cardiomyopathy have ended up with abnormal LV function because of the occurrence of coronary vascular events. Unless pharmacologic agents prevent the occurrence of further ischemic events it would seem logical that regardless of progress in the pharmacologic treatment of heart failure and rhythm disturbances that the presence of uncorrected coronary stenoses still threatens the survival of patients with ischemic cardiomyopathy. For patients with myocardium jeopardized by the presence of coronary stenoses and at risk for future coronary events, why would we not expect bypass grafting to improve the survival rate? There appear to be three situations where surgery might not benefit. The first would be if the operative risk outweighed the long-term benefit. The second would be if there was a high incidence of mortality that was unrelated to ischemia, or if ischemia did not pose risk, and the third if bypass grafting was ineffective in preventing ischemia.

In regard to the first issue, although there is an incremental risk during bypass surgery produced by abnormal LV function, with modern myocardial protection that increment is small. The in-hospital risk of bypass surgery, even for those with severe LV dysfunction, represents a relatively small proportion of the total risk of patients with ischemic cardiomyopathy. Review of 14,075 Cleveland Clinic Foundation patients undergoing primary isolated bypass surgery during the years 1990–1999 showed in-hospital mortality rates according to preoperative LV function to be normal ($n = 7203$) 1.5%, mild impairment ($n = 3378$) 0.8%, moderate impairment ($n = 2132$) 2.5%, and severe impairment ($n = 1362$) 3.2%, respectively. Other centers have also demonstrated a low procedure-related mortality for operations for ischemic cardiomyopathy.

Second, there is evidence that ischemic events do contribute in a major way to the mortality of patients with ischemic cardiomyopathy. Investigators from the Assessment of Treatment with Lisinopril and Survival (ATLAS) trial reported a detailed study of autopsy data. In ATLAS, 1083 deaths occurred and 188 postmortem examinations were performed [18]. Thirty-three patients who underwent postmortem examinations were judged to have died from non-cardiac causes and of the 155 judged to have died from heart disease, 56 had acute coronary pathology noted at autopsy. Furthermore, 54% of patients undergoing sudden death exhibited acute coronary findings. Because of ischemia-induced arrhythmias could result from ischemia not caused by new vascular occlusion and postmortem examinations might not always identify new changes in coronary anatomy for patients with diffuse atherosclerosis, these figures for the impact of new ischemic events on death rate have to be considered minimum figures. Studies based on clinical judgements of cause of death cannot be relied upon to identify deaths related to ischemic events. In ATLAS, 26% of the patients who underwent autopsy were found to have died of myocardial infarction but only 4% of patients who did not have a postmortem examination were judged to have died of myocardial infarction on clinical grounds. Studies of patients without abnormal LV function who have asymptomatic ischemia (Asymptomatic Cardiac Ischemia Pilot (ACIP) Trial) have shown that myocardial ischemia predicts mortality despite current medical therapy [19]. Why would we think that ischemia is benign for patients with abnormal LV function?

Third, can coronary bypass surgery prevent fatal ischemic events? We know that coronary bypass surgery does not totally prevent ischemic events of all magnitude. There is relatively little evidence that coronary bypass surgery over the long term lowers the rate of diagnosis of myocardial infarction. However, it does appear from the randomized trials of the past that coronary surgery lowers the risk of fatal myocardial infarction and we have already noted the data from the CASS registry clearly showing a decreased risk of sudden death after bypass surgery for patients with symptoms of CHF [6]. In addition, there are more recent data from the SOLVD (Studies of Left Ventricular Dysfunction) studies that the mortality rate from ischemic cardiomyopathy

is decreased by bypass surgery despite treatment with modern pharmacologic therapy. One of the SOLVD studies was designed to test the impact of Anapril on the survival of patients with ischemic cardiomyopathy (left ventricular ejection fraction, LVEF ≤ 0.35). Thirty-five percent of the 5410 patients in this study had undergone previous bypass surgery a mean of 1.8 years prior to entry into the study [20]. During a 3-year follow-up, those patients had a 26% lower mortality rate than the patients who did not have a history of bypass surgery, and this decreased risk of death was mostly due to a decreased risk of sudden death. Further work from the SOLVD trial found that diabetic patients strongly benefitted from bypass surgery in terms of survival [21]. It is important to note that patients with unstable angina or myocardial infarction within a month of entry were excluded from the SOLVD trial, meaning that the patients that were included would not have been considered clinically to be at a particularly high risk for ischemic events.

The authors of SOLVD have made the observation that the effect of bypass surgery in decreasing the risk of sudden death may be a possible explanation for the inability to demonstrate a positive effect of implanted cardioverter defibrillators (ICD) on survival rate in the Coronary Artery Bypass Graft (CABG) Patch Trial. The CABG Patch Trial involved patients with ischemic cardiomyopathy who all underwent bypass surgery and tested ICD implantation against pharmacologic management for the prevention of mortality. There did not appear to be a benefit from ICD implantation [22]. One explanation for the lack of improvement with ICD implantation was that the mortality rate in CABG Patch for the patients who had bypass surgery and pharmacologic treatment was only 6% per year. Thus, bypass surgery may have lowered the mortality rate to a level where improvement was difficult to demonstrate even with ICD implantation.

In the anti-arrhythmic versus implantable defibrillator (AVID) trial, patients with life threatening ventricular arrhythmias received either anti-arrhythmic drugs (AAD) or ICD implantation, and while 80% of patients had ischemic cardiomyopathy only 30% had undergone bypass surgery [17]. In AVID, patients with EF <0.34 had an improved survival rate with ICD implantation. However, this improvement was based on a particularly bad outcome for the AAD patients with survival rates of only 64% and 72% at 2 years of follow-up for patients with EF <0.20 and 0.20–0.34, respectively. Although the ICD patients did have an improved survival rate, those survival rates still were not very good with 2 year survival rates of 72%, 82%, and 83% for patients with EF of <0.20, 0.20–0.34, and >0.34, respectively. Thus, the patients in the AVID trial had high mortality rates despite ICD implantation. It is true that the AVID patients appeared to be at a greater arrhythmic risk than those that were included in the CABG Patch trial but these data also suggest that ICD implantation is not a substitute for revascularization.

Patients with ischemic cardiomyopathy are heterogeneous in regard to coronary anatomy, ischemic jeopardy, and myocardial viability. It is probable that there are patients who can be categorized as having ischemic cardiomyopathy that will benefit very little from revascularization and some that will benefit a lot. There are now available imaging modalities that appear to be able to help identify these patient subsets. There are multiple techniques available and the information they provide concerning myocardial viability differs. Single photon emission tomography (SPECT) using thallium-21 or technetium-99 perfusion tracers examines cell membrane integrity. Metabolic activity can be identified using positron emission tomography (PET) and dobutamine stress echocardiography addresses the issue of contractile reserve. All of these techniques have been tested with clinically based trials in regard to their prediction of long-term clinical outcomes after revascularization and appear to have some predictive value. Magnetic resonance imaging (MRI) also may be used to predict viability and outcomes although few data have correlated that technique with long-term clinical outcomes. In general, SPECT and PET tomography are quite sensitive, that is to say, very few viable cells are necessary for them to be identified as viable. However, the strategies do not appear to be as specific in terms of recovery of regional myocardial function after revascularization. Dobutamine stress echocardiography is not as sensitive but appears to be more specific for the ability of myocardium to improve its function after revascularization.

Meta-analysis of 24 studies correlating myocardial viability assessment and survival with or without revascularization for patients with ischemic cardiomyopathy was performed by Allman and colleagues [23]. There were 3088 patients in the studies included in the meta-analysis with EFs of 32 ± 8%. Patients were followed for 25 ± 10 months after the diagnostic studies. For patients who exhibited myocardial viability revascularization decreased the risk of death by about 80%. There was a 3.2% annual mortality for the revascularized group compared with a 16% annual mortality for patients who did not undergo revascularization. Patients who did not demonstrate myocardial viability had a worse annual mortality in the revascularized group (7.7% per year) and a relatively better survival rate for patients treated medically (6.2% per year). Patients without myocardial viability did not exhibit an improved survival rate in any subgroup based on ventricular function. Patients with myocardial viability exhibited more benefit from revascularization as the EF decreased. Although the individual studies contain smaller patient numbers than the meta-analysis, the findings of the individual studies were consistent. The authors were unable to identify an advantage for any particular type of viability study in terms of the accuracy of prediction of outcomes.

Studies of myocardial viability can also be of value in predicting the functional recovery of abnormal myocardium after revascularization. Thallium SPECT has been shown to predict improvement of EF if large areas of viability are demonstrated. Dobutamine echocardiography also has been shown to be of value in predicting improvement in measurements of global LV function.

More recent data indicate that identification of viability myocardium preoperatively can predict improved function class postoperatively [24]. Marwick et al. correlated improvement in exercise capacity after revascularization with viable myocardium of >20% of the LV mass as identified by PET correlating with improvement in rate pressure product [25]. Further Cleveland Clinic Foundation studies have shown that PET appeared to be more accurate in improvement of exercise capacity than was dobutamine echo.

Based on the previous randomized trials of bypass surgery versus medical treatment, the improvements in the short- and long-term outcomes of bypass surgery, the confirmatory data from more modern trials that we have discussed, the continued high risk of patients with ischemic cardiomyopathy despite non-surgical treatments, and data showing the benefit of surgery for patients with myocardial viability, it does not seem to me that randomized trials testing revascularization versus non-surgical treatment for patients with ischemic cardiomyopathy and myocardial viability are either needed or justified. However, there are many other questions that are as yet unanswered.

First, what is the optimum role of percutaneous procedures (PCT) in the revascularization of patients with ischemic cardiomyopathy? Most revascularization studies have involved revascularization via bypass surgery for the overwhelming majority of patients with ischemic cardiomyopathy. Even with the use of coronary stenting, all comparative trials of surgery versus PCT revascularization have documented less consistent revascularization with PCT. On the other hand, PCT has shown to have been effective at least over the short-term, for some high-risk patient subsets [25]. The importance of complete revascularization for a patient with ischemic cardiomyopathy has also been a deterrent to the routine use of PCT for these patients. For patients with coronary vascular anatomy suitable for stenting, second generation (drug-coated) stents may provide more consistent and long lasting revascularization than previous PCT technologies.

Second, patients with ischemic cardiomyopathy are often post-bypass surgery. Reoperation for patients with recurrent ischemia based on progression of atherosclerosis who also have abnormal LV function is not a strategy that has been tested with randomized trials.

Third, for patients without jeopardy of viable myocardium there is not a great deal of evidence that operation improves survival rate compared with medical management.

However, despite the existence of these and other questions, bypass surgery has a central role in the treatment of ischemic cardiomyopathy and is the best long-term strategy for the majority of these patients.

References

1 The VA Cooperative Study Group. Eighteen-year follow-up in the Veterans Affairs Cooperative Study of coronary artery bypass surgery for stable angina. *Circulation* 1992; **86**: 121–130.

2 Passamani E, Davis KB, Gillespie MJ et al. A randomized trial of coronary artery bypass surgery. Survival of patients with a low ejection fraction. *N Engl J Med* 1985; **312**: 1665–1671.

3 Alderman EL, Bourassa MG, Cohen LS et al. Ten year follow-up of survival and myocardial infarction in the randomized Coronary Artery Surgery Study. *Circulation* 1990; **82**: 1629–1646.

4 Myers WO, Gersh BJ, Fisher LD et al. Medical versus early surgical therapy in patients with triple-vessel disease and mild angina pectoris: a CASS registry study of survival. *Ann Thorac Surg* 1987; **44**: 471–486.

5 Kaiser GC, Davis KB, Fisher LD et al. Survival following coronary artery bypass grafting in patients with severe angina pectoris (CASS). An observational study. *J Thorac Cardiovasc Surg* 1985; **89**: 513–524.

6 Holmes Jr. DR, Davis KB, Mock MB et al. The effect of medical and surgical treatment on subsequent sudden cardiac death in patients with coronary artery disease: a report from the Coronary Artery Surgery Study. *Circulation* 1986; **73**: 1254–1263.

7 Bell MR, Gersh BJ, Schaff HV et al. Effect of completeness of revascularization on long-term outcome of patients with three-vessel disease undergoing coronary artery bypass surgery: a report from the Coronary Artery Surgery Study (CASS) Registry. *Circulation* 1992; **86**: 446–457.

8 Sharma GV, Deupree RH, Khuri SF et al. Coronary bypass surgery improves survival in high-risk unstable angina. Results of a Veterans Administration Cooperative Study with an 8-year follow-up. Veterans Administration Unstable Angina Cooperative Study Group. *Circulation* 1991; **84(Suppl III)**: III-260–III-267.

9 Gavaghan TP, Gebski V, Baron DW. Immediate post-operative aspirin improves vein graft patency early and late after coronary artery bypass graft surgery. A placebo-controlled, randomized study. *Circulation* 1991; **83**: 1526–1533.

10 Flaker GC, Warnica JW, Sacks FM et al. Pravastatin prevents clinical events in revascularized patients with average cholesterol concentrations: Cholesterol and Recurrent Events (CARE) Investigators. *J Am Coll Cardiol* 1999; **34**: 106–112.

11 The Post-Coronary Artery Bypass Graft Trial Investigators. The effect of aggressive lowering of low-density lipoprotein cholesterol levels and low-dose anticoagulation on obstructive changes in saphenous-vein-coronary-artery bypass grafts. *N Engl J Med* 1997; **336**: 153–162.

12 Loop FD, Lytle BW, Cosgrove DM, Stewart RW, Goormastic M, Williams GW, Golding LAR, Gill CC, Taylor PC, Sheldon WC, Proudfit WL. Influence of the internal-mammary-artery graft on 10-year survival and other cardiac events. *N Engl J Med* 1986; **314**: 1–6.

13 Lytle BW, Blackstone EH, Loop FD, Houghtaling PL, Arnold JH, Akhrass R, McCarthy PM, Cosgrove DM. Two internal thoracic artery grafts are better than one. *J Thorac Cardiovasc Surg* 1999; **117**: 855–872.

14 Gibbons RJ, Chatterjee K, Daley J, Douglas JS, Fihn SD, Gardin JM, Grunwald MA, Levy D, Lytle BW, O'Rourke RA, Schafer WP, Williams SV. ACC/AHA/ACP-ASIM guidelines for the management of patients with chronic stable angina: a report of the American College of Cardiology/American Heart Association Task Force on Practice Guidelines (Committee on Management of Patients with Chronic Stable Angina). *J Am Coll Cardiol* 1999; **33**: 2092–2197.

15 Eagle KA, Guyton RA, Davidoff R, Ewy GA, Fonger J, Gardner TJ, Gott JP, Herrmann HC, Marlow RA, Nugent WC, O'Connor GT, Orszulak TA, Rieselbach RE, Winters WL, Yusuf S. ACC/AHA guidelines for coronary artery bypass graft surgery: a report of the American College of Cardiology/American-Heart Association Task Force on Practice Guidelines (Committee to Revise the 1991 Guidelines for Coronary Artery Bypass Graft Surgery). *J Am Coll Cardiol* 1999; **34**: 1262–1347.

16 Pitt B, Zannad F, Remme WJ *et al.* The effect of spironolactone on morbidity and mortality in patients with severe heart failure. *N Engl J Med* 1999; **341**: 709–717.

17 Domanski MJ, Sakseener SI, Epstein AE *et al.* Relative effectiveness of the implantable cardioverter-defibrillator and antiarrhythmic drugs in patients with varying degrees of left ventricular dysfunction who have survived malignant ventricular arrhythmias. *J Am Coll Cardiol* 1999; **34**: 1090–1095.

18 Uretsky BF, Thygesen K, Armstrong PW *et al.* Acute coronary findings at autopsy in heart failure patients with sudden death. Results from the assessment of treatment with lisinopril and survival (ATLAS) trial. *Circulation* 2000; **102**: 611–616.

19 Davies RF, Goldberg AD, Forman S *et al.* Asymptomatic Cardiac Ischemia Pilot (ACIP) Study two-year follow-up. Outcomes of patients randomized to initial strategies of medical therapy versus revascularization. *Circulation* 1997; **95**: 2037–2043.

20 Veenhuyzen GD, Singh SN, McAreavey D *et al.* Prior coronary artery bypass surgery and risk of death among patients with ischemic left ventricular dysfunction. *Circulation* 2001; **104**: 1489–1493.

21 Dries DL, Sweitzer NK, Drazner MH *et al.* Prognostic impact of diabetes mellitus in patients with heart failure according to the etiology of left ventricular systolic dysfunction. *J Am Coll Cardiol* 2001; **38**: 421–428.

22 Bigger Jr. JT. Prophylactic use of implanted cardiac defibrillators in patients at high risk for ventricular arrhythmias after coronary-artery bypass graft surgery. Coronary Artery Bypass Graft (CABG) Patch Trial Investigators. *N Engl J Med* 1997; **337**: 1569–1575.

23 Allman KC, Shaw LJ, Hachamovitch R, Udelson JE. Myocardial viability testing and impact of revascularization on prognosis in patients with coronary artery disease and left ventricular dysfunction: a meta-analysis. *J Am Coll Cardiol* 2002; **39**: 1151–1158.

24 Marwick TH. Use of standard imaging techniques for prediction of postrevascularization functional recovery in patients with heart failure. *J Cardiac Fail* 1999; **5**: 334–346.

25 Morrison DA, Sethi G, Sacks J *et al.* Percutaneous coronary intervention versus repeat bypass surgery for patients with medically refractory myocardial ischemia (AWESOME randomized trial registry experience with post-CABG patients). *J Am Coll Cardiol* 2002; **40**: 1951–1954.

CHAPTER 10

Valve surgery for patients with left ventricular dysfunction

Patrick M. McCarthy

Introduction

Clinicians are frequently faced with patients with heart failure, or severely impaired ventricular function, who have clinically significant valve lesions. In a recent study from the University of Michigan a search of their echocardiographic database illuminated the problem and the poor prognosis of these patients [1]. Of the patients with a 35% or less left ventricular ejection fraction (LVEF), 48.6% had either 3 or 4+ mitral regurgitation (MR), and 34.5% had 3 or 4+ tricuspid regurgitation (TR). By univariable and multivariable analysis severe MR and TR regurgitation both were shown to be significant predictors of mortality (Figure 10.1). Additional studies from the Mayo Clinic confirm the frequent finding of MR and TR in congestive heart failure (CHF) patients, and the poor prognosis of patients with significant MR and TR [2].

Historically, clinicians were taught that mitral valve replacement in patients with a 40% or less EF and low cardiac index was extremely high risk, and that "the risk of operative mortality becomes prohibitive" [3]. However, these words of wisdom from 1980 reflected the state of the art at that point in time. The standard of care at that time was to replace the mitral valve, with a ball-in-cage prosthesis and the subvalvular components impeded prosthetic valve function (Figure 10.2). In addition, the entire valve, including the papillary muscles and subvalvular apparatus, were removed. We now know, these "valvular–ventricular" interactions are important to maintain ventricular function [4,5]. After removal of the papillary muscles and their chordal attachments to the valve and to the valve annulus, the ventricle dilates and becomes more dysfunctional. The high operative mortality in 1980 was compounded by the lack of

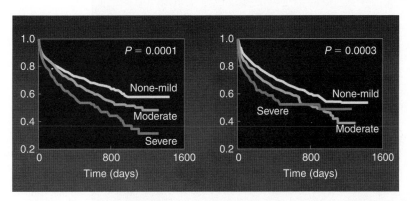

Figure 10.1 In a study from the University of Michigan, 3 or 4+ MR (left panel) was present in 48.6% of patients with an EF of 35% or less, and 3 or 4+ TR was present in 34.5%. By univariable and multivariable analysis MR and TR predicted reduced survival (reprinted with permission from [1]).

sophisticated methods of myocardial protection, and more limited capabilities for peri-operative care.

There are several other sources of information indicating that MR portends a poor prognosis in those with ischemic disease. The presence of MR

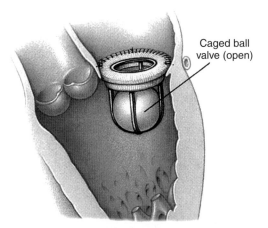

Caged ball valve (open)

Figure 10.2 In the 1970s and 1980s valve replacement, rather than repair, was performed in most patients with MR. During those operations the entire subvalvular apparatus, along with the leaflets and chords, were removed to avoid impingement on the ball-in-cage valve. This lead to reduced ventricular function associated with a high operative and late mortality. Mitral valve surgery for patients with LV dysfunction was high risk during that time period.

was shown to indicate a poor long-term outcome in patients post myocardial infarction (MI) [6]. In a study from the Cleveland Clinic, patients who underwent percutaneous coronary intervention had a significantly worse prognosis if there was 3 or 4+ MR, compared to those without MR [7]. Even those with 1 or 2+ MR, had reduced survival (Figure 10.3). This was especially true for patients with an EF less than 40%. Several other papers document the poor prognosis of MR in patients with LV dysfunction [8–10].

Surgical treatment of MR in patients with severe LV dysfunction

Since 1980, when mitral valve replacement in patients with LV dysfunction was high risk, surgical outcomes have improved considerably. Much has been learned about the mechanisms of MR, intra-operative and post-operative management, and the type of procedure and ring prosthesis to be employed for valve repair. Bolling published a series of patients who underwent mitral valve repair (not replacement) with severe LV dysfunction [11]. Surgeons were first struck by the low operative mortality (2%). The concept of the "pop-off" mechanism had been circulated for decades to explain the high mortality of patients

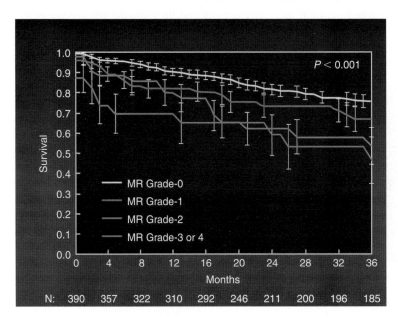

Figure 10.3 Patients who underwent percutaneous coronary intervention had a significantly worse prognosis if they had MR. This was even true for those with only 1 or 2+ MR (reprinted with permission from [7]).

who underwent surgery for MR with severe LV dysfunction. According to this concept, MR was somewhat beneficial, in that the ventricle was unloaded into the low-pressure left atrium. By removing this pop-off mechanism with a competent mitral valve, afterload was increased on the ventricle (which now had to eject solely into the systemic circulation). This increased workload led to early peri-operative death. Therefore, Bollings' successful surgical series was remarkable because it refuted this pop-off concept. Equally remarkable, 3-year survival was approximately 75%, considerably better than they expected for patients with heart failure with severe LV dysfunction and MR (Figure 10.4). Further studies from the University of Michigan also showed that by removing the volume overload caused by MR the ventricles remodeled, end-diastolic and end-systolic volumes decreased, forward stroke volume and cardiac output improved, and EF improved [12] (Table 10.1).

These results were reproduced in one of our studies from the Cleveland Clinic [13]. Also, in our series we investigated hospital admissions for CHF. All patients had been admitted with heart failure at least once, with a range of 1–6 times before surgery, and a mean of 2 admissions. In addition to similar favorable survival like Bollings' report, freedom from hospital readmission for heart failure was very high in our series (Figure 10.5). Furthermore, we also observed late changes in ventricular volumes and structure, and an improvement in ventricular function (Figure 10.6).

The recently completed Acorn Clinical Trial was a multi-center-randomized prospective trial of patients with low LVEF (mean 24%) and MR. After just mitral valve surgery they found favorable changes in LV volumes and exercise capacity, quality of life, and New York Heart Association (NYHA) class [14]. Notably, this was the first randomized surgical study of patients with severe MR and severe LV dysfunction, and it confirmed a low operative

Table 10.1 Changes after mitral valve replacement in patients with severe LV dysfunction (reproduced with permission from [12]).

Echocardiographic parameter	Pre-operative	Post-operative (24 months)	P-value
End-diastolic volume (mL)	281 ± 86	206 ± 88	<0.001
EF (%)	16 ± 5	26 ± 8	0.008
Regurgitant fraction (%)	70 ± 12	13 ± 10	<0.001
Cardiac output (L/min)	3.1 ± 1.0	5.2 ± 0.8	0.001
Sphericity index (D/L)	0.82 ± 0.10	0.74 ± 0.07	0.005

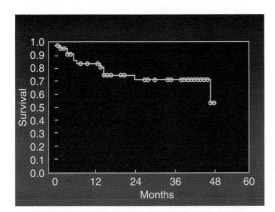

Figure 10.4 Bolling and colleagues reported a series of patients who underwent mitral valve repair, instead of replacement, and found a low early mortality, and acceptable late mortality for a group of patients with LV dysfunction and heart failure. Other surgeons began to adopt this more aggressive strategy in patients with LV dysfunction (reproduced with permission from [11]).

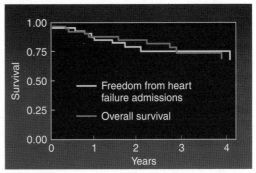

Figure 10.5 In a study of mitral valve surgery patients with severe LV dysfunction from the Cleveland Clinic, early and late mortality were low. Also freedom from heart failure readmission was high considering that all patients had been hospitalized from 1 to 6 times for heart failure before the operation, with a mean number of pre-operative admissions of 2.1 ± 1.5 (reproduced with permission from [13]).

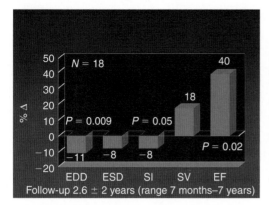

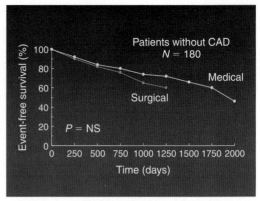

Figure 10.6 After mitral valve surgery in patients with severe LV dysfunction in the Cleveland Clinic study we also observed improvement in ventricular volumes and function (reproduced with permission from [13]). EDD: end-diastolic diameter; ESD: end-systolic diameter; SI: sphericity index; SV: sphericity volume.

Figure 10.7 A retrospective, propensity matched, study from the University of Michigan showed no difference in survival for medically or surgically treated patients with low EF and severe MR. Although the study had flaws, and reported Dr. Bolling's earliest results using a flexible mitral repair ring which was prone to failure, it points out the need for a prospective-randomized trial of this patient population (reproduced with permission from [8]). CAD: coronary artery disease.

mortality (1.6%) with favorable changes in ventricular function for both control (mitral valve surgery only) or treated patients (mitral valve surgery with CorCap™).

These studies have demonstrated in patients with severe LV dysfunction and MR that contemporary surgical results offer a low mortality, improved LV volumes and function, improved exercise capacity, quality of life and NYHA class, low need for re-hospitalization for heart failure, and good mid-term survival. Is survival better than for those patients being treated with contemporary medical therapy that includes beta-blockers, biventricular pacing, and defibrillators? The answer is not clear. A recent report from the University of Michigan showed no survival advantage for those treated with surgery [8]. This retrospective, but propensity matched, analysis (Figure 10.7) had the usual flaws of all retrospective studies (such as determining retrospectively that a patient *could* have been a surgical candidate) and also compared to the earliest mitral valve surgery results using flexible rings that later studies found to have a high risk for late MR recurrence (see next section on Ischemic MR). A randomized prospective trial of medical therapy versus surgical treatment would be the ideal solution. Grant applications for such a study have been submitted. The ACC/AHA Practice Guidelines suggest that such surgery can be considered, and is a Class IIb [15].

Ischemic MR

Ischemic MR (IMR) is different from functional MR caused by idiopathic dilated cardiomyopathy for several reasons. First, IMR is more common, so surgeons and cardiologists outside of major heart failure programs frequently encounter these patients and have to make decisions on how best to treat them. Idiopathic cardiomyopathy patients are not common outside transplant centers and, as yet, uncommonly referred for surgery. Based on data from the Cleveland Clinic with percutaneous coronary interventions, patients with MR had a worse prognosis than those with no MR and, therefore, coronary bypass with mitral valve repair may be the preferred approach [7]. Second, many patients are encountered who need coronary artery bypass (CAB) who have mild or moderate MR and the decision has to be made whether the mitral valve should be treated or not at the time of CAB. Finally, the unique pathophysiologic characteristics of IMR, and the complexity of the MR jet, make it more challenging to successfully repair. Fortunately new data can help the surgeon provide a successful IMR repair.

A common surgical myth is that CAB alone will consistently reduce or eliminate IMR. Sometimes this will be true for the patient who has active ischemia with a non-transmural MI and regional wall motion

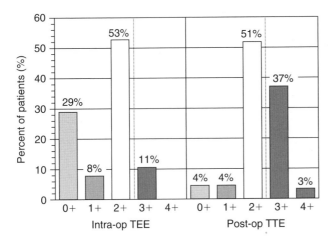

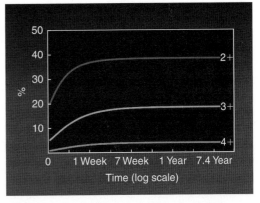

Figure 10.8 Patients with 3+ MR who underwent CAB alone had persistent MR in follow-up. Intra-operative downgrade of MR grade by TEE should be ignored by surgeons (reproduced with permission from [16]).
TEE: trans-esophageal echocardiography;
TTE: transthoracic echocardiography.

abnormalities. However, the majority of patients who have had a transmural infarct have a more fixed defect, with geometric changes of the ventricle (remodeling), and therefore coronary bypass alone would not be expected to eliminate MR. The group at Brigham and Women's Hospital studied patients with 3+ MR and found that after CAB alone, the MR continued [16,17] (Figure 10.8). At the Cleveland Clinic, we looked at patients who had 2+ IMR which was left untreated at the time of CAB [18]. A majority of the patients either stayed at 2+ MR during follow-up, or progressed to 3 or 4+ MR (Figure 10.9). Furthermore, in a propensity-matched group, the survival was worse for patients who had MR who underwent coronary bypass, than for those who underwent CAB but who had no MR (Figure 10.10). Similar findings were reported from the University of Toronto [19,20]. They did not find reduced survival in those with mild or moderate MR, but they found decreased event free survival, and worse late functional status [19] (Figure 10.11).

Papers have indicated that if IMR is corrected at the time of CAB, then late survival is better [20,21]. Not all studies would agree with this, however. A recent study from Washington University indicated no difference in survival in patients with 3–4+ MR who were left untreated [22]. However, patients with untreated MR were generally sick patients undergoing emergency surgery and the survival was limited. Other retrospective studies found no difference in survival [23–25].

A randomized, prospective, surgical trial to determine whether there are survival benefits,

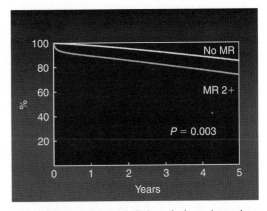

Figure 10.9 Cleveland Clinic data demonstrated that patients with 2+ MR before coronary bypass typically had persistent 2+ MR, or developed 3 or 4+ MR during follow up (reproduced with permission from [18]).

Figure 10.10 In a Cleveland Clinic study the patients who had untreated 2+ MR at CAB had worse survival than matched patients that had CAB but who did not have MR (reproduced with permission from [18]).

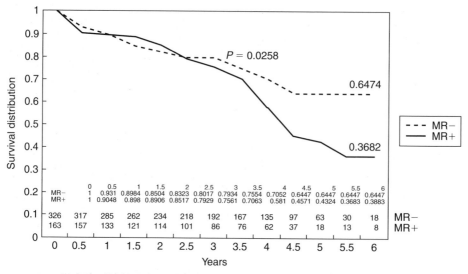

	0	0.5	1	1.5	2	2.5	3	3.5	4	4.5	5	5.5	6
MR−	1	0.931	0.8984	0.8504	0.8323	0.8017	0.7934	0.7554	0.7052	0.6447	0.6447	0.6447	0.6447
MR+	1	0.9048	0.898	0.8906	0.8517	0.7929	0.7561	0.7063	0.581	0.4571	0.4324	0.3683	0.3883
	326	317	285	262	234	218	192	167	135	97	63	30	18
	163	157	133	121	114	101	86	76	62	37	18	13	8

Figure 10.11 From the University of Toronto, late event free survival was better in patients without MR undergoing CAB, than in those with 1 or 2+ MR (reproduced with permission from [19]).

improved ventricular function benefits, decreased re-hospitalization, or improved quality of life in patients who undergo mitral valve repair along with coronary bypass, instead of just CAB alone, has not yet been performed, but is underway. The evidence now is accumulating, however, that in today's era, in experienced hands, the mortality of adding mitral valve repair to CAB is low. CAB itself will likely add significant survival benefit to patients with low EF and viable muscle [26–30]. The results of the prospective multi-center Acorn CorCap™ study indicate that removing or correcting the volume overload from MR led to improvement in ventricular function and size. Therefore, the weight of the evidence seems to be favoring a lower threshold for mitral valve repair with CAB than surgeons were taught years ago. Prospective trials will help us sort this out. The ACC/AHA Guidelines do not answer this question [15].

IMR surgery

What is the mechanism of IMR, and therefore, how is it best repaired? In some patients, would mitral valve replacement be a better option than mitral valve repair?

The mechanisms of chronic IMR are complex. Most often, there is a posterior infarction with ventricular scar in the distribution of the circumflex or right coronary artery. This leads to localized regional

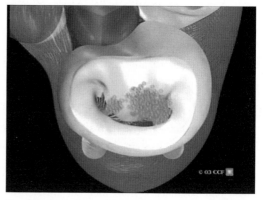

Figure 10.12 Patients with IMR frequently have a complex jet of MR that arises from the medial commissure (P3 area according to Carpentier's classification). The jet is secondary to numerous factors including ventricular remodeling that tethers the posterior papillary muscle (see animation at http://cvbook.nmh.org).

wall motion abnormalities frequently associated with ventricular dilation, a drop in EF, increase in ventricular volumes, and remodeling to a globular-shaped heart (change in sphericity) [32,33,34]. Papillary muscle tethering restricts closure (Carpentier type IIIB), especially involving the medial commissure (P3 area) creating a complex jet that is predominantly from the medial commissure, but that also may originate from the lateral commissure [32,33,34] (Figure 10.12). The valve leaflets and chordae appear to be "normal," but recent studies have shown that they are

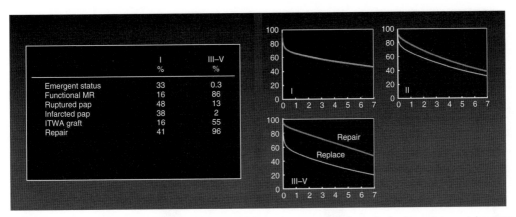

	I %	III–V %
Emergent status	33	0.3
Functional MR	16	86
Ruptured pap	48	13
Infarcted pap	38	2
ITWA graft	16	55
Repair	41	96

Figure 10.13 In most patient groups mitral valve repair leads to a better survival than mitral valve replacement, however, in some subsets (usually the sickest patients) no benefit could be demonstrated because survival was reduced in both groups (reproduced with permission from [41]).

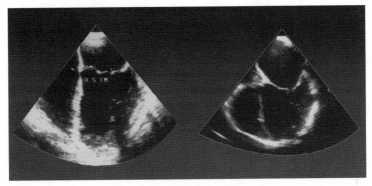

Figure 10.14 When the mitral valve is severely tethered due to ventricular dilation (right panel vs. normal on left) the mitral valve leaflets are pulled toward the apex. A variety of echocardiographic measurements have been used to quantify this, including mitral valve tent height (reproduced with permission from [44]).

stiffer than normal leaflets and have a different biochemical composition [35]. It should be noted that in rare circumstances there is severe acute MR from papillary muscle rupture, or there is infarction and fibrosis with elongation of the papillary muscles that causes prolapse, but both of these are much less common than the classic restriction of the leaflets in patients with ventricular dilation from chronic ischemic cardiomyopathy. Mitral annular motion is reduced, and the typical three-dimensional annular shape is distorted [34,36]. Historically, the medical profession has believed that the "skeleton" of the heart is fixed and therefore the inter-trigone area cannot dilate. However, several recent reports indicate that with idiopathic and ischemic cardiomyopathy the inter-trigone area dilates as well as the posterior annulus [37–40].

In summary, chronic IMR typically is caused by ventricular infarction and remodeling that leads to leaflet tethering (primarily at the medial commissure, P3), dilation involving both the posterior and anterior (inter-trigone) annulus, and changes of leaflet stiffening. The MR jet is complex and eccentric and may vary in intensity depending on factors such as preload and afterload.

In most circumstances, the literature indicates that mitral repair is associated with a lower mortality than mitral valve replacement [17,41–43]. However, there are subsets when mitral valve repair shows no survival advantage over mitral valve replacement [41] (Figure 10.13). Furthermore, Calafiore demonstrated that with severe mitral valve tethering, which is reflected with an increased mitral valve coaptation depth or "tent height" (Figure 10.14), that the leaflets

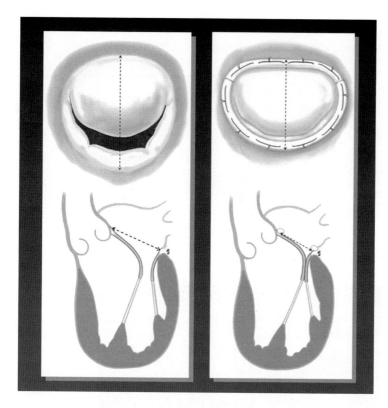

Figure 10.15 In a series of experiments from Stanford University they found that fixing the septal-lateral dimension (or anterior–posterior dimension) is the most important aspect to maintain valvular competence with IMR.

are so severely tethered that repair using annular reduction may not be sufficient to restore adequate coaptation of the leaflets [44]. This then would lead to residual, or later recurrent, MR. However, it should be noted that these surgeons were using a suture-only annuloplasty technique for mitral valve repair. In this study, chord-sparing mitral valve replacement was better. Modern techniques of chord-sparing mitral valve replacement may reduce the deleterious effects of removing the subvalvular apparatus [45]. In a small series of our patients, we found no difference in survival of repair versus replacement for patients with severe LV dysfunction [13].

In summary, in almost all patients, in almost all studies, mitral valve repair seems to be better than replacement because of improved early survival. For those with the most severe tethering of the leaflets, then chord-sparing mitral valve replacement may be an acceptable alternative.

The choice of which mitral repair annuloplasty ring and technique has been controversial. Three recent pieces of evidence help in this decision-making process. First, experimental evidence from Millers' laboratory at Stanford University indicate that fixing the septal-lateral dimension (anterior–posterior) is the most important aspect to maintain valvular competence [40,43,46] (Figure 10.15). A complete remodeling ring that will fix the septal-lateral dimension of the annulus best accomplishes this goal [43]. Second, human studies from Brazil (Figure 10.16), as well as experimental studies from Stanford and the University of Pennsylvania, indicate that the inter-trigone area dilates [37–40]. A flexible ring is a less desirable treatment for patients with cardiomyopathy because it can become distorted by inter-trigone dilation. Finally, studies using three-dimensional echos in humans have shown that the pattern of annular dilation and tethering of the mitral leaflets is asymmetric in patients with ischemic cardiomyopathy [34]. Tethering of the leaflets in patients with idiopathic dilated cardiomyopathy is uniform across medial, central, and lateral (corresponding to P1, P2, and P3), but the tethering predominates at the medial aspect (P3) in ischemic cardiomyopathy (Figure 10.17). From clinical observation and with these studies confirming the unique aspects of ischemic cardiomyopathy, we concluded that the ideal ring for annuloplasty in patients

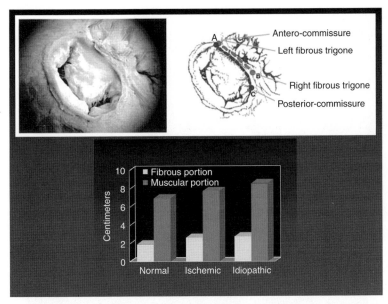

Figure 10.16 Autopsy studies from Brazil, and subsequently animal and human studies, have documented that the inter-trigone area dilates in patients with ischemic and idiopathic cardiomyopathy. This has implications regarding the use of a complete remodeling ring versus a partial band (reproduced with permission from [37]).

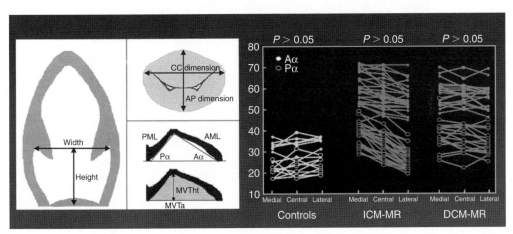

Figure 10.17 IMR is asymmetric in that the jet predominantly originates at the medial aspect. This is due to tethering of the valve leaflets at that area, which is markedly different from patients with normal symmetric closure of the valve, and patients with idiopathic dilated cardiomyopathy also have symmetric tethering (reproduced with permission from [34]).

with ischemic cardiomyopathy would be a complete remodeling ring that was rigid, reduced the septal-lateral dimension, and further reduced the P3 region (the site of the most extensive tethering) and conformed to the three-dimensional annular shape caused by tension on the annulus at the P3 region. A new ring was released in 2004; the Carpentier–McCarthy–Adams IMR ETlogix ring

(see disclosure at end of the book (page 305)). Animation of the concept of IMR and reduction with an annuloplasty ring (Figures 10.12 and 10.18] can be viewed at http://cvbook.nmh.org. Early results are encouraging [47].

The size of the ring used for IMR or idiopathic cardiomyopathy is generally much smaller than for patients with myxomatous mitral valve disease.

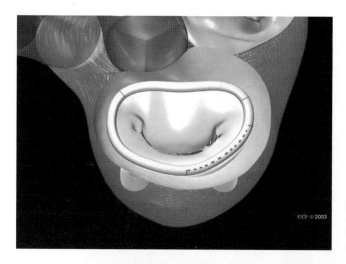

CCF © 2003

Figure 10.18 Animation of the repair of IMR using a new asymmetric three-dimensional annuloplasty ring can be viewed at http://cvbook.nmh.org.

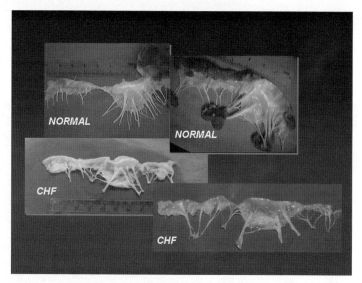

Figure 10.19 While patients with heart failure from idiopathic or ischemic cardiomyopathy may have leaflets that appear "normal" in terms of the morphology of the leaflet, studies have shown that there is extensive stiffening of the leaflets due to changes in their biochemical properties. Since the leaflets are not elongated, however, generally IMR patients are treated with small rings (26 or 28 mm) (reproduced with permission from [35]).

Patients with myxomatous mitral valve disease have elongated leaflet length involving both the anterior and posterior leaflet, especially when that leaflet is flail [48]. On the other hand, patients with ischemic or idiopathic cardiomyopathy have valves that appear "normal" (Figure 10.19). While patients with myxomatous disease may need large rings (32–36 mm are common), patients with ischemic functional MR generally require small or normal-size rings (26–28 mm). While using a small ring in patients

with myxomatous disease may contribute to systolic anterior motion with LV outflow tract obstruction (especially with a normal or small LV cavity), in the setting of cardiomyopathy (usually with a dilated LV) this is not a clinical concern.

The underlying problem in ischemic cardiomyopathy, however, is the changes in the ventricular geometry that lead to tethering of the leaflets. Operations have been suggested to relieve this tethering such as: by moving the papillary muscles with

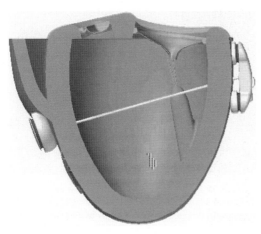

Figure 10.20 The Coapsys™ device developed by Myocor was designed to change both the septal-lateral dimension of the mitral annulus, as well as move the underlying pathology; the enlarged and remodeled LV. The animation can be viewed at http://cvbook.nmh.org.

sutures [49]; reconstructing the ventricular wall posteriorly for a posterior infarct [50]; placing a balloon-inflated device outside the LV that pushes the wall of the ventricle back to a more normal shape [51]; or extending leaflets with pericardium [52].

One device to treat IMR is already in human use undergoing clinical trials. The Coapsys™ device (Myocor Inc., Minneapolis, MN) is a generation beyond the Myosplint™ device (see Chapter 11 on LV reconstruction). The device includes a single trans-ventricular splint and pads on the outer surface of the LV. Another pad is placed on the right ventricle (RV) (Figure 10.20). The procedure is performed off-pump with echo guidance. With continuous echo monitoring, the pads are tightened until MR reduces, and is eventually eliminated [53–56]. One pad on the LV is positioned at the level of the mitral valve annulus. This pad, during tightening, pulls the posterior annulus toward the anterior leaflet, thereby decreasing the septal-lateral dimension. The second pad, on the free wall of the LV, is near the posterior papillary muscle. This pad, when tightened, will change the ventricular shape and decrease the distance of the posterior papillary muscle to the mitral annulus. The concept can be viewed in three-dimensional animation at the website http://cvbook.nmh.org. The Coapsys concept addresses both the septal-lateral annular dilation and the lateral displacement of the posterior papillary muscle. The Coapsys™ device is being studied (Phase II) in the Randomized Evaluation of a Surgical Treatment for Off-pump Repair of the Mitral Valve (RESTOR-MV) trial, which is ongoing in the United States [56]. The non-randomized TRACE trial was performed outside the United States [55]. This device is the first of its kind that will treat both the annular problems of patients with cardiomyopathy and ventricular remodeling that was the initial cause of MR.

In summary, mitral valve surgery for patients with severe LV dysfunction and MR historically was high risk and with only limited effectiveness. The outcomes and hence that reputation, however, are changing. Several centers are now reporting mitral valve repair in these patients with acceptable mortality, late improvements in ventricular function and volumes, improved quality of life for the patient, and improved NYHA class [57]. Three- and five-year survival appear to be quite good compared to patients with MR, severe LV dysfunction, and only medical therapy. The recently completed CorCap™ study further emphasized these points in a multi-center, prospective, randomized surgical trial [14]. These reports should help lead to wider adoption of mitral valve surgery for patients with LV dysfunction. In general, repair is preferable to valve replacement. Because of inter-trigone dilation, and the desire to maintain the septal-lateral dimension, complete remodeling rings that are rigid and hold their shape appear to be the best solution for patients with IMR, otherwise recurrent MR may appear [58,59]. An asymmetric ring that optimizes closure of the medial commissure shows encouraging early results for IMR patients. Ventricular solutions either through direct surgical reconstruction, or with new devices that are being developed, should add to the effectiveness and durability of repair. Finally, for patients with excessive tethering in whom annuloplasty would not be able to maintain mitral valve competence, then, chord-sparing mitral valve replacement (almost always using a tissue valve) is a reasonable alternative.

Tricuspid valve surgery

The tricuspid valve is frequently overlooked when we discuss patients with valve disease. However, TR is very common in patients with heart failure

(3–4+ occurred in 34.5% of patients) and predicts mortality [1,2,60]. Very little is written about the tricuspid valve in the literature, especially surgical [61]. Only about 10% as many papers are written about tricuspid valve surgery as are written about mitral valve surgery.

We investigated the Cleveland Clinic database to understand unrepaired TR in patients who underwent mitral valve surgery. From 1993 until 2000, 5589 patients underwent mitral valve surgery *without* tricuspid valve surgery at the Cleveland Clinic. Preoperative echocardiography showed that 845 patients (15.8%) had either 3 or 4+ TR; therefore, in almost 16% of patients, the tricuspid valve was not repaired despite significant pre-operative TR. Retrospectively this may reflect the preconceived notion that following mitral valve surgery, pulmonary artery pressures will drop and therefore TR will resolve. It may also have reflected intra-operative downgrade. The pre-discharge echo after mitral valve surgery showed that 9.0% still had 3 or 4+ TR. Therefore, TR does not consistently resolve with mitral valve surgery. Furthermore, in the most recent follow-up echos, TR had increased to 11.4%, so it persists after mitral valve surgery. However, re-operation for tricuspid valve disease was very rare (0.7%). Part of this may be due to the high risk of performing tricuspid valve surgery in this setting. Studies from our institution and others showed an operative mortality of 30–39% for patients who underwent re-operation surgery for TR after prior repair [61–63]. In summary, from our database study and others, we concluded that TR is not repaired as often as it should be and it frequently persists if unrepaired [61,64–66].

Studies from our institution and others also showed that functional TR is similar to functional MR in that following successful tricuspid valve surgery, the RV will remodel and RV function will improve [67,68]. In a group of Cleveland Clinic patients who underwent isolated TR surgery, there was improvement in RV volumes (Figure 10.21) and function (Figure 10.22), after correction of isolated TR [61].

Functional TR also is similar to functional MR in that effective consistent repair has been elusive. We reported on 795 patients who underwent repair for functional TR from 1990 to 1991 [61]. Overall, 14% of patients had 3 or 4± TR on pre-discharge echo, and by 1 year, this had increased significantly (Figure 10.23). We then analyzed the experience to

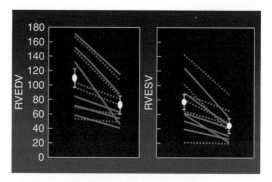

Figure 10.21 Following isolated tricuspid valve surgery for TR RV end-systolic and end-diastolic volume (RVESV and RVEDV, respectively) dropped. These are similar to the changes seen following mitral valve repair for patients with severe LV dysfunction (reproduced with permission from [67]).

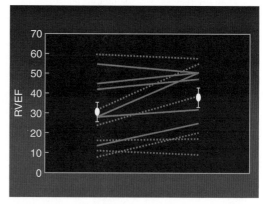

Figure 10.22 Following isolated tricuspid valve surgery for patients with TR the RVEF improved. This was associated with a drop in RV volumes (reproduced with permission from [67]).

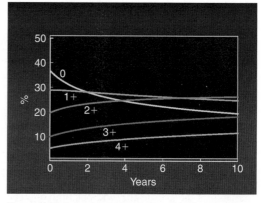

Figure 10.23 Following isolated tricuspid valve repair for functional TR pre-discharge TR persisted, approximately 14% at discharge and 3 or 4+ tricuspid rose with time (reproduced with permission from [61]).

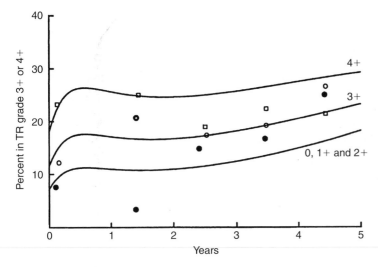

Figure 10.24 Patients who had severe TR (4+) were more likely to redevelop TR following repair, and 3+ TR patients were also more likely (reproduced with permission from [61]).

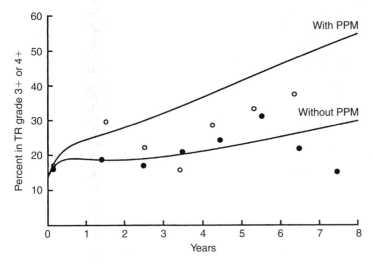

Figure 10.25 Patients who had a permanent transvenous pacemaker (PPM) wire that crossed the tricuspid valve were far more likely to redevelop TR following valve repair. By 8 years approximately 60% of patients had recurrent TR (reproduced with permission from [61]).

determine what were the risk factors for failure. Preoperative 3 and 4+ TR patients were more likely to redevelop TR (Figure 10.24). Not surprisingly, but never analyzed before, patients who had a permanent transvenous pacemaker that crossed the tricuspid valve were also far more likely to redevelop TR (Figure 10.25). Patients that had suture annuloplasty (DeVega technique) also were prone to have a very high recurrence of TR (Figure 10.26). On the other hand, patients that had a classic Carpentier tricuspid repair ring (rigid near-complete ring) had no increase over time (Figure 10.27). Patients who had a flexible band (Cosgrove–Edwards) were more stable than those who had the DeVega repair, but also developed recurrent TR during follow-up (Figure 10.28). Risk factors for early failure were *not* pulmonary

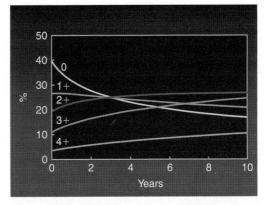

Figure 10.26 Patients who had suture tricuspid annuloplasty (the Devega technique) were very likely to redevelop 3 or 4+ TR over time (P = blank) (reproduced with permission from [61]).

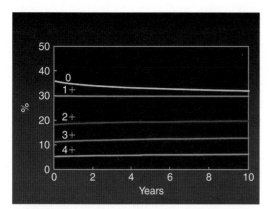

Figure 10.27 The most stable group of patients had a classic Carpentier tricuspid repair ring (rigid near-complete ring) and had no significant change in TR over time (reproduced with permission from [61]).

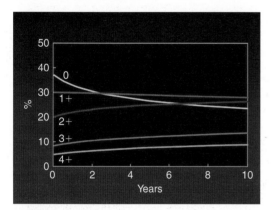

Figure 10.28 Patients who had a flexible band (Cosgrove–Edwards) were more stable than those who had a Devega repair, but also developed recurrent TR during follow up (P = 0.05) (reproduced with permission from [61]).

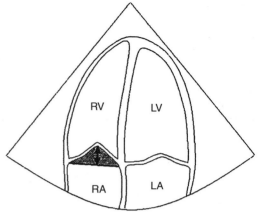

Figure 10.29 In an echocardiographic study the most significant predictor of recurrent TR was extreme tethering of the tricuspid valve leaflets due to a dilated RV (reproduced with permission from [69]). RA: right atrium: LA: left atrium.

hypertension, advanced NYHA functional class, need for mitral surgery, or ring size. Since this paper, additional echo studies indicate very similar results to ischemic mitral repair; extreme tethering of the tricuspid leaflets due to a dilated RV was a significant risk factor for failure (Figure 10.29) [69,70].

Today our approach to TR has evolved, in large part based on these recent studies and our experience treating patients with heart failure. For patients undergoing conventional surgery (or LV assist device (LVAD) implant), we perform tricuspid repair if there has been ≥2+ TR on pre-operative studies. We ignore intra-operative TR down grades. Tricuspid surgery is typically performed on the beating heart (after assuring there is no PFO or ASD), after the other components of the surgery are completed, and just before weaning from cardiopulmonary bypass. If there is a transvenous pacemaker (or implantable cardioverter-defibrillators, ICD) wire it is pushed into a commissure (typically the postero-septal) and this commissure is closed with suture. If there is 4+ TR, and/or extensive tethering from RV dilation, then we perform bicuspidization of the tricuspid valve by using suture to exclude the posterior leaflet before ring repair. Finally a rigid, near-complete ring designed for the unique three-dimensional anatomy of the tricuspid valve is placed (see disclosure at end of the book (page 305)). Rarely (<5%) we would do a chord-sparing tricuspid valve replacement for extreme RV dilation and tethering. The ACC/AHA Practice Guidelines recommend tricuspid valve surgery (Class I or IIa) for severe symptomatic disease, and Class IIb if the patient is undergoing mitral valve surgery and has pulmonary hypertension or a dilated annulus [15].

Aortic valve surgery in patients with LV dysfunction

Clinicians frequently see patients with severe LV dysfunction who have either severe aortic insufficiency or severe aortic stenosis. These two groups of patients have historically been considered high risk for surgery. Again, recent data indicate that surgery can play a major role for this group of patients.

Similar to patients with MR and LV dysfunction, patients with severe aortic insufficiency and LV dysfunction suffer from volume overload, ventricular

Table 10.2 Characteristics of patients undergoing aortic valve replacement for aortic insufficiency unmatched.

	Study group LVEF ≤ 30%	Control group LVEF > 30%	P-value
Number	88	636	
Mean age	56 ± 12	52 ± 15	0.001
%Female	9%	23%	0.002
FC III	33%	16%	<0.0001
FC IV	8%	4%	<0.0001
BUN	20 ± 9.5	18 ± 8	<0.0001
Mean F/U	8.2 ± 6.5 years	6.4 ± 5.6 years	

FC: functional class.

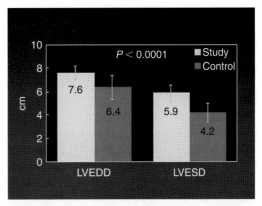

Figure 10.30 Patients with a low EF from aortic insufficiency were found to have significantly dilated LV end-diastolic and end-systolic dimensions compared to the control group that had higher EFs.
LVEDD: LV end-diastolic diameter; LVESD: LV end-systolic diameter.

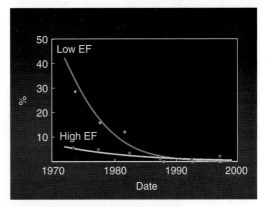

Figure 10.31 Patients who had surgery for a low EF with severe aortic insufficiency had a high operative mortality during the 1970s and early 1980s. However, by the mid-1980s this had been reduced and the operative mortality since then was zero at the Cleveland Clinic, and not statistically significantly different from patients with a normal EF and severe aortic insufficiency.

dilation, and reduced EF [71,72]. This can contribute to ventricular fibrosis and collagen deposition. Patients presenting with very advanced LV dysfunction and heart failure have been considered for cardiac transplantation because conventional wisdom has been that this group of patients have irreversible LV dysfunction, operative mortality is about 10%, long-term mortality is high, and only a few will have a meaningful recovery of LV function post-operatively [73]. Because of this perception, and our observation that this no longer appeared to be true, we reviewed the Cleveland Clinic experience in patients who had severe isolated aortic insufficiency who underwent surgery [72,74].

From 1972 until 1998, 88 patients were identified who had LVEF ≤30%, and 636 patients were the control group with LVEF >30% [72,74]. As expected, the patients who had low EF had more advanced symptoms, and these were also older patients (Table 10.2). This group of patients also had more severely dilated end-diastolic and end-systolic dimensions than the control group (Figure 10.30). Overall, the hospital mortality for patients with severe LV dysfunction was quite high during the 1970s but significantly decreased over time (Figure 10.31). In fact, there had not been a death in this group since 1986. Like the situation with severe MR and LV dysfunction this historically was a very high-risk group of patients. But we were now able to neutralize those risk factors. Propensity matching was used to determine survival. Survival for the matched group was lower for the group with severe LV dysfunction (Figure 10.32). However, since the date of operation had such a significant impact on early survival, two groups

were created. One showed projected survival for the matched patients if they had had surgery in 1980, and the other if they had had surgery in 2000 (Figure 10.33). The survival curve for the patients operated in 2000 indicates that the early, and 5-year survival, would be similar to patients with better LV function. Studies also showed post-operative improvement in EF, reduction in LV mass, and an improvement in LV end-systolic dimension over time (Figure 10.34).

From these studies, we concluded that patients with advanced LV dysfunction secondary to severe aortic insufficiency should be offered aortic valve surgery and not transplantation. Their operative mortality is no longer prohibitive. Early and mid-term survival should be similar to the group of patients with better LV function. However even though the risk is low, ideally these patients will be referred for surgery early because there could be late

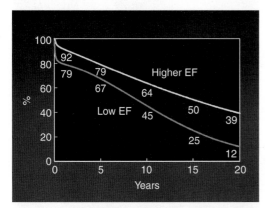

Figure 10.32 By propensity matching survival in the low EF group was lower, but this included the entire time period.

effects on their survival, and we do not expect ventricular function will return to normal even though it typically improves.

At the other extreme are the patients with severe LV dysfunction and severe aortic stenosis. This group of patients may not be able to generate a high gradient across the aortic valve. This group should be studied with dobutamine echocardiogram to determine whether this is a "pseudo-stenosis" of the aortic valve, or a true aortic stenosis [72]. Patients with pseudo-stenosis usually increase the aortic valve area with the administration of dobutamine as ventricular function improves. On the other hand, patients with severe calcific stenosis will not change aortic valve area with the infusion of dobutamine (Figure 10.35). These patients also have been considered to be high risk, but a recent study indicated that this is not as dangerous as thought before.

We reviewed the outcomes of patients seen from 1990 to 1998 at the Cleveland Clinic who had severe aortic stenosis with severe LV dysfunction [72,75,76]. Propensity matching was performed. The in-hospital

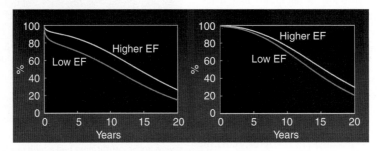

Figure 10.33 Based on matching, if a patient had surgery in 1980 there would be a difference in early and late survival, but projected outcome for surgery in 2000 showed no significant early difference in survival, including at 5 years.

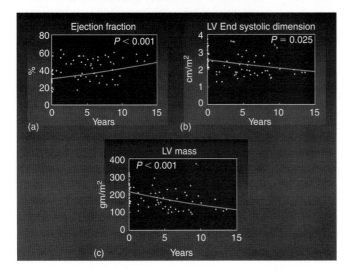

Figure 10.34 The group of patients that had aortic valve surgery for severe LV dysfunction showed an improvement in EF over time, a reduction in LV end-systolic dimension, and a reduction in LV mass.

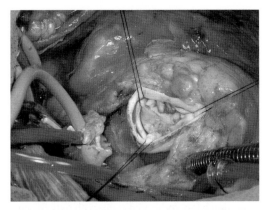

Figure 10.35 This patient had very severe aortic stenosis from a bicuspid aortic valve, with severe LV dysfunction and a very low gradient. In fact, the patient had originally been listed for heart transplant. Further studies documented the extreme calcification of the valve and the patient successfully underwent aortic valve replacement instead of cardiac transplantation.

operative mortality for patients who underwent aortic valve replacement (AVR) with severe LV dysfunction and a low gradient was 8%. A third group was identified from the database who were not offered surgery who had the same low EF, low-gradient characteristics (Table 10.3) [75]. This group followed the "natural history" of patients with unoperated aortic stenosis. Figure 10.36 shows the late survival for the three groups of patients. The group of patients who underwent AVR who had a low gradient with severe LV dysfunction did not have as high a survival as the group that had high-gradient aortic stenosis and better LV function. However, the survival for medically treated patients was abysmal. In follow-up the majority of low EF AVR patients had returned to NYHA Functional Class I or II (Figure 10.37). The message from this study is that patients with severe LV dysfunction and true aortic stenosis can undergo

Table 10.3 Propensity-matched patients who underwent AVR for AS (reproduced with permission from [75]).

	AVR group (n = 39)	Control group (n = 56)	P-value
Clinical data			
Age, in years (range)	73 ± 9 (44–86)	75 ± 6 (58–90)	0.66
Male/female (%)	77/23	73/27	0.68
Body surface area (m²)	1.89 ± 0.22	1.84 ± 0.21	0.51
NYHA Functional Class III/IV	29 (74%)	40 (71%)	0.75
CCS Class III/IV	12 (31%)	14 (25%)	0.54
Syncope	5 (13%)	8 (14%)	0.84
Previous MI	20 (51%)	23 (41%)	0.33
Previous CABG	14 (36%)	20 (36%)	0.99
Diabetes mellitus	15 (38%)	19 (34%)	0.65
Systemic hypertension	22 (56%)	33 (59%)	0.81
Creatinine level (mg/dL)	1.7 ± 1.3	1.7 ± 1.3	0.44
Multivessel CAD on angiogram	27 (69%)	18 (62%)	0.5
	(*n* = 39)	(*n* = 29)	
Echocardiographic data			
Aortic valve area (cm²)	0.60 ± 0.12	0.60 ± 0.09	0.66
Mean TVG in mmHg (range)	24 ± 5 (11–30)	24 ± 4 (14–30)	0.60
Peak TVG (mmHg)	41 ± 8	41 ± 8	0.83
Moderate to severe MR	23 (59%)	33 (59%)	1.0
Pulmonary artery systolic pressure (mmHg)	47 ± 13	52 ± 13	0.04
	(*n* = 25)	(*n* = 34)	
LVEF (%)	22 ± 6	23 ± 8	0.36
LV end-diastolic diameter (cm)	6.2 ± 0.6	6.1 ± 0.7	0.08
LV end-systolic diameter (cm)	5.0 ± 0.8	5.0 ± 0.7	0.40
Moderate to severe RV dysfunction	22 (56%)	35(63%)	0.55

Data are presented as the mean value ± SD or number (%) of patients.
CABG: CAB graft; CAD: coronary artery disease; CCS: Canadian Cardiovascular Society; TVG: transvalvular gradient.

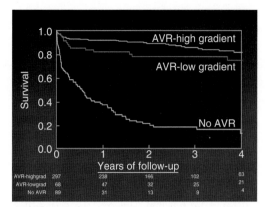

Figure 10.36 We investigated patients who had severe LV dysfunction, with severe aortic stenosis and a low gradient. A comparison group were those who had aortic valve surgery who had a high gradient and normal LV function, and finally a third group were identified who had a low EF, low gradient, but who were treated with medical therapy instead of AVR. The group treated with medical therapy had a strikingly poor prognosis. There was a decrease in survival in the group that had low EF with low gradient, but generally an acceptable early and late mortality (reproduced with permission from [72]).

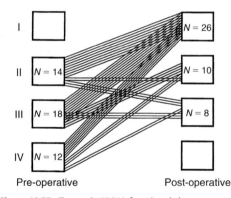

Figure 10.37 Change in NYHA functional class symptoms in 44 of 46 late survivors in the AVR group ($P \leq 0.001$ for change in NYHA Functional Class III/IV symptoms, pre-operatively and post-operatively. N = number of patients (reproduced with permission from [75]).

surgery with an acceptable early and late mortality. AVR for this condition, and for those with (AI) and severe LV dysfunction, are both Class I indicators for surgery in the ACC/AHA Practice Guidelines [77].

Why is valve surgery safer today for patients with LV dysfunction and heart failure?

Cardiac surgery has advanced through a series of stepwise improvements over the past decades. There

are no single changes that can be identified as the major breakthrough that led to better survival than reported from studies in the 1970s–1980s. However, for most of us who have been performing cardiac surgery during this time, it appears that many factors play a role. First, intra-operative cardiac protection is much better today for patients with valvular and coronary disease. Antegrade and retrograde cardioplegia became routine at the Cleveland Clinic in the early 1990s [78]. In addition to using cold blood cardioplegia, many surgeons use a "hot shot" of cardioplegia before removing the cross clamp. Cardiac protection has become predictable with only the rare need for an intra-aortic balloon pump. The surgeon must be very meticulous about giving cardioplegia to be sure that the heart is fully arrested. Frequent, repeated doses of cardioplegia in this group are warranted, especially if there is severe LV hypertrophy. Second, peri-operative monitoring and the use of inotropes in this group have improved. The introduction of the phosphodiesterase inhibitor, milrinone, ushered in a new era for the management of these patients. The use of this drug may cause systemic vasodilation requiring norepinephrine, or occasionally vasopressin (rarely methylene blue) (see Chapter 14 on post-operative care). These drugs have added a potent new treatment to our arsenal. Finally, compared to two decades ago our options for valve repair versus replacement, and the prostheses themselves, are better. The Starr–Edwards ball-in-cage valve was common then and it does not have the favorable hemodynamic characteristics of today's low-gradient biologic valves, or bi-leaflet mechanical valves. Poor hemodynamic performance by the valve in the early post-operative phase may have contributed to the early morbidity and mortality observed in the early days of valve surgery in this population.

Conclusion

Despite these advances, and publications in both the cardiology and cardiac surgery literature, operations for valve disease in patients with LV dysfunction are still relatively rare considering the large population of patients at risk. Modern techniques yield a low peri-operative morbidity and mortality with improved long-term ventricular function and improved patient functional class. Many patients referred for transplants are now instead able to be treated with valve operations or, if they are already on a transplant list, may be de-listed following valve surgery [79]. Also, inadequate results of valve repair for IMR and functional TR have been identified as a problem and new annuloplasty rings, concepts, and use of chord-sparing valve replacement should decrease recurrent or residual regurgitation. With more publications addressing the topic of valve surgery in patients with LV dysfunction, and as the prospective-randomized trial data from the Coapsys and Acorn trials are published, then referrals for this type of surgery should increase.

References

1 Koelling TM, Aaronson KD, Cody RJ, Bach DS, Armstrong WF. Prognostic significance of mitral regurgitation and tricuspid regurgitation in patients with left ventricular systolic dysfunction. *Am Heart J* 2002; **144**(3): 524–529.

2 Patel JB, Borgeson DD, Barnes ME, Rihal CS, Daly RC, Redfield MM. Mitral regurgitation in patients with advanced systolic heart failure. *J Card Fail* 2004; **10**(4): 285–291.

3 Braunwald E. Valvular heart disease. In: *Heart Disease: A Textbook of Cardiovascular Medicine*. W.B. Saunders Co., Philadelphia, PA, 1980.

4 David TE, Uden DE, Strauss HD. The importance of the mitral apparatus in left ventricular function after correction of mitral regurgitation. *Circulation* 1983; **68**(**Suppl II**): II-76–II-82.

5 Sarris GE, Miller DC. Valvular–ventricular interaction: the importance of mitral chordae tendineae in terms of global left ventricular systolic function. *J Card Surg* 1988; **3**(3): 215–234.

6 Grigioni F, Enriquez-Sarano M, Zehr KJ, Bailey KR, Tajik AJ. Ischemic mitral regurgitation: long-term outcome and prognostic implications with quantitative Doppler assessment. *Circulation* 2001; **103**(13): 1759–1764.

7 Ellis SG, Whitlow PL, Raymond RE, Schneider JP. Impact of mitral regurgitation on long-term survival after percutaneous coronary intervention. *Am J Cardiol* 2002; **89**(3): 315–318.

8 Wu AH, Aaronson KD, Bolling SF, Pagani FD, Welch K, Koelling TM. Impact of mitral valve annuloplasty on mortality risk in patients with mitral regurgitation and left ventricular systolic dysfunction. *J Am Coll Cardiol* 2005; **45**(3): 381–387.

9 Robbins JD, Maniar PB, Cotts W, Parker MA, Bonow RO, Gheorghiade M. Prevalence and severity of mitral regurgitation in chronic systolic heart failure. *Am J Cardiol* 2003; **91**(3): 360–362.

10 Trichon BH, Felker GM, Shaw LK, Cabell CH, O'Connor CM. Relation of frequency and severity of mitral regurgitation to survival among patients with left ventricular systolic dysfunction and heart failure. *Am J Cardiol* 2003; **91**(5): 538–543.

11 Bolling SF, Pagani FD, Deeb GM, Bach DS. Intermediate-term outcome of mitral reconstruction in cardiomyopathy. *J Thorac Cardiovasc Surg* 1998; **115**(2): 381–386; discussion 387–388.

12 Badhwar V, Bolling SF. Mitral valve surgery in the patient with left ventricular dysfunction. *Semin Thorac Cardiovasc Surg* 2002; **14**(2): 133–136.

13 Bishay ES, McCarthy PM, Cosgrove DM *et al.* Mitral valve surgery in patients with severe left ventricular dysfunction. *Eur J Cardiothorac Surg* 2000; **17**(3): 213–221.

14 Acker MA, Bolling S, Shemin R, *et al.* Mitral valve surgery in heart failure: insights from the Acorn Clinical Trial. *J Thorac Cardiovasc Surg* 2006; **132**(3): 568–77.

15 Bonow RO, Carabello BA, Chatterjee K *et al.* ACC/AHA 2006 guidelines for the management of patients with valvular heart disease: a report of the American College of Cardiology/American Heart Association Task Force on practice guidelines. *J Am Coll Cardiol* 2006; **48**: e64–e71.

16 Aklog L, Filsoufi F, Flores KQ *et al.* Does coronary artery bypass grafting alone correct moderate ischemic mitral regurgitation? *Circulation* 2001; **104**(**12 Suppl 1**): I-68–I-75.

17 Adams DH, Filsoufi F, Aklog L. Surgical treatment of the ischemic mitral valve. *J Heart Valve Dis* 2002; **11**(**Suppl 1**): S21–S25.

18 Lam BK, Gillinov AM, Blackstone EH *et al.* Importance of moderate ischemic mitral regurgitation. *Ann Thorac Surg* 2005; **79**(2): 462–470.

19 Mallidi HR, Pelletier MP, Lamb J *et al.* Late outcomes in patients with uncorrected mild to moderate mitral regurgitation at the time of isolated coronary artery bypass grafting. *J Thorac Cardiovasc Surg* 2004; **127**(3): 636–644.

20 Paparella D, Mickleborough LL, Carson S, Ivanov J. Mild to moderate mitral regurgitation in patients undergoing coronary bypass grafting: effect on operative mortality and long-term significance. *Ann Thorac Surg* 2003; **76**(4): 1094–1100.

21 Prifti E, Bonacchi M, Frati G, Giunti G, Babatasi G, Sani G. Ischemic mitral valve regurgiation grade II–III: correction in patients with impaired left ventricular function undergoing simultaneous coronary revascularization. *J Heart Valve Dis* 2001; **10**(6): 754–762.

22 Diodato MD, Moon MR, Pasque MK *et al.* Repair of ischemic mitral regurgitation does not increase mortality or improve long-term survival in patients undergoing coronary artery revascularization: a propensity analysis. *Ann Thorac Surg* 2004; **78**(3): 794–799.

23 Tolis Jr. GA, Korkolis DP, Kopf GS, Elefteriades JA. Revascularization alone (without mitral valve repair) suffices in patients with advanced ischemic cardiomyopathy and mild-to-moderate mitral regurgitation. *Ann Thorac Surg* 2002; **74**(5): 1476–1481.

24 Thourani VH, Weintraub WS, Guyton RA *et al.* Outcomes and long-term survival for patients undergoing mitral valve repair versus replacement: effect of age and concomitant coronary artery bypass grafting. *Circulation* 2003; **108**(3): 298–304.

25 Wong DR, Agnihotri AK, Hung JW *et al.* Long-term survival after surgical revascularization for moderate ischemic mitral regurgitation. *Ann Thorac Surg* 2005; **80**(2): 570–577.

26 Allman KC, Shaw LJ, Hachamovitch R, Udelson JE. Myocardial viability testing and impact of revascularization on prognosis in patients with coronary artery disease and left ventricular dysfunction: a meta-analysis. *J Am Coll Cardiol* 2002; **39**(7): 1151–1158.

27 Lytle BW. The role of coronary revascularization in the treatment of ischemic cardiomyopathy. *Ann Thorac Surg* 2003; **75**(6 Suppl): S2–S5.

28 Bonow RO. Myocardial viability and prognosis in patients with ischemic left ventricular dysfunction. *J Am Coll Cardiol* 2002; **39**(7): 1159–1162.

29 Chareonthaitawee P, Gersh BJ, Aaoz PA, Gibbons RJ. Revascularization in severe left ventricular dysfunction: the role of viability testing. *J Am Coll Cardiol* 2005; **46**: 567–574.

30 Tarakji K, Brunken R, McCarthy PM *et al.* Myocardial viability testing and the effect of early intervention in patients with advanced left ventricular systolic dysfunction. *Circulation* 2006; **113**(2): 230–237.

31 Kumanohoso T, Otsuji Y, Yoshifuku S *et al.* Mechanism of higher incidence of ischemic mitral regurgitation in patients with inferior myocardial infarction: quantitative analysis of left ventricular and mitral valve geometry in 103 patients with prior myocardial infarction. *J Thorac Cardiovasc Surg* 2003; **125**(1): 135–143.

32 Otsuji Y, Handschumacher MD, Leil-Cohn N *et al.* Mechanism of ischemic mitral regurgitation with segmental left ventricular dysfunction: three-dimensional echocardiographic studies in models of acute and chronic progressive regurgitation. *J Am Coll Cardiol* 2001; **37**(2): 641–648.

33 Enriquez-Sarano M, Schaff HV, Frye RL. Mitral regurgitation: what causes the leakage is fundamental to the outcome of valve repair. *Circulation* 2003; **108**: 253–256.

34 Kwan J, Shiota T, Agler DA *et al.* Geometric differences of the mitral apparatus between ischemic and dilated cardiomyopathy with significant mitral regurgitation: real-time three-dimensional echocardiography study. *Circulation* 2003; **107**(8): 1135–1140.

35 Grande-Allen KJ, Barber JE, Klatka KM *et al.* Mitral valve stiffening in end-stage heart failure: evidence of an organic contribution to functional mitral regurgitation. *J Thorac Cardiovasc Surg* 2005; **130**(3): 783–790.

36 Ahmad RM, Gillinov AM, McCarthy PM *et al.* Annular geometry and motion in human ischemic mitral regurgitation: novel assessment with three-dimensional echocardiography and computer reconstruction. *Ann Thorac Surg* 2004; **78**(6): 2063–2068.

37 Hueb AC, Jatene FB, Moreira LF, Pomerantzeff PM, Kallas E, de Oliveira SA. Ventricular remodeling and mitral valve modifications in dilated cardiomyopathy: new insights from anatomic study. *J Thorac Cardiovasc Surg* 2002; **124**(6): 1216–1224.

38 McCarthy PM. Does the intertrigonal distance dilate? Never say never. *J Thorac Cardiovasc Surg* 2002; **124**(6): 1078–1079.

39 Gorman 3rd JH, Gorman RC, Jackson BM, Enomoto Y, St John-Sutton MG, Edmunds Jr LH. Annuloplasty ring selection for chronic ischemic mitral regurgitation: lessons from the ovine model. *Ann Thorac Surg* 2003; **76**(5): 1556–1563.

40 Tibayan FA, Rodriguez F, Langer F *et al.* Annular remodeling in chronic ischemic mitral regurgitation: ring selection implications. *Ann Thorac Surg* 2003; **76**(5): 1549–1555.

41 Gillinov AM, Wierup PN, Blackstone EH *et al.* Is repair preferable to replacement for ischemic mitral regurgitation? *J Thorac Cardiovasc Surg* 2001; **122**(6): 1125–1141.

42 Grossi EA, Goldberg JD, LaPietra A *et al.* Ischemic mitral valve reconstruction and replacement: comparison of long-term survival and complications. *J Thorac Cardiovasc Surg* 2001; **122**(6): 1107–1124.

43 Miller DC. Ischemic mitral regurgitation redux – to repair or to replace? *J Thorac Cardiovasc Surg* 2001; **122**(6): 1059–1062.

44 Calafiore AM, Gallina S, Di Mauro M *et al.* Mitral valve procedure in dilated cardiomyopathy: repair or replacement? *Ann Thorac Surg* 2001; **71**(4): 1146–1153.

45 Reardon MJ, David TE. Mitral valve replacement with preservation of the subvalvular apparatus. *Curr Opin Cardiol* 1999; **14**(2): 104–110.

46 Tibayan FA, Rodriguez F, Langer F *et al.* Does septa-lateral annular cinching work for chronic ischemic mitral regurgitation? *J Thorac Cardiovasc Surg* 2004; **127**(3): 654–663.

47 Daimon M, Fukuda S, Adams DH, *et al.* Mitral valve repair with Carpentier-McCarthy-Adams IMR ETlogix annuloplasty ring for ischemic mitral regurgitation: early echocardiographic results from a multi-center study. *Circulation* 2006; **114 (I Suppl)**: I588–93.

48 Malkowski MJ, Guo R, Orsinelli DA *et al.* The morphologic characteristics of flail mitral leaflets by transesophageal echocardiography. *J Heart Valve Dis* 1997; **6**(1): 54–59.

49 Peeler BB, Kron IL. Suture relocation of the posterior papillary muscle in ischemic mitral regurgitation. *Op Tech Thorac Cardiovasc Surg* 2005; **10**(2): 113–122.

50 Levine RA, Schwammenthal E. Ischemic mitral regurgitation on the threshold of a solution from paradoxes to unifying concepts. *Circulation* 2005; **112**: 745–758.

51 Hung J, Guerrero JL, Handschumacher MD, Supple G, Sullivan S, Levine RA. Reverse ventricular remodeling reduces ischemic mitral regurgitation: echo-guided device application in the beating heart. *Circulation* 2002; **106**(20): 2594–2600.

52 Kincaid EH, Riley RD, Hines MH, Hammon JW, Kon ND. Anterior leaflet augmentation for ischemic mitral regurgitation. *Ann Thorac Surg* 2004; **78(2)**: 564–568.

53 Fukamachi K, Inoue M, Popovic ZB *et al.* Off-pump mitral valve repair using the Coapsys device: a pilot study in a pacing-induced mitral regurgitation model. *Ann Thorac Surg* 2004; **77(2)**: 688–693.

54 Fukamachi K, Inoue M, Popovic Z *et al.* Optimal mitral annular and subvalvular shape change created by the Coapsys device to treat functional mitral regurgitation. *ASAIO J* 2005; **51(1)**: 17–21.

55 Mishra YK, Mittal S, Jaguri P, Trehan N. Coapsys mitral annuloplasty for chronic functional ischemic mitral regurgitation: 1-year results. *Ann Thorac Surg* 2006; **81(1)**: 42–46.

56 Grossi EA, Saunders PC, Woo YJ *et al.* Intraoperative effects of the Coapsys annuloplasty system in a randomized evaluation (RESTOR-MV) of functional ischemic mitral regurgitation. *Ann Thorac Surg* 2005; **80(5)**: 1706–1711.

57 Geidel S, Lass M, Schneider C *et al.* Downsizing of the mitral valve and coronary revascularization in severe ischemic mitral regurgitation results in reverse left ventricular and left atrial remodeling. *Eur J Cardiothorac Surg* 2005; **27(6)**: 1011–1016.

58 McGee EC, Gillinov AM, Blackstone EH *et al.* Recurrent mitral regurgitation after annuloplasty for functional ischemic mitral regurgitation. *J Thorac Cardiovasc Surg* 2004; **128(6)**: 916–924.

59 Tahta SA, Oury JH, Maxwell JM, Hiro SP, Duran CM. Outcome after mitral valve repair for functional ischemic mitral regurgitation. *J Heart Valve Dis* 2002; **11(1)**: 11–19.

60 Nath J, Foster E, Heidenreich PA. Impact of tricuspid regurgitation on long-term survival. *J Am Coll Cardiol* 2004; **43**: 405–409.

61 McCarthy PM, Bhudia SK, Rajeswaran J *et al.* Tricuspid valve repair: durability and risk factors for failure. *J Thorac Cardiovasc Surg* 2004; **127**: 674–685.

62 King RM, Schaff HV, Danielson GK *et al.* Surgery for tricuspid regurgitation late after mitral valve replacement. *Circulation* 1984; **70**: I-193–I-197.

63 Bernal JM, Morales D, Revuelta C, Llorca J, Gutiérrez-Morlote J, Revuelta JM. Reoperations after tricuspid valve repair. *J Thorac Cardiovasc* 2005; **130(2)**: 495–503.

64 Frater R. Tricuspid insufficiency. *J Thorac Cardiovasc Surg* 2001; **122(3)**: 427–429.

65 Dreyfus GD, Corbi PJ, Chan KM, Bahrami T. Secondary tricuspid regurgitation or dilatation: which should be the criteria for surgical repair. *Ann Thorac Surg* 2005; **79(1)**: 127–132.

66 Matsunaga A, Duran CM. Progression of tricuspid regurgitation after repaired functional ischemic mitral regurgitation. *Circulation* 2005; **112(Suppl I)**: I-453–I-457.

67 Mukherjee D, Nader S, Olano A, Garcia MJ, Griffin BP. Improvement in right ventricular systolic function after surgical correction of isolated tricuspid regurgitation. *J Am Soc Echocardiogr* 2000; **13(7)**: 650–654.

68 Sugimoto T, Okada M, Ozaki N, Kawahira T, Fukuoka M. Influence of functional tricuspid regurgitation on right ventricular function. *Ann Thorac Surg* 1998; **66(6)**: 2044–2050.

69 Fukuda S, Song JM, Gillinov AM *et al.* Tricuspid valve tethering predicts residual tricuspid regurgitation after tricuspid annuloplasty. *Circulation* 2005; **111(8)**: 975–979.

70 Fukuda S, Gillinov AM, McCarthy PM, *et al.* Determinants of recurrent or residual functional tricuspid regurgitation after tricuspid annuloplasty. *Circulation* (**Suppl**) (in press).

71 Bonow RO, Carabello B, de Leon A *et al.* Guidelines for the management of patients with valvular disease: executive summary. A report of the American College of Cardiology/American Heart Association Task Force on Practice Guidelines (Committee on Management of Patients with Valvular Disease). *Circulation* 1998; **98**: 1949–1984.

72 McCarthy PM. Aortic valve surgery in patients with left ventricular dysfunction. *Semin Thorac Cardiovasc Surg* 2002; **14(2)**: 137–143.

73 Bonow RO, Nikas D, Elefteriades JA. Valve replacement for regurgitant lesion of the aortic or mitral valve in advanced left ventricular dysfunction. *Cardiol Clin* 1995; **13(1)**: 73–83, 85.

74 McCarthy PM, Kumpati GS, Blackstone EH *et al.* Aortic valve surgery for chronic aortic regurgitation with severe LV dysfunction: time for reevaluation? *Circulation* 2001; **104(Suppl, abstr)**: II-684.

75 Pereira JJ, Lauer MS, Bashir M *et al.* Survival after aortic valve replacement for severe aortic stenosis with low transvalvular gradients and severe left ventricular dysfunction. *J Am Coll Cardiol* 2002; **39(8)**: 1356–1363.

76 Pereira JJ, Asher CR, Blackstone EH *et al.* Long-term survival replacement after aortic valve replacement in patients with low gradient severe aortic stenosis and significant left ventricular dysfunction. *J Am Coll Cardiol* 2000; **35(Suppl I)**: 533A.

77 Bonow RO, Carabello BA, Chatterjee K *et al.* ACC/AHA 2006 guidelines for the management of patients with valvular heart disease: a report of the American College of Cardiology/American Heart Association Task Force on practice guidelines. *J Am Coll Cardiol* 2006; **48**: e25–e37.

78 Loop FD, Foster R, Ogella D, Teplitsky D. Integrated pump switch for antegrade/retrograde cardioplegia. *Ann Thorac Surg* 1991; **52(2)**: 320–321.

79 Mahon NG, O'Neill JO, Young JB *et al.* Contemporary outcomes of outpatients referred for cardiac transplantation evaluation to a tertiary heart failure center: impact of surgical alternatives. *J Card Fail* 2004; **10(4)**: 273–278.

CHAPTER 11

Ventricular reconstruction and device therapies for cardiomyopathy patients

Patrick M. McCarthy & Edwin C. McGee, Jr.

Introduction

Ischemic cardiomyopathy is the most common cause of heart failure and systolic left ventricular (LV) dysfunction in industrialized nations. The chapters on coronary artery bypass surgery, valve surgery, and this chapter on ventricular surgery, address the three components of the surgical approach to patients with ischemic cardiomyopathy. The chapters on viability testing and coronary artery bypass surgery address the most common surgical therapy of heart failure, revascularization to viable yet jeopardized segments of myocardium. The chapter on valve disease addresses surgery for functional mitral and tricuspid regurgitation associated with ventricular volume overload. This chapter deals with surgery for dyskinetic and akinetic ventricular segments in selected patients who have survived transmural infarcts and have gone on to develop significant heart failure. Furthermore, we will discuss the more nascent field of direct ventricular approaches to non-ischemic dilated cardiomyopathy using external devices.

Migrino and colleagues in the Global Utilization of Streptokinase and Tissue plasminogen activator (t-PA) for Occluded coronary arteries (GUSTO I) trial, demonstrated that within minutes following a myocardial infarction 17% of patients develop ventricular dilation [1]. They also showed that ventricular dilation is a marker for poor late outcome. In patients with a left ventricular end systolic volume index (LVESVI) of 40–50 mL/m^2, mortality at 1 year was 16% as compared to 33% when LVESVI > 60 mL/m^2. The process of pathologic LV remodeling begins as infarcted necrotic myocytes are replaced by fibrosis and collagen.

Ventricular dilation leads to several physiologic and *mechanical* disadvantages including increased myocardial wall stress, subendocardial hypoperfusion, increased myocardial oxygen consumption, afterload mismatch, and activation of compensatory neurohormonal mechanisms [2]. Systolic wall stress correlates with myocardial oxygen consumption and may stimulate myocyte hypertrophy, increased myocyte apoptosis, altered matrix metalloproteinase or collagen turnover, and altered myocyte calcium handling [3–8]. LV remodeling may progress over a period of time to a stage of extensive transmural scar formation with subsequent ventricular wall thinning and systolic expansion, leading to a dyskinetic segment, and the formation of a true ventricular aneurysm. Alternatively, and more commonly in the current era of aggressive early treatment for myocardial infarction including thrombolytics and percutaneous coronary intervention, the infarction may be halted before it leads to transmural necrosis. As such, scar is often mixed with viable muscle. At surgery the appearance of the myocardium is marbled, with scar and muscle intertwined. Most of these segments are akinetic, with variable amounts of thinning depending on the amount of remaining viable muscle, and the time since infarction.

The surgeon should be aware that the epicardial surface of the ventricle is frequently different than the endocardial layer. Ventricular dilation causes

(a)

(b)

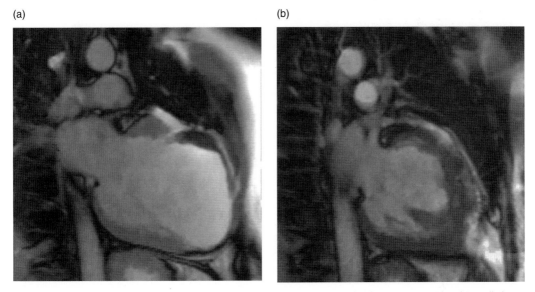

Figure 11.1 A dynamic MRI scan before and after left ventricular reconstruction (LVR) in a patient with a thin-walled aneurysm. (The cine version can be viewed at http://cvbook.nmh.org)

endocardial hypoperfusion, and there may be well-developed extensive endocardial scar, but little in the way of visible epicardial scar. In these patients there is no systolic bulging involving the infarcted segment, but rather an area of akinesis.

Preoperative imaging is helpful in distinguishing ventricular scar from viable myocardium. In our experience magnetic resonance imaging (MRI) has been the most useful study to assess viability (Figure 11.1). Often patients have pre-existing pacing and defibrillator hardware and are unable to get an MRI. Positron emission tomography (PET) is a good second choice for these individuals.

The remodeled pathologic ventricular scar leads to impaired ventricular function and progressive heart failure by several mechanisms. The thin-walled dyskinetic scar often creates dysfunction in the areas of myocardium remote from the scar. In the most common circumstance, an anterior aneurysm from a left anterior descending artery (LAD) infarct leads to progressive dysfunction in the territories perfused by the circumflex and right coronary artery [9]. This dysfunction can occur even though there is no atherosclerotic burden in either the circumflex or right coronary arteries and is related to increased wall stress in the viable areas adjacent to the aneurysm. Ventricular dysfunction is also associated with the

development of ventricular tachyarrhythmias, which are initiated from the border zone of infarcted and viable myocardium. Finally, aneurysms may lead to embolization from endocardial LV thrombus.

The goal of surgical therapies for LV aneurysm, therefore, is to reconstruct the dilated aneurysm such that wall stress improves in the remote dysfunctional area with improved function and myocardial efficiency [9–12]. Cryoablation can also be used to eliminate foci of tachyarrhythmias, and all ventricular thrombus is removed.

The modern era of LV aneurysm surgery began when Dr. Denton Cooley resected an anterior aneurysm using cardiopulmonary bypass [13]. For many years aneurysm repairs consisted of "linear" repairs that removed the thin-walled scar lateral to the LAD. Many surgeons continue to use this type of repair. However, in the 1980s more complete reconstructions that included the infarcted septum were conceived and carried out with various techniques described by Cooley, Jatene, and Dor [14,15]. Most of these surgeons reconstructed the septum using a patch of Dacron or pericardium, although Jatene did not use patch reconstruction routinely. More contemporary descriptions of left ventricular reconstruction (LVR) have been published both with and without a patch [16–18].

(a)   (b)

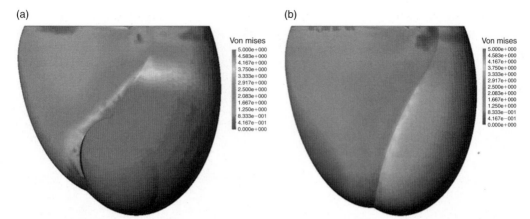

Figure 11.2 Mathematical modeling can be used to approximate changes in wall stress in patients with an LV aneurysm before (a), and after (b) reconstruction. Red depicts areas of high stress, blue are areas of low stress, green are intermediate. (Complete images can be viewed at http://cvbook.nmh.org)

There are theoretical, mathematical, and observational data to support reconstruction of an LV aneurysm to reverse heart failure and improve wall stress and cardiac function. Mathematical modeling predicts that resection of a dyskinetic scar will lead to a net improvement in cardiac function [11]. Following aneurysm reconstruction, improvements are seen both in myocardial oxygen consumption and myocardial efficiency which leads to an improvement in the neurohormonal milieu of heart failure [9–12,19–21]. These changes also directly lead to a net reduction of ventricular wall stress (Figure 11.2). However, resection of an akinetic scar may lead to an equivocal result and depends on the properties of the scar and the adjacent muscle. Not all patients who undergo reconstruction of an akinetic area will improve [11].

Indication for LVR surgery in ischemic cardiomyopathy

Reconstructing an LV aneurysm, or thin-walled akinetic segment, should decrease ventricular wall stress and therefore reduce myocardial oxygen consumption leading to an increase in myocardial efficiency. As a result, an improvement in the heart failure neurohormonal feedback loop occurs [20,21]. The classic indications for LV aneurysm repair include congestive heart failure, cerebral or systemic embolism originating from thrombus contained in the aneurysm, and persistent malignant ventricular arrhythmias despite medical therapy. In a practical sense, however, many patients undergo reconstruction because the surgeon is already committed to surgery because of other indications such as left main coronary artery disease, three vessel disease with positive viability studies, or severe mitral regurgitation (MR).

In our practice, reconstruction is performed if there is a discreet thin-walled aneurysm that collapses with venting the aorta or left atrium. Frequently there are adhesions from the transmural infarct to the pericardium. Most often these aneurysms are in the distribution of the distal LAD. If there is diffuse scar mixed with muscle in all three coronary territories, no reconstruction is undertaken as there is not a discreet area to reconstruct. In our experience, wall thinning is as important as the presence of scar. We do not resect areas that are thick walled without visible scar or without scar that is apparent by MRI. This approach differs from that taken by others [17,19]. As viability studies are only 80–90% accurate we do not reconstruct areas that are, upon direct inspection in the operating room (OR), thick-walled muscle even though preoperative studies indicated non-viable scarred myocardium. If there is any question as to viability we err on the side of revascularization and forego reconstruction. Most often reconstruction is performed for a true dyskinetic aneurysm, but if there is transmural scar with

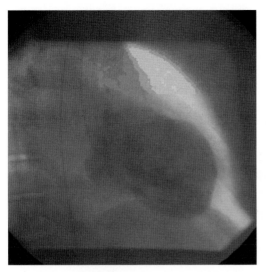

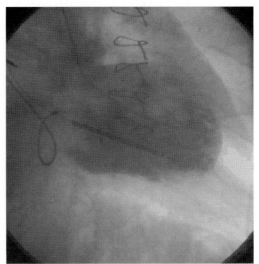

Figure 11.3 This left ventriculogram depicts an anterior aneurysm that responded well to LVR (see the cine image at http://cvbook.nmh.org).

Figure 11.4 This patient was not a candidate for LVR in our opinion, due to diffuse global akinesia caused by infarction in all three coronary territories. (The cine version can be viewed at http://cvbook.nmh.org).

thinning then an akinetic area will be reconstructed. Akinetic regions that are amenable to reconstruction are most often found in patients who have a rim of marbled epicardial muscle and scar overlying dense subendocardial scar.

The contraindications to LVR are the usual contraindications to performing surgery for heart failure. Patients who have stage D inotrope dependent heart failure usually do not benefit from LVR. If major comorbidities that would impair late survival and quality of life do not exist, we think that introppe dependent patients are best served by transplantation or ventricular assistance as destination therapy. Representative ventriculograms of candidates with discreet scar that can be safely resected (Figure 11.3) versus patients with diffuse scar secondary to multiple vessel infarct with no apparent resectable area can be viewed at http://cvbook.nmh.org (Figure 11.4).

Techniques for LVR
Double cerclage ventriculoplasty

The majority of our patients are reconstructed using direct suture approaches without the use of a prosthetic or autologous patch [18]. Most patients (89% in our experience) also undergo coronary artery bypass surgery, and almost 50% undergo concomitant mitral valve (MV) surgery. The operation is performed through a full sternotomy. If the LAD target vessel is graftable, then a bypass graft (usually the left internal mammary artery (LIMA)) is placed to this vessel. If there is a true thin-walled LV aneurysm and a diffusely diseased and occluded LAD vessel, then the LAD is either not grafted or is grafted with a vein, and the LIMA used to revascularize the circumflex system. An attempt is made to graft the LAD if possible since it supplies septal perforators that can carry collateral flow to other coronary vessels.

After establishing cardiopulmonary bypass the cross-clamp is applied and arrest is achieved with antegrade and then retrograde cold blood cardioplegia. Myocardial standstill is maintained between bypass grafts by giving cardioplegia retrograde and down the vein, or radial artery bypass grafts. If the right coronary artery needs to be grafted, it is revascularized first so that cardioplegia can be given intermittently through the graft during the remainder of the cross-clamp time. Retrograde cardioplegia inconsistently protects the right heart, but by performing the right coronary bypass first, protection of the right heart is optimized by delivering cardioplegia both retrograde and down the right coronary graft. The MV is repaired for those with 2+ or greater MR on preoperative studies. The technique for MV repair is covered in Chapter 10. If

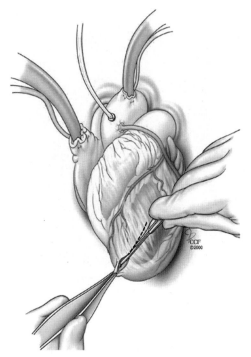

Figure 11.5 The incision for LVR is typically 2 cm left of the LAD and extends 3–5 cm parallel to the LAD. This is routinely performed with the heart beating and empty.

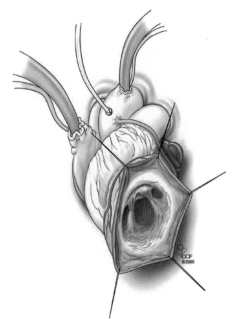

Figure 11.6 The thin LV walls are retracted with stay sutures to facilitate exposure of the septum, the papillary muscles, and the border zone of infarcted and normal appearing muscle.

there is a history of atrial fibrillation then a Maze procedure or a modified Maze procedure may also be performed. The left atrial appendage is closed or excised. The left atrium is closed and the LIMA to LAD and proximal anastomoses are performed. A terminal dose of warm substrate enhanced cardioplegia (Hot shot) is given first retrograde then antegrade. The aortic cross-clamp is released and the LVR is performed on the beating heart. The aortic vent is left on active suction during the ventricular surgery, and the heart is allowed to reperfuse.

The LV scar is opened approximately 2 cm lateral to the LAD. The incision is extended perpendicular for 3–4 cm (Figure 11.5). Any underlying LV thrombus is carefully removed. 2-0 retention sutures are used to retract the edges of the scar to facilitate exposure into the left ventricle (Figure 11.6). A subendocardial resection is undertaken down to the border zone of normal and scarred myocardium for patients with a history of ventricular tachycardia or with a calcified layer of subendocardial scar. Cryolesions at −60° centigrade are placed along the entire

border zone for 2 min at each application site for those with a history of ventricular arrhythmias.

The ventricle is reconstructed in the majority of patients using a double cerclage technique with ventriculoplasty (Figure 11.7). The border zone between contracting and infarcted myocardium is determined by a combination of visual inspection and palpation. For those with true dyskinetic scar usually the border zone is quite visible. For patients with an akinetic area of mixed muscle and scar, palpation can be very valuable in determining the border zone. The distribution of the scar can vary considerably. In some patients the majority of the scar is on the anterior free wall of the left ventricle with only about 20% of the scar involving the septum. Other patients will have a significantly different pattern with much of the scar involving the septum and little anterior free wall involvement.

While the heart is beating, a purse string of 0-polypropylene suture is placed in the border zone. Each bite is buried deeply into the scar tissue within millimeters of the border zone (Figure 11.7). The suture is tied tightly to create a "neck." The orifice is typically 1–3 cm. The classic Dor procedure

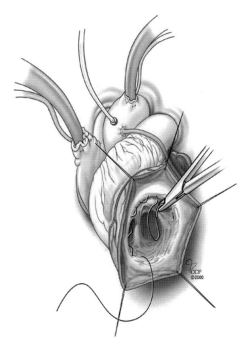

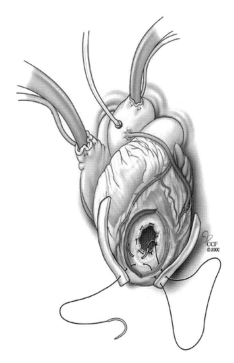

Figure 11.7 Reconstruction begins with a O-polypropylene suture placed at the border zone, with the suture slightly into the scar (which will hold sutures well).

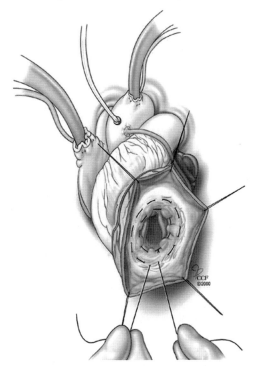

Figure 11.8 The first purse-string suture is tied at the border zone. A second purse-string is placed 3–5 mm above this into the scar.

Figure 11.9 When the second purse-string suture is tied the neck of the aneurysm is usually 1–3 cm. Rarely a patch is used because of heavy calcium on the septum that can not be removed safely, or concern that the remaining LV cavity will be very small and contribute to diastolic dysfunction. Two strips of felt are positioned on either side of the ventriculotomy. These are sewn in place with horizontal mattress sutures of 2-0-polypropylene. Along the septum the sutures are placed carefully so that they exit the LV free wall 0.5–1 cm to the left of the LAD. The mattress sutures should extend all the way down to the prior purse-string sutures. This obliterates the cavity between the aneurysm neck and the LV free wall, and minimizes the chances for bleeding.

(endoventricular circular patch plasty) would consist of sewing a patch over this opening [14]. In over 95% of our patients, however, we simply close the opening using a second purse string suture of 0-polypropylene a few millimeters above the previous suture (Figure 11.8). After tying this suture, the neck is usually only 1 cm, and sometimes is completely obliterated. Two strips of felt are then placed on the epicardial surface (Figure 11.9). Horizontal mattress sutures of 2-0-polypropylene sutures are then used to approximate the border zone between normal and infarcted myocardium. The sutures are passed through the free wall of the LV with the needle passing all the way down to the level of the

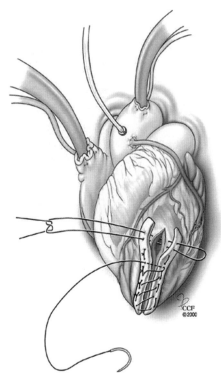

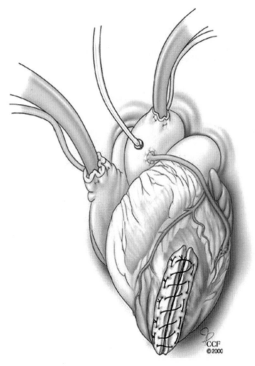

Figure 11.10 The horizontal mattress sutures are tied tightly, alternating from top to bottom of the suture line so that the middle (area of highest tension) is tied last (this does not correspond to the illustration).

Figure 11.11 The ventriculomy is oversewn superficially in two layers with 2-0-polypropylene as a final hemostatic layer.

purse string sutures. For the second bite the needle is passed up along the septum and is brought out the free wall of the left ventricle staying just to the lateral side of the LAD. Care is taken not to obliterate the LAD, and the sutures are not passed underneath the LAD which may occlude septal perforators. Usually only 4–6 horizontal mattress sutures are required. These are then tied while the assistant holds pressure on the free edge of the left ventricle (Figure 11.10). If there is a very thin-walled LV aneurysm then part of the scar (occasionally a large portion of scar) is excised. For akinetic areas there is less resection of the mixed scar and muscle. The ventricular cavity beneath the purse string sutures then is almost completely surrounded by normal myocardium except for the small rim of scar where the first purse string suture was placed. The ventriculoplasty is then closed with a hemostatic layer of running 2-0-polypropylene, typically in two layers with care taken to incorporate felt with each bite

(Figure 11.11). Bleeding has been very rare with this technique. The technique can be viewed at http://cvbook.nmh.org (Figure 11.12).

If the patient has a QRS duration >120 ms then LV epicardial pacing wires are placed on the lateral left ventricle midway between the base and apex of the heart. Prior to decannulation these leads are evaluated for pacing and sensing thresholds, and later after protamine has been given they are tunneled to a small pocket underneath the left clavicle where they are available for later biventricular synchronous pacing if the patient has recurrent heart failure. Intraoperative echocardiography is used to assess any remaining air in the LV cavity, to assess the presence of MR, and to evaluate overall LV function while the patient is weaned from cardiopulmonary bypass. We frequently employ a low dose inotropic infusion such as epinephrine to wean off bypass. Occasionally, we use milrinone but are cautious with its utilization given its significant vasodilatory properties. Rarely is an intra-aortic balloon pump (IABP) required. We feel that doing the LVR

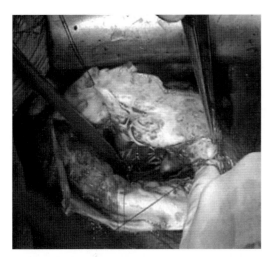

Figure 11.12 The LVR operation can be viewed at http://cvbook.nmh.org for both a classic LV aneurysm, and an akinetic infarct.

with the heart beating is advantageous in two regards. The transition zone between scar and viable tissue may be indistinct on inspection of the arrested heart. When the heart is beating the transition zone becomes more obvious and in addition, palpation can be used to further delineate non-contractile scar from contracting viable myocardium. Furthermore, myocardial recovery, in these already compromised ventricles, may be enhanced by doing the reconstruction on an empty beating perfused heart and allow for a more expeditious wean from cardiopulmonary bypass.

The technique for reconstruction of an akinetic infarct is essentially the same (Figure 11.12) (see video on http://cvbook.nmh.org). In our experience over 95% of patients can be closed primarily without using a prosthetic patch. In concept, the prosthetic patch simply replaces one akinetic segment with another smaller akinetic patch. There are rare exceptions, however, which do require patch closure. Occasionally patients with a heavily calcified LV aneurysm are best treated with a patch. For most patients, however, the calcified area is removed with the electrocautery. For other patients with scattered calcium throughout the septum, resection of the calcified areas cannot be completed without creating a ventricular septal defect. In patients with remaining calcium tying the purse string sutures may not reduce the neck of the aneurysm. In these patients, we place

one purse string suture and then close the aneurysm with a patch as per the classic Dor procedure. We also perform a classic Dor when we are concerned that, without a patch, the reconstructed left ventricle would be too small. Although the ejection fraction appears high, a small LV cavity leads to a decreased stroke volume, and manifests clinically with tachycardia and elevated pulmonary artery pressures secondary to diastolic dysfunction. A reconstructed small left ventricle can also create distortion of the papillary muscles causing MR. This is a very unusual circumstance. Balloon "mannequins" and other devices are available that can be used to "size" the ventricular cavity. We try to leave a remaining ventricular cavity (left ventricular end diastolic volume (LVEDV)) of approximately 100 mL, and with experience have found that sizing with a balloon is rarely required.

Recent variations on the technique of ventricular reconstruction have been reported by Mickleborough and the RESTORE Group (Reconstructive Endoventricular Surgery Returning Original Radius Elliptical Shape to the LV) [16,17]. It should be noted that all contemporary techniques reconstruct the infarcted septum either with suture or some variation of patching. The most important concept is to exclude the infarcted thin-walled area.

Early and late results following LVR for ischemic cardiomyopathy
Cleveland Clinic results

In the contemporary period, LVR can be performed with an acceptably low mortality, even for those with advanced heart failure. We presented 84 patients with class III or IV heart failure who underwent LVR [22]. Thirty-day survival in that group was 100%, and 1-, 2- and 3-year survival were 90%, 85%, and 83%, respectively (Figure 11.13). Mean New York Heart Association (NYHA) class decreased from 3.4 to 1.4 ($P = 0.0001$; Figure 11.14). These results in patients with advanced heart failure were not significantly different from our overall group of 223 patients. Our 5-year experience included 223 patients with a mean age of 62 years; 69% were dyskinetic aneurysms and 31% were akinetic. Thirty-day survival in this group was 98%, with 1- and 3-year survival of 92% and 86%, respectively.

Measuring ventricular function before and after ventricular reconstruction is difficult with

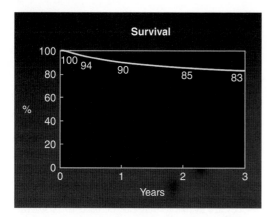

Figure 11.13 Survival for 84 patients with class III (63%) or class IV (37%) congestive heart failure (CHF) who underwent LVR at Cleveland Clinic. True dyskinetic aneurysms accounted for 63%, and akinetic segments 37%. Thirty-day survival was 100%, in hospital mortality was 2.4%; 1-year survival was 90%; and 3-year survival was 83%.

Table 11.1 Improvement in ventricular volume and ejection fraction after LVR as demonstrated by intraoperative and postoperative 3-D echocardiography.

	Before IE (n = 30)	After IE (n = 30)	Follow-up (n = 22)
EDV (mL)	196 ± 81	133 ± 53*	139 ± 50* **
ESV (mL)	143 ± 75	79 ± 42*	82 ± 36* **
SV (mL)	53 ± 22	55 ± 22	57 ± 18
FSV (mL)	22 ± 12	53 ± 24*	58 ± 21* **
EF	0.29 ± 0.11	0.43 ± 0.13*	0.42 ± 0.09* **

FSV indicates forward SV (determined in the 16 patients with preoperative MR); SV: total LV stroke volume; EF: ejection fraction; EDV: end diastolic volume; ESV: end systolic volume; IE: infarct exclusion.
*$P < 0.01$ versus before IE; **$P < 0.01$ by ANOVA.
Reprinted with permission from [23].

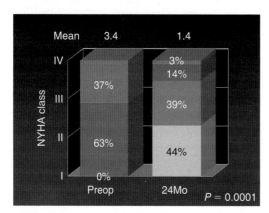

Figure 11.14 Mean NYHA class decreased from 3.4 to 1.4 at 24-month follow-up.

two-dimensional (2-D) echo. Since the anterior wall is frequently reconstructed, but not resected, the akinetic scar may still be visible by 2-D echo. Underestimation of the improvement in ventricular function may occur. We have used quantitative data with three-dimensional (3-D) reconstruction ideally from cardiac cine-MRI or 3-D echocardiography. An example of an MRI before and after LVR is available at http://cvbook.nmh.org (Figure 11.1). The 3-D echocardiography has been used to document a significant improvement in left ventricular ejection fraction (LVEF) from 29% preoperatively to 43% predischarge and 42% at follow-up [23]. The

change in ejection fraction corresponds with a significant drop in ventricular volumes (Table 11.1, 11.2 and 11.3, Figure 11.15).

However, occasional patients are found to have a combination of recurrent MR and ventricular dilation. It is not clear whether this subgroup of patients had some residual low level of MR that led to volume overloading and subsequent ventricular dilation, or whether the ventricular remodeling process continued and subsequently caused MR. Similar findings have been described by Dr. Dor's group [12]. Because of this finding of recurrent MR and ventricular dilation we have been diligent in our use of MV repair for patients undergoing LVR, in particular in our more recent experience. We have a very low threshold for performing mitral repair ($\geq 2+$).

In a subgroup of patients we were able to show the changes that one would expect in neurohormones with the reversal of LV dilation and heart failure [22]. In this study, neurohormones significantly improved in a subgroup of 10 patients who were prospectively studied (Figure 11.16).

In the Cleveland Clinic experience survival following LVR was not influenced by the addition of concomitant MV repair (Figure 11.17). This is interesting because most studies indicate that patients with MR have a worse prognosis [16,17]. One of the few markers for poor prognosis and re-admission to the hospital following LVR was a QRS duration $>120\,ms$

Table 11.2 Test results at 3- and 6-month follow-up intervals.

	Changes at 3 months after implant				Changes at 6 months after implant			
	Pretreatment	3 months	n	P	Pretreatment	6 months	n	P
LVEDD (mm)	74.0 ± 2.1	68.4 ± 1.6	9	<0.02	72.9 ± 1.8	64.7 ± 3.2	7	<0.06
LVESD (mm)	65.5 ± 2.2	62.8 ± 1.7	8	0.17	65.8 ± 2.7	58.6 ± 5.3	5	0.31
LVEF (%)	21.7 ± 1.5	27.6 ± 3.2	9	<0.04	21.6 ± 1.6	32.8 ± 4.9	8	<0.04
MR, 0–4+	1.3 ± 0.3	0.7 ± 0.2	9	0.05*	1.1 ± 0.2	0.07 ± 0.2	7	**
Peak $\dot{V}o_2$ (mL/kg/min)	14.7 ± 1.5	14.8 ± 1.4	7	0.84	14.4 ± 1.2	16.8 ± 2.1	9	0.15
Heart rate (bpm)	82 ± 4.1	82 ± 3.9	9	0.98	84 ± 4.1	76 ± 2.6	9	<0.05
Systolic BP (mmHg)	113 ± 5.2	118 ± 5.2	8	0.40	113 ± 4.6	120 ± 8.1	9	0.44
Diastolic BP (mmHg)	78 ± 2.6	82 ± 3.0	8	0.12	78 ± 2.3	78 ± 3.0	9	0.83
NYHA class	2.5 ± 0.2	1.6 ± 0.2	9	0.005*	2.5 ± 0.2	1.7 ± 0.2	9	0.025*
MN living with HF	28.8 ± 7.3	24.4 ± 7.7	5	**	43.0 ± 10.4	25.8 ± 6.4	5	0.05*
Uniscale	3.8 ± 0.5	6.4 ± 1.1	5	<0.1*	3.9 ± 0.8	6.9 ± 1.0	5	0.05*

Data are mean ±SE. n indicates number of patients. Patient cohorts may differ for each parameter and time point on the basis of available data and follow-up duration. Reprinted with permission from [56].

LVEDD: left ventricular end diastolic dimension; LVESD: left ventricular end systolic dimension; peak $\dot{V}o_2$: peak oxygen consumption; BP: blood pressure; MN living with; HF: Minnesota living with heart failure quality of life questionnaire (a higher score indicates worse quality of life and daily functioning); and Uniscale, quality of life assessment (a higher score indicates better quality of life).

*Wilcoxon signed-rant test; other P-values are paired t-test.

**Insufficient data.

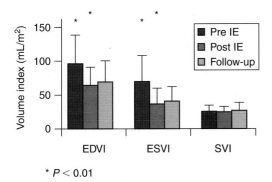

* $P < 0.01$

Figure 11.15 Improvement in ventricular volume and ejection fraction after LVR as demonstrated by intraoperative and postoperative 3-D echocardiography (reprinted with permission from [23]).
EDVI: end diastolic volume index; ESVI: end systolic volume index; IE: infarct exclusion; SVI: stroke volume index.

(Figure 11.18). Patients with a QRS duration >120 ms had decreased survival compared to those with shorter durations, and this was more pronounced for the most prolonged QRS duration. It is not known yet whether our practice of placing LV epicardial pacing wires in these patients with subsequent biventricular synchronous pacing will effect their late survival. In the COMPANION (Comparison of Medical Therapy, Pacing and Defibrillation in Heart Failure) trial, patients with biventricular synchronous pacing not only had a better quality of life and functional class, but better survival than those with untreated left bundle branch block and severe LV dysfunction [24]. Patients with preoperative implantable cardioverterdefibrillators (ICDs) also had a worse prognosis than patients without an ICD [25]. The proper strategy for how to manage these patients post-LVR is not yet determined from a standpoint of their ventricular arrhythmias. For patients who have severe ischemic cardiomyopathy an ICD may be warranted. In a retrospective study from the Cleveland Clinic Foundation, it appeared that postoperative EP testing was able to determine patients who were at high risk for events, and this may be a worthwhile strategy in the future to determine which patients following LVR require an ICD [26].

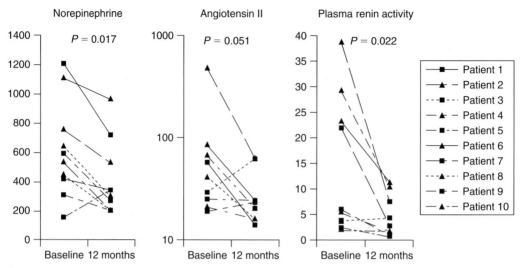

Figure 11.16 Improvement in neurohormonal profile following LVR (reprinted with permission from [20]).

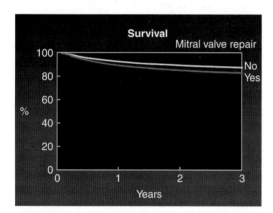

Figure 11.17 There was no difference in early or late survival for 84 patients with class III or IV CHF who underwent LVR with or without MV repair.

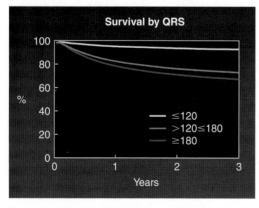

Figure 11.18 Survival after LVR was significantly reduced for those patients with a QRS duration >120 ms.

Other contemporary results are also good. The RESTORE Group reported on 662 patients who underwent the LVR. Hospital mortality was 7.7% and MV repair was performed in 22% [17,27]. Postoperative ejection fraction increased from 30% to 40% and left ventricular end systolic volume (LVESV) decreased from 96 to 62 mL/m^2. Three-year survival was 89.4%. Mickleborough also reported a low hospital mortality of 2.6% in 196 patients [16]. One and 5-year survival were 91% and 84%; 80% of survivors were in NYHA class I or II. As in our series, ventricular tachycardia was noted to be a preoperative risk factor for poor outcome. In contradistinction to our series where MR was not a prognostic factor, 2+ or greater MR was associated with poor outcome following LVR. Lundblad reported an 8.7% operative mortality in 149 patients with a 5-year cumulative survival of 77%[28]. They also identified history of ventricular arrhythmia as a risk factor for a poor late result as well as a linear repair technique. Balooki and colleagues described a very long-term, 22 year, experience with LV aneurysm repair using a variety of techniques [24]. Their best results were in the most recent experience with repairs similar to those described by Dor. However, their perioperative mortality was high, in part because they operated on patients in cardiogenic shock [30]. Finally, similar to our experience, late survival of patients with resection for dyskinetic true aneurysms was a little better but not necessarily statistically significantly better than patients with akinetic segments in most series [24,31]. These studies confirm the effectiveness of reconstructing akinetic segments in centers with experience in this surgical population. Late survival appears to be worse for patients with linear repair than more complete repair [29,30].

The STICH (Surgical Treatment of Ischemic Heart Failure) trial is a prospective randomized multicenter clinical trial of medical therapy only, medical therapy plus coronary artery bypass graft (CABG), and medical therapy plus CABG and LVR [32]; 2800 patients with heart failure, LVEF <35%, and coronary anatomy suitable for surgical revascularization will be studied. The primary endpoint for medical versus surgical therapy will be survival, and the primary endpoint for CABG alone versus CABG plus ventricular reconstruction will be survival free of hospitalization. The expected completion date of the study is 12/2008.

Summary

There are theoretical reasons why reconstruction of a dyskinetic LV segment, or discreet akinetic thin-walled segment, should lead to improved myocardial function. Clinical experience has shown that these operations can be performed with an acceptable operative mortality, and lead to an improvement in ejection fraction, New York Heart Functional class, and good 3- and 5-year survival. In our experience, a relatively simple technique that does not require patch placement can be performed in approximately 15–25 min without prolonging the ischemic time of the surgery. Patients at risk for late death include those with a long QRS duration, and a history of ventricular tachycardia. Whether these are markers for more severely impaired ventricles that will not respond, or whether the use of biventricular synchronous pacing/ICDs may improve survival in this subgroup, has yet to be determined. No randomized trial comparing survival in LVR to medical therapy alone or CABG alone has been completed.

LVR and devices for patients with dilated cardiomyopathy

Introduction

Randas Batista MD, a cardiac surgeon practicing in Brazil, was frustrated by the lack of therapy for patients with Chagas disease and dilated cardiomyopathy [33]. Knowing about the success of LV aneurysm surgery, and reasoning that ventricular dilation itself decreased efficiency, he embarked upon a series of operations to remove a portion of the ventricular wall in patients with dilated cardiomyopathy. The partial left ventriculectomy (PLV) (Batista Procedure) was undertaken typically in the lateral wall between the papillary muscles and was closed with a single layer of running suture. The heart was then smaller, had less wall stress, and better systolic function. Surgeons in the United States heard of this approach when Dr. Batista discussed this approach during the discussion of a lung volume reduction paper [34]. Subsequently several physicians went to Brazil to witness this operation. When two of us from the Cleveland Clinic Foundation (McCarthy and Starling) went to Brazil in May of 1995, Dr. Batista had operated on, 250–300 patients with an operative mortality of around 10%, and most survivors were clinically improved.

During 1995, United States and British centers began performing the Batista procedure with mixed results. We began offering the procedure as an alternative to transplantation. As experience grew, and our initial results appeared favorable, three non-transplant candidate patients also received the Batista procedure. Our results have been reported [35–37]. By 1998, we elected to abandon this procedure because it was unpredictable, and because we thought there were other options on the horizon that may be more effective. Though we no longer perform the Batista procedure, our experience with the operation is briefly summarized here.

Theory behind PLV

The operation was designed to reduce ventricular radius and therefore directly decrease ventricular wall stress through the Law of LaPlace. Improvement in ejection fraction and systolic function was observed by several other investigators [38–41]. We also in small studies showed improvement of wall stress as determined by echocardiographic and non-invasive hemodynamic measurements [42,43]. Mathematical modeling and finite element analysis showed a leftward shift of pressure volume loops, but at the expense of a counteracting effect in diastole, potentially leading to significant diastolic dysfunction [44–46]. In essence, the Batista procedure improved systolic function, but worsened diastolic function, with a net effect of little benefit on overall LV pumping capacity [11,45–47]. The heterogeneity

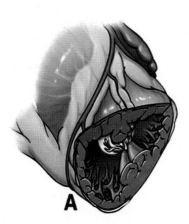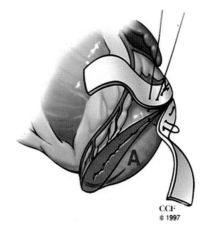

Figure 11.19 The Batista procedure (PLV) excised the lateral wall of the left ventricle, generally between the two papillary muscles. Following reconstruction LV volumes, dimension, wall stress, and ejection fraction improved. Unfortunately, the decreased diastolic compliance offset the benefits in many patients.

of diastolic dysfunction, we have postulated, may be related to underlying ventricular fibrosis and possibly explains why some patients demonstrate a clinical benefit and others showed no improvement or even worsened after surgery.

Cleveland Clinic indications for the Batista procedure

We initially offered this procedure to patients who were awaiting heart transplantation. We reasoned that if surgery was successful the patient could come off the transplant list. If the therapy were only transiently successful then the patient would have postponed the adverse events and comorbidities of transplantation and immunosuppression for some period of time. If the therapy was unsuccessful or the patient got worse, mechanical assistance could be used as a bridge-to-transplantation. By definition all patients had class III or IV heart failure and had tried and failed conventional medical therapy. Of 62 patients, 23 were on inotropic agents before surgery, three patients were on IABP counter pulsation, and one patient was on a left ventricular assist device (LVAD). All patients had dilated left ventricles, with a left ventricular end diastolic dimension (LVEDD) >7 cm as determined by echocardiography. Patients with ischemic cardiomyopathy were excluded since these patients could undergo more accepted ventricular aneurysm resection or reconstruction for akinetic segments.

PLV surgical technique

Our technique was a modification of Batista's original report and has been published [35]. In brief, MV repair was performed in 61 of the 63 patients, and consisted of an Alfieri edge-to-edge leaflet approximation with insertion of a flexible annuloplasty band. A wedge shaped portion of the left ventricle supplied by the circumflex artery was then resected between the papillary muscles (Figure 11.19). In 33 patients (53%) one or both papillary muscles were also resected and then resuspended which allowed for a larger resection. The goal of the operation was to try to have an LVEDD of approximately 6 cm following resection. The ventriculotomy was reconstructed with strips of felt using horizontal mattress sutures and a running suture.

Cleveland Clinic results

Two patients died resulting in a hospital mortality of 3.2% (37), 11 patients (18%) received LVAD as rescue therapy, 32 patients returned to class IV heart failure. Three-year survival was 60% (Figure 11.20), LVEF increased from 16 ± 7.6 to 31.5 ± 10.9 ($P = <0.0001$). Changes in ventricular volume and ejection fraction were relatively stable over time. Increased pulmonary artery systolic pressure was a predictor of poor survival. Reduced maximum exercise oxygen consumption predicted a rapid return to class IV heart failure, and higher left atrial pressure was associated with a lower event free

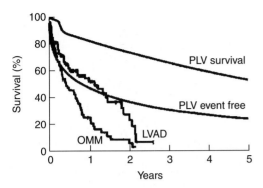

Figure 11.20 While the Batista procedure was largely abandoned in the USA due to its unpredictable failure rate, when taken into perspective versus the published REMATCH results it is less of a disappointment.

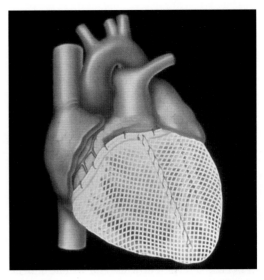

Figure 11.21 The Acorn CorCap™ is a mesh that is placed around both ventricles, snugged to reduce volume a small amount, and then secured to the base of the heart.

survival. Preoperative MR was not a risk factor for any outcome after the Batista procedure. Other surgeons, notably Suma and Frazier, have continued to use the Batista procedure or a modification for selected patients. Suma has reported 2-year survival of 71% and Frazier continues to work toward identifying proper patient selection criteria [41,48]. The PLV Second International Registry analyzed a pool of data on 287 patients from 48 institutions and found that event free survival was reduced when PLV was performed as an emergent rather than elective procedure [49]. Also, NYHA class IV patients had an event free survival of only 39% at 2 years, versus 59% for those with NYHA class less than IV.

Summary of the Batista procedure

The Batista experience is an interesting example of a "failed" surgical procedure. The media portrayed this operation as a simple cure for many patients with heart failure which led to the very unfortunate dissemination of the procedure to programs, centers, and surgeons with little experience in the care of heart failure patients. Many patients did poorly early after the procedure and ultimately died if they were not salvaged by transplantation. Others improved, only to return to heart failure after a period of years. Transplantation trades the chronic disease of heart failure for the chronic disease of immunosuppression. Many of our patients, who subsequently were transplanted, benefited from the Batista procedure as they were able to avoid immunosuppression for a period of time. At 5-year follow-up 26% of patients

were still alive and free of heart failure. Indeed, our first patient is alive 10 years after surgery. Some of these patients had been inotrope dependent and hospitalized for weeks or months awaiting a heart (such as our first patient). When compared to the results of the REMATCH (Randomized Evaluation of Mechanical Assistance for the Treatment of Congestive Heart Failure) trial the results actually look favorable (Figure 11.20). PLV could potentially help some patients with dilated cardiomyopathy if we could identify the characteristics of the subpopulation that benefit. Unfortunately, preoperative our ability to determine ventricular fibrosis and quantify diastolic dysfunction are limited. Furthermore, other medical devices were developed that target patients with dilated cardiomyopathy and the surgery should be much less morbid than the Batista procedure.

Device therapies for dilated cardiomyopathy
Acorn device

The Acorn Corcap™ is a polyester mesh jacket that is placed around the ventricles of the heart [50] (Figure 11.21). The mesh is compliant so that it does not interfere with diastolic function, and it also conforms to the surface of the heart. The mesh acts similar to cardiomyoplasty, in which the latissimus dorsi muscle is wrapped around the heart. The device is designed to prevent further dilation, and can actually lead to a mild reduction in ventricular volume.

Animal studies with the Corcap™ have shown a lowered end diastolic and end systolic volume, and shifted the end systolic pressure–volume relationship (ESPVR) [51–53]. Sabbah reported downregulation of stretch-mediated P21 RAS (renin–angiotensin system) plasmic reticulum indicating that early reverse remodeling alters gene expression [54]. In an ovine model placement of the CorCap™ following anterior myocardial infarction was shown to lead to a diminished area of akinesis in the treated group [55].

Early non-randomized trials in 27 patients showed an improvement in NYHA functional class, a decrease in LVEDD and left ventricular end systolic dimension (LVESD) and an improvement in ejection fraction [56]. Similar findings were reported by Raman in five patients undergoing CorCap™ with concomitant CABG [57].

The pivotal clinical trial performed was a multicenter randomized trial comparing CorCap™ to medical therapy, or CorCap™ with MV repair versus MV repair only. The endpoint of the trial was the effect of the CorCap™ on heart failure. Enrollment in the trial was completed in June of 2003 and reports of the data were presented at the American Heart Association meeting in November 2004; 38% in the CorCap™ group improved (versus 27% control) and 37% worsened (versus 45% control; $P < 0.05$). The CorCap™ group required fewer procedures like transplant or LVAD when compared with control, manifested a greater reduction in LVEDV and LVESV, and had a greater improvement in sphericity index and quality of life scores [58]. The data on CorCap™ with MV repair versus MV repair only were also favorable, and are awaiting publication. Clinical trials to use CorCap™ for patients early post acute myocardial infarction to prevent dilatorious remodeling are being planned. Food and Drug Administration (FDA) review is pending.

Myocor Myosplint

The theory behind the Batista procedure was based on the Law of LaPlace. A reduction of the ventricular radius would lead to a reduction in ventricular wall stress [59]. The Myocor Myosplint device was designed to change the shape of the ventricle into a

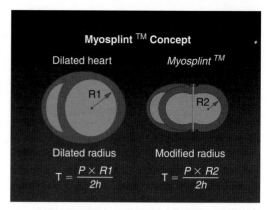

Figure 11.22 The Myocor Myosplint™ device used transventricular splints to reduce LV size, and hence wall stress. It was not fully investigated because the Coapsys™ device was designed by the same company to address MR as well as the remodeled LV.

bi-lobe configuration, with each lobe having a reduced radius and therefore reduced wall stress (Figure 11.22). Since the ventricular wall is not removed (as with the Batista procedure) the effects upon diastolic dysfunction should be less marked. Finite element analysis indicates that the net effect of the shape change induced by the Myosplint should lead to an improvement in cardiac function and an improvement in stroke volume [60], unlike predictions for the Batista procedure. Computational model analysis of the same concept, but using a different device, came up with similar conclusions [61].

Three-dimensional echocardiography performed in a porcine heart failure model with the Myosplint showed there is reduced end diastolic and end systolic volume, improved ejection fraction, decreased wall stress, and that the changes were sustained after 1 month of pacing [59]. In this animal model, however, there were no associated changes in cardiac output or end diastolic pressure. A phase I study was initiated in the United States and Germany. Changes in ventricular volume and ejection fraction from initial patients showed the expected changes. However, the company developed a new product, Coapsys™, that is designed to achieve off-pump MV repair along with some ventricular volume reduction (see Chapter 10). The fate of the Myosplint device, therefore, is uncertain and the device may be set aside in favor of the device more focused on the reduction of MR.

Summary

For patients with non-ischemic delated cardiomyopathy systolic function can be improved via resection (the Batista procedure), or device based therapy (Myosplint). However, the diastolic dysfunction created by the Batista procedure, and clinically unpredictable outcomes, greatly reduced initial enthusiasm. The CorCap™ passively constrains the ventricles and has successfully completed clinical trials. As of this time (2005), those trials are not yet published and the FDA has not yet approved this device.

References

1 Migrino RQ, Young JB, Ellis SG, White HD, Lundergan CF, Miller DP, Granger CB, Ross AM, Califf RM, Topol EJ. End-systolic volume index at 90 to 180 minutes into reperfusion therapy for acute myocardial infarction is a strong predictor of early and late mortality. *Circulation* 1997; **96**: 116–121.

2 Mann DL. Mechanisms and models in heart failure: a combinatorial approach. *Circulation* 1999; **100**: 999–1008.

3 Weber KT, Janicki JS. Myocardial oxygen consumption: the role of wall force and shortening. *Am J Physiol Heart Circ Physiol* 1977; **233**: H421–H430

4 Bavaria JE, Furukawa S, Kreiner G et al. Myocardial oxygen utilization after reversible global ischemia. *J Thorac Cardiovasc Surg* 1990; **100**: 210–220.

5 Pimentel DR, Amin JK, Xiao L et al. Reactive oxygen species mediate amplitude-dependent hypertrophic and apoptotic responses to mechanical stretch in cardiac myocytes. *Cir Res* 2001; **89**: 453–460.

6 Spinale FG, Coker ML, Thomas CV, Walker JD, Mukherjee R, Hebbar L. Time-dependent changes in matrix metalloproteinase activity and expression during the progression of congestive heart failure: relation to ventricular and myocyte function. *Cir Res* 1998; **82**: 482–495.

7 Gomez AM, Valdivia HH, Cheng H et al. Defective excitation-contraction coupling in experimental cardiac hypertrophy and heart failure. *Science* 1997; **276**: 800–806.

8 Grossman W, Jones D, McLaurin LP. Wall stress and patterns of hypertrophy in the human left ventricles. *J Clin Invest* 1975; **56**: 56–64.

9 DiDonato M. Sabatier M. Toso A et al. Regional myocardial performance of non-ischemic zones remote from anterior wall left ventricular aneurysm. *Eur Heart J* 1995; **16**: 1285–1292.

10 Dang AB, Guccione JM, Zhang P, Wallace AW, Gorman RC, Gorman III JH, Ratcliffe MB. Effect of ventricular size and patch stiffness in surgical anterior ventricular restoration: a finite element model study. *Ann Thorac Surg* 2005; **79**: 185–193.

11 Artrip JH, Oz MC, Burkhoff D. Left ventricular volume reduction surgery for heart failure: a physiologic perspective. *J Thorac Cardiovasc Surg* 2001; **122**: 775–782.

12 DiDonato M, Sabatier M, Dor V, Gensini GF, Toso A, Maioli M, Stanley AW, Athanasuleas C, Buckberg G. Effects of the Dor procedure on left ventricular dimension and shape and geometric correlates of mitral regurgitation one year after surgery. *J Thorac Cardiovasc Surg* 2001; **121**: 91–96.

13 Cooley DA, Collins HA, Morris GC, Chapman DW. Ventricular aneurysm after myocardial infarction. Surgical excision with the use of temporary cardiopulmonary bypass. *J Am Med Assoc* 1958; **167**: 557–560.

14 Dor V, Kreitmann P, Jourdan J et al. Interest of physiological closure (circumferential plasty on contractile areas) of left ventricle after resection and endocardectomy for aneurysm or akinetic zone. Comparison with classical technique about a series of 209 left ventricular resections. *J Cardiovasc Surg* 1985; **26**: 73.

15 Jatene AD. Left ventricular aneurysmectomy. Resection or reconstruction. *J Thorac Cardiovasc Surg* 1985; **89**: 321–331.

16 Mickleborough LL, Carson S, Ivanov J. Repair of dyskinetic or akinetic left ventricular aneurysm: results obtained with a modified linear closure. *J Thorac Cardiovasc Surg* 2001; **121**: 675–682.

17 Athanasuleas C, Stanley AWH, Buckberg G et al. Surgical anterior ventricular endocardial restoration (SAVER) for dilated ischemic cardiomyopathy. *Semin Thorac Cardiovasc Surg* 2001; **13(4)**: 448–458.

18 Caldeira C, McCarthy PM. A simple method of left ventricular reconstruction without patch for ischemic cardiomyopathy. *Ann Thorac Surg* 2001; **72**: 2148–2149.

19 Buckberg GD. Early and late results of left ventricular reconstruction in thin-walled chambers: is this our patient population? *J Thorac Cardiovasc Surg* 2004; **128**: 21–26.

20 Schenk S, McCarthy PM, Starling RC, Hoercher KJ, Hail MD, Ootaki Y et al. Neurohormonal response to left ventricular reconstruction surgery in ischemic cardiomyopathy. *J Thorac Cardiovasc Surg* 2004; **128**: 38–43.

21 Dor V. Left ventricular reconstruction: the aim and the reality after twenty years. *J Thorac Cardiovasc Surg* 2004; **128**: 17–20.

22 McCarthy PM, Young JB, Hoercher KJ, Smedira NG, Secic M, Starling RC. Surgical LV reconstruction for end-stage heart disease: outcomes and effect on NYHA class and hospitalizations for heart failure. *Circulation* 2001; **104**: II-358 (A-1706).

23 Qin JX, Shiota T, McCarthy PM et al. Real-time three-dimensional echocardiographic study of left ventricular function after infarct exclusion surgery for ischemic cardiomyopathy. *Circulation* 2000; **102(Suppl III)**: III-101–III-106.

24 Salukhe TV, Francis DP, Sutton R. Comparison of medical therapy, pacing and defibrillation in heart failure (COMPANION) trial terminated early; combined biventricular pacemaker-defibrillators reduce all-cause mortality and hospitalization. *Int J Cardiol* 2003; **87**: 119–120.

25 Lee R, Hoercher KJ, McCarthy PM. Left ventricular reconstruction and the surgical treatment of the failing heart. In Sellke FW, del Nido PJ, and Swanson SJ (eds). *Surgery of the Chest*, 7th edn. Elsevier Saunders, Philadelphia, 2005: pp. 1685–1709.

26 O'Neill JO, Starling RC, Khaykin Y, McCarthy PM, Young JB, Hail M, Albert NM, Smedira N, Chung MK. Residual high incidence of ventricular arrhythmias despite left ventricular reconstructive surgery. *PACE* 2003; **26**: 988.

27 Athanasuleas CL, Buckberg GD, Stanley AW, Siler W, Dor V, DiDonato M, Menicanti L, Almeida de Oiveira S, Beyersdorf F, Kron IL, Suma H, Kouchoukos NT, Moore W, McCarthy PM, Oz MC, Fontan F, Scott ML, Accola KA; RESTORE group. Surgical ventricular restoration in the treatment of congestive heart failure due to postinfarction ventricular dilation. *J Am Coll Cardiol* 2004; **44**: 1439–1445.

28 Lunblad R, Abdelnoor, M, Svennevig JL. Surgery for left ventricular aneurysm: early and late survival after simple linear repair and endoventricular patch plasty. *J Thorac Cardiovasc Surg* 2004; **128**: 449–456.

29 Bolooki H, DeMarchena E, Mallon SM *et al.* Factors affecting late survival after surgical remodeling of left ventricular aneurysms. *J Thorac Cardiovasc Surg* 2003; **126**: 374–383; discussion 383–385.

30 McCarthy PM. Ventricular aneurysms, shock, and late follow-up in patients with heart failure. *J Thorac Cardiovasc Surg* 2003; **126**: 323–325.

31 Couper GS, Bunton RW, Birjiniuk V, DiSesa VJ, Fallon MP, Collins Jr JJ, Cohn LH. Relative risks of left ventricular aneurysmectomy in patients with akinetic scars versus true dyskinetic aneurysms. *Circulation* 1990; **82(Suppl 5)**: IV248–IV256.

32 Jones RH. Is it time for a randomized trial of surgical treatment of ischemic heart failure? *J Am Coll Cardiol* 2001; **37**: 1210–1213.

33 Batista RJ, Santos JL, Takeshita N, Bocchino L, Lima PN, Cunha MA. Partial left ventriculectomy to improve left ventricular function in end-stage heart disease. *J Card Surg* 1996; **11**: 96–98.

34 Miller, Jr JI, Lee RB, Mansour KA. Lung volume reduction surgery: Lessons learned. *Ann Thor Surg* 1996; **61(5)**: 1464–1469.

35 McCarthy PM, Starling RC, Wong J, Scalia GM, Buda T, Vargo RL, Goormastic M, Thomas JD, Smedira NG, Young JB. Early results with partial left ventriculectomy. *J Thorac Cardiovasc Surg* 1997; **114**: 755–763; discussion 763–765.

36 McCarthy JF, McCarthy PM, Starling RC, Smedira NG, Scalia GM, Wong J, Kasirajan V, Goormastic M, Young JB. Partial left ventriculectomy and mitral valve repair for end-stage congestive heart failure. *Eur J Cardiothorac Surg* 1998; **13**: 337–343.

37 Franco-Cereceda A, McCarthy PM, Blackstone EH, Hoercher KJ, White JA, Young JB, Starling RC. Partial left ventriculectomy for dilated cardiomyopathy: is this an alternative to transplantation? *J Thorac Cardiovasc Surg* 2001; **121**: 879–893.

38 Angelini GD, Pryn S, Mehta D, Izzat MB, Walsh C, Wilde P *et al.* Left-ventricular-volume reduction for end-stage heart failure. *Lancet* 1997; **350**: 489.

39 Gradinac S, Miric M, Popovic Z, Popovic AD, Neskovic AN, Jovovic L *et al.* Partial left ventriculectomy for idiopathic dilated cardiomyopathy: early results and six months follow-up. *Ann Thorac Surg* 1998; **66**: 1963–1968.

40 Moreira LFP, Stolf NAG, Bocchi EA, Bascal F, Giorgi MCP, Parga JR, Jatene AD. Partial left Ventriculectomy with mitral valve preservation in the treatment of patients with dilated cardiomyopathy. *J Thorac Cardiovasc Surg* 1998; **115**: 800–807.

41 Frazier OH, Gradinac S, Segura AM, Przybylowski P, Popovic Z, Vasiljevic J *et al.* Partial left ventriculectomy: which patients can be expected to benefit? *Ann Thorac Surg* 2000; **69**: 1836–1841.

42 Wong J, Garcia M, McCarthy PM, Starling R, Buda T, Vargo T *et al.* Alterations in left ventricular wall stress after left ventricular remodeling surgery. *Circulation* 1997; **96(Suppl)**: I-344.

43 Fukamachi K, McCarthy PM, Smedira NG, Buda T, Wong J, Starling RC *et al.* Effects of ventriculectomy on left ventricular performance: one year follow up. *Circulation* 1998; **68(Suppl I)**: I-1201.

44 Dickstein ML, Spotnitz HM, Rose EA, Burkhoff D. Heart reduction surgery: an analysis of the impact on cardiac function. *J Thorac Cardiovasc Surg* 1997; **113**: 1032–1040.

45 Ratcliffe MB, Hong J, Salahieh A, Ruch S, Wallace AW. The effect of ventricular volume reduction surgery in the dilated, poorly contractile left ventricle: a simple finite element analysis. *J Thorac Cardiovasc Surg* 1998; **116**: 566–577.

46 Burkhoff D. New heart failure therapy: the shape of things to come? *J Thorac Cardiovasc Surg* 2003; **125**: S50–S52.

47 Schreuder JJ, Steendijk P, van der Veen FH, Alfieri O, van der NT, Lorusso R *et al.* Acute and short-term effects of partial left ventriculectomy in dilated cardiomyopathy: assessment by pressure-volume loops. *J Am Coll Cardiol* 2000; **36**: 2104–2114.

48 Suma H, Isomura T, Horii T, Sato T, Kikuchi N, Iwahashi K, Hosokawa J. Nontransplant cardiac surgery for end-stage cardiomyopathy. *J Thorac Cardiovasc Surg* 2000; **119**: 1233–1245.

49 Kawaguchi AT, Suma H, Konertz W, Popovic Z, Dowling RD, Kitamura S, Bergsland J, Linde LM, Koide S, Batista RJ. Partial left ventriculectomy: the 2nd international registry report 2000. *J Card Surg* 2001; **16(1)**: 10–23.

50 Starling RC, Jessup M. Worldwide clinical experience with the CorCap™ cardiac support device. *J Cardiac Failure* 2004; **10**: S225–S233.

51 Saavedra WF, Tunin RS, Mishima T *et al*. Reverse remodeling and enhanced adrenergic reserve from a passive external ventricular support in experimental dilated heart failure. *Circulation* 2000; **102(Suppl II)**: II-501.

52 Chaudry PA, Mishima T, Sharov VG *et al*. Passive epicardial containment prevents ventricular remodeling in heart failure. *Ann Thorac Surg* 2000; **70**: 1275–1280.

53 Power J, Raman J, Byrne M. Passive ventricular constraint is a trigger for a significant degree of reserve remodeling in an experimental model of degenerative heart failure and dilated cardiomyopathy. *Circulation* 2000; **102(Suppl II)**: II-502.

54 Sabbah HN, Gupta RC, Sharov VG *et al*. Prevention of progressive left ventricular dilation with the Acorn Cardiac Support Device (CSD) down regulates stretch-mediated P21ras, attenuates myocardial hypertrophy, and improves sarcoplasmic reticulum calcium cycling in dogs with heart failure. *Circulation* 2000; **102(Suppl II)**: II-683.

55 Pilla JJ, Blom AS, Brockman DJ, Bowen F, Yuan Q, Giammarco J, Ferrari VA *et al*. Ventricular constraint using the acorn cardiac support device reduces myocardial akinetic area in an ovine model of acute infarction. *Circulation* 2002; **106(12 Suppl 1)**: I-207–I-211.

56 Konertz WF, Shapland JE, Hotz H *et al*. Passive containment and reverse remodeling by a novel textile cardiac support device. *Circulation* 2001; **104(Suppl 1)**: I-270–I-275.

57 Raman JS, Hata M, Storere JM, Buxton BF, Alferness C, Hare D. The mid-term results of ventricular containment (Acorn Wrap) for end-stage ischemic cardiomyopathy. *Ann Thorac Cardiovasc Surg* 2001; **7**: 278–281.

58 Mann DL, Acker MA, Jessup M *et al*. ACORN investigators and study coordinators. Rationale, design, and methods for a pivotal randomized clinical trial for the assessment of a cardiac support device in patients with New York Health Association class III–IV heart failure. *J Card Fail* 2004; **10**: 185–192.

59 McCarthy PM, Takagaki M, Ochiai Y, Young JB, Tabata T, Shiota T, Qin JX, Thomas JD, Mortier TJ, Schroeder RF, Schweich Jr CJ, Fukamachi K. Device-based change in left ventricular shape: a new concept for the treatment of dilated cardiomyopathy. *J Thorac Cardiovasc Surg* 2001; **122**: 482–490.

60 Guccione JM, Salahieh A, Moonly SM, Kortsmit J, Wallace AW, Ratcliffe MB. Myosplint decrease wall stress with out depressing function in the failing heart: a finite element model study. *Ann Thorac Surg* 2003; **76**: 1171–1180.

61 Melvin DB. Ventricular radius reduction without resection: a computational analysis. *ASAIO J* 1999; **45**: 160–165.

CHAPTER 12

Mechanical circulatory support

José Luis Navia

The gold-standard therapeutic option and last resort for patients with end-stage heart failure is heart transplantation. Unfortunately, this therapy that could provide an excellent quality of life and long-term survival is limited purely by availability. In the United States, the shortage of available donor hearts has resulted in an increased waiting list of approximately 7000 patients per year [1], while the number of heart transplant procedures performed annually remains relatively consistent (2500/year). This recognized donor shortage has a domino effect: the expanding number of patients on the transplant waiting list greatly increases the risk of mortality in these patients up to 30%. This vast expanse between possible recipients and available donors generates an urgent, realistic need for a device that would provide mechanical cardiac support until eventual transplantation. The number of people with congestive heart failure (CHF) who could benefit from cardiac support with a mechanically assisted device is estimated to be between 35,000 and 70,000 a year in the United States. Since the need for patients to undergo cardiac transplantation is not expected to diminish, long-term mechanical support offers the best hope for patients with end-stage CHF.

Over the last two decades, many devices were developed that offered patients cardiac support for a period of time (e.g. bridge-to-transplant). Only during the past decade, has mechanical circulatory support (MCS) gained increased acceptance in the treatment of patients with CHF who were unresponsive to conventional medical treatment. With the alternative of MCS patients who had little hope of survival received the cardiac support necessary until transplantation was possible.

MCS encompasses a variety of devices either connected to the heart or placed within the heart to assume some degree of cardiac function. These devices range from a total artificial heart (TAH) (completely replacing the natural heart with a mechanical pump) to a small catheter-mounted pump that moderately augments cardiac function. This chapter reviews the current state of the art of implantable MCS systems, focusing on short- and long-term support, new axial flow pumps, and the TAH.

Background

In the early 1960s, Drs. DeBakey and Spencer [2] were the first to observe that allowing the heart to rest and beat on cardiopulmonary bypass (CPB), the ventricle could recover. It made operations possible on many difficult and even hopeless cases. It also opened a realm of possibilities. Rapid developments in assist device technologies ensued over the next three decades. As early as 1961, a new circulatory assist device, the intra-aortic balloon pump (IABP), was developed and introduced by Moulopoulus *et al.* [3]. Seven years later, Kantrowitz *et al.* [4] reported the first survival of a patient with post-infarction cardiogenic shock using the IABP. In 1962 Dennis and colleagues were the first to use a roller pump as a left ventricular assist device (LVAD) [5]. The following year, DeBakey [6] implanted the first intrathoracic LVAD designed for long-term use. Unfortunately, the patient suffered neurologic damage pre-implant and the pump had to be discontinued after 4 days. In 1966, however, DeBakey [7] reported successful use of the LVAD, connected between the left atrium and the axillary artery, after a double valve replacement. It was removed without opening the chest. The patient was maintained 10 days and eventually discharged home. This case substantiated and initiated

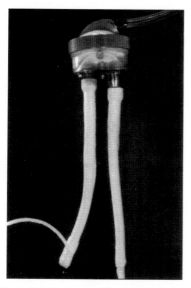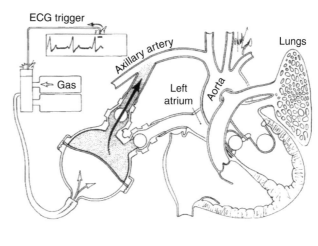

Figure 12.1 The DeBakey blood pump, the Baylor left ventricular device was successfully used for post-cardiotomy in 1966.

the use of LVADs for post-cardiotomy support (Figure 12.1).

The intense focus and rapid development of MCS systems led the National Heart Institute (later renamed The National Heart, Lung and Blood Institute (NHLBI)) to create the Artificial Heart Program. Founded in 1964, this program promoted multicenter research studies by actively offering grant supports for the study of short- and long-term MCS systems, including research for a TAH. When heart transplantation was temporarily abandoned due to immunologic rejection, the research for long-term assist support was intensified. By the early 1970s, the Artificial Heart Program set broader long-term goals:

1 to develop an emergency cardiac assist system;
2 to develop a cardiac assist system to provide temporary circulatory support;
3 to develop a permanent heart assist system; and
4 to develop a totally implantable artificial heart [8,9].

The immense response to the NHLBI laid the foundation for the formulation of LVAD programs. One of the earliest LVADs was developed by the Texas Heart Institute in the early 1970s. Designed for use in post-cardiotomy cardiogenic shock, the MCS was a pneumatic abdominal LVAD (ALVAD) with an external pneumatic console and a percutaneous driveline. Later, in 1978, the LVAD was first used as a bridge-to-transplantation as part of a clinical trial. For 7 days, the device supported a patient who had irreversible stone heart. This was a milestone in the research on the physiologic effect of LVADs on cardiac function. It demonstrated the device could reduce all indices of cardiac work and maintain systemic perfusion and coronary flow.

Better prosthetic materials, engineering advances and increasing clinical experience contributed to the evolution of LVADs. With NHLBI support, new generations of MCS systems (e.g. HeartMate, Thoratec, and Novacor) were designed to use for long-term support. During the 1990s, these devices were approved by the Food and Drug Administration (FDA) for use as a bridge-to-transplantation. Eventually, the electric HeartMate was shown to provide superior survival to medical therapy of advanced heart failure patients, and chronic MCS was approved for non-transplant patients. The Randomized Evaluation of Mechanical Assistance for the Treatment of Congestive Heart Failure (REMATCH) trial pointed to a new future for the field [10].

Indications for MCS

MCS is indicated when the heart can no longer provide the body's perfusion requirements. Regardless of the primary process leading to cardiac failure, the

Table 12.1 Hemodynamic and clinical criteria for initiating mechanical support.

Cardiac output	<2.0 L/min/m^2
Systolic blood pressure	<90 mmHg
Left atrial or wedge pressure	>20 mmHg
Right atrial pressure	>20 mmHg
Urine output	<30 mL/h
Systemic vascular resistance	>2100 dynes/s/cm^5
Metabolic acidosis	
Pulmonary edema	
Decreased mental status	

Table 12.2 Contraindicates criteria for MCS.

- Chronic renal failure
- Severe peripheral vascular disease
- Symptomatic cerebral vascular disease
- Severe hepatic
- Pulmonary disease
- Malignancy
- Significant blood dyscrasias
- Uncontrollable infection

hemodynamic criteria for mechanical cardiac assistance are generally based on the characteristics of cardiogenic shock, first proposed by Norman and colleagues [11]. The proper time to initiate mechanical support is often difficult to define given that a patient may not be able to recover after a certain level of clinical decompensation. Generally, accepted hemodynamic and clinical criteria for initiating mechanical support are outlined in Table 12.1.

Mechanical ventilation is frequently required if severe cardiac dysfunction and symptomatic pulmonary edema develop, despite maximum pharmacologic support. A temporary measure to stabilize the patient is IABP counterpulsation. If implemented early, this will often successfully provide adequate support. Patients who typically require MCS demonstrate a low cardiac index, elevated filling pressures, and minimal cardiac reserve. Patients with chronic heart failure usually become progressively ill, often decompensating over time (or abruptly) and require pharmacologic and mechanical assist support to re-establish hemodynamic stability.

Criteria that contraindicate MCS have also been established and are included in Table 12.2.

Sepsis, particularly, has the potential to produce rapid deterioration and, since active infection is a relative contraindication to MCS, an aggressive culture and antibiotic therapy should be initiated early in all patients. After antibiotic therapy, signs of clinical improvement and a negative culture may reduce the need for MCS; however, if the patient fails to respond quickly, a device should be placed and antibiotic therapy continued postoperatively. Another important factor that requires careful assessment is the patient's neurologic status. Critically ill patients

may exhibit serious irreversible neurologic deficits. Any evidence of permanent central neurosystem injury may eliminate a patient's eligibility for MCS. Thorough evaluation of a patient's neurocognitive status is imperative as part of the decision-making process for MCS placement.

Individual patient selection undoubtedly remains the basis of clinical outcome. Despite extensive investigations and clinical outcome data, no formal criteria have been introduced for the placement of LVADs. LVAD placement versus continuing medical therapy requires clinical judgment to weigh the estimated risk of perioperative complication associated with LVAD with the assumed risk of death without surgical intervention. Timing is critical to a good outcome. Patients who are considered for LVAD placement late in their clinical decompensation may develop associated multi-organ failure and sepsis. This dramatically increases the risk of death. While LVAD support is capable of reversing organ dysfunction, it must be instituted before the onset of permanent damage. For example, in patients with refractory heart failure, surgeons should be encouraged to make an early decision to implant an assist device that has the capability of supporting higher flows and allows the heart to rest. This may greatly improve the recovery of the heart and the end-results, or waiting for heart transplantation. Clinical studies have demonstrated that earlier LVAD implantation decreases morbidity and mortality, improves rehabilitation, improves post-transplant survival and can lead to hospital discharge.

A second key factor in determining the use of LVADs is the extent of myocardial dysfunction; a patient may require left, right, or biventricular support. The cause and extent of myocardial dysfunction influence the duration of support. While there is a wide range of indications for acute mechanical support, the primary goal is rapid restoration of the circulatory system and quick stabilization of the patient's hemodynamics.

Many patients present acutely in cardiogenic shock and the luxury of an extensive evaluation with repeated assessment of the trends in the patient's clinical course is not available. Examples include patients with left main occlusion or other massive myocardial infarction, or post-cardiotomy patients. In these cases, "bridge-to-bridge" support with another MCS may be appropriate, or simply MCS until other issues can be sorted out such as transplant candidacy, neurologic status, or other medical issues. Frequently, these patients receive the extracorporeal Abiomed BVS-5000 system, but at The Cleveland Clinic we generally prefer extracorporeal membrane oxygenation (ECMO). We have used ECMO more often because it can be rapidly placed by a variety of team members (residents, fellows, and cardiologists), usually percutaneously via femoral vessels. It provides biventricular support, it oxygenates the patient and the heparin-coated system and cannula can be run without systemic anticoagulation [12]. Once ECMO is in place and the patient is stabilized, periodic evaluations of the extent of native heart recovery and the patient's neurologic status are made. Simultaneously, evaluation for cardiac transplantation is carried out. Patients who do not have a major contraindication to transplant (i.e. malignancy, occult untreated infection, or neurologic deficit), who indicate no sign of cardiac recovery, and who meet all other criteria are selected for cardiac transplantation. The usual strategy is to maintain ECMO support between 48 and 72 h to stabilize the patient. If the patient maintains good neurologic function but cannot be weaned from ECMO, the transition is made to a chronic ventricular assist device (VAD) until a donor heart becomes available. If, however, a patient shows improvements in heart function, the device is gradually weaned from the patient and ultimately removed.

An ideal MCS device

An ideal MCS system should be capable of successfully supporting patients in clinical settings ranging from post-cardiotomy cardiogenic shock to chronic heart failure. In addition, the device should be able to provide adequate flow, maximize hemodynamics and have the ability to unload the ventricles for any patient, regardless of size. Therefore, to support patients with varying body surface areas (BSAs), an available selection of small-sized diameter cannulas and pumps are requirements. The "ideal" MCS device would also include the following parameters:

1 Easily inserted.
2 Adaptable for patients who require biventricular support.
3 Supports the use of an oxygenator as needed, particularly in patients with acute lung injury.
4 Requires minimal or no anticoagulation.
5 Constructed of a biocompatible surface that does not promote thrombus formation.
6 Results in minimal destruction of blood or plasma components.
7 Allows for ambulation and physical rehabilitation.
8 Easily converted to a long-term implantable device.

Temporary MCS

The introduction of temporary MCS in the treatment of heart failure has made survival possible for many patients. For patients with post-cardiotomy cardiogenic shock, temporary MCS can be used days to weeks; patients with dilated cardiomyopathy can be supported weeks to months. In both cases, optimum outcomes are recovery of cardiac function.

Occasionally, temporary MCS is used as a back-up for high-risk conventional operations such as coronary artery bypass surgery, valve surgery, aneurysm resection, etc. Temporary support must meet the same criteria as those first listed under *The Ideal Mechanical Circulatory Support Device*.

Of critical value for temporary support mechanisms is easy implantability. For example, in a post-cardiotomy clinical setting, with access to the great vessels, the device should allow for versatility in choosing any inflow or outflow side that is clinically indicated. Another situation may be in active resuscitation as in the catheterization laboratory. If a patient goes into cardiac arrest during a cardiac catheterization, time is critical. Time may not allow transporting the patient to the operating room and the only viable option would be percutaneous cannulation insertion for MCS.

Indications for support and patient selection

Indications for use of MCS encompass a wide range. Foremost, when the heart no longer safely meets the perfusion requirements of the body, MCS is the only alternative. At this time, the two acute goals are rapid restoration of circulation and stabilization of hemodynamics.

The key is timing. Defining what constitutes optimum timing is often difficult and it is generally better to err on the side of early implantation versus late implantation. If MCS is initiated after a certain point, the heart may not be able to recover, and MCS is associated with a lower rate of patient survival.

The decision to implant MCS is dependent on the patient's clinical status. These include: post-cardiotomy pump failure, acute myocardial infarction, decompensated heart failure, post-cardiac transplantation allograft dysfunction, acute myocarditis, deterioration during cardiac catheterization, right ventricular failure during LVAD placement, cardiac arrest, and massive pulmonary embolism. Of these, the two major acute indicators for a VAD are post-cardiotomy shock syndrome and myocardial infarction.

Patients undergoing cardiac surgery procedures are at risk for myocardial injuries caused by ischemia either iatrogenic (such as vein graft artheroemboli), or during aortic cross-clamping, during reperfusion or from cardiac arrhythmia or metabolic abnormalities. Post-cardiotomy cardiogenic shock is defined as either cardiac failure that results from the inability to be weaned from CPB or cardiac failure that occurs in the immediate postoperative period. It results from myocardial compromise related to stunning, infarction or poor myocardial preservation, and carries extensive morbidity and mortality rates. For patients in post-cardiotomy cardiogenic shock, hemodynamic instability in the absence of mechanical support is associated with a >50% mortality. It has been reported that early MCS implantation that is capable of supporting higher flows and allowing the heart to unload and rest may improve results and allow for recovery of stunned myocardium [13]. For patients unable to be weaned from CPB due to either marginal preoperative cardiac function or a large intraoperative myocardial infarction, the insertion of temporary MCS is often appropriate.

Patients in post-cardiotomy shock who are put on temporary MCS can be divided into two groups: those with persistent or exacerbation of perioperative dysfunction who are unable to be weaned from support and those with adequate preoperative ventricular function who sustain a myocardial insult and will be able to tolerate device removal. In the latter group, a few days of temporary MCS usually assists in the reversibility of the myocardial insult, especially if the myocardial injury is limited, determined by cardiac enzymes, electrocardiography, and echocardiography.

Cardiogenic shock usually occurs when more than 40% of the ventricular mass is lost to infarction. Treating patients in cardiogenic shock after acute myocardial infarction is difficult and survival may depend on rapid institution of circulatory support. Early myocardial revascularization of ischemic myocardium has shown to improve survival. Some patients have been supported by a percutaneous ECMO or by standard CPB until angioplasty or coronary artery bypass surgery could be performed. It may be impossible to wean patients without hemodynamic stabilization from temporary mechanical support; therefore, these patients should be converted to bridge-to-transplant support with the implantation of a long-term device (e.g. HeartMate or Novacor). This technique is also advisable for patients younger than 65 without permanent organ dysfunction who prove difficult to wean from temporary mechanical support. Utilizing a long-term LVAD for bridge-to-transplant could be the best option for these patients.

Early *implantation of* mechanical assistance is favored in the experience of The Cleveland Clinic, using an IABP as the first step in mechanical support. Furthermore, new pharmacologic agents, such as phosphodiesterase inhibitors (e.g. milrinone), nitric oxide, and vasopressin have helped to optimize hemodynamics during this critical initial period and reduces the need for right ventricular support [14,15]. Once mechanical assistance has been instituted, the patient can undergo periodic evaluation to assess native heart recovery, end-organ function, and neurologic status. In this subgroup, transition is generally made to a chronic LVAD until an organ donor becomes available. Patients who demonstrate gradual improvement in myocardial function may be weaned from the device and the device ultimately removed. Although early implantation of a mechanical device before the onset of irreversible organ failure is ideal, in reality, this is not always possible. Many patients will present in a moribund state with heart failure symptoms and severe biventricular failure.

Types of mechanical support

Intra-aortic balloon pump

Today, almost 30 years since the first clinical trial, the IABP is the most frequently used cardiac assist device. Primarily, it is selected for patients in acute cardiogenic shock and refractory to medical therapy. IABP has established its role in the management of acute left ventricular dysfunction and has become a standard tool in facilities performing coronary care and cardiac surgery. Initial clinical experience with IABP was obtained from medical patients with ischemic heart disease; however the technology was soon adopted by cardiac surgeons for use in patients who could not be weaned from CPB. IABP has also been successfully implemented as a short-term device for bridge-to-transplantation in patients with acute decompensation due to progressive chronic heart failure. The main physiologic effect of IABP is in support of the failing heart. This is accomplished via increasing the diastolic aortic root coronary perfusion pressure while decreasing ventricular afterload during systole. Increased coronary blood flow, coupled with a reduction in the pre- and afterload, improves myocardial contractility and, thus, results in increased cardiac output. In addition, decreased left ventricular stroke work affected by systolic balloon deflation results in a reduction of myocardial oxygen consumption by 10–20% [16].

Several variables are known to affect the physiologic performance of IABP in clinical practice. These include insertion, location, timing, heart rhythm, and blood pressure. The position of the balloon should be downstream to the left subclavian artery; the balloon should fit the aorta so that during inflation it nearly occludes the vessel. Experimental work indicates that in adults, greater balloon volumes of 30–40 mL are preferable over smaller volumes because the higher volumes significantly improve both the left ventricle unloading and the diastolic coronary perfusion pressure. Inflation should be timed to coincide with the closure of the aortic valve. Clinically, this is the dicrotic notch of aortic blood pressure trace. Deflation should occur as late as possible to maintain the duration of the augmented diastolic blood pressure, but before the aortic valve opens and the ventricle ejects. For practical purposes, deflation is timed to occur with the onset of the electrocardiogram (ECG) R-wave.

IABP is both the least invasive and the least complex mechanical cardiac assist device available. Being both easy and quick for percutaneous insertion, without requiring a surgical procedure for removal, it is popular. IABP reduces afterload, left ventricular work and myocardial oxygen consumption during systole; it augments diastolic pressure and coronary blood perfusion. Despite these positive effects, the balloon neither displaces a significant volume nor decompresses nor unloads the left ventricle, and results in only modest improvement in cardiac output. Furthermore, whether or not it actually improves coronary perfusion beyond the critical stenosis and benefits patients with non-ischemic shock are uncertain.

IABP is usually inserted into the common femoral artery, most commonly by percutaneous Seldinger technique or occasionally by surgical cut down. Direct insertion into the ascending aorta is used for intraoperative insertion in patients with severe aortoiliac or femoral occlusive disease that prevents passage of the balloon catheter from below. Weaning the patient from IABP requires a change in the ratio of assisted heartbeats from 1:1 to 1:3. Removing a percutaneously placed IABP requires an attempt to flush out any thrombus as the balloon catheter is being removed. Pressure should then be applied to the insertion site for at least 30 min to obtain hemostasis.

In spite of improvements in IABP design and insertion techniques, peripheral vascular complications may occur. These include arterial thrombosis, embolization, and hemorrhage. Other complications that may occur are balloon rupture, thrombosis within the balloon, sepsis, insertion site infection, false aneurysm formation, atrioventricular (A-V) fistula, and femoral neuropathy. Several reports have documented potential risk factors that may contribute to limb ischemia during IABP placement: namely, peripheral vascular disease, diabetes, smoking, advanced age, obesity, female gender, and

cardiogenic shock [17]. Another potential complication is balloon rupture, easily recognized by the
appearance of blood within the balloon catheter.
Indicators for IABP removal are leg ischemia, balloon
rupture, and sepsis. If, however, a patient is balloon
dependent, a replacement balloon can be inserted
into a new site.

Several disadvantages limit the use of IABP in
patients with heart failure. First, particularly for
patients with right ventricular heart failure, IABP is
not as effective as other, more sophisticated support
devices. Second, for patients with non-ischemic
cardiogenic shock, there may be less positive effects.
Third, many patients in cardiogenic shock will
remain refractory low cardiac output, despite IABP
support. For these patients, a more effective method
of ventricular assistance is imperative to prevent
multiple organ failure and/or death. Devices like
centrifugal and pneumatic pumps have proven to
be more effective.

Extracorporeal centrifugal pump

Centrifugal pump assist device systems are familiar
primarily due to their routine use during CPB. They
are also frequently used as a VAD because of their
widespread availability, low cost and simplicity of
implantation and operation. One advantage of the
centrifugal pump is its variety in design. A specific
choice of pump design can be made for a specific
purpose. This makes them ideal for short-term left
ventricular support as well as for use in ECMO systems or therapy for right heart failure after LVAD
placement or cardiac transplantation. All centrifugal pumps work on the principle of generating a
rotary motion by virtue of moving blades, impellers,
or concentric cones. Most pumps consist of a single
moving part and can be manufactured cheaply.

Centrifugal pumps are usually positioned external to the patient. The pump has an acrylic pump
head with inlet and outlet ports, oriented at right
angles to each other. The impeller, composed of a
stack of parallel cones, is driven through a magnetic
coupling by an external motor and console [18,19]
(Figure 12.2). Rotation of the impeller creates a
constrained vortex which drives blood flow in proportion to the rotational speed. These pumps can
provide a high flow rate with a relatively modest
increase in pressure and are particularly sensitive to
afterload. The rate of flow depends on the revolutions

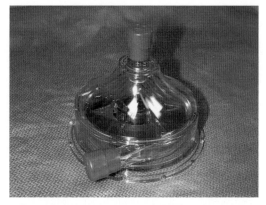

Figure 12.2 Centrifugal Pump, Bio-Medicus Bio-Pump consists for valveless rotator cones, which are made to impart
a circular motion to the blood, generating centrifugal
force, pressure, and flow.

per minute (rpm) imparted to the pump head
(inflow); it is pumped from the side of the pump
head through a second cannula (outflow) to the
great vessels. Due to the centrifugal nature of the
blood flow, the extracorporeal centrifugal pumping
system is less traumatic to blood elements. The
amount of flow generated by a roller pump is proportional to the outflow resistance and the filling
pressure [20,21]. Centrifugal blood flow, however, is
very sensitive to change in volume so that volume
infusion is common early to maintain the desired
flow rate. Design differences in commercially available pump heads are found in the number of
impellers, the shape and angle of the blade, and the
amount of prime in volume. The only exception is
the Medtronic bio-pump (Medtronic Biomedicals,
Inc., Minneapolis, MN), based on two concentric
cones generating the rotary motion. The pump
heads are disposable and collectively inexpensive to
manufacture. They are mounted on a magnetic
motorized unit that generates power studies document that centrifugal pumps compared to roller
pumps have superior performance regarding the
extent of mechanical injury to red blood cells [22].

Different surgical techniques are employed for
cannulation and device placement. For left ventricular assistance, a 28 French or 32 French cannula is
placed for uptake in the left atrium via the left atrial
appendage, the left interatrial groove, the left atrial
free wall, the right superior pulmonary vein, or
the left ventricle apex; the arterial return cannula is
placed on the ascending aorta. Right or biventricular

assistance is achieved by placing a medium–large cannula into the right atrium via the free wall or right atrial appendage; the return cannula is placed into the pulmonary artery or right ventricular outflow track. Pump cannulas are usually inserted through a median sternotomy with the patient on CPB. The cannula should be placed through a stab wound in the chest so the sternal incision can be closed. Special effort should be taken to search for air bubbles, especially those trapped inside the pump head. Purse string sutures should be tightly secured around the cannula so air is not sucked up into the left atrium.

During prolonged support, the pump head should be changed every several days to avoid thrombus formation. There is a significant limitation of centrifugal pump support if frequent pump malfunction occurs or thrombus is generated on the pump head that requires a pump exchange. In addition, there is no possibility for ambulation or rehabilitation for patients who must remain sedated and on mechanical ventilation.

As stated earlier, one of the major advantages of the centrifugal pump over more complicated assist devices is its simplicity of operation. If the cannulas have been properly placed so they drain well, without kink or occlusion against the atrial or ventricle walls, flow is generally easy to adjust. The speed (rpm) of the impeller can be increased or decreased to adjust the flow, measured by the in-line sensor. To minimize blood trauma and avoid the creation of air via cavitation, rpm's should be maintained at the lowest acceptable level. As the centrifugal system is non-occlusive, if flow ceases, one of the lines must be clamped. Otherwise, blood will flow from the high-pressure chamber to the low-pressure chamber. When adequate flow cannot be obtained at the appropriate rpm, the problem is usually hypovolemia. This is manifested by line chatter, low central venous pressure (CVP), and low left atrial pressure and should respond to volume replacement. If CVP is high and left atrial pressure is low, right heart failure is likely and the patient should be treated with pulmonary vasodilation and inotropic support. If both CVP and left atrial pressure are high and flow is down, the problem may be cardiac tamponade that requires emergency re-exploration.

Heparin should be administered during weaning from the device, as pump flow is progressively reduced. Transesophogeal echocardiogram (TEE) is used to assess cardiac function.

Significant morbidity is associated with the use of the centrifugal pump, particularly when in use more than 48 consecutive hours. Complications include bleeding, coagulopathy, renal insufficiency, infection, and thromboembolism.

The centrifugal pump is generally associated with an acceptable weaning rate (46–52%) and survival rate (20–41%) [23–26].

Extracorporeal life support: ECMO system

When drugs and an IABP aren't enough, other means of cardiac support may be appropriate. Extracorporeal life support (ECLS), or extracorporeal membrane oxygenation (ECMO), refers to a system that provides both cardiac and pulmonary support. Although many different systems exist, the basic configuration of an ECMO system is a centrifugal pump coupled with a hollow fiber membrane oxygenator and oxygen blender. ECMO not only circulates and oxygenates the blood, it also acts as a temporary substitute for the entire circulatory system. ECMO, as a short-term assist device or for ECLS, functions under the same principles as CPB. The most important difference between ECMO and CPB is duration of support. CPB is typically employed for hours during cardiac surgery while ECMO is designed to support life for longer durations using low doses of heparin. To avoid bleeding complications associated with traditional CPB on centrifugal pump, ECMO uses heparin-coated circuits combined with oxygenator support. This heparin-coated process involves a covalent bonding of heparin to the internal surfaces of the circuits and the oxygenator, reducing both the inflammatory response and the use of high doses of systemic heparinization. In addition, reversing the heparin does not become an issue. The heparin-coated process involved inside the ECMO cannulas and connectors and the tubing circuitry system, pump head and oxygenator, protects against the CPB-induced inflammatory response, and reduces or eliminates the systemic heparinization which would otherwise be necessary to avoid clotting in the system.

Initially, in 1978, ECLS was primarily used for respiratory support. The simplicity, versatility, portability, and familiarity of its design, as well as its ease of cannulation, began resulting in a wide range of uses. Reported by Hill *et al.* [27] in 1972, the first successful use of prolonged ECMO support was for a young man with traumatic aortic rupture who was successfully managed on venoarterial extracorporeal support for 3 days. Since the reporting of this case, ECMO has been incorporated for a wide range of support: neonatal cardiopulmonary support, adult post-cardiotomy support, adult respiratory support, and as a bridge-to-left-ventricular device or heart lung transplantation. ECMO unloads the right ventricle but does not completely unload the left ventricle, even though the left ventricle preload is reduced.

The first successful use of ECLS on a neonate was done by Barllet *et al.* [28] in 1972. The small volume of prime required for ECLS made it the only form of cardiopulmonary support available for neonates. This immediate success led to an increased use of ECMO. By 1990, 65 centers were routinely using ECLS to treat severe respiratory failure in newborn infants, with an overall survival rate >83% [29].

The venoarterial ECMO mode is used primarily for cardiac support or cardiac respiratory support while the venovenous mode is used for pulmonary support. The current system consists of a pump console (550 Bio-Console 7 with TX 50 Bio-Pro Flow transducer), an integrated heat exchanger system (Bio-Cal 370 Blood Temperature Control Model), a pump cart (Bio-Medicus 7 PBSJ Cabinets) (Medtronic Bio-Medicos, Inc., Eden Prairie, MN), and a centrifugal blood pump (Bio-Pump 7 BP-80, Medtronic Bio-Medicus, Inc., Minneapolis, MN) in conjunction with the oxygenator (Maxima Plus PRSJ (hollow fiber oxygenator), Medtronic Cardiac Surgery, Medrontic, Inc., Cardiopulmonary Division, Anaheim, CA) and an oxygen blender (Sechrist Industries, Inc., Anaheim, CA) (Figure 12.3). The cannulas and connector are heparin coated (Duraflo 7 (Baxter-Bentley 7, Irvine, CA)); the pump tubing, pump head, and oxygenator are also heparin coated (Carmeda 7 BioActive Surface (Medtronic Block System, Inc., Anaheim, CA)), reducing heparin requirements but not eliminating the need for systemic heparinization during support. This can be an important factor in postoperative patients with coagulopathy. On the other hand, prolonged

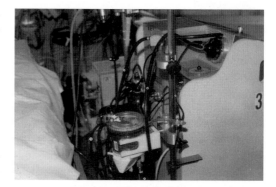

Figure 12.3 The current ECMO system used at the Cleveland Clinic: a centrifugal pump, oxygenator, and heat exchanger.

support without heparinization results in a 20% incidence of ventricular thrombus and a 6% incidence of pump head thrombus [30]. So, after surgery is completed, observation for any bleeding is carefully made. The patient is heparinized to an active clotting time of 180–200 s. The pump function is monitored by specially trained intensive care unit (ICU) nurses and perfusionists and maintained daily by perfusionists. Any evidence of clotting in the pump head or tubing requires a change in the pump. Leakage of plasma across the membrane, from the blood face to the gas face, continues to be a problem. Leakage gradually decreases the efficiency of the oxygenator and increases the system's flow for adequate oxygenator exchanges.

ECMO cannula insertion and patient management

The versatility of ECMO support enables it to be used for univentricular, biventricular, or cardiopulmonary support sometimes without thoracic cannulation. This unique feature allows rapid restoration of circulation by peripheral cannulation during acute resuscitation (e.g. acute cardiac arrest or cardiogenic shock). For venoarterial ECMO support, No. 16–20 French (F) arterial cannulas (Duraflo7, Baxter-Bentley 7, Irvine, CA; Fen Flex 2, Research Medical Inc., Midvale, UT) are inserted percutaneously into the common femoral artery either by the Seldinger technique or by a cut down to expose the artery. In the femoral vein, No. 18F to 28F venous cannulas (Duraflo 7, Baxter-Bentley 7, Irvine, CA;

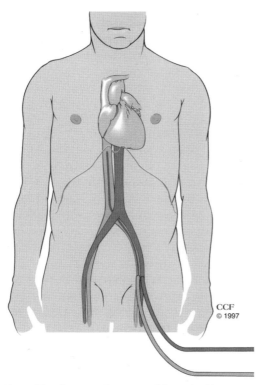

Figure 12.4 The set-up for venoaterial ECMO with cannulation of the left femoral artery and vein.

Fen Flex 2, Research Medical Inc., Midvale, UT) are advanced into the right atrium via the common femoral vein. To avoid lower limb ischemia, a 10F pediatric aortic cannula (Medtronics Bio-Medicus, Inc., Anaheim, CA) is connected to the arterial line and is inserted into the superficial femoral artery (Figure 12.4). Percutaneous femoral insertion may not be feasible. Catastrophic arterial or venous complications may occur from forceful placement of the cannula and result in vessel transaction, perforation, or dissection. In addition, many patients have small arterial lumens and those who receive high doses of vasopressors may experience arterial spasm. In these cases, the safest approach is vessel isolation by cut down rather than by percutaneous cannulation.

Transthoracic ECMO cannula insertion may be used in patients who require post-cardiotomy support. Arterial cannulation is usually placed into the ascending aorta and a long venous cannula inserted into the femoral vein. Other options for cannulation are the right axillary artery to allow chest closure (Figure 12.5) [31]. During cannulation, all air must be evacuated from the system. ECMO flows of 4–6 L/min are frequently possible at pump speeds of 3000–3200 rpm. Higher pump speeds

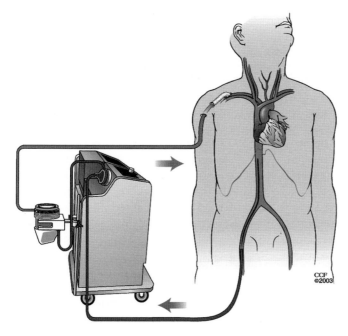

Figure 12.5 ECMO axillary circuit: venous inflow through the right femoral vein, centrifugal blood pump with oxygenator, arterial inflow through interposition graft over the right axillary artery, and exteriorization by a small second incision.

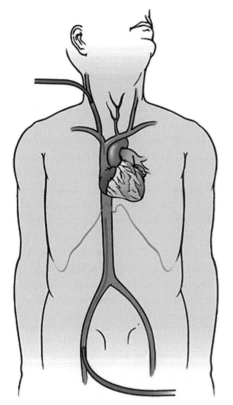

Figure 12.6 Venovenous ECMO: right internal jugular vein and right common femoral vein cannulation.

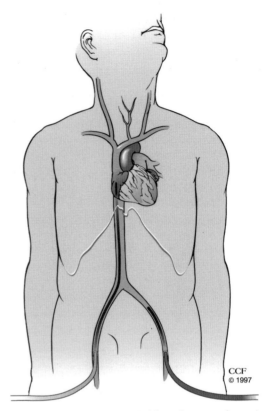

Figure 12.7 Venovenous ECMO: bilateral common femoral vein cannulation.

should be avoided to minimize mechanical trauma to the blood cells.

Cannulas tunneled through the chest wall require an operative procedure for removal; those placed in the axillary artery or the femoral vein can be removed at the bedside. The benefit of this latter, non-operative approach is reduced bleeding and less risk of infection for these critically ill patients. When larger cannulas are used, repair of the vessel may be required when the cannula is removed.

For venovenous ECMO support mode, cannulation is used routinely in one of two methods. Either the common jugular vein and common femoral vein (Figure 12.6) are used or the bilateral common femoral vein (Figure 12.7). Insertion of the cannula is achieved via a percutaneous Seldinger technique. Short-term venovenous ECLS can be run without systemic heparinization; long-term support requires systemic heparinization to obtain an active clotting time of 160–200 s.

Patient management weaning from ECLS post-cardiotomy support

The ultimate goal of post-cardiotomy support is to maintain optimum perfusion of all organs during the body's recovery from an acute hemodynamic insult, to prevent further deterioration of end-organ function, and to allow the heart to (ideally) recover. ECLS is usually continued 24–72 h, although longer periods are possible.

Patients on ECMO receive intravenous inotropic doses adequate to maintain ventricular ejection. Ventricular ejection is confirmed by a pulse on the arterial waveform, or by observing the aortic valve opening on the TEE. If a mechanical valve is present, then maintaining opening and closing of the valve avoids thrombus formation. Patients with severe ventricular dysfunction such that the heart is not ejecting ideally, should have an left ventricle vent to prevent ventricular distention or thrombosis. For the majority of patients, we also use an IABP that decreases afterload that can adversely affect the injured heart, and it adds pulsatility to the continuous flow generated by the centrifugal pump [32].

Patients undergo vigorous diuresis or hemofiltration to remove excess third-space fluid. Luer locks are placed in the arterial and venous connectors during ECMO insertion to allow easy hemofiltration. This technique is reported by Noon and colleagues [33], who used it in over 36% of their patients.

Continuous venovenous hemodialysis (CVVHD) permits control of fluid balance by continuous ultrafiltration that can be adjusted for volume removal and also allows for dialysis as needed.

During ECMO support, a mixed venous oxygen saturation >70% is ideal to ensure adequate systemic flow. The centrifugal pump speed can be adjusted to control flow and allow some degree of cardiac ejection to decrease the potential for intracardiac thrombus formation. Monitoring central venous and pulmonary artery diastolic pressures, along with pump flow, are critical to assess hemodynamic support. The most common problem is a decrease in venous drainage, usually manifested by "chugging" of the venous line with respiratory variations in flow. This could be indicative of hypovolemia but is also caused by cannula kinking, mal-positioning, mal-positioned (partly occluded) cannula, pneumothorax, or pericardial tamponade. Fluid administration to increase intravascular volume is often required in the first 24 h after ECMO is begun.

Standard critical care therapy to maintain a patient's normal status includes sedation, neuromuscular block, and continued ventilation. For ventilatory support, pressure-controlled ventilation is used to maintain peak inspiratory pressure below 35 cmH$_2$O at tidal volumes of 8–10 mL/kg. Inspired oxygen is initially set at 100% with a positive end-expiratory pressure of 5 cmH$_2$O. Fractional inspired oxygen is then gradually decreased as possible to <50% to maintain a PO$_2$ between 85 mmHg. These measurements are instituted to diminish the effect of high intrapulmonary pressure and oxygen toxicity due to a lung injury or acute respiratory distress syndrome (ARDS). Several adjustments may be necessary before ECMO oxygenation and gas sweep rate, along with the ventilator (FIO$_2$), achieve normal arterial blood gases. Blood gases drawn from a left atrial line quantify the effectiveness of the lungs in gas

exchange. Oxygenation or ECMO flow, or both, can be decreased until approximately 75% of arterial blood gases are supported by the patient alone.

Anticoagulation is started when bleeding slows (<100 mL/h) by systemic heparinization with continuous infusion, starting at 8–10 unit/kg/h and titrated to maintain a prothrombin time (PTT) between 45 and 55 s or an activated clotting time (ACT) between 180 and 200 s. This maintains a balance that reduces both the rate of bleeding and clot formation inside the head pump and in the heart cavity. Most post-cardiotomy patients placed on ECMO should be started on heparin infusions within 24 h; patients placed on ECMO by percutaneous placement should be started on heparin infusion earlier. ECMO reduces platelet levels, therefore, platelet counts should be checked every 8 h and patients transfused, when necessary, to maintain counts over 50,000/mm^3. Fresh frozen plasma and cryoprecipitate are given as needed to control coagulopathy.

When recovery is unlikely or uncertain, transplant screening is initiated. Echocardiogram is used to assess the degree of myocardial recovery. If improvement is not noted in 48–72 h of support, the heparin is increased while ECMO flows are temporarily reduced to 500–1000 mL/min. TEE is performed. Inotropic support can also be increased to assess ventricular function recovery. Improvements in wall motion suggest support may be weaned. If a patient has persistent left ventricular dysfunction, is neurologically intact and a candidate for transplantation, conversion to an implantable LVAD as a bridge-to-heart transplantation as the usual option.

It is critical to allow time for myocardial as well as end-organ recoveries before considering weaning a patient from support. The principle of weaning patients from support (common to all devices) is reducing the flow to transfer a greater workload to the heart. The flow is gradually reduced in increments of 0.5–1 L/min. Adequate anticoagulation is important during this low flow to prevent thrombosis. Reducing the flow to <1 L/min for longer periods is not generally recommended. Heparinization is increased to maintain an ACT of 300 s. With optimal pharmacologic support and continuous TEE assessment of ventricle functions, flows are reduced while monitoring systemic blood pressure, cardiac output, pulmonary pressure, and valve function. A patient who maintains cardiac output and low pulmonary pressure with preservation of the left ventricular function suggests weaning will be successful. If weaning fails, resumption of ECMO flow should follow. Patients who show no signs of recovery undergo full evaluation for cardiac transplantation. If there are contraindications, then the patient is usually left on support several days, inotropes and IABP are optimized, and ECMO is removed. Survival is rare in this group.

Complications

The most common complications of ECMO for post-cardiotomy patients are bleeding, renal failure, neurologic injuries, and leg ischemia.

Reoperation for bleeding was required in 61% of patients; renal failure occurred in 30% and neurologic injuries in 11% [33]. The incidence of leg ischemia has been significantly reduced by insertion of a No. 10F pediatric cannula directed distally into the superior femoral artery to increase blood flow toward the distal limb and has become common practice.

Neurologic complications remain a challenge. These occur from various preoperative, intraoperative, and postoperative etiologies: hypoxemia, ischemia, micro- or macro-thromboembolic event or intracerebral bleeding with thrombocytopenia. Prolonged support increases these risks. Early conversion to an implantable LVAD is generally recommended within 48–72 h, if the heart does not recover and before these complications appear. ECMO complications include: oxygenator "wetting" or failure; tubing fracture or rupture; pump failure or cracking; cannula dislodgement with catastrophic bleeding; thrombus formation in cannulas or pump head; air or particulate embolus; and vascular injury, venous obstruction or arterial ischemia.

Published reports state that 45–60% of all patients can be successfully weaned from support, but overall survival, however, is <30% with only 50% of weaned patients discharged alive from the hospital. Risk factors associated with increased mortality include age >60 years, emergency operation, reoperations, renal insufficiency, and left ventricular dysfunction [34,35].

At the Cleveland Clinic Foundation, from September 1992 to July 1999, 202 patients in cardiac failure were supported with ECMO [36]. Mean age

was 55 years. One hundred and seven patients (53%) underwent post-cardiotomy support. Of these, 60 (56%) had isolated coronary revascularizations; 19 (18%), coronary artery bypass graft (CABG) and valve operations; 15 (14%), isolated valve operations and 13 (12%), other procedures. Risk factors for death included older age, reoperation, and thoracic aortic repair. Survival at 3 days, 30 days, and 5 years were 76%, 38%, and 24%, respectively. Patients who survived 30 days had a 63% 5-year survival. Failure for patients to be bridged to transplant or weaned from support were associated with renal and hepatic failure while on ECMO support, neurologic event, and presence of infection. Complications during support were infection in 49%, requirement of dialysis in 40%, neurologic events in 33%, and limb complications in 25% (Figure 12.8). The dominant predictors of death during ECMO were cardiac failure and multisystem organ failure (Figure 12.9).

In our experience, ECMO support was converted to an implantable LVAD in 42 patients and directly as a bridge-to-transplantation in 6 patients. Survival rates were 85%, 67%, 54%, and 44% at 7 days, 30 days, 1 year, and 5 years, respectively, after

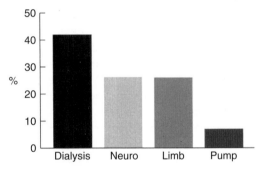

Figure 12.8 Complication during ECMO support.

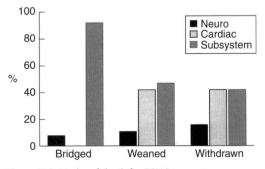

Figure 12.9 Modes of death for ECMO support.

cessation of ECMO support. Patient survival to transplantation was 67% with 92% of patients alive 6 months after transplantation [36] (Figure 12.10).

The majority of patients supported with ECMO were younger than 55 years of age and aggressively managed. In the older patients, survival was markedly reduced, especially those associated with pre-ECMO renal or hepatic dysfunction or post-ECMO neurologic injury. ECMO support should be initiated if renal or hepatic dysfunction is present only in very selected patients with a high likelihood of recovery. If ECMO is initiated and rapid clinical improvement is not seen, early ECMO termination is warranted.

ECMO is a versatile form of portable cardiopulmonary support. The ease of direct percutaneous cannulation to correct acute physiologic failure has increased its use. ECMO technology should continue to improve post-cardiotomy patient survival, allowing the patient to recover or transfer to an implantable device for bridge-to-transplantation or perhaps to a permanent destination therapy LVAD.

Extracorporeal pneumatic pulsatile device pump

The extracorporeal pneumatic pulsatile device pump is a pneumatically driven external pulsatile assist device used for univentricular or biventricular support for patients with post-cardiotomy cardiogenic shock or as a bridge-to-transplantation. As the power source is external, patient mobility is limited. Currently, two different systems are available. They differ in degrees of complexity and desirability for

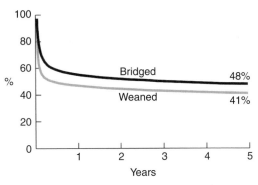

Figure 12.10 Survival after discontinuing ECMO (time zero) stratified according to the outcomes of ECMO: bridged or weaned.

short- and long-term support, but are similar in ability to support either or both ventricles and in the requirements for anticoagulation therapy. These two devices are Abiomed BVS-5000 (Abiomed Cardiovascular Inc., Danvers, MA) and the Thoratec (Thoratec Corp., Pleasanton, CA).

Abiomed BVS-5000

The Abiomed BVS-5000 is an extracorporeal, pneumatically driven, pulsatile VAD clinically introduced in 1988 and approved by the FDA in 1992. It was the first extracorporeal device designed to provide pulsatile univentricular or biventricular support. Used in both Europe and the United States, this device provides temporary support for post-cardiotomy patients [37]. It is estimated that more than 1500 patients are currently being supported with this system.

The Abiomed BVS-5000 is a vertical pump housing two individual polyurethane chambers. One gravity-filled atrial chamber and one air-driven ventricular chamber pneumatically pump the blood to the outflow cannula. Having three-leaflet polyurethane valves, continuous systemic heparinization is necessary to achieve an ACT of 180 s after surgical bleeding is controlled. The system provides approximately 5 L/min of pulsatile flow to either the right or left side of the heart, or both. The pneumatic system uses compressed air to drive the blood pump. There are no gas cylinders. The console is highly automatic and consists of an on/off switch and weaning modes; minimal operator intervention is required. The pump chamber itself consists of a collapsible polyurethane bladder with a capacity of 100 mL and a maximum output of 5.5 L/min. The atrial chamber operates on a fill-to-empty mode and can be affected by changes in the height of the pump relative to the patient or by volume status. Blood drains passively from the patient's atrium into the atrial chambers of the blood pump. Passive flow of blood into the atrial chamber is dependent on gravity and is related to the height of the patient's atrium, the CVP (preload) and the central venous capacity. The top of the blood pump should be between zero and 10 inches below the patient's atrium. When the pump is filling (absence of negative pressure generation), it is designed to prevent atrial collapse with each pump cycle and to prevent suction of air into the circuit. As the pump is

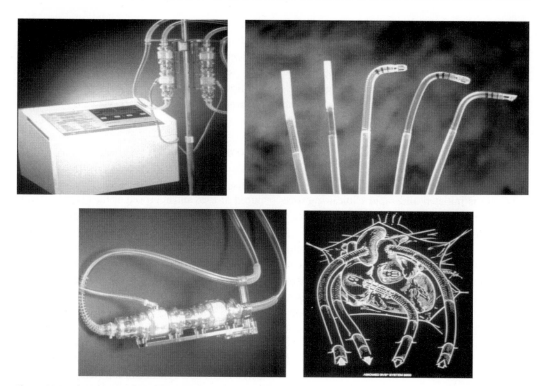

Figure 12.11 The Abiomed BVS-5000, a paracorporeal, pulsatile system for temporary left, right or biventricular support, different cannulas, and cannulation strategies.

transparent, filling can be assessed visually. When the atrial chamber of the blood pump is full and the pressure inside the atrial chamber exceeds the pressure inside the ventricular chamber, the three-leaflet valves open, allowing blood to flow into the ventricular chamber of the blood pump. While the ventricular bladder is filling with blood, the air surrounding the bladder is displaced and delivered through the driveline to the BVS-5000 console. The console monitors the return air flow as the ventricular bladder is filled and sends compressed air into the ventricular chamber around the outflow bladder to eject 80 mL of blood. The ventricular chambers require active pulsatile pumping by a pneumatic driveline. During diastole the air is vented to the atmosphere, allowing refilling of the chamber during the next cycle. The rate of pumping and the duration of pump systole and diastole are adjusted by the pump microprocessor that operates asynchronously to the native heart rate. The pump automatically makes adjustments to account for pre- and afterload changes and delivers a constant stroke volume of approximately 80 mL (Figure 12.11).

The BVS-5000 console monitors two parameters: flow through the blood pump and driveline pressure. Low flow usually means the blood pump is placed too high or there is inadequate blood volume. High pressure means the driveline or blood pump tubing is kinked or occluded or the systemic vascular resistance (SVR) may have increased. Low-pressure implies a possible leak in the driveline or disconnection in the driveline. A foot pump, stored in the rear of the console, acts as a back-up if the BVS-5000 system should completely fail.

For right heart support, a right atrial cannula is placed into the free wall of the right atrium, and the arterial cannula is anastomosed usually to main pulmonary artery. For left heart support, an atrial cannula is placed in the left atrium via the interatrial groove, the left atrial dome, or the left atrial appendage. An alternative method for left heart support is a cannula placed in the left ventricle apex. The arterial graft-cannula return is anastomosed to the ascending aorta. Atrial cannulas can be a 46F wire-reinforced light-house-tipped cannula or the new 32F and 42F bend-tipped cannulas. Outflow and arterial cannulas are 42F and 46F with either 12 or 14 mm Dacron grafts attached for anastomosis to the pulmonary artery or ascending aorta. The cannulas are usually passed through stab wounds in the chest wall and tunneled into the mediastinum to permit sternum closure.

After postoperative bleeding is controlled, systemic heparinization is required to maintain an ACT of 180–200 s. Weaning from the system involves reducing the flow in small increments and waiting to see if the ventricle will eject enough stroke volume on its own to maintain adequate cardiac output. The process continues in the same manner as for ECMO support. TEE monitoring is essential for assessing the amount of recovery in cardiac function. Heparinization is usually increased to an ACT of 300 s. Inotropic support may be increased as weaning progresses. The flow is then reduced incrementally to 0.5 L/min. In biventricular support, the right pump flow should be weaned before the left pump.

The primary advantage of the Abiomed is its ability to provide prolonged univentricular or biventricular support. The device has not been demonstrated to cause significant hemolysis and the pulsatile flow may have some degree of physiologic benefit. This device has become one of the most commonly used means of short-term mechanical support for shock from post-cardiotomy and for myocardial infarction, myocarditis, right ventricular support in conjunction with long-term LVAD support [37,38].

This system is best used as a bridge-to-recovery. It has become popular in community hospitals because it is safe, easy to operate and requires minimal bedside monitoring without the need of a full-time perfusionist. The system functions reliably for several days with an average support duration of 5–9 days. The patient can be transferred to a transplant center for further treatment [39]. The advantage of this system versus the centrifugal pump and ECMO is increased mobility for the patient (e.g. moving from bed to a chair, dangling of the legs, and limited ambulation). The patient can be extubated, which is an added advantage. Disadvantages include continuous systemic anticoagulation, limited mobility (compared with an implantable LVAD), and the need for the patient to remain in the ICU.

Although patients have been supported as long as 90 days, the device is best suited for short-term use, <10 days [34].

Thoratec VAD

The Thoratec VAD is an extracorporeal pneumatic device that can be used for univentricle or biventricle support. It has three components: the blood pump, the cannula, and the dual drive console.

The pump itself consists of a rigid polycarbonate housing that contains a flexible blood sack actuated by alternating positive and negative air pressures. The blood pump, or VAD, is placed on the anterior abdominal wall and acts as a prosthetic ventricle. It consists of a smooth seamless pumping chamber enclosed in a rigid case. The blood sack is manufactured from a proprietary polyurethane developed to improve thromboresistance, flex-life, and strength [40]. Mechanical valves maintain unidirectional flow to the blood pump; sensors detect when the sack is full of blood and automatically signal the console to eject blood from the pump. The external pneumatic drive console provides alternating positive and negative air pressures which empty and fill the prosthetic ventricle with a stroke volume of 65 mL and a maximum flow rate of 7 L/min [41]. The device may be set in one or three modes: asynchronous (fixed grade), volume (fill to empty), and synchronous (timed to ECG) [42] (Figure 12.12).

In the asynchronous mode, the VAD rate is fixed and is useful for initiating VAD support. It is then switched to the volume mode. In the commonly applied volume mode, the device's pumping rate is adjusted according to the rate of the patient's venous return, so the VAD and output rates vary with the changes in preload delivered to the pump. Thoratec recommends this mode of operation for most patients. The synchronous mode is synchronized to the heart rate with a VAD ejection, triggered by R-wave of the ECG. Pump filling coincides during systole, followed by pump ejection during diastole. This mode can also be used to wean patients from support following recovery of cardiac function. It is important that the VAD fills completely and ejects completely to prevent stasis and possible VAD thrombus formation.

The prosthetic ventricle is placed extracorporeal on the anterior abdominal wall. The cardiac chambers and great vessel communicate via a polyurethane cannula through the chest wall. An inflow cannula is placed in the left atrium or left ventricular apex; an outflow cannula is attached to a 14 mm

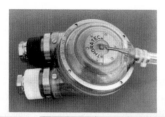

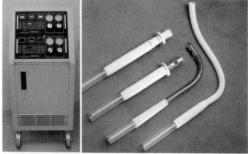

VAD blood pump
- LVAD, RVAD, BiVAD
- Max output = 7.2 L/min
- Pneumatic
- Prosthetic valves
- 65 mL stroke volume
- Rigid/clear *polysulfone* housing

Dual drive console cannulae
- Inflow: atrial or ventricular
- Outflow: arterial

Figure 12.12 The Thoratec left and/or right VAD, a paracorporeal, pneumatically powered system configured univentricular or biventricular support, system components. BiVAD: biventricular assist device; RVAD: right ventricle assist device.

outflow graft sewn to the ascending aorta. When the VAD is used as a right ventricular assist system, similar cannulas are used for the right atrium and pulmonary artery cannulation [43,44] (Figure 12.13).

Complete anticoagulation is required to reduce the risk of thrombus formation in the pump and in the native ventricle. Long-term anticoagulation requires Coumadin with an International Normalized Ratio (INR) of 2.5–3.

Patients supported on the Thoratec dual drive console can ambulate within the hospital making it possible for them to be transferred from a critical care unit to a general ward after extubation. There are, however, two major limitations of the Thoratec System: its limited mobility and its limited rehabilitation. Both of these are due to the system's large drive console.

New TLC-II, portable VAD drivers that feature a lightweight battery, or line-operated biventricular pneumatic drive unit should improve this situation, promoting greater mobility, self-care, and possible hospital discharge [45,46] (Figure 12.14). One of the most important advantages of this system is its ability to provide long-term support including longer waiting periods for transplantation. Weaning from biventricular support proceeds in the usual fashion.

Complications of the Thoratec VAD are similar to other temporary circulatory support stems. These include bleeding, device malfunction, renal failure, infection, and thromboembolic event. Multisystem

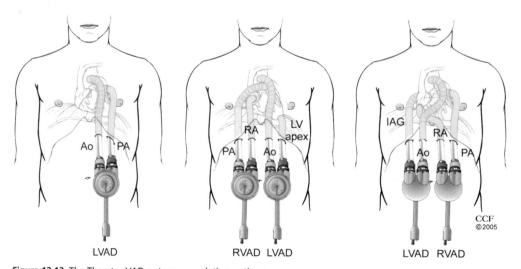

Figure 12.13 The Thoratec VAD system: cannulation options.
Ao: aorta; IAG: interatrial groove; LV: left ventricle; PA: pulmonary artery; RA: right atrium; RVAD: right VAD.

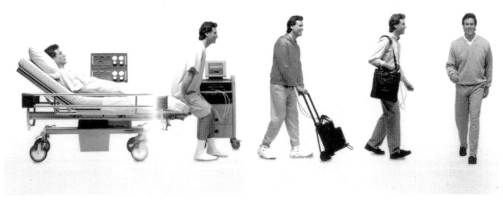

Figure 12.14 The Thoratec TCL-II portable VAD driver, permit patient greater mobility and ambulation.

organ failure and sepsis are the most frequent causes of death while patients are on mechanical support.

The Thoratec voluntary registry reported that the Thoratec VAD was used in 1376 heart failure patients until May 2000, bridging to transplantation (B to Tx) in 828 patients, and 195 for post-cardiotomy support. The remaining 353 implants involve incomplete information or hybrid device configuration and there were excluded for analysis. In the 828 (B to Tx), the Thoratec was used as a biventricular assist device in 472 cases, left ventricular assistance in 326 cases, and right ventricular assistance in 30 cases up to 512 days of support; 60% of the 828 patients underwent cardiac transplantation, and the post-transplant survival rate was 86%. In the 195 cases of post-cardiotomy support, 38% were weaned from support, and 59% of those were discharged from the hospital; 49 post-cardiotomy patients were considered for transplantation, and of those 32 received transplant and 23 were discharged [47]. The Thoratec VAD system's ability to provide short- or long-term univentricular or biventricular support makes it a valuable adjunct to the cardiac assist device family.

Implantable VAD support

The introduction of mechanical circulatory support systems for heart failure has made it possible for many patients to survive who otherwise would have died. Over the last two decades, many devices have been developed which allow patients to be supported for periods of time.

Although a variety of ventricular assist device support (VADS) have been used to support the

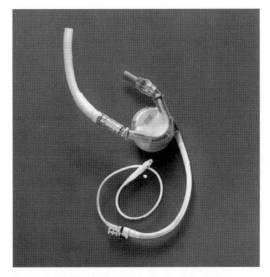

Figure 12.15 The VE HeartMate implantable LVAD.

failing heart as a bridge to myocardial recovery or transplantation, the ultimate goal is the development of a totally portable implantable system that provides long-term support for end-stage of heart disease, allowing the patient to be maintained as an out-patient. Currently, the most promising long-term implantable left ventricular assist device systems for patients succumbing to end-stage heart failure are Novacor LVAS (WorldHeart Corporation, Novacor LVAS, Oakland, CA), and HeartMate LVAD (Thoratec Laboratories Corp., CA)[48,49]. Both devices are implantable, long-term, univentricular cardiac assist devices. (Fig. 12.15 and 12.16). The implantable left ventricular

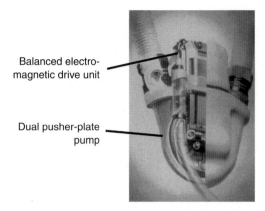

Balanced electro-magnetic drive unit

Dual pusher-plate pump

Figure 12.16 The Novacor N1000PC implantable LVAD.

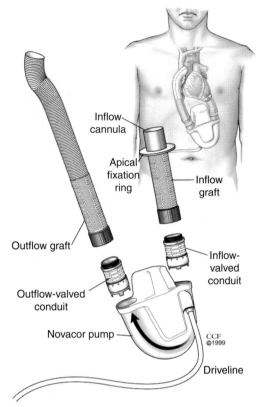

Inflow cannula

Apical fixation ring

Inflow graft

Outflow graft

Inflow-valved conduit

Outflow-valved conduit

Novacor pump

CCF ©1999

Driveline

Figure 12.17 The Novacor system components.

assist device has shown to be extremely effective hemodynamically and allows 'resurrection' of moribund patient. The next section will discuss in depth the spectrum of devices currently in use, the role of the totally artificial heart and the results of the Cleveland Clinic's LVAD program.

LVAD: device descriptions

Currently, Novacor (Worldheart Novacor, Ottawa, Canada, formerly Baxter-Novacor, Oakland, CA) and HeartMate (Thoratec HeartMate, Pleasanton, CA; originally TCI, Woburn, MA) are the two FDA approved implantable LVADs. The HeartMate LVAD is implantable, pulsatile and easy to operate. It is available in pneumatic or electrical design. Introduced in 1986, the original HeartMate 1000 IP was a pneumatic pump, fabricated from titanium [50]. It housed a flexible, textured polyurethane diaphragm bonded to a rigid pusher-plate actuated pneumatically from a portable external console. In 1991, the HeartMate was redesigned to a portable, battery powered electric model. The basic difference from the original design is a low-speed torque motor that pushes the same plate through a pair of nested helical cams. An external vent equalizes the air pressure and permits emergency pneumatic operation. The blood contacting surfaces are textured to encourage the deposition of circulating cells minimizing thrombus formation.

The pump is positioned below the left hemidiaphragm, usually in a preperitoneal pocket. The Novacor, IP HeartMate and Ventricular Electric

HeartMate each work by drawing blood from the inflow cannula in the left ventricular apex, passing the blood through the pump located outside the heart and ejecting the blood through the outflow cannula anastomosed to the ascending aorta, by passing the left ventricle. All devices have porcine valves in the inflow and outflow conduit positions to ensure unidirectional blood flow (use www.video). HeartMate devices have a short titanium inflow cannula attached to the inflow conduit as one unit (Figure 12.18). Novacor has a longer inflow conduit made of a gelatin-sealed graft attached to a separate valve-inflow conduit. The valve-outflow conduit is attached to a low-porosity graft sewn to the aorta (Figure 12.17). All three devices have a long, percutaneous driveline that connects to the power pack for venting the Novacor and Ventricular Electric HeartMate or for the pneumatic actuation of the IP HeartMate. The driveline attaches to the left side of the pump, passes through a subcutaneous tunnel, and exits the body to the right of the umbilicus. The HeartMate blood pump is composed of a blood

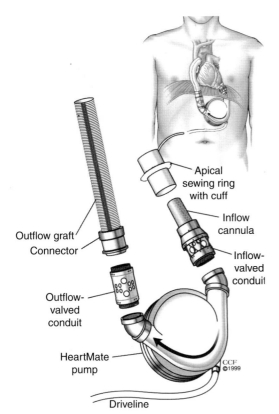

Figure 12.18 The HeartMate system components.

Labels in figure: Apical sewing ring with cuff; Inflow cannula; Inflow-valved conduit; Outflow graft Connector; Outflow-valved conduit; HeartMate pump; Driveline; CCF ©1999

chamber and an air/motor chamber. A polyurethane diaphragm attached to a pusher-plate divides the chambers. Activation of the pusher-plate is done by pressurized air in the pneumatic device and by a bearing roll driven by a motor in the electric version. The blood chamber titanium shell is textured by sintered titanium microspheres; the diaphragm has an integrally textured surface. This textured surface stimulates the formation of a neointimal-like lining, which, in turn, prevents thrombus formation. The driveline containing the electric cable and an air vent exit the skin to attach to the external drive console. Both models use 25 mm porcine xenograft valves (Medtronic-Hancock, Minneapolis, MN) within the inflow and outflow Dacron graft conduits. They are capable of a maximum stroke volume of 85 mL and a maximum pump output of approximately 11 L/min. Novacor has a lightweight fiberglass-epoxy housing and a blood chamber of seamless polyurethane. The two pusher-plates are connected by a solenoid that controls blood injection [51].

HeartMate and Novacor devices use different modes of operation. HeartMate can be operated in a fixed-rate or automatic mode and works asynchronously to the left ventricular contraction and ECG. The pneumatic device can be synchronized with the ECG. To reduce blood stasis, the LVAD usually functions automatically. Ejection occurs when the device chamber reaches 90% of the total LVAD chamber volume. Thus, the device operates asynchronously from the native heart in a fill-to-empty mode and is capable of changing the LVAD output according to venous return. During exercise, the device works parallel with the left ventricle, contributing systemic cardiac output through ejection across the aortic valve. While Novacor can run asynchronously, it is generally operated in a synchronous counterpulsation mode. The pump fills passively during left ventricular systole and ejects during diastole. This helps lower left ventricular afterload and, in large ventricles, causes ejection through the aortic valve, which may facilitate left ventricular recovery. Novacor has a stroke volume of 65 mL and generates flows 6–8 L/min.

Novacor has always had an electric power source. The Vented Electric (VE) HeartMate replaced the bulky external consul with the portability of batteries. Both electric devices give patients the freedom of hospital discharge and extended periods of a tether-free existence. This greatly improves the patient's quality of life.

Operative technique

Early during surgery, a TEE is performed to assess the presence of patent foramen ovale or atrial septal defect. If present, these require closure before LVAD actuation to prevent paradoxical embolism or right-to-left shunting when the left side is unloaded by the LVAD. This right-to-left shunt can generate severe systemic arterial desaturation [52]. Also, TEE is useful to assess left ventricle thrombus and competency of the aortic and tricuspid valves aortic regurgitation. AI ≥2+ should be repaired, and tricuspid regurgitation ≥3+ is also be repaired. When the LVAD is functioning correctly, the left ventricle is completely unloaded with usually no ejection through the aortic valve, which remains closed. As LVAD-supported patients with mechanical aortic valves can thrombose and embolize to the

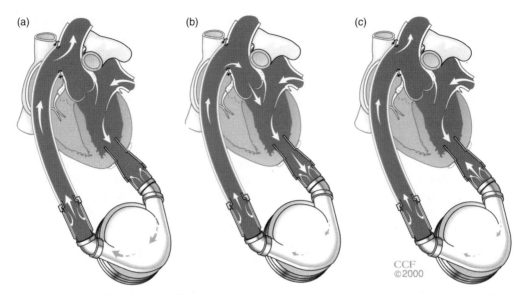

Figure 12.19 (a) Blood flows from the left atrium through the completely unloaded left ventricle and the pump inflow conduit into the HeartMate and is pumped back to the aorta, with the aortic valve closed. (b) In presence of aortic insufficiency, some blood ejected into the aorta flows back to the left ventricle, increasing the left ventricle pressure, and reducing forwards pump flows. (c) In presence of inflow conduit valve insufficiency, blood regurgitates into the left ventricle during LVAD ejection, creating same previous situation.

coronary arteries or systemically, mechanical valves should be replaced by tissue valves or homografts. Likewise, severe aortic insufficiency causes a cycle of blood flow through the pump and the left ventricle that significantly reduces systemic forward flow. Therefore, aortic insufficiency in the native aortic valve requires repair or replacement with a tissue valve.

A similar hemodynamic result is observed when the inflow conduit valve becomes insufficient. Part of the LVAD ejected blood regurgitates to the left ventricle, increasing left ventricle pressure and reducing systemic blood flow. If this occurs, the device needs to be changed [53] (Figure 12.19). Mitral regurgitation is not usually repaired as it reduces with the initiation of left ventricle unloading.

The midline incision is extended to the mid-point between the tip of the xyphoid and the umbilicus. A pocket is created in the left upper quadrant of the abdominal wall between the posterior rectus fascia and the peritoneum or the pocket can be created between the rectus muscle and the posterior rectus fascia [54]. The pump can also be implanted in the intra-abdominal position, avoiding the creation of a pocket and the associated complications, such as pump pocket infection. This technique

may be also chosen for patients expected to have long-term implants (i.e. those highly sensitive to human leukocyte antigens (HLAs), have a large body mass or type O blood or destination therapy). The disadvantage of intra-abdominal implantation lies in a more demanding operation at the time of explant due to the adherence of abdominal contents to the pump, intra-abdominal driveline, and the pump pocket cannulas. After the pump pocket is created, the pump is seated into the pocket with the driveline tunneled subcutaneously from the pocket and exiting through a stab wound created on the right flank. CPB is instituted with standard cannulation and the aorta is cross-clamped. Infusion of cardioplegic solution is started. When cardiac arrest is accomplished, a left ventricular apical ventriculotomy is performed using a coring knife. Caution must be taken at the time of the ventriculotomy to avoid the section of the distal left anterior descending coronary artery or a diagonal coronary artery branch or damage the interventricular septum. Braided polyester pledgetted sutures are passed through the edge of the ventriculotomy. These sutures are then passed through the sewing cuff of the inflow cannula and tied. The cannula is placed in the left ventricle and secured. Although not very much tension is applied to these sutures (due to unloading of the left ventricle), the edge of the ventriculotomy should be reinforced with a strip of felt to avoid tearing of the surrounding myocardium, when the myocardium is very friable due to acute myocardial infarction. The outflow cannula (Dacron graft) is cut to the proper length and sewn to the ascending aorta. A fragment of the aorta must be excised at the site of the anastomosis to lower resistance of blood flow that is being ejected from the pump. Consequently, this decreases the amount of stress applied to the inflow valve during pump systole. The outflow cannula is deaired and clamped.

The ventricle is filled and deaired; the aortic cross-clamp is released, allowing the heart to start beating. This maneuver forces blood through the pump, deairing the pump itself. TEE helps determine that no residual air is present. The outflow cannula is then connected to the pump. With a needle placed in the graft, the device is hand-pumped, deairing the system. When satisfactory deairing is achieved, the outflow graft is unclamped and the driveline connected to the controller and power source. The device is set to a fixed rate of 50 bpm; pulmonary artery and left atrial lines are placed and the patient weaned from CPB. It is imperative to keep the left atrial pressure >10 mmHg to avoid air being sucked into the pump through the connections in the inflow conduit. Heparin is reversed and the patient decannulated.

Unless concomitant conditions exist, for example, atrial fibrillation, patients with HeartMate LVADs do not require anticoagulation therapy. For routine LVAD anticoagulation during the postoperative period, patients are treated with aspirin (325 mg/day). This protects against platelet aggregation and embolization; it also reduces sensitization during long-term support. In patients with gastritis or another bleeding disorder, aspirin is withheld or stopped [55].

Patients on Novacor pumps require full anticoagulation therapy during LVAD support. As soon as postoperative bleeding is under control, systemic heparinization is started for a target ACT of 180–200 s, or to achieve a PTT of 50–70 s. Some centers suggest using low-molecular-weight dextran infusion in the operating room. Anticoagulation is changed to warfarin at 1–2 weeks, along with aspirin to keep the INR of 2.5–3.5.

Several conditions need to be considered before implanting a LVAD. Many patients (about 50% in our series) have had previous surgery; therefore, a reoperation will make LVAD implant more demanding, time consuming, and prone to bleeding. Also, patients with biventricular failure will have a congested liver with abnormal liver function, and the patient may have coagulopathy. We give vitamin K for 3 days before (if possible) the operation and 3 days after surgery. Aprotinin is standard during surgery to reduce the risk of postoperative bleeding. Other blood products are given as needed. Patent coronary bypass grafts should be left intact to avoid arrhythmias, angina, and right ventricular dysfunction.

Patients with a BSA <1.5 m^2 may not be able to accommodate the LVAD implant as it may cause abdominal compression, early satiety, gastric obstruction, or abdominal wound dehiscence. In smaller patients, it may be better to use paracorporeal VADs like Thoratec.

Cleveland Clinic experience with implantable LVADs

Our LVAD bridge-to-transplant program (B to Tx) was analyzed for morbidity and mortality; for device-related complications, and for risk factors for death. Focus was on three major complications during device support: infection, stroke, and device failure. At the Cleveland Clinic, LVAD implants began in December 1991. By December 2001, a total of 264 patients received 277 LVADs. Of these, 137 were electric HeartMates; 81, pneumatic; 57, Novacor (16 Vascutek inflow conduit types); 2, Micromed DeBakey (Houston, TX); and 1, Jarvik 2000 (Jarvik Inc, NY, NY). Nine patients received two devices; and two patients received three devices. Patient characteristics, medical and ventricular support, and type of LVAD device is shown in Table 12.3.

Temporal trends

The temporal prevalence of various LVAD devices is illustrated in Figure 12.20. The number of pre-LVAD temporary VADs has gradually climbed. The IABP remains dominant; however, like ECMO, its use has declined. Over the last few years, Abiomed support has seen an increase due to a number of patients

Table 12.3 Patient characteristics and medical and temporary device support before LVAD insertion.

Variable	n*	Number	Percent of n
Demography			
Women	264	41	16
Age (mean ± SD)	264	55 ± 11.1	
BSA (m², mean ± SD)	261	1.99 ± 0.24	
Hemodynamics			
P_{RA} (mmHg, mean ± SD)	179	18.1 ± 6.3	
P_{PA} systolic (mmHg, mean ± SD)	255	50 ± 15.2	
P_{PA} diastolic (mmHg, mean ± SD)	255	28 ± 7.9	
Cardiac index (L/min/m², mean ± SD)	238	1.83 ± 0.47	
Myopathy	264		
Ischemic		171	65
Idiopathic dilated		79	30
Other		14	5
Comorbidity			
Serum creatinine (mg/dL, median, quartiles)	263	1.5	1.2–2.0
Total bilirubin (mg/dL, median, quartiles)	263	1.5	1.0–2.6
Prior thoracic surgery	264	130	49
Infection within 7 days of LVAD insertion	264	24	9
Ventricular tachycardia within 3 days of LVAD insertion	264	82	31
Ventricular fibrillation within 3 days of LVAD insertion	264	14	5
Pre-LVAD medical and temporary device support			
Length of ICU stay (days, median, and quartiles)	257	5	2–14
Intubated	264	149	56
Inotropes	264	248	94
IABP	264	202	77
Abiomed	264	7	3
ECMO	264	51	19
AICD	264	37	14

P_{RA}: mean right atrial pressure; P_{PA}: pulmonary artery pressure; AICD: automatic implantable cardioverter defibrillator.

*Number of patients for whom data were available.

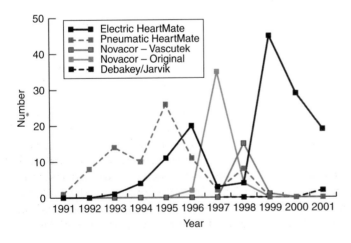

Figure 12.20 The temporal prevalence of various LVAD devices at the Cleveland Clinic.

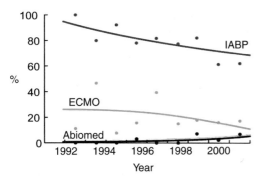

Figure 12.21 Temporal trends of use pre-LVAD temporary ventricular assistance over time.

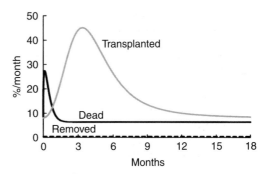

Figure 12.22 Competing risks of mortality, transplantation, and removal of LVAD for survival. Hazard Function driving the competing risk.

transferred to our institution for further treatment, already on Abiomed support (Figure 12.21).

Ischemic cardiomyopathy has been the main cause of extracorporeal support, reaching 70%, and has remained stable over time; 24% of all patients had creatinine levels >2; and 20% had a total bilirubin >3.

Univariate Cox Proportional Hazard Regression analysis was used to identify predictors of mortality while patients remained on support. Risk factors included the requirements of pre-LVAD/ECMO, low pulmonary artery systolic pressure, reoperation, higher total bilirubin, smaller patient size, and women. However, the LVAD type was *not* a risk factor for death before transplantation, regardless of the number of device-related complications. Of 264 patients mechanically supported, 180 (68%) successfully underwent cardiac transplantation; 79 (30%) patients died on support. Mean support duration was 89 days. Two patients underwent explant: the first underwent a partial left ventriculectomy during device explantation and died of heart failure a year later; the second patient did well for a year, but gradually deteriorated to New York Heart Association Functional Class III, and eventually expired.

Competing independent rates for risk of transplantation, risk of death on support, LVAD removal for survival and their progression over time is shown in Figures 12.22 and 12.23. The transition from LVAD to transplantation peaks at 3 months. Nearly 50% of patients are transplanted at this time, after which it slowly decreases.

Risk of death before transplant peaks within the first week of device implantation and then falls to a constant risk of 5.2% per month. Despite the different risks for complications among LVAD devices,

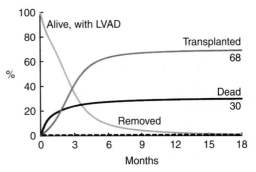

Figure 12.23 Prevalence at each moment in time of patients in each category: (1) alive with LVAD, (2) death before transplantation, (3) transplanted, and (4) LVAD removal.

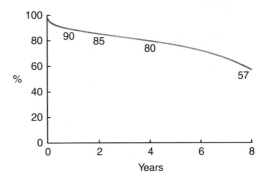

Figure 12.24 Overall survival after transplantation.

there were *no* statistically significant differences between devices and survival before transplantation. Survival from the time of LVAD insertion to 30 days, 3 months, 1 year, and 4 years were 84%, 74%, 64%, and 55%, respectively. Comparing survival after transplantation to devices, no significant differences were found. Overall 1-year survival rates after transplantation were 90% at 1 year, 85% at 2 years, 80% at 4 years, and nearly 60% at 8 years (Figure 12.24).

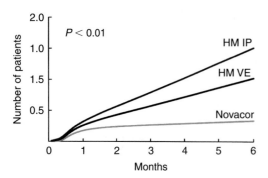

Figure 12.25 Driveline infections during LVAD support.

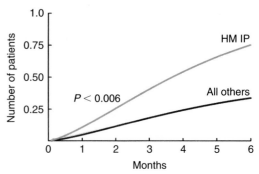

Figure 12.26 Cumulative number of pump pocket infections according to type of LVAD.

Time-related complications

Positive blood cultures, skin infections at the drive-line exit sites and infections in the pump pocket were common complications among patients on LVAD support [56, 57]. Data from the Cleveland Clinic experience reports 54% of the HeartMate patients and 30% of the Novacor patients had positive blood cultures after pump implantation [58]. Some sources of infection may be the result of pre-existing vascular lines, urinary catheters, and prolonged ventilatory support.

Driveline infections were present in 25% of the HeartMate implant patients and in 10% of the Novacor patients. Infections were primarily caused by staphylococcus and were managed with local care and systemic antibiotics. In 10% of HeartMate patients and in 4% of Novacor patients, the device itself was the host for infection in the pump pocket. These infections were treated with antibiotics until heart transplantation could be performed. Infections may also be managed with local debridement followed by drainage and irrigation with povidone–iodine and antibiotics.

Examination of cumulative numbers of driveline infections per patient, according to device type over time, demonstrated significant differences between HeartMate and Novacor systems ($P < 0.04$). Figure 12.25, shows the most significant incidence of driveline infections were attributed to the pneumatic HeartMate. Every patient supported by this device presented with at least one driveline infection at 4 months. The incidence of pump pocket infections were similar, with the pneumatic HeartMate showing more significant rates of infection than other devices ($P < 0.006$) (Figure 12.26). HeartMate devices were also more prone to blood stream infections than the

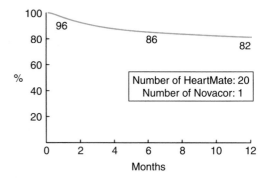

Figure 12.27 Device failure for HeartMate LVAD Hazard Function.

Novacor devices. At 2 months of support, patients assisted with HeartMates presented with at least one blood infection. This incidence increased across time.

Device failure

Device failure occurred in 21 patients, with a greater incidence in HeartMate patients than in Novacor patients. Failure rates were similar for pneumatic and VE HeartMates, although no pneumatic devices were used beyond 6 months. Freedom from failure for HeartMate was 96%, 86%, and 82% at 1, 6, and 12 months, respectively.

Figure 12.27 shows the pattern of failure by Hazard Function. Failure peaked within the first month of use and then declined. This overall pattern of risk, however, obscures the observations that prior to 1995, only 1 failure occurred in 39 implants; from 1995 to the end of 1997, 16 failures occurred in 74 implants, with a particularly prominent number of failures in 1995 (10 in 37). From 1998 to 2001, the

VE HeartMate became almost as reliable as Novacor, with only 2 failures in 105 implants.

Neurologic complications during LVAD support

In our experience, the frequency of thromboembolic events has been significantly higher with Novacor, even though all patients received warfarin and antiplatelet agents as recommended.

The incidence of early (<7 days) postoperative strokes was similar for both HeartMate and Novacor devices (>10%). The incidence of ischemic strokes during the late postoperative period was significantly different. Novacor was much higher at 39% than HeartMate at 1.5%.

Early strokes are often related to preoperative problems such as cardiac arrest or left ventricular thrombi from myocardial infarction; therefore, neurologic status must be carefully assessed before LVAD implantation. Conversely, late strokes are predominantly thromboembolic and device related.

The magnitude of risk of thromboembolic event was substantially different by device. Novacor had a statistically higher cumulative number of embolic events per patient than HeartMate ($P = 0.0001$). These differences in thromboembolic rates may be related to the interior surfaces of the devices. Novacor originally used a long, corrugated, Dacron inflow graft, entirely proximal to the inflow valve. In our experience, this inflow conduit frequently showed extensive thrombus and a poorly adherent pseudointima. Since FDA approval, the inflow conduit has been shortened and changed to a gelatin-sealed graft (Vascutek), or more recently Gore-tex. This change has reduced the incidence of stroke rate, but still shows a higher risk of embolic event than HeartMate ($P < 0.04$) (Figure 12.28). Even though the Novacor device required total anticoagulation therapy during support, no significant differences in the number of cerebral bleeding complications per patient were demonstrated over time between these devices.

Destination therapy LVADs

The ultimate goal in the development of the implantable LVAD was to create a clinical alternative to cardiac transplantation or medical therapy for end-stage cardiomyopathy patients who were not transplant candidates. LVAD soon became the

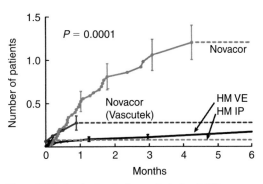

Figure 12.28 Cerebral embolic events during LVAD support, cumulative number of events per patient for each type of device.

standard approach as a bridge-to-transplantation, but was never extensively studied as a permanent support device until the REMATCH trial. This trial was designed to test the efficacy and safety of the HeartMate VE LVAD as "destination therapy" for patients with end-stage heart failure who were not considered candidates for cardiac transplantation.

One hundred and twenty-nine patients with end-stage heart failure were randomized 1:1 to receive optimal medical treatment for heart failure or HeartMate LVAD implantation. This landmark study was conducted from 1998 through 2001 in 20 centers across the United States [10]. The primary end-point was death by any cause. Secondary end-points included serious adverse events, quality-of-life indices, symptoms of depression, functional status, and number of days of hospitalization. Sixty-eight patients received LVADs; 61 patients underwent medical treatment. Overall survivors showed a 48% reduction in the risk of death by any cause in the LVAD group compared to the medical therapy group ($P = 0.001$). The Kaplan–Meier estimates of survival at 1 year were 52% for the LVAD group and 25% for the medical therapy group ($P = 0.002$). After 2 years, the survival rate was 23% for the LVAD group and 8% for the medical therapy group ($P = 0.09$) (Figure 12.29).

Terminal heart failure caused the majority of deaths in the medical treatment group. The most common cause of death in the LVAD group was sepsis (41%), followed by device failure (17%). The probability of infection was 28% after 3 months. Most infections were at the driveline site or at the pump pocket. There were no reported device failures

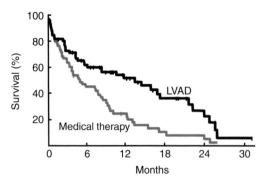

Figure 12.29 REMATCH study. Kaplan–Meier analysis of survival in the group that received LVAD and the group that received optimal medical therapy.

at 12 months; at 24 months, the probability of LVAD failure was 35%. In spite of this, the results of the clinical trial showed superior survival benefits offered by LVAD versus optimal medical therapy.

Morbidity and mortality associated with the device were considerable. Device failure due to infection was the most important adverse event that occurred within 30 days of device implantation. Risk factors that predisposed infection included the percutaneous driveline site and the clinical status of the patient at the time of LVAD implantation. Other significant limiting factors were mechanical failure, inflow valve insufficiency, and neurologic event. Patients supported with HeartMate in the REMATCH Trial did experience improvements in hemodynamics and in functional class. The information provided by the REMATCH Trial established the realistic feasibility of destination therapy. This suggests a tremendous opportunity for improvement, not only with patient management, but also for changes in the device design to improve clinical results. Both quality of life and survival advantage can be extended or maximized by making the system more durable, reliable, and reducing the propensity for infection. With these changes, the indication for destination therapy could become a reality for patients with end-stage heart failure.

LVAD as a bridge-to-recovery

During extended use of LVAD as a bridge-to-transplantation in patients with myocarditis or dilated cardiomyopathy, some patients experience significant improvement in left ventricular function.

Many show various grades of heart failure reversal at structural, cellular, molecular, and clinical levels [59, 60].

Some patients who received long-term support for cardiomyopathy showed reasonable or nearly normal myocardial function for extended periods of time when the device was turned off or explanted due to complications. Authors have reported this reversal lasting several years [61, 62]. This supports the hypothesis that the LVAD could be used as a bridge for cardiac recovery. Unfortunately, there is limited successful clinical experience.

Many patients with LVADs experience multiple hemodynamic changes and improved native left and right ventricular functions. This occurs due to a decrease in left ventricle end-diastolic diameter (LVEDD) that demonstrates a reduction in loading pressure. left ventricle geometry and related physiologic measurements and ejection fractions improve. Pulmonary capillary wedge pressure and pulmonary vascular resistance decrease [63]. Peak oxygen consumption during maximal exercise (MVO_2) improves over time. LVAD support helps reverse the remodeling process, at all levels, and leads to functional recovery. These factors substantiate its importance as a bridge-to-recovery [64, 65]. In a German study by Mueller and Hetzer, 105 patients with dilated cardiomyopathy received LVAD support [66–68]. Of these, 24 patients were weaned from the device; 14 continued in stable cardiac function from 3 months to 4.5 years. Heart failure recurred in seven patients from 4 to 24 months. Patients whose conditions remained stable were compared with those whose conditions deteriorated. The latter group had a longer duration of heart failure pre-VAD and, therefore, needed longer periods of support to meet the criteria for LVAD removal. They also had a larger chamber size and a lower ejection fraction. Another finding in their study was that improvements in cardiac function for patients on LVAD support disappeared if support remained more than 6 months. It has been postulated that prolonged LVAD support may lead to atrophy and fibrosis of the myocardium [69]. Based on the definition of cardiac remodeling, this process can be modified in the course of time and is actually bidirectional.

Yacoub and colleagues [70, 71] explored the strategy of using a selective β-2-adrenergic receptor antagonist (Clenbuterol) to produce maximum "reverse remodeling" by inducing physiologic cardiac hypertrophy in combination with LVAD support.

To date, the most consistent weaning from assist devices were found in patients with acute but reversible injuries. Patients with myocarditis seem to fare better than those with dilated or ischemic cardiomyopathy [64]. With the realization that LVADs can be successfully explanted, their use as a bridge-to-recovery opened new frontiers for an alternative therapy for end-stage heart failure. Other adjuncts for LVAD support to improve cardiac function are emerging: Clenbuterol and other therapies such as gene therapy and cell transplantation or a combination. These new concepts in the treatment of CHF could reduce the number of patients needing cardiac transplantation and reduce the current donor organ shortage. Results from these early studies encourage continued exploration of this strategy for patients with end-stage heart failure.

Future directions of assist devices

Total artificial heart

TAH implantation provides complete support of the circulatory system but requires removal of the native heart. Although TAH has been used to provide permanent support, its most important role has been a bridge-to-transplantation for patients who desperately need biventricular support and in whom an LVAD is inadequate therapy. Clinical devices are the CardioWest 70 TAH (formerly Jarvik-70) and AbioCor TAH (Abiomed Inc., Bainbridge, MA) [72, 73].

The CardioWest C-70 (CardioWest Technologies Inc., Tucson, AZ) is a pneumatically driven, pulsatile biventricular cardiac replacement system. The prosthetic ventricles are made of polyurethane. Medtronic-Hall mechanical valves provide unidirectional flow. A diaphragm, which retracts during diastole, separates blood and air, and is displaced forward during systole by compressed air to propel blood out of the TAH. Flows reach up to 15 L/min.

The TAH is implanted in the mediastinum after the ventricles have been excised; the atrial cuffs are retained. Drivelines are external by percutaneous insertion and attached to the console. Full systemic anticoagulation is necessary (Figure 12.30).

The AbioCor implantable replacement heart (IRH) is the first implantable TAH. It has used for

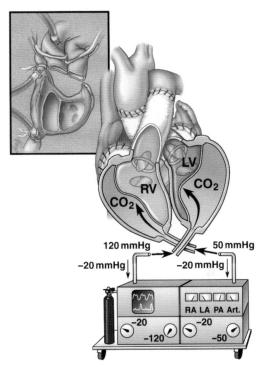

Figure 12.30 TAH, The CardioWest TAH, implantable pump and external console.

destination therapy for patients with irreversible biventricular end-stage heart failure with no other therapeutic options and a life expectancy <30 days. It is the first electrohydraulic artificial heart system that use a transcutaneous energy transmission system, providing power across the skin. It is a fully implantable system with two pumping chambers and three-leaflet valves that provide continuous, unidirectional hydraulic flow motion via an electrically driven centrifugal pump [74]. It provides a range of flows from 4 to 8 L/min. All blood-conducting surfaces of the AbioCor thoracic unit, including the three-leaflet valve (24 mm internal diameter), is polyether urethane (Angioflex, AbioMed, Inc., Bainbridge, MA) that forms a smooth and continuous blood-conducting surface from the inflow cuffs to the outflow grafts (Figures 12.31 and 12.32).

The four external components consist of an external transcutaneous energy transfer (TET) coil, batteries, TET module, and a bedside console. The external TET coil transfers energy across the skin to the internal TET coil and is secured over the internal coil with an adhesive dressing. It can be connected to

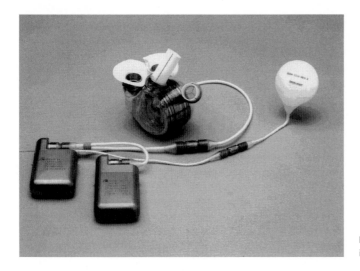

Figure 12.31 The Abiomed AbioCor: internal system components.

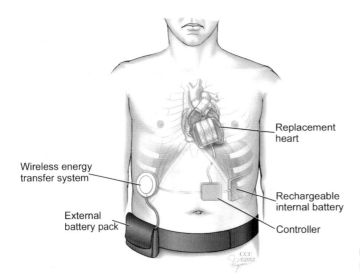

Wireless energy transfer system

Replacement heart

External battery pack

Rechargeable internal battery

Controller

Figure 12.32 The Abiomed AbioCor: implantable replacement heart.

either the bedside console or the portable TET module. During patient ambulation, the external TET coil is connected to the portable TET module. This module delivers energy to the internal coil from external batteries. The bedside console is used during implantation, recovery, and hospitalization. The bedside console provides a clinician with a graphic user interface for control and monitoring of the implanted system via radio frequency (RF) communication. The external batteries, lithium-ion based, are able to provide 1 h of support per pound of battery and can be carried in a vest, handbag or attached to a velcro belt [75].

Results

After a series of successful, extensive animal research studies, preclinical implants and *in vitro* studies, the FDA granted approval in January 2001 for a multicenter trial. Seven male patients were implanted with the AbioCor IRH system. The multicenter clinical trial was designed for patients with severe irreversible biventricular failure who were not candidates for other types of therapy, including heart transplantation, who were on maximum medical therapy and dependent on inotropic agents. All patient-candidates had a 30-day predicted mortality of more than 70%, based on the AbioCor prognostic model or acute myocardial infarction shock scores [76].

Exclusion criteria included active infections, severe peripheral vascular disease, blood dyscrasia, recent stroke, or transient ischemic attack (TIA) due to arteriolosclerosis. All potential recipients underwent a complete psycho-social evaluation. If clearly indicated that a patient was a potential candidate, a variety of digital thoracic images of the patient's chest were performed, such as computerized tomography scan and magnetic resonance imaging. A sophisticated software program allowed for *in vitro* surgery implantation of the AbioCor thoracic unit.

The primary end-point was mortality, from any cause, in patients with severe heart failure and a predicted life expectancy of <30 days despite optimized medical management. The second end-point was any adverse event, device malfunction or complications related to the presence of the device. Quality of life was also a determinant.

Age range was 51–79 years. Six patients were ischemic and one had idiopathic cardiomyopathy. Four patients had previous coronary artery bypass surgery; all patients were dependent on inotropic agents. Three patients were not considered transplant candidates because of age (>70 years); four were excluded due to high pulmonary vascular resistance and two had significant renal dysfunction. BSA ranged from 1.83 to 2.17 mol/L. CPB time ranged from 125 to 240 min. Four patients lived beyond the 60-day study end-point, twice their predicted life expectancy. There were two intraoperative deaths (due to intraoperative bleeding or aprotinin reactions). Four late deaths were recorded: one from multisystem organ failure and three from cerebrovascular accident (CVA). One patient is alive on support. Despite strict anticoagulation protocols, thromboembolic events were a devastating phenomenon, arising from the support struts within the atrial cuffs. Nevertheless, the AbioCor showed a high degree of reliability. There were no serious device-related infections; quality of life was significantly improved in four of seven patients [75].

In summary, the AbioCor system is the first totally implantable artificial heart. Early results from the multicenter trial demonstrated a high degree of reliability but high morbidity and mortality

rates. Regardless, important goals were achieved. TAH technology will continue to evolve.

Continuous-flow systems

The next generation of devices is continuous flow pumps. These are either axial (straight) or centrifugal (right angle inflow and outflow relationship) miniature pumps that generate flow through high-speed revolutions of an impeller blade. There are smaller and nonpulsatile pumps that deliver a constant blood flow, which accommodates with variable preload and afterload hemodynamic situations. The advantages of these pumps are a much smaller size devices, about 100 gm (suitable for both pediatric and small adult patients), can be placed with a limited surgical dissection to create a pump pocket, do not require vent line and the drive line is smaller than the pulsatile one, reducing the risk of pump pocket and drive line infections. This new generation is a silent system, without valves, reducing the risks of infection and valve malfunctions, and can be easier to convert to a completely implantable design.

Jarvik 2000

The Jarvik 2000 Heart (Jarvik Heart Inc., New York, NY) is a silent compact axial flow impeller pump that produces flow by means of a rotating, vaned impeller [77] (Figure 12.33).The blood pump is small, lightweight (2.5 cm × 5.5 cm, 90 g, displacement volume 25 mL) biocompatible, valveless, and contains a single moving part (the rotor) with a high rotational speed to promote blood that continuously washes the tiny bearing and prevents thrombus formation. A brushless direct current motor contained within the housing creates the electromagnetic force necessary to rotate the impeller. The blood contacting surfaces within the pump are manufactured with titanium. Due to the axial flow design, no internal compliance chamber or vent is needed. The pump is implanted through a left thoracotomy or sternotomy. The outflow graft can be placed on the ascending or descending aorta. The pump is positioned within the left ventricle (Figure 12.34). Either a percutaneous cable connected to a manually operated controller or a totally implantable system can power this pump. The percutaneous power cable is externalized through the right side of the abdomen or, alternatively, through

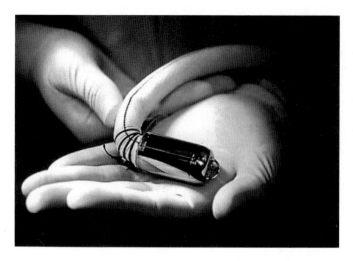

Figure 12.33 Continuous flow pumps: the Jarvik 2000 heart.

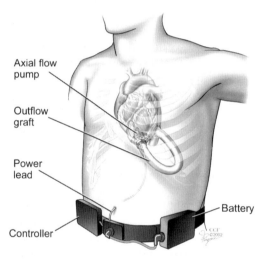

Axial flow pump

Outflow graft

Power lead

Battery

Controller

Figure 12.34 The Jarvik 2000: heart, implantable system components.

a skull-mounted pedestal [77]. The power cable is connected to the controller which controls and monitors the impeller speed. Continuous power at 12 V is provided to the controller and pump by either lithium-ion or lead-acid batteries.

The impeller rotates at speeds of 8000–12,000 rpm, providing blood flow of up to 8 L/min. Power consumption is <12 W. At 8000 rpm, against a mean pressure of 60 mmHg, the Jarvik 2000 produces flows of slightly more than 2 L/min, quite sufficient to improve the performance of a chronic failing heart. In addition, the smaller transabdominal or post-auricular power delivery driveline is less prone to infection than the larger and stiffer lines of the pulsatile LVADs [78, 79].

During implantation, serial echocardiograms with simultaneous blood pressure measurements are useful to determine the appropriate Jarvik 2000 pump speed setting. Some ejection of the blood from the left ventricle through the aortic valve is desirable to avoid blood stasis and thrombus formation in the aortic root. The pump speed is adjusted from 8000 to 12,000 rpm (in 1000 rpm increments) when the aortic valve is observed. The guideline is an optimal speed setting of 1000 rpm less than the speed at which the aortic valve remains closed.

One complication that occurs with the axial flow pump is thrombosis within the left ventricle, around the inflow conduit, which may generate inflow obstruction. Partial or complete inflow obstruction can be determined by an acute increase in power requirements of the pump motor. This needs to be confirmed by echocardiogram. Systemic or intradevice thrombolytic therapy is the treatment for this complication. Thrombosis of the device may result in device failure or infarction in other organs. Typically a combination of low-molecular-dextran, heparin, warfarin, dipyridamole, and aspirin is used for anticoagulation and to suppress platelet function.

Clinical studies of the Jarvik 2000 are now being conducted in eight centers in the United States and in five centers in Europe. In the United States, the study involved only a temporary use of the Jarvik

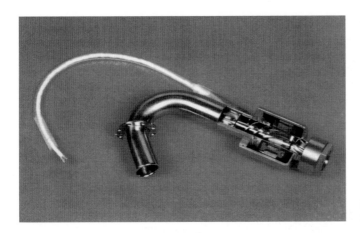

Figure 12.35 The Micromed DeBakey VAD system.

2000 in heart transplant candidates. In Europe, however, the system is being used as both a bridge-to-transplantation and destination therapy. Indication criteria of the study are New York Heart Association Functional Class (NYHAFC) IV, cardiac index <2 L/min, maximum medical therapy with IABP support and no other significant morbidities.

Between March 2000 and October 2002, the Jarvik 2000 was implanted in 45 patients worldwide. In Europe, 11 of 15 patients were supported as destination therapy. Average duration of support was 285 days. The United States patient population averaged support of 59 days. The first patient supported with Jarvik used as destination therapy was implanted in June of 2000, more than 3.5 years later, the patient remains alive. In the United States, three centers have implanted the Jarvik 2000 in 29 patients as a bridge-to-transplantation [79, 80]. Fourteen patients (52%) were supported to heart transplantation; five patients (17%) continue on support awaiting transplantation. Average post-transplantation follow-up period for surviving patients is 15 months (range: 1.5–28 months). Average duration of support was 68.5 days (range: 3–214 days). On support, patients' hemodynamic function improved rapidly and inotropic agents became unnecessary in most cases. Serious complications during support occurred in 18 of 45 patients. Patient deaths were five from sepsis and multiple organ failure, four from myocardial ischemia, one from coagulopathy, and three from right heart failure. Two destination therapy patients died of severe subdural hematomas. The hematomas resulted from complications associated with the skull-mounted pedestal in one case and from a fall in the other case. There were three device-related deaths attributed to device thrombosis, stroke, and improper power cable disconnection by the patient. Non-lethal complications included left ventricle thrombus, coronary thrombosis, and gastrointestinal bleeding. Three patients were treated successfully with tissue plasminogen activator (tPA) for lysis of left ventricle thrombi. No important infections were observed.

MicroMed DeBakey

The MicroMed DeBakey VAD (Micromed, Houston, TX), is an axial flow pump being studied clinically. The LVAD consists of three systems: a miniaturize titanium axial flow pump, an external controller, and a clinical data acquisition system. The device is electromagnetically actuated, miniaturized, and fully implantable. A titanium inflow cannula connects the pump to the apex of the left ventricle. A Vascutek Gelweave vascular graft (outflow conduit) connects the pump to the ascending aorta. An ultrasonic flow probe is placed around the outflow conduit. Together, with the flow probe wiring, the pump motor cable is tunneled externally, above the right iliac crest, and attached to the LVAD external controller system. This pump produces a flow of 4–5 L/min against 100 mmHg pressure with the inducer–impeller spinning at about 10,000 rpm. It requires >10 W of input power. The pump is 1.2 inches in diameter and 3 inches in length. The priming volume of the pump, including the inflow cannula, is 35 mL [80, 81] (Figure 12.35).

For optimal mobilization of the patient and freedom of movement, the electrical power is delivered by one of two 12-V batteries. Each battery lasts 6–8 h. The entire system weighs 2.5 kg. The pump is implanted through a median sternotomy incision. This incision extends a few centimeters below the xiphoid. A small abdominal wall pocket is created below the rectus muscle sheath.

The common recommendation for anticoagulation is to begin intravenous heparin or subcutaneous low-molecular-weight heparin as soon as postoperative bleeding is minimal and any coagulopathy is controlled. It is then converted to coumadin, aspirin, and clopidogrel as a standard regimen for anticoagulation.

Clinical results presented by Noon et al. [82], showed 51 patients (44 males/7 females) implanted with a MicroMed DeBakey LVAD system in September 2000. A detailed account of the first 32 patients has been completed. Support duration ranged up to 133 days; 21 patients were supported more than 30 days and 13 patients were supported more than 60 days. Median time to transplant was 74.5 days with a median support ratio of 47 days. The cumulative number of patient-days of support was 1876 days. Fifty percent of the patients enrolled in the clinical trial had idiopathic dilated cardiomyopathy; 38% had ischemic cardiomyopathy. Mean cardiac index of patients was 1.7 L/min/m^2 and an average mean pulmonary pressure of 25 mmHg. Using these data, the probability of survival of 30 days after MicroMed LVAD implant was 81%. Eleven of the 32 patients were transplanted; 10 of 32 patients died on support. Death in most patients occurred as a result of multisystem organ failure. There were few incidences of late bleeding, most occurring more than 5 days after implantation. These appeared to be related to anticoagulation. There was also a small incidence of hemolysis. The MicroMed is a continuous axial flow pump with an output that is determined by the pump's rpm and the delta pressure between the inflow and the outflow cannula sites. At a fixed rpm, the pump output in patients varies depending on the ventricular pressure changes during cardiac and central aortic pressures. Continuous flows produced by the pump may be steady or pulsatile, depending on the delta pressure. Pump flow may decrease when the rpm is increased above a certain level because of progressive ventricular loading lowering the ventricular pressure. This could be, in part or in total, the result of complete ventricular collapse. In this stage, the only way to improve flow is to reduce the rpm or increase preload, or both.

The initial clinical experience with the MicroMed DeBakey VAD as a bridge-to-transplantation showed that the pump was capable to provide good hemodynamic performance and reliable circulatory support, with low incidence of major complications.

Comments

During the last decade, LVAD has become a widely accepted option as temporary MCS. LVADs have been successfully used in patients with severe heart failure who are unresponsive to conventional treatment or who are awaiting cardiac transplantation. By preventing further cardiac deterioration and by improving end-organ function, LVADs have proven helpful for these critically ill patients. The LVAD provides effective hemodynamic support and an infrequent need for mechanical right ventricular assistance. It allows patients to exercise with the probability of being discharged from the hospital. These results are far better than the results for patients treated medically [49, 55, 83, 84]. There are, however, adverse events attributed to chronic MCS. Predominant are the risks of infection, stroke, and device failure that need further investigation. In our experience, both HeartMate and Novacor implantable LVADs provided good hemodynamic support and a good quality of life for patients awaiting heart transplantation. These devices are reliable. Novacor originally posed a much higher risk of thromboembolic events, but recent design changes have reduced these risks. Unfortunately, LVADs carry significant risks of infection. These are due to pre-existing illness, a vulnerable percutaneous connection and immunologic deficiencies related to prolonged circulatory support. Patients who develop driveline or device infections may be able to undergo heart transplantation, but infections remain a serious limitation to widespread long-term LVAD support. Chronic infections decrease quality of life, increase the overall cost of therapy and may require pump replacement with a negative impact on clinical outcomes.

LVAD success as a viable therapy for end-stage CHF was confirmed by REMATCH [10]. The results showed better survival and quality of life in patients supported by LVADs despite a high incidence of device failures and complications. These results will improve with new generations of devices. The value of the study is its ability to demonstrate that long-term support is not only feasible, but also desirable in this chronically ill group of patients. Continued investigation and research will ultimately produce a device for permanent implant. Blood pumps of the future will be small, totally implantable, efficient, reliable, and durable. As technology evolves, improved LVADs and, perhaps, improved TAHs, will open new frontiers along with new problems. The key will be how promptly the problems are recognized and how rapidly they are overcome.

References

1 Evans RW. *Cardiac Replacement: Estimation of Need, Demand, and Supply in Management of End-Stage Heart Disease.* Lippincott-Raven, New York, NY, 1998: 169–179.

2 Spencer FC, Eiseman B, Trinkle JK *et al.* Assisted circulation for cardiac failure following intracardiac surgery with cardiorespiratory bypass. *J Thorac Cardiovasc Surg* 1965; **49**: 56–73.

3 Moulopoulus SD, Topaz SR, Kolff WJ. Extracorporeal assistance to the circulation and intraaortic balloon pumping. *Trans Am Soc Artif Intern Organs* 1962; **8**: 86.

4 Krantrowitz A, Tjonneland S, Freed PS, Phillips SJ, Butner AN, Sherman Jr JL *et al.* Initial clinical experience with intraaortic balloon pumping in cardiogenic shock. *J Am Med Assoc* 1968; **203**: 113–118.

5 Dennis C. Left-heart bypass. In: *Mechanical Devices to Assist the Failing Heart.* Publication No. 1283. National Academy of Sciences-National Research Council, Washington DC, 1966: 27.

6 Hall CW, Liotta D, Henly WS *et al.* Development of artificial intrathoracic circulatory pumps. *Am J Surg* 1964; **108**: 685–692.

7 DeBakey ME. Left ventricular bypass pump for cardiac assistance. Clinical experience. *Am J Cardiol* 1971; **27**: 3–11.

8 Department of Health and Human Services, National Institutes of Health, National Heart, Lung, and Blood Institute: Left heart assist blood pumps (request for proposal). Bethesda, MD, 1977.

9 Department of Health and Human Services, National Institutes of Health, National Heart, Lung, and Blood Institute: Development of electrical energy converters to power and control left assist devices (request for proposal). Bethesda, MD, 1977.

10 Rose EA, Gelijns AC, Moskowitz AJ, Heitjan DF *et al.* Long term use of a ventricular assist device for end-stage heart failure. *New Eng J Med* 2001; **345(20)**: 1435–1443.

11 Norman JC, Cooley DA, Igo SR. Prognastic indices for survival during postcardiotomy intraaortic balloon pumping. *J Thoracic Cardionas Surg* 1977; **74**: 709–714.

12 Barlett RM, Roloff DW, Coster JR *et al.* Extracorporeal life support: the University of Michigan experience. *J Am Med Assoc* 2000; **283**: 904–908.

13 Jett GK. Abiomed BVS 5000: experience and potential advantages. *Ann Thorac Surg* 1996; **61**: 301–304.

14 Argenziano M, Choudmri AF, Moazami N *et al.* A prospective randomized trial of arginine vasopressin in the treatment of vasodilatory shock after left ventricular assist device placement. *Circulation* 1997; **96(Suppl)**: 286–270.

15 Argenziano M, Choudmri AF, Moazami N *et al.* Randomized, double-blind trial of inhaled nitric oxide in LVAD percipients with pulmonary hypertension. *Ann Thorac Surg* 1998; **65**: 340–345.

16 Alderman JD, Gabliani GI, McCabe CH, Brewer CC, Loreu BH, Pasternak RC *et al.* Incidence and management of limb ischemia with percutaneous wire-guided intraaortic balloon catheters. *J Am Coll Cardiol* 1987; **9**: 524–530.

17 Alcan KE, Stertzer SH, Wallsh E, Bruno MS, DePasquale NP. Current status of intra-aortic balloon counterpulsation in critical care cardiology. *Crit Care Med* 1984; **12**: 489–495.

18 Golding LAR, Steward RW, Loop FD. Centrifugal pumps in clinical practice. In: Unger F, ed. *Assisted Circulation.* Springer-Verlag, Berlin, 1989: 160–166.

19 Pennington DG, Merjavy JP, Swartz MT, Willman VL. Clinical experience with a centrifugal pump ventricular assist device. *ASAIO Trans* 1982; **28**: 93–99.

20 Hoerr HR, Kraemer MF, Williams JL. *In-vitro* comparison of the blood handling by the constrained vortex and twin roller blood pumps. *J Extra-Corpor Technol* 1987; **19**: 316–321.

21 Iatridis E, Chan T. An evaluation of vortex, centrifugal and roller pump systems. *Proceedings: International Workshop on Rotary Blood Pumps*, Vienna, Austria, September 1991.

22 Hoerr HR, Kraemer MF, Williams JL *et al. In vitro* comparison of the blood handling by the constrained vortex and twin roller blood pumps. *J Extra-Corpor Technol* 1987; **19**: 316–321.

23 Golding LA, Crouch RD, Stewart RW *et al.* Postcardiotomy centrifugal mechanical ventricular support. *Ann Thorac Surg* 1992; **54**: 1059–1064.

24 Mehta SM, Aufiero TX, Pae WE *et al.* Results of mechanical ventricular assistance for the treatment of postcardiotomy cardiogenic shock. *ASAIO J* 1996; **42**: 211–218.

25 Magovern GJ, Park SB, Maher TD. Use of a centrifugal pump without anticoagulants for postoperative left ventricular assist. *World J Surg* 1985; **9**: 25–36.

26 Noon GP, Ball JW, Short HD. Biomedicus centrifugal ventricular support for postcardiotomy cardiac failure: a review of 129 cases. *Ann Thorac Surg* 1996; **61**: 291–295.

27 Hill JD, O'Brien TG, Murray JJ *et al.* Extracorporeal oxygenation for acute posttraumatic respiratory failure (shocklung syndrome): use of the Bramson membrane lung. *N Engl J Med* 1972; **286**: 629–634.

28 Bartlett RH, Gazzaniga AB, Jefferies R *et al.* Extracorporeal membrane oxygenation (ECMO) cardiopulmonary support in infancy. *ASAIO Trans* 1976; **22**: 80–88.

29 Stolar CJ, Snedecor SS, Bartlett RH. Extracorporeal membrane oxygenation and neonatal respiratory failure: experience from the extracorporeal life support organization. *J Pediatr Surg* 1991; **26**(5): 563–571.

30 Muehrcke DD, McCarthy PM, Stewart RW. Complications of extracorporeal life support systems using heparin-bound surfaces: the risk of intracardiac clot formation. *J Thorac Cardiovasc Sur* 1995; **110**: 843–851.

31 Navia JL, Atik FA, Beyer EA. Extracorporeal membrane oxygenation with right axillary artery perfusion. *Ann Thorac Surg* 2005; in press.

32 Bavaria JE, Furukawa S, Kreiner G. Effect of circulatory assist devices on stunned myocardium. *Ann Thorac Surg* 1990; **49**: 123–128.

33 Muehrcke DD, McCarthy PM, Stewart RW *et al.* Extracorporeal membrane oxygenation for postcardiotomy cardiogenic shock. *Ann Thorac Surg* 1996; 684–691.

34 Goldstein DJ, Oz MC. Mechanical support for postcardiotomy cardiogenic shock. *Semin Thorac Cardiovasc Surg* 2000; **12**: 220–228.

35 Peek GJ, Firmin RK. The inflammatory and coagulative response to prolonged extracorporeal membrane oxygenation. *ASAIO J* 1999; **45**: 250–263.

36 Smedira NG, Moazami N, Golding CM *et al.* Clinical experience with 202 adults receiving extracorporeal membrane oxygenation for cardiac failure: survival at 5 years. *J Thorac Cardiovasc Surg* 2001; **122**(1): 92–102.

37 Jett Gk. Abiomed BVS 5000: experience and potential advantages. *Ann Thorac Surg* 1996; **61**: 301–304.

38 Wassenberg PA. The Abiomed BVS 5000 biventricular system. *Perfusion* 2000; **15**: 369–371.

39 Hellman DN, Morales DL, Edwards NM, Mancicni DM *et al.* Left ventricle assist device bridge-to-transplant network improves survival after failed cardiotomy. *Ann Thorac Surg* 1999; **68**: 1187–1194.

40 Farrar DJ, Litwak P, Lawson JH *et al. In vivo* evaluation of a new thromboresistant polyurethane for artificial heart blood pumps. *J Thorac Cardiovasc Surg* 1998; **95**: 191–200.

41 Rowles JR, Mortime BJ, Olsen DB. Ventricular assist and total artificial heart devices for clinical use in 1993. *ASAIO J* 1993; **39**: 840–855.

42 Farrar DJ, Hill JD. Univentricular and biventricular Thoratec VAD support as bridge to transplantation. *Ann Thorac Surg* 1993; **55**: 276–282.

43 Pae WE, Lundblad O. Thoratec paracorporeal pneumatic ventricular assist device. *Oper Tech Thorac Cardiovasc Surg* 1999; **4**: 352–362.

44 Arabia FA, Paramesh V, Toporoff B *et al.* Biventricular cannulation for the Thoratec ventricular assist device. *Ann Thorac Surg* 1998; **66**: 2119–2120.

45 Farrar DJ, Buck KE, Coulter JH *et al.* Portable pneumatic biventricular driver for the Thoratec ventricular assist device. *ASAIO J* 1997; **43**: 631–634.

46 von Segesser LK, Tkebuchava T, Leskosek B *et al.* Biventricular assist using a portable driver in combination with implanted devices: preliminary experience. *Artif Organs* 1997; **21**: 72–75.

47 Farrar DJ. The Thoratec ventricular assist device: a paracorporeal pump for treating acute and chronic heart failure. *Sem Thorac Cardiovasc Surg* 2000; **12**(3): 243–250.

48 Portner PN, Oyer PE, Pennintong G *et al.* Implantable electric left ventricular assist system: bridge to transplantation and future. *Ann Thorac Surg* 1989; **47**: 142–150.

49 McCarthy PM, Savage RM, Fraser CD, Vargo R, James KB, Goormastic M, Hobbs RE. Hemodynamic and physiologic changes during support with an implantable left ventricular assist device. *J Thorac Surg* 1995; **109**: 409–418.

50 McCarthy PM, Sabik JF. Implantable circulatory support devices as a bridge-to-transplantation. *Sem Thorac Cardiovasc Surg* 1994; **6**: 174–180.

51 McCarthy PM, Portner Pm, Oyer PE *et al.* Clinical experience with the Novacor ventricular assist system: bridge to transplant and the transition to chronic application. *J Thorac Cardiovasc Surg* 1992; **102**: 578–587.

52 Rao V, Slater JP, Edwards NM, Oz MC. Surgical management of valvular disease in patients requiring LVAD support. *Ann Thorac Surg* 2001; **71**(5): 1448–1453.

53 Vigneshwar K, McCrathy PM, Hoercher KJ *et al.* Clinical experience with long term use of implantable left ventricular assist device: indication, implantation, and outcomes. *Sem Thorac Cardiovasc Surg* 2000; **12**(3): 229–237.

54 McCarthy PM, Wang N, Vargo R. Preperitoneal insertion of the HeartMate 100 IP left ventricular assist device. *Ann Thorac Surg* 1994; **57**: 634–638.

55 McCarthy PM, Smedira NG, Vargo RL, Goormastic M, Hobbs R, Starling R, Young J. One hundred patients with HeartMate left ventricular assist device: evolving concepts and technology. *J Thorac Cardiovasc Surg* 1998; **115**: 904–912.

56 McCarthy PM, Schmitt SK, Vargo R *et al.* LVAD infections: implications for permanent use of the device. *Ann Thorac Surg* 1996; **61**: 359–365.

57 Argenziano M, Catanese KA, Moazami N *et al.* The influence of infection on survival and successful transplantation

in patients with left ventricular assist devices. *J Heart Lung Transplat* 1997; **16**: 822–831.

58 Navia JL, McCarthy PM, Hoercher KJ, Smedira NG, Banbury MK, Blackstone EH. Do left ventricular assist device (LVAD) bridge to transplantation outcomes predict the results of permanent LVAD implantation. *Ann Thorac Surg* 2002; **74**: 2051–2062; discussion 2062–2063.

59 Pennington DG, Bernahard WF, Golding LR *et al.* Long term follow-up of postcardiotomy patients with profound cardiogenic shock treated with ventricular assist device. *Circulation* 1985; **72**: 216–226.

60 Kurrelmeyer K, Kaira D, Bozkurt B *et al.* Cardiac remodeling as a consequence and cause of progressive heart failure. *Clin Cardiol* 1998; **21(Suppl I)**:I14–I19.

61 Goldstein S, Ali AS, Sabbah H. Ventricular remodeling-mechanism and prevention. *Cardiol Clinics* 1998; **16**: 623–631.

62 Kapadia S, Dibbs Z, Kurrelmeyer K *et al.* The role of cytokines in the failing human heart. *Cardiol Clinics* 1998; **16**: 645–656.

63 Frazier OH, Beneditic CR, Radovancevic B *et al.* Improve ventricular function after chronic left ventricular unloading. *Ann Thorac Surg* 1996; **62**: 675–682.

64 Jaski BE, Kim J, Maly RS *et al.* Effects of exercise during long-term support with a left ventricular assist device. *Circulation* 1997; **95**: 2401–2406.

65 Hoel R, Vermes E, Tixier DB *et al.* Myocardial recovery after mechanical support for acute myocarditis: Is sustained recovery predictable? *Ann Thorac Surg* 1999; **68**: 2177–2180.

66 Hetzer R, Muller J, Weng Y *et al.* Cardiac recovery in dilated cardiomyopathy by unloading with a left ventricular assist device. *Ann Thorac Surg* 1999; **68**: 742–749.

67 Hetzer R, Muller J, Weng Y *et al.* Midterm follow-up of patients who underwent removal of a left ventricular assist device after cardiac recovery from end-stage dilated cardiomyopathy. *J Thorac Cardiovasc Surg* 2000; **120**: 843–855.

68 Muller J, Loebe M, Weng Y *et al.* Weaning from mechanical support in patients with dilated cardiomyopathy. *Circulation* 1997; **96**: 542–549.

69 Dipla K, Mattielo JA, Jeevananvam V *et al.* Myocyte recovery after mechanical circulatory support in humans with end-stage heart failure. *Circulation* 1998; **97**: 2316–2322.

70 Yacoub MH. A novel strategy to maximize the efficacy of left ventricular assist devices as a bridge to recovery. *Eur Heart J* 2001; **22**: 534–540.

71 Yacoub MH, Tansley P, Birks EJ *et al.* A novel combination therapy to reverse end stage heart failure. *Transplant Proc* 2001; **33**: 2762–2764.

72 Frazier OH. History of mechanical cardiac assistance. *Sem Thorac Cardiovasc Surg* 2000; **12(3)**: 207–220.

73 Frazier OH. Future directions of cardiac assistance. *Sem Thorac Cardiovasc Surg* 2000; **12**: 251–257.

74 Dowling RD, Gray LA, Etoch SW *et al.* Initial experience with the AbioCord implantable replacement heart system. *J Thorac Cardiovasc Surg*, in press.

75 Dowling RD, Gray LA, Etoch SW, Laks H, Marelli D, Samuels L, Enwistle J, Couper G, Vlahakes G, Frazier OH. The AbioCord implantable replacement heart. *Ann Thorac Surg* 2003; **75**: S93–S99.

76 Hochman JS, Sleeper LA, Webb JG *et al.* Early revascularization in acute myocardial infarction complicated by cardiogenic shock. SHOCK Investigators. Should we emergently revascularize occluded coronary arteries for cardiogenic shock. *N Engl J Med* 1999; **341**: S325–S334.

77 Westaby S, Banning AP, Jarvik RK *et al.* First permanent implant of the Jarvik 2000 Heart. *Lancet* 2000; **356**: 900–903.

78 Westaby S, Katsumata T, Houel R, Pigott D, Frazier OH, Jarvik RK. Jarvik 2000 Heart; potential for bridge to myocyte recovery. *Circulation* 1998; **98**: 1568–1574.

79 Westaby S, Frazier OH, Pigott D, Saito S, Jarvik RK. Implantable technique for the Jarvik 2000 Heart. *Ann Thorac Surg* 2002; **73**: 1337–1340.

80 Frazier OH. Future direction of cardiac assistance. *Sem Thorac Cardiovasc Surg* 2000; **12(3)**: 251–257.

81 Vitali E, Lanfranconi M, Ribera E, Bruschi G, Colombo T *et al.* Successful experience in bridging patients to heart transplantation with the MicroMed DeBakey ventricular assist device. *Ann Thorac Surg* 2003; **75**: 1200–1204.

82 Noon G, Morley DL, Irwin S, Abdelsayed SV, Benkowki RJ *et al.* Clinical experience with the Micro-Med DeBakey assist device. *Ann Thorac Surgery* 2001; **71**: S133–S138.

83 Frazier OH, Rose EA, Oz MC, Dembitsky W, McCarthy PM, Radovancevic B, Poirer VL, Dasse KA. Heartmate LVAD investigators left ventricular assist system. Multicenter clinical evaluation of the HeartMate vented electric left ventricular assist system in patients awaiting heart transplantation. *J Thorac Cardiovasc Surg* 2001; **122**: 1186–1195.

84 Jaski BE, Lingle RJ, Kim J *et al.* Comparison of functional capacity in patients with end-stage heart failure following implantation of a left ventricular assist device versus heart transplantation: results of the experience with the left ventricular assist device with exercise trial. *J Heart Lung Transplant* 1999; **18**: 1031–1040.

CHAPTER 13

The role of heart transplantation

David O. Taylor

Introduction

Despite the latest advances in the treatment of chronic heart failure described in prior chapters, many patients continue to progress to advanced, end-stage failure. For those that are candidates, cardiac transplantation is the only proven therapy to offer improved survival and quality of life. Current survival rates for cardiac transplantation approach 88–90% at 1 year for many US transplant centers with survival rates approaching 50–60% at 10 years – a marked improvement over the survival rates with conventional medical therapy alone. In the REMATCH (Randomized Evaluation of Mechanical Assistance for the Treatment of Congestive Heart Failure) trial [1], patients with severe, end-stage inotrope-dependent heart failure were randomized to left ventricular assist device (LVAD) or continued maximal medical therapy, including intravenous inotropes. In order to be enrolled in this trial, patients had to be deemed ineligible for cardiac transplantation, thus these patients may not be representative of similar patients listed for transplantation. However, age alone was a common reason for transplant exclusion. The survival in the medical management arm was dismal. Only 25% survived to 1 year, while 52% of the LVAD group survived to 1 year. Thus, even with the limitations noted above, end-stage heart failure patients requiring continuous inotropic therapy (and perhaps the current generation of LVADs) are at extreme risk of death and would be better served with cardiac transplantation assuming, of course, they are candidates. Patients with slightly less severe, but ambulatory heart failure (New York Heart Association (NYHA) class IIIA, IIIB, early IV) not requiring inotropic therapy represent a bigger dilemma. For patients with ambulatory but advanced heart failure (NYHA class III, early IV) on angiotensin-converting enzyme (ACE) inhibitors and beta-blocking agents, the short-term (<3 years) mortality approaches 9–15%/year, comparable over this time period to cardiac transplantation [2–4]. However, the longer-term (>3 years) mortality exceeds transplantation, thus for many of these patients transplantation offers the best long-term treatment option. For these ambulatory but ill patients, careful risk/benefit analysis is needed to identify patients at higher risk for early death without transplantation or at higher risk for death post-transplantation.

In addition to improving the quantity of life in these patients, cardiac transplantation has been associated with a marked improvement in quality of life, despite the rigors of post-transplant care. At 5 years post-operatively, 65% of US cardiac transplant recipients are working full time, part time, or retired [5]. Many of the remaining 35% are probably capable of returning to work but are unable to do so because of various societal factors. At 5 years post-transplant, 91% of US cardiac transplant recipients report no physical limitation in their daily activities [5].

Unfortunately, because of the current donor organ shortage, this useful therapy for heart failure is available to only a limited number of potential candidates. While perhaps as many as 50,000 individuals in the United States with end-stage heart failure could potentially benefit from transplantation each year, around 2200 procedures are performed annually in this country. As of July 31, 2002, there were just over 4000 patients on the US heart transplant waiting list and in 2001 only 2202 cardiac transplant procedures were performed [6].

The yearly cardiac transplant volume in the United States has not increased in over 10 years despite the current public education campaigns and utilization of "higher-risk" donor organs. While cardiac transplant is generally thought to be "cost-effective" despite its relatively high costs, its overall impact on health care expenditures is quite small. In 1994, O'Connell and Bristow [7] concluded that of an estimated 38 billion dollars spent annually on heart failure care in this country, only 270 million dollars were spent on cardiac transplantation (0.7%). Thus from both a numerical and economical viewpoint, cardiac transplant has a very small role in the overall treatment of heart failure in this country. However, for the few who do undergo transplantation, the impact can be profound.

Selecting patients for transplantation

Candidate selection criteria are often divided into those which identify patients who would benefit from transplantation (inclusion or indication criteria) and those patients who are at very high risk for death with, or in spite of, transplantation (exclusion or contraindication criteria). In reality these two categories are somewhat overlapping.

Simply put, the general indication for cardiac transplantation is an end-stage heart disease (not necessarily heart failure) associated with an estimated survival significantly less than that expected with cardiac transplantation for that individual. Table 13.1 lists examples of common indications. However, cardiac transplantation in never indicated simply because of *past* episodes of severe heart failure, an isolated low ejection fraction (regardless of how low), or "inoperable" coronary or valvular heart disease. It is of utmost importance that patients being considered for cardiac transplantation have exhausted all other medical, surgical, and device options. Even patients with severely reduced ejection fractions should be considered for revascularization and/or valve surgery if there is a reasonable chance for stabilization or improvement. Perhaps these types of high-risk surgery would best be performed at transplant centers where ventricular assist devices are available if needed. In the current era, all patients (except those in shock or requiring inotropes) should have failed a trial of

Table 13.1 Indications for cardiac transplantation.

Cardiogenic shock
- Severe heart failure requiring continuous inotropic therapy
- Severe heart failure (NYHA class III–IV) with poor short-term prognosis despite maximal medical therapy
- Restrictive or hypertrophic cardiomyopathy with NYHA class III–IV symptoms
- Refractory angina pectoris with documented cardiac ischemia despite maximal medical therapy, not amenable to revascularization, with an estimated poor short-term prognosis
- Recurrent or refractory ventricular arrhythmias despite maximal medical and/or device therapy
- Complex congenital heart disease with ventricular (systemic or venous) failure that is progressive and not amenable to surgical or percutaneous repair.
- Hypoplastic left heart syndrome
- Low-grade tumors confined to the myocardium, unresectable and without evidence of metastasis

beta-blocker therapy or have a clear contraindication to their use prior to being transplanted. Often times, even stable patients on the cardiac transplant list who have failed prior attempts at beta-blockade can be successfully titrated onto therapy with close and meticulous follow-up and subsequently be safely removed from the "waiting list."

Predicting which patients are at high risk for poor outcome without transplantation is actually quite difficult. Clearly those in cardiogenic shock or truly inotrope dependent are at very high risk and would likely benefit from transplantation. As noted earlier, determining risk in the group of ambulatory heart failure patients is problematic. Historical data suggests that several factors can predict poor outcome in ambulatory heart failure patients (Table 13.2) but many of these factors were identified before the widespread use of ACE-inhibitors and very few of these factors have been re-examined in the current beta-blocker era. Nonetheless, of these, NYHA class IV symptoms, peak oxygen consumption measured by metabolic exercise test <12–14 mL/kg/min or <50% predicted, and elevated left and right cardiac filling pressures, and/or low cardiac index despite maximal medical therapy identify a subgroup of ambulatory patients at high risk for early mortality who should be strongly

Table 13.2 Factors predictive for mortality in patients with heart failure.

Coronary artery disease as etiology of heart failure
- Idiopathic restrictive cardiomyopathy as etiology of heart failure
- Left ventricular ejection fraction
- Right atrial pressure
- Pulmonary capillary occlusive pressure
- Cardiac index
- Stroke work index
- NYHA class
- Peak oxygen consumption measured at metabolic exercise testing
- 6-min walk distance
- History of syncope
- Plasma norepinephrine
- Plasma atrial natriuretic peptide
- Plasma brain natriuretic peptide
- Serum sodium

considered for transplantation. Likewise, peak oxygen consumption >18 mL/kg/min or 70% predicted, normal resting hemodynamics, and beta-blocker therapy identify a subgroup of patients at lower risk for early mortality who, in general, do not require listing for transplantation.

One often sees "transplant contraindications" divided into the "absolute" and the "relative"; however, most, if not all, of the so-called "absolute" contraindications have been successfully breached in individual cases. Therefore, it makes more sense to consider all such exclusion criteria as "relative" contraindications or more appropriately, "risk factors for poor outcome" which must be weighed in the context of other factors. Table 13.3 lists a wide variety of potential risk factors and the general magnitude of their effect on post-transplant survival based on prior registry data and expert panel recommendation [5,8–15]. Table 13.4 lists specific risk factors with odds ratios for mortality after transplantation from the Registry of the International Society for Heart and Lung Transplantation (ISHLT) [10].

At most transplant centers, candidacy decisions are made by a panel or committee of heart failure and transplantation professionals including cardiologists, cardiac surgeons, social workers, transplant nurse specialists, psychologists, psychiatrists, and

ethicists by carefully weighing the risks and benefits. In addition to the risk/benefit consideration for the individual patients, the committee must also weigh the relative risk of said transplantation on those patients already on the list and those soon to be listed. Given the severe donor organ shortage, theoretically, each transplant procedure deprives another potential recipient on the list of the same chance at better survival. While advocating for their individual patient, the transplant selection committee must remain a wise and thoughtful shepherd of this very limited resource.

Management of patients on the waiting list

It is vitally important that patients awaiting transplantation be maintained in as optimal health as possible. Close follow-up and a low threshold for hospitalization to intensify heart failure management are important to prevent deterioration to such a point that transplantation becomes too high risk. Patients on the transplant waiting list often deteriorate to the point of becoming beta-blocker intolerant and inotrope dependent. While some centers allow inotrope-dependent patients to wait outside the hospital (particularly if they have an implantable cardioverter defibrillators (ICD)), in our experience, patients with this severe degree of heart failure require almost daily surveillance to prevent or minimize complications that could prevent transplantation. Thus in our institution, inotrope-dependent candidates remain in the hospital and on telemetric monitoring for the duration of their wait. Likewise, mechanical circulatory support should be considered *early* in the course of inotrope-dependent patients, prior to the onset of severe renal or hepatic impairment which make mechanical support surgery much higher risk. In fact, data from a small series at the University of Michigan [16] and a larger series from the Cardiac Transplant Research Database [17] suggest that mechanical circulatory support may be preferable to prolonged inotropic support.

All patients on the waiting list, including the inotrope dependent, should participate in cardiac rehabilitation and physical therapy programs as their condition allows. Ambulatory patients on the waiting list should undergo routine "risk stratification" with repeat metabolic exercise testing and right

Table 13.3 Patient characteristics increasing the risk of morbidity and mortality after cardiac transplantation.

Criterion	Increase in risk
PVR > 6 wood units, unresponsive to vasodilators	Marked
PVR > 6 wood units, decreasing in response to vasodilators but not below 3–4 wood units	Moderate
PVR > 3 wood units, decreasing below three wood units in response to vasodilators	Minimal
Pulmonary artery systolic pressure >70 mmHg, unresponsive to treatment	Marked
Transpulmonic gradient (mean PAP − PCWP) > 15–20 mmHg	Moderate
Transpulmonic gradient (mean PAP − PCWP) 10–15 mmHg	Minimal
Active, untreated infection	Marked
Treated infection currently controlled on antibiotics	Moderate
Recent resolved infection	Minimal
Irreversible, severe hepatic disease	Marked
Moderate hepatic dysfunction not clearly related to cardiac congestion	Moderate
Mild hepatic enzyme elevations likely related to cardiac congestion	Minimal
Irreversible, severe renal disease	Marked
Moderate renal dysfunction not clearly related to low cardiac output	Moderate
Mild renal dysfunction likely related to low cardiac output	Minimal
Irreversible pulmonary disease with FEV-1 <1 L or FVC <50% predicted	Marked
Irreversible pulmonary disease with FEV-1 ⩽1.5 L or FVC <65% predicted	Moderate
Mild/moderate pulmonary disease, FEV-1 >1.5 L or FVC >65% predicted	Minimal
Recent pulmonary infarction	Moderate
Age 50–60 years	Minimal
Age 60–70 years	Moderate
Age >70 years	Marked
Age 1–5 years	Moderate
Diabetes mellitus with significant end-organ damage	Moderate to marked
Diabetes mellitus without end-organ damage	Moderate
Cerebrovascular disease, severe, symptomatic	Marked
Cerebrovascular disease, mild to moderate, asymptomatic	Minimal
Peripheral vascular disease, severe, symptomatic	Marked
Peripheral vascular disease, mild to moderate, asymptomatic	Minimal
Gastrointestinal bleeding, active	Marked
Peptic ulcer disease, treated	Minimal
Diverticulitis recent	Moderate
Chronic active hepatitis	Moderate to marked
Chronic Hepatitis C with low viral load and benign liver biopsy	Minimal
Malignancy, recent	Marked
Malignancy, remote	Minimal
Myocardial infiltrative disease	Marked
Myocardial inflammatory disease	Moderate
Major affective disorder or schizophrenia with poor control	Marked
Major affective disorder or schizophrenia with good control	Moderate
Personality disorders	Moderate
Cigarette abuse	Moderate
Substance abuse, active unresolved	Marked
Substance abuse, resolved albeit recent	Moderate
Medical noncompliance	Marked
Obesity, moderate (120–1140%; IBW or BMI 30–35)	Minimal to moderate
Osteoporosis	Minimal to moderate
Lack of social support	Minimal to moderate

PVR: pulmonary vascular resistance; wood units (mmHg/L/min); PAP: pulmonary artery pressure; PCWP: pulmonary capillary wedge pressure; FEV-1: 1 s forced expiratory volume; FVC: forced vital capacity; IBW: ideal body weight; BMI: body mass index (weight in kg divided by height in m^2).

Modified with permission from Renlund DG, Taylor DO. In: Topol EJ, ed. *Cardiac Transplantation in Textbook of Cardiovascular Medicine*, 2nd edn. Lippincott Williams & Wilkins, 2002: 1917.

Table 13.4 Risk factors for mortality after heart transplantation in adults.

Variable	1 year (n = 37,257)		5 years (n = 23,684)	
	Odds ratio	P-value	Odds ratio	P-value
Repeat heart transplantation	2.27	<0.0001	2.36	<0.0001
Ventilator use	1.94	<0.0001	1.28	0.01
Congenital heart disease	1.47	0.001	–	–
Non-CAD, Non-IDC diagnosis	1.25	<0.0001	1.22	<0.0001
VAD implanted	1.25	0.0003	1.35	0.002
Female donor	1.23	<0.0001	1.14	0.0002
Recipient age (linear analysis)	1.0 + 0.025/year for each year over age of 50 years	<0.0001	1.0 + 0.025/year for each year over age of 50 years	<0.0001
Donor age (linear analysis)	1.0 + 0.025/year for each year over age of 30 years	<0.0001	1.0 + 0.02/year for each year over age of 30 years	<0.0001
PVR (linear analysis)	1.0 + 0.13/wood unit for each wood unit over 1.0 wood unit	<0.0001	1.0 + 0.07/wood unit for each wood unit over 1.0 wood unit	0.03
Ischemic time (linear analysis)	1.0 + 0.26/h for each hour over 3 h	<0.0001	1.0 + 0.26/h for each hour over 3 h	<0.0001

CAD: coronary artery disease; IDC: idiopathic dilated cardiomyopathy; VAD: ventricular assist device; PVR: pulmonary vascular resistance in wood units (mean pulmonary artery pressure in mmHg minus mean pulmonary capillary wedge pressure in mmHg divided by the cardiac output in liters/minute) (adapted from [10] with permission).

heart catheterization (every 3–6 months), to identify patients at high risk for deterioration as well as those who may have improved to such a degree that they can be removed from the waiting list. Periodic right heart catheterizations are also useful to identify patients with progressive pulmonary hypertension who can be aggressively treated prior to developing fixed or high-risk pulmonary artery pressures. Occasionally ambulatory patients who are otherwise not inotrope dependent require continuous intravenous inotropes and/or vasodilators to maintain acceptable pulmonary artery pressures and allow successful cardiac transplantation. Many patients with borderline or even unacceptable pulmonary artery hypertension, unresponsive to aggressive intravenous agents will respond dramatically to mechanical circulatory support and become transplantable.

Selecting donor hearts

By the very nature of the circumstances leading to brain death and the subsequent hemodynamic and metabolic changes associated with brain death itself, a potential donor heart is rarely "normal" at the time of organ donation. One must weigh the risk of acute and chronic allograft failure against the potential recipient's risk of survival without that particular organ. While a high-risk donor may be unacceptable for a young, stable outpatient on the waiting list, it may perfectly acceptable for a patient in extremis who cannot be otherwise stabilized to await a better donor. In addition, one may attempt to justify the listing of high-risk candidates by allocating only "marginal" donor organs that would not be utilized otherwise and allocating the "better" donor organs for the more suitable candidates on the list. While this "alternate list" [18] approach has its ethical strengths, the risk for poor post-operative outcome is increased accordingly when one uses a higher-risk donor organ in a higher-risk recipient.

All organ donors are screened carefully for acute and chronic infectious diseases. Usually donors with chronic transmittable infectious diseases, such as HIV, Hepatitis B and C are considered for donation only to recipients already infected with these. While the risk of transmission for Hepatitis C from an antibody positive donor is relatively high (perhaps as high as 50%), given the generally slow course of the disease, the risk may be acceptable in a marginal candidate without other options or a patient in extremis who is likely not to live until a "better" organ becomes available. Active malignancy in the potential donor usually excludes organ donation except in the case of primary brain malignancies, which have a very low incidence of metastasis, particularly cardiac metastasis. However, the presence of a ventriculoperitoneal shunt or recent brain surgery increases the risk of hematologic spread.

Evaluation of the donor heart usually involves electrocardiography, echocardiography, and at times invasive hemodynamics and coronary arteriography. Echocardiography is used to exclude current or pre-existing valvular or myocardial dysfunction that would preclude transplantation. However, this data, particularly the echocardiographic data, must be viewed within the context of the overall donor situation. While brain death can be associated with massive catecholamine release and subsequent myocardial necrosis, many echocardiographic wall motion abnormalities represent "stunning" and are reversible with correction of the donor hemodynamic and metabolic perturbations, or removal from the uncorrectable milieu with transplantation. In general, hearts with echocardiographic or visual evidence of moderate to severe left ventricular hypertrophy, particularly if associated with an anticipated long ischemic time, are not considered acceptable donor organs. Even in the absence of risk factors for coronary artery disease (CAD), coronary arteriography is generally recommended in male donors >45 years of age and female donors >50–55 years of age. Risk factors for CAD may warrant angiography in even younger donors. While donor hearts with significant CAD or valvular disease have been successfully transplanted after concomitant surgical correction, this practice is not standard of care and should be reserved for the "alternate list" type patient. Donor factors which increase the risk for early and late post-transplant mortality include donor age (linear risk), using a cytomegalovirus (CMV) positive donor heart in a CMV negative recipient, using a female donor heart in a male recipient, and longer donor heart ischemic time (linear) [5,8,10,13]. Even though most centers try to match donor/recipient size to within 80% (donor weight range 80–120% of recipient), most large multicenter registries have failed to identify size matching or mismatching as a significant predictor of outcome. Recipient size (height, weight, and body mass index (BMI)) is predictive of poorer

outcomes but donor size or size matching has not been [5]. Over-sizing (larger donor than recipient) is generally only a problem if the recipient has a small mediastinal space, such as a small adult, adolescent or child, or the recipient has a non-dilated cardiomyopathy. Under-sizing can be a particular problem in the setting of recipient pulmonary hypertension where the undersized right ventricle is unable to generate the systolic pressure required to overcome the high pulmonary artery pressure. As noted above, using a small female donor in a male recipient is higher risk, but it does not appear to be due only to the size mismatch. However, under-sizing with an adult male donor is generally acceptable, because a normal heart from an average-sized male donor can usually support even the largest recipients.

Cardiac transplant surgery

There are three donor heart implantation techniques used currently: the traditional Lower–Shumway or bi-atrial orthotopic technique [19], the bi-caval or "anatomic" orthotopic technique [20], and the rarely used heterotopic or "piggyback" technique [21]. Concerns about the development of significant tricuspid valve regurgitation, sinus node dysfunction, and atrial arrhythmias with the traditional bi-atrial technique led to the development and application of the bi-caval technique. While the bi-caval technique may result in slightly longer ischemic times (20 min or less on average), there appears to be less atrial arrhythmias, sinus node dysfunction, and tricuspid valve regurgitation [22].

In the traditional bi-atrial technique, the recipient heart is transected at the mid-atrial level, leaving behind the cuff of the right atrium containing the vena cava and the cuff of the left atrium containing the pulmonary vein ostia. The donor heart left atrial cuff is created by removing a matching area of the left atrium containing the pulmonary vein ostia. The donor and recipient left atria are then anastomosed with running suture ending with the atrial septum. The donor right atrium is opened from the inferior vena cava (IVC) toward the atrial appendage and away from the sinus node. The donor and recipient atria are then anastomosed with running suture beginning with the atrial septum, overlapping the left atrial side of the septal anastomosis.

The great vessels are trimmed to fit and anastomosed end-to-end with running suture.

In the bi-caval technique, the recipient left atrial cuff is prepared just as in the bi-atrial technique. The recipient right atrium is excised leaving only small atrial cuffs around the vena cava for sizing. The donor left atrium is prepared and anastomosed to the recipient left atrium similar to the bi-atrial technique. The donor atrial/caval cuffs are anastomosed end-to-end to the recipient atrial/caval cuffs. The great vessels are trimmed to fit and anastomosed end-to-end just as in the bi-atrial technique.

The heterotopic technique involves leaving the native heart in place and placing the donor heart in such a position to create a parallel circuit or "piggy-backing" as it is sometimes referred to. The donor heart is placed into the right chest with anastomoses between the donor and recipient left atria, donor right atrium and/or superior vena cava (SVC) and recipient right atrium and/or SVC, the donor and recipient aortas (end-to-side), and donor pulmonary artery and recipient pulmonary artery via a prosthetic conduit or directly into the recipient right pulmonary artery. The heterotopic technique is rarely used today (<1% of heart transplant procedures). Two situations where it was most often employed included: (1) large recipients with significant pulmonary hypertension when the available donor heart is small and (2) use of a small donor heart as a "biologic" left or right ventricular assist device. In the current era, mechanical assist devices can safely support patients with significant pulmonary hypertension providing enough time for significant "reversal" of the supposedly fixed hypertension, thus allowing successful transplantation even with smaller donor organs. In addition, mechanical assist devices have progressed enough in reliability and efficacy to replace the heterotopic transplant as an "assist" device.

Post-operative cardiac allograft function

The early post-operative allograft function is dependent on a variety of concomitant factors including pre-operative donor heart function, donor inotrope/vasoconstrictor use, donor heart ischemic time, effectiveness of cardiac preservation techniques, and acute cardiac denervation. The donor heart usually requires 2–5 days of low-dose inotropic and/or chronotropic agents, such as isoproterenol, dopamine, dobutamine, milrinone, or epinephrine. As ischemic injury is often associated with significant diastolic dysfunction as well, the donor heart may require higher than normal cardiac filling pressure to maintain adequate cardiac output. When a small heart with acutely limited contractile reserve is unable to maintain adequate cardiac outputs, it may be helpful to temporarily pace or use chronotropic agents to keep the heart rate (HR) 100–130, thus raising cardiac output. Right ventricular failure is an ominous post-operative sign and the result of pre-existing recipient pulmonary artery hypertension, acute post-operative pulmonary arteriolar vasoconstriction, or donor heart ischemic injury. The treatment includes pulmonary artery vasodilators, such as milrinone, prostaglandins, nitroprusside or nitric oxide (if available), and inotropic agents. Occasionally temporary mechanical right ventricular assistance is required. The best treatment for post-operative right ventricular failure is *prevention* by careful attention to pre-operative pulmonary artery pressures in those on the waiting list, avoidance of long ischemic times and small donor hearts in patients with known pulmonary artery hypertension, and meticulous hemostasis to avoid large volume transfusions which can precipitate acute pulmonary artery hypertension.

Cardiac denervation causes important changes in drug responsiveness. Due to vagal denervation, digoxin, atropine, edrophonium, and quinidine will not affect aortic valve (AV) nodal conduction. Later post-operatively, supersensitivity to adenosine and direct-acting catecholamines, such as epinephrine, isoproterenol, and dobutamine, can be seen due to adenosine receptor and adrenergic receptor upregulation. Sympathomimetic drugs that act indirectly through the cardiac nerve terminals such as dopamine and ephedrine are less effective as inotropes or chronotropes in the denervated heart.

Immunosuppressive therapy

While primary allograft dysfunction and surgical complications account for approximately 80% of the early mortalities (<30 days), issues related to immunosuppression, either "too much" or "too little", account for 50–70% of mortalities after 30 days [8]. With the current 30-day mortality rates of

<10%, the overwhelming majority of the post-transplant deaths occur after 30 days. Thus, the "perfect" immunosuppressive regimen would save many more lives that the "perfect" surgical technique or donor organ.

Immunosuppressive regimens have changed significantly since the first human heart transplant in 1967. The early days of azathioprine, high-dose corticosteroids, and later anti-thymocyte globulin (ATG) gave way to the "cyclosporine era" in the early 1980s. Cyclosporine, in combination with lower doses of corticosteroids and azathioprine became the standard cocktail in the mid-1980s and was often referred to as "triple-drug therapy". The addition of antilymphocyte preparations back into the regimen, using ATG or OKT3, became popular but failed to demonstrate superiority over "triple therapy" alone. The 1990s saw the introduction of tacrolimus as an alternative to cyclosporine in heart transplantation and the introduction of mycophenolate mofetil as an alternative to azathioprine. In recent years, we have seen the introduction of rapamycin and a derivative of rapamycin and new humanized, monoclonal antilymphocyte preparations (namely the anti-interleukin-2 receptor antagonists) into clinical heart transplantation. There are several new immunosuppressive agents and strategies ready to be tested in the upcoming years (Table 13.5).

An "ideal" regimen must, by definition, be free of significant side effects, highly effective and relatively cost-effective – a far cry from our current regimens. In fact, the only "perfect" chronic immunosuppressive drug regimen would be a NO-drug regimen, that is, complete and permanent allograft acceptance without the need for ongoing immunosuppressive drugs, so-called "allograft tolerance." Tolerance has been demonstrated in many animal models, including primate models and on a limited basis in unique human situations.

Cardiac allograft rejection
Basic mechanisms of allograft rejection
A working knowledge of the basic immunobiology of allograft rejection is crucial to understanding the rationale for immunosuppressive strategies. It is currently believed that the immune system–allograft interaction begins when a variety of immune cells, including T-lymphocytes and antigen presenting cells (APC), adhere to the vascular endothelium of the transplanted organ. An interaction between so-called "adhesion molecules" on the immune cells and their ligands on the endothelial cell surface begins the process. Quiescent endothelial cells are induced to express adhesion molecules by ischemia, surgical manipulation or cytokines, resulting in leukocyte adhesion, and transmigration. Thus, the adhesion molecule/ligand interaction plays a pivotal role in the immune response, and offers a potential target for attenuating the overall immunologic response. Transplanted organs undergo damage from anoxia or surgical manipulation and consequently upregulate endothelial adhesion molecules. Thus, prophylactic blockade employing antibodies against one or more of these components may attenuate initial T-cell responses during engraftment. The major adhesion molecule–ligand pairs involved are CD2–LFA3 (leukocyte function associated antigen-3) and ICAM1 (intercellular adhesion molecule-1)–LFA1, which enhance the interaction of T-cells with both endothelium and APC. Blockade of these interactions has been shown to attenuate immune response in a wide variety of animal models, and initial clinical experience is encouraging.

It is generally believed that T-cells become activated against alloantigen by one of two pathways: (1) a "direct" interaction with foreign antigens presented by endothelial cells, myocytes or passenger dendritic cells in association with donor major histocompatibility complex (MHC) antigens and (2) "indirect" interaction with foreign peptides processed and presented by recipient APC. This presentation of antigen leads to a series of intracellular events resulting in an "activated" T-cell which secretes various cytokines, including interleukin-2 (IL-2). Amplification of this T-cell response occurs due to the self-expression of IL-2 receptor, occupancy by IL-2, and stimulation of T-cell proliferation. Other cytokines secreted (interferon-gamma (IFN-gamma), tumor necrosis factor-alpha (TNF-alpha), IL-4, IL-5, and IL-6) stimulate the activation and proliferation of macrophages, B-cells, and other cells involved in the inflammatory response. The immune cascade, involving helper T-cells, cytotoxic T-cells, natural killer (NK) cells, B-cells, antibodies and complement, ultimately leads to damage of the donor endothelial cells, vascular

Table 13.5 Pharmacology of common immunosuppressive agents.

Agent	Identification	Mechanism of action	Administration	Toxicity	Drug interactions/uses
Cyclosporine*	Cyclic e-decapeptide produced by the fungus *Tolypocadium inflatum Gams*	Binds to cyclophilin, inhibits calcineurin dependent transcription and translation of cytokine genes, particularly IL-2	PO or IV, oral to IV dose adjustment is 3:1, marked individual variation in bioavailability, oral dose 6–8 mg/kg/day, targeted to level or toxicity	Renal, hypertension, gingival hyperplasia, hirsutism, tremor, headache, parasthesias, flushing	Metabolism decreased by: ketoconazole, diltiazem, verapamil, erythromycin, cimetidine, grapefruit; Metabolism increased, by: dilantin, phenobarbital, isoniazid, rifampin, carbamazepine; used in chronic maintenance immunosuppression
Tacrolimus	Macrolide isolate of *Streptomyces tsukubaensis*	Binds to FKBP, inhibits calcineurin-dependent transcription and translation of cytokine genes, particularly IL-2	PO or IV, oral to IV dose adjustment is 5:1, marked individual variation in bioavailability, oral dose 0.05–0.15 mg/kg/day, targeted to level or toxicity	Renal, hypertension, tremor, headache, flushing, parasthesias, glucose intolerance	Metabolism decreased by: ketoconazole, diltiazem, verapamil, erythromycin, cimetidine, grapefruit; Metabolism increased by: dilantin, phenobarbital, isoniazid, rifampin, carbamazepine; used in chronic maintenance immunosuppression, may substitute for cyclosporine to treat rejection
Azathioprine	Pro-drug of 6-mercaptopurine	Inhibits purine ring biosynthesis, decreasing synthesis of DNA and RNA	PO or IV, no significant oral to IV adjustment, 1–2 mg/kg/day, WBC count to remain >4500/mm^3	Macrocytic anemia, leukopenia, pancreatitis, cholestatic jaundice, hepatitis	Allopurinol slows metabolism by inhibiting xanthine oxidase. When used with allopurinol, azathioprine dose is decrease by two-thirds and WBC monitored, used in chronic maintenance immunosuppression
Mycophenolate mofetil	Morpholinoethylester of mycophenolic acid	Inhibits IMPDH, inhibiting the *de novo* pathway for guanine nucleotide biosynthesis	PO or IV, no significant oral to IV adjustment, 2000–6000 mg/day	Gastrointestinal distress, leukopenia	No significant interactions; used in chronic maintenance immunosuppression, may substitute for azathioprine to treat rejection

(Continued)

Table 13.5 (Continued)

Agent	Identification	Mechanism of action	Administration	Toxicity	Drug interactions/uses
Sirolimus (rapamycin)	Macrocyclic triene antibiotic produced by *Streptomyces hygroscopicus*	Binds to FKBP, inhibits IL-2 and IL-6 driven events	Sirolimus: PO, loading dose 5–6 mg, then 1–2 mg/day, based on toxicity and/or levels	Hypertriglyceridemia, thrombocytopenia, leukopenia	Metabolism decreased by diltiazem and ketoconazole; Metabolism increased by rifampin; interactions likely similar to cyclosporine; used in chronic maintenance and treatment of rejection
Everolimus (SDZ-RAD)	Derivative of rapamycin	Same as rapamycin	Everolimus: (not FDA approved for solid organ transplantation. In heart trial doses of 0.75 and 1.5 mg orally bid were used)	Same as rapamycin	Same as rapamycin
Cyclophosphamide	Type of nitrogen mustard	Activated by a cytochrome P-450-catalyzed reaction in the liver to form alkylating species, crosslinks DNA preventing lymphocyte proliferation	PO or IV, oral to IV dose adjustment is 1.4:1. Oral dose is 0.5–1.0 mg/kg/day, WBC to remain >4500/mm^3	Pancytopenia, hemorrhagic cystitis, alopecia	Additive effect with other inhibitors of lymphocyte proliferation, may substitute in the short term to treat vascular rejection
Methotrexate	Folic acid analogue	Inhibits dihydrofolate reductase, inhibiting purine biosynthesis	PO or IV, oral to IV dose adjustment is 1.4:1. Oral dose is 7.5–15 mg/week, WBC to remain >4500/mm^3	Pancytopenia, mucositis, alopecia, cirrhosis	Additive effect with other inhibitors of lymphocyte proliferation, may be used in recurring or refractory rejection
Corticosteroids	Synthetic or semi-synthetic analogues of adrenocorticotropic hormones	Lymphocytolysis, inhibits release and action of various IL, interferes with antigen-receptor interactions	PO or IV with methyl-prednisolone and hydrocortisone (no significant oral to IV dose adjustment), PO with prednisone, prednisone 1 mg = hydrocortisone 4 mg =	Pituitary–adrenal suppression, cushingoid habitus, glucose intolerance, hyperlipidemia, hypertension, posterior subcapsular cataracts, myopathy,	Multiple drug interactions, none clinically significant; used in chronic maintenance immunosuppression and in the treatment of established rejection episodes

(Continued)

Table 13.5 (Continued)

Agent	Identification	Mechanism of action	Administration	Toxicity	Drug interactions/uses
			methylprednisolone 0.8 mg; maintenance dose prednisone 0.0–0.1 mg/kg/day	osteoporosis, skin fragility, PUD	
Muromonab-CD3 antibody (OKT3)	IgG$_{2A}$ murine monoclonal immunoglobulin molecule	Binds to the CD3 surface antigen of lymphocytes, inhibits antigen recognition, opsonizes lymphocytes	IV only, 2.5–5 mg/day	Fever, chills, gastrointestinal distress, pulmonary edema, HAMA formation	No interactions; used in early rejection prophylaxis and in the treatment of rejection
ATG	Equine polyclonal antibodies to human thymocytes	Opsonizes lymphocytes	IV only, 10–20 mg/kg/day	Fever, chills, serum sickness, leukopenia, thrombocytopenia	No interactions; used in early rejection prophylaxis and in the treatment of rejection
Thymoglobulin	Rabbit polyclonal antibodies to human thymocytes	Opsonizes lymphocytes	IV only, 1.5 mg/kg/day	Fever, chills, serum sickness, leukopenia, thrombocytopenia	No interactions; used in early rejection prophylaxis and in the treatment of rejection
Daclizumab	Chimeric monoclonal IgG1 antibody	Blocks the IL-2 receptor alpha chain	1 mg/kg IV once before transplant repeated an additional four times at 2-week intervals	Gastrointestinal distress	No interactions; used in early rejection prophylaxis
Basiliximab	Chimeric monoclonal IgG$_{1K}$ antibody	Blocks the IL-2 receptor alpha chain	20 mg IV 2 h before transplant and repeated 4 days after	Gastrointestinal distress	No interactions; used in early rejection prophylaxis

*Cyclosporine is available in two formulations, oil based and microemulsion based. The latter is associated with better bioavailability.

IL: interleukin; PO: by mouth; IV: intravenous; WBC: white blood cell count; PUD: peptic ulcer disease; HAMA: human antimouse antibody; FKBP: FK binding protein; IMPDH: inosine monophosphate dehydrogenase; SDZ-RAD: sirolimus (rapamycin) and its derivative, everolimus; FDA: Food and Drug Administration.

Modified with permission from Renlund DG, Taylor DO. In: Topol EJ, ed. *Cardiac Transplantation in Textbook of Cardiovascular Medicine*, 2nd edn. Lippincott Williams & Wilkins, 2002: 1923–1924.

smooth muscle cells, myocytes, and intracellular matrix manifesting as "allograft rejection."

The T-cell response is initiated by the direct or indirect presentation of the alloantigen and binding to the T-cell receptor (TCR)/CD3 complex. This leads to activation of several tyrosine kinases such as p56-Lck, p59-Fyn, and ZAP-70. The ensuing phosphorylation-activation of phospholipase C (PLC) leads ultimately to a rise in intracellular calcium. Calcium along with calmodulin activates the serine-threonine phosphatase calcineurin. Calcineurin dephosphorylates the cytoplasmic subunit of nuclear factor of activated T-cells (NFAT-c), enabling its translocation to the nucleus, where it complexes with the nuclear subunit (NFAT-n). This complex binds to the promoter regions of various cytokine genes, especially the IL-2 promoter, upregulating transcription. IL-2, in both an autocrine and paracrine fashion, activates the proliferative pathways in the activated T-cells, as well as other immune cells. Cyclosporine and tacrolimus (formerly FK506), in complex with their cytoplasmic binding proteins, cyclophilins, and FK binding proteins (FKBP), respectively, inhibit the function of calcineurin and thus downregulate expression of IL-2 and other cytokines. Helper T-cells utilize the CD4 molecule which is closely associated with the TCR, and plays a major role in immune amplification. Blocking the function of the CD4 molecule can selectively block the response of a helper T-cell to MHC class II-alloantigen complex.

Once IL-2 binds to its receptor on the T-cell, a series of intracellular events occur via activation of various cyclin kinases. These kinases are important cell cycle regulatory proteins. In order for the cell to proliferate and the immune response amplify, the activated T-cell must progress through the cell cycle. As in most dividing cells, the cell must pass from the G1 state to the synthetic (S) phase which is dependent on nucleic acid synthesis in preparation for mitosis. Antimetabolites, like azathioprine, cyclophosphamide, and methotrexate act to inhibit DNA synthesis during this crucial phase of cell replication. Lymphocytes are primarily dependent on the *de novo* pathway of purine and pyrimidine synthesis unlike other cells capable of rapid division, where the "salvage" pathways can contribute to a significant extent. Mycophenolate mofetil, by inhibiting a key enzyme of the *de novo* pathway,

inosine monophosphate dehydrogenase (IMPDH), blocks the proliferative response of T-cells. Sirolimus (rapamycin) and its derivative, everolimus (formerly SDZ-RAD) acts to block several events downstream of the IL-2 receptor. This drug binds to the same binding proteins as tacrolimus (primarily FKBP-12), but rather than inhibiting calcineurin, it inhibits cytoplasmic proteins collectively termed target of rapamycin (TOR) proteins. These proteins are required for cell cycle progression in response to IL-2 stimulation, and hence sirolimus and everolimus are able to block the proliferative response of T-cells after immune activation. Sirolimus and everolimus inhibits 70 kD S6 kinase (p70s6k), preventing the phosphorylation of S6 ribosomal protein, which is thought to be involved in translation of cell cycle regulatory proteins. The IL-2 receptor itself can be blocked or inactivated by monoclonal antibodies directed against specific components of the receptor complex. Two such agents, basiliximab and daclizumab, are currently in human trials and appear promising.

Another critical event in T-cell activation involves the "co-stimulatory" signals, which are antigen-independent pathways that significantly enhance the T-cell responses. It is currently believed that these "co-stimulatory" signals are necessary for full activation of the T-cell. Activation of the TCR without a co-stimulatory signal leads to programmed cell death or anergy, rather than activation. The CD28 and CD40 molecules and their ligands are the two best studied co-stimulatory signals to date. The CD28 molecule, found on T-cells, interacts with its ligand (B7-1 (CD80), B7-2 (CD86), and B7-3) on activated APCs. This interaction amplifies the T-cell response by downregulating IκBα which leads to enhanced translocation of a CD28 response element (c-Rel) to the nucleus, where it upregulates IL-2 gene expression. The second co-stimulatory signal involves the interaction between CD40 on the APC with its ligand on activated T-cells CD154 (gp 39), a member of the TNF family. This interaction has effects on both T- and B-cells. In the B-cell, this signal leads to direct activation. In B-cells and other APCs the signal causes upregulation of the expression of B7-1, B7-2, and B7-3. Upregulation of B7 molecules will lead to an increased CD28/B7 signal, amplifying the immune response as noted above. In small and large animal models, blockade of these co-stimulatory

Table 13.6 ISHLT cardiac biopsy grading scale [23].

ISHLT grade	Histopathologic findings	Original "Billingham" grade
0	No evidence of rejection	No rejection
1A	Focal (perivascular or interstitial) infiltrates without myocyte necrosis	Mild rejection
1B	Diffuse but sparce infiltrates without myocyte necrosis	Mild rejection
2	Only one focus of aggressive lymphocytic infiltration and/or myocyte damage	Focal moderate rejection
3A	Multifocal aggressive infiltrates and/or myocyte damage	Moderate rejection
3B	Diffuse inflammatory infiltrates with myocyte damage	Borderline severe
4	Diffuse aggressive polymorphous inflammatory infiltrates with myocyte necrosis. May include edema, hemorrhage, or vasculitis	Severe rejection

pathways markedly attenuates the immune response to the transplanted organ. Sirolimus is also thought to interfere with this pathway by inhibiting the down-regulation of IκBα.

In summary, current immunosuppressive agents and strategies attempt to:

1 prevent the initial activation of the T-cell by interfering with the TCR complex;
2 prevent activation of the co-stimulatory pathways by blockade of these receptors;
3 interfere with the downstream effects of TCR activation, namely IL-2 production;
4 prevent activation of the IL-2 receptor;
5 interfere with the downstream effects of IL-2 receptor activation, namely cell cycling and proliferation.

Classification of cardiac allograft rejection

Traditionally rejection was often classified (temporally) as hyperacute (occurring minutes to hours after transplantation), acute (days to months), and chronic (months to years). The most ominous form of rejection, hyperacute rejection, generally caused by preformed anti-human leukocyte antigen (HLA) antibodies, has been greatly reduced by pre-operative screening for allo-reactive antibodies and prospective, donor-specific crossmatching in sensitized recipients, and nowadays is an extremely rare event. Acute cellular rejection remains a significant problem in solid organ transplantation and has at its core, the T-lymphocyte-mediated immune response. Acute vascular rejection involves both the cellular and humoral immune systems and is often associated with severe allograft dysfunction and mortality. Allograft vasculopathy or "chronic rejection" is a complex process that involves both immunologic injury and vascular proliferative responses.

Cardiac allograft rejection is now most often classified histologically. Table 13.6 shows the current ISHLT classification scheme [23]. In addition to their histologic grade, a clinical qualifier is often added such as "with or without hemodynamic compromise," "treated with augmented immuno-suppression or untreated," etc. While changes in cardiac function can be associated with significant rejection and can be demonstrated by invasive hemodynamic monitoring or echocardiography, the "gold-standard" for the diagnosis of rejection remains the endomyocardial biopsy. It is performed percutaneously generally via the right internal jugular or femoral vein using a specially designed bioptome. It is felt that the ability to diagnose early rejection, before irreversible graft damage occurs, justifies the use of endomyocardial biopsy as a surveillance technique. Since the great majority of acute rejection episodes occurs in the first 6 months post-operatively (actually, the first 3 months), the frequency of biopsies is greatest early on. A typical protocol would involve weekly biopsies for the first 4–6 weeks, every other week for the next 4–6 weeks, every 3–4 weeks for the next 6–12 weeks, every 4–6 weeks for the next 6–12 weeks, every 6–8 weeks until 1 year post-operatively. Thereafter the frequency decreases with rare programs eliminating surveillance biopsies altogether after year 1, but the majority of programs decreasing the frequency to every 3–6 months. The benefit of surveillance biopsies in asymptomatic long-term survivors (>5 years) is unclear. Surveillance for "chronic rejection" or allograft CAD is generally performed with yearly coronary angiography (see allograft vasculopathy paragraph below).

Basic immunosuppressive regimens

Currently, the "standard" maintenance immunosuppression protocols for heart transplantation (so-called "triple therapy") include: (1) a calcineurin inhibitor (CNI) such as cyclosporine or tacrolimus, (2) an antiproliferative agent such as azathioprine (AZA), mycophenolate mofetil (MMF), or rarely cyclophosphamide, and (3) corticosteroids such as prednisone or prednisolone. Many centers also add an antilymphocyte antibody such as ATG, OKT3, or an IL-2 receptor blocker (basiliximab or daclizumab) to create a "quadruple-drug" regimen. In the setting of pre-transplant renal insufficiency, a popular protocol involves delaying the initiation of the CNIs for 4–10 days post-operatively to allow for recovery of renal function and using antilymphocyte antibody therapy in the interim, so-called "sequential therapy." Significant controversy remains regarding which agent within each of the first two categories is preferred, whether corticosteroids are required long term, and the role of the antilymphocyte antibody therapies. According to the most recent data from the Registry of ISHLT [8], approximately 47% of patients transplanted from 1999–2001 received perioperative antilymphocyte antibody therapy, approximately half of these receiving ATG, the rest divided equally between OKT3 and IL-2 antibodies. Approximately 72% of these patients were receiving cyclosporine at year 1 as their CNI, compared to 25% receiving tacrolimus. Approximately 70% of these patients were receiving mycophenolate mofetil at year 1 as their antiproliferative agent, compared to 15% receiving azathioprine, and only 3% receiving rapamycin; 82% of patients were receiving some dose of corticosteroids at 1 year.

CNIs: cyclosporine versus tacrolimus therapy

Two single center (University of Pittsburgh [24] and University of Munich [25]) and two multicenter (US [26] and European [27]) trials have suggested at least equivalent and perhaps better anti-rejection properties of tacrolimus when compared with cyclosporine with significantly less hyperlipidemia, hirsutism, and hypertension associated with tacrolimus use. The incidence of renal dysfunction

is similar between the two agents and the incidence of new or worsening diabetes is only minimally higher with tacrolimus use. Likewise, the costs and need for blood level monitoring is similar between the two agents. Currently the choice of agents seems to be dictated by institutional preference, individual patient efficacy, and side-effect profile.

The antiproliferatives: azathioprine versus mycophenolate mofetil therapy versus rapamycin

In the largest, randomized controlled trial in heart transplantation to date, MMF was compared to azathioprine in combination with cyclosporine and corticosteroids. In this study, reported by Kobashigawa *et al.* [28], 650 primary heart transplant recipients were randomized equally between the two study groups. Intent-to-treat analysis of all 650 randomized patients revealed no significant differences between the two study groups with regards to survival, rejection, or safety parameters. As intravenous MMF was not available during the time of this study, 72 patients unable to take oral medications by the sixth day after surgery were withdrawn without ever receiving study drug and three-fourths were placed on open-label azathioprine. These 72 patients experienced a high mortality or retransplant rate (56% by 1 year) and had more MMF assigned patients (38 versus 34). These facts, coupled with the 11% early cross-over rate (primarily in one direction) significantly affected the discriminatory power of the study. When the data were analyzed for only those 578 patients receiving at least one dose of the study drug (a more clinically relevant group), the MMF group experienced an 11% (2–22%, 95% confidence intervals) reduction in treated rejection episodes and a 34% (1–56%, 95% confidence intervals) reduction in biopsy-proven rejection episodes associated with severe hemodynamic compromise. In addition, the MMF-treated group experienced less mortality during the first 12 months post-transplant (6.2% versus 11.4%, $P = 0.031$). Of particular interest is the observation that during the 12 months post-transplant there were no deaths in the 19 patients in the MMF group who experienced an episode of severe hemodynamically compromising rejection as compared with 12 deaths (32%) in the 38 such patients in the AZA group. The whole of these data suggest that

MMF may be superior to AZA in preventing (and successfully treating) the more severe forms of allograft rejection. The adverse events in the two groups were similar except for more diarrhea, esophagitis, and opportunistic infection (primarily herpes virus) in the MMF group and more leukopenia in the AZA group.

SDZ-RAD have muddied the "antiproliferative" waters. They are potent antiproliferative agents and have made a major breakthrough in the field of coronary stenting where the introduction of rapamycin-eluting stents has almost eliminated re-stenosis in stented segments. However, the introduction of these drugs into solid organ transplantation has probably led to more questions than answers. It is unclear whether these agents are best used in place of the CNI, with mycophenolate and corticosteroids (as part of a so-called, "CNI-free" protocol) or with a CNI, in the place of mycophenolate or aza-thioprine. The currently completed and ongoing clinical trials in renal transplantation include both of these approaches. For heart transplantation, only the latter approach has been tried. In the Everolimus trial [29], 634 heart transplant recipients were randomized between two doses of everolimus (3.0 and 1.5 mg/day) and azathioprine (1–3 mg/kg/day) along with cyclosporine and corticosteroids. At 6 months, the two everolimus groups had significantly fewer efficacy failures (acute rejection 3A or higher, hemodynamically compromising rejection, death, graft loss, or lost-to-follow-up) than the AZA group (27% in 3 mg/day RAD group and 36.4% in the 1.5 mg/day RAD group versus 47.7% in the AZA group). The survival rates were not significantly different between the groups. The incidence of viral infections, primarily CMV, was significantly lower in the two RAD groups than the AZA group, and the incidence of bacterial infections was slightly higher in the RAD groups than the AZA group. Arguably the more exciting results of the trial is the effect on allograft vasculopathy, measured in this trial by 12-month intravascular ultrasound (IVUS) [29]. In a subgroup of 211 patients, post-operatively and 12-month IVUS images were compared. There was a significant difference in the primary IVUS endpoint (change in average maximal intimal thickness) between the AZA group and the two RAD groups (0.10 mm in AZA versus 0.03 mm in RAD 3 mg/day, and 0.04 mm

in RAD 1.5 mg/day). Similar differences were found in the secondary endpoints of average intimal area and volume. When allograft vasculopathy was defined as a maximal intimal thickness increase ≥ 0.5 mm, 52.8% of the AZA group, 35.7% of the RAD 1.5 mg/day group, and 30.4% of the RAD 3 mg/day group developed vasculopathy at 1 year.

A similar, but smaller trial comparing sirolimus to azathioprine has reported similar findings. Keogh *et al.* [30,31] randomized 136 heart transplant recipients to two doses of sirolimus (3 and 5 mg/day) versus azathioprine (2.5 mg/kg/day). At 6 months the incidence of acute rejection was significantly lower in the two SRL groups (29.4% in 3 mg/day and 36.2% in the 5 mg/day) when compared to the AZA group (61.4%). The mean maximal proximal coronary stenosis increased 41% in the AZA group as compared to only 4% in the combined SRL groups. Similarly, the maximal mid-vessel stenosis increased by 56% in the AZA group but increased only 5% in the combined SRL groups.

Whether these changes in IVUS-defined vasculopathy will translate into better long-term outcomes remains to be seen. However, given the good correlation between 1-year IVUS parameters and long-term outcome in prior studies, these results are quite encouraging. However, both of these studies compared sirolimus and everolimus to azathioprine rather than mycophenolate mofetil. The magnitude of difference in rejection rates between the groups was greater in the sirolimus/everolimus studies than the mycophenolate study [28]. Likewise, mycophenolate was not associated with a significant decrease in IVUS-defined vasculopathy at 12 months when compared to azathioprine [28].

In summary, it appears that mycophenolate mofetil has eclipsed azathioprine as the principle antiproliferative agent in heart transplantation, but, given these most recent study results, the role of sirolimus and everolimus should be expanding in the near future.

Chronic corticosteroid therapy

The role of corticosteroids in *chronic* immunosuppressive protocols remains unsettled. There has never been an appropriately sized, randomized controlled trial addressing this issue; however, there is much single center data supporting the use of corticosteroid-free maintenance protocols, at least in a substantial subgroup of patients. Few programs currently use a true corticosteroid-free protocol (double therapy with cyclosporine and azathioprine), but most programs attempt to wean corticosteroids completely off during the first 4–12 months, primarily in those patients who experience little or no acute allograft rejection. Most programs utilizing triple-drug protocols without antilymphocyte antibody induction therapy attempt to completely withdraw corticosteroid no sooner than 4–6 months post-transplant, whereas the programs with the earliest corticosteroid withdrawal (2 days to 2 months) use "quadruple-drug" protocols (standard triple therapy plus antilymphocyte antibody therapy). While it is arguable whether patients experiencing multiple rejection episodes early after transplant should be weaned completely off corticosteroids late after transplant, it seems clear that patients who experience little or no acute allograft rejection episodes can be safely maintained without corticosteroids. Taylor *et al.* [32] reported outcomes in 374 patients who received antilymphocyte antibody therapy (primarily OKT3) along with cyclosporine and azathioprine and tapering doses of corticosteroid until discontinued over a 5–6-week period post-operatively. Early mild or moderate rejection episodes were treated with augmented corticosteroids followed by another weaning attempt. Early corticosteroid weaning was abandoned if a severe cellular rejection, vascular rejection, or more than two treated mild–moderate rejection episodes occurred. One hundred and eleven (30%) patients were successfully weaned early from corticosteroids and experienced an excellent long-term survival (82%, 10-year actuarial) which was significantly better than the remaining patients (36%, 10-year actuarial). While these data do not suggest that it was the lack of corticosteroids that led to the excellent survival, it seems unlikely that the addition of corticosteroids back to the regimen of these patients could have improved survival further.

Combination therapy

With prednisone, two CNI's, at least three antiproliferative agents, and at least four antilymphocyte antibodies, the number of possible combinations is quite large. In small, case control reports just about every possible combination has been tried. However, in the larger clinical trials (including those discussed above) the combinations have included primarily:

1 cyclosporine, AZA, and prednisone;
2 cyclosporine, MMF, and prednisone;
3 tacrolimus, AZA, and prednisone;
4 cyclosporine, everolimus, and prednisone;
5 cyclosporine, sirolimus, and prednisone.

Protocols 1–4 have included anti-thymocyte antibodies OKT3 or ATG in selected patients. These combinations have proved safe and effective in heart transplantation. Several other combinations are now undergoing evaluation.

A small, single center study from the University of Munich [25] suggests that the combination of tacrolimus, MMF, and corticosteroids may be more effective than cyclosporine, MMF, and corticosteroids especially when MMF dosing is adjusted to blood levels rather than administered as a fixed dose. The infection risks associated with this combination seemed acceptable. It appears that equivalent doses of MMF are associated with higher MPA levels when combined with tacrolimus as compared to cyclosporine. Preliminary evidence suggests that cyclosporine decreases the MPA level slightly by affecting intestinal absorption and enterohepatic recirculation of MPA whereas tacrolimus has a neutral effect on MPA pharmacokinetics.

The treatment of acute rejection

The treatment of acute cardiac rejection depends on the histologic grade, the clinical situation and the prior rejection history. In general, mild rejection episodes (ISHLT grade 1A, 1B, low-grade 2) are often treated only by optimizing the current immunosuppression. Moderate rejections episodes (advanced 2, 3A, low-grade 3B) are usually treated with significantly augmented immunosuppression, such as an oral or intravenous pulse of corticosteroids and optimization of background immunosuppression. Severe rejection (ISHLT grade 4) is generally treated with high-dose intravenous corticosteroids, anti-thymocyte antibodies (such as OKT3 or ATG) and optimization of background immunosuppression. Due to the contribution of the humoral immune system (B-lymphocytes, plasma cells, and anti-allograft antibodies), acute vascular rejection is generally treated with high-dose intravenous corticosteroids, pulsed oral or intravenous cyclophosphamide, anti-thymocyte antibody, and plasmapheresis. Hemodynamically compromising rejection, regardless of the biopsy grade, is associate with poor short- and long-term outcomes and must be treated aggressively. Those associated with minimal cellular infiltrates (ISHLT 0, 1) are often presumed to be a "vascular type" and treated accordingly, whereas those associated with moderate cellular infiltrates (ISHLT 3) are usually treated as outlined above for "severe (ISHLT 4)."

Patients with recurrent rejection despite optimal drug doses/levels often require conversion to the alternative CNI, conversion to an alternative antiproliferative, addition of another immunosuppressive agents, and even total lymphoid irradiation in refractory cases. For example, tacrolimus can be substituted for cyclosporine, mycophenolate mofetil substituted for azathioprine, sirolimus substituted for or added to mycophenolate mofetil or azathioprine, etc.

The future: new agents, gene therapy, and creating tolerance

While most of the current clinical investigative effort is focused on better utilizing the immunosuppressive agents we have available, there a few new agents in animal studies and early clinical trials. None, however, seem at this stage to be "breakthrough" drugs. Gene therapy is a promising technique that is currently being investigated. The ability to genetically alter a donor organ could 1 day revolutionize organ transplantation. Attempts at "humanizing" xenografts are well underway primarily using transgenic pig models. Genetic manipulation of these pigs to express human complement regulatory proteins has led to marked attenuation of the typical hyperacute xenograft rejection. Genetic manipulation utilizing gene transfection (both viral and non-viral) has been successfully performed in animals. A variety of genes have been targeted. Over-expression of both TGF-b1 and IL-10 has been associated with improved murine allograft survival. Likewise over-expression of CTLA4-Ig in murine liver transplantation is associated with mononuclear infiltrates but no parenchymal damage (suggestive of local T-cell anergy). Causing apoptosis of the infiltrating allo-reactive immune cells by over-expression of Fas-ligand in the graft would seem like a potentially successful approach. However, experimental trials of this method have generally failed. The major limitation of the current transfection technology is the durability of the transfection. Unlike transgenic organs, transfected organs would require repeated treatments to maintain gene expression. Despite its limitations, gene therapy will likely play a significant role in the future of transplantation.

Allograft tolerance: the Holy Grail

Simply put, the best immunosuppressive agent is *no* immunosuppressive agent. Unless an immunosuppressive agent is capable of affecting *only* the allo-reactive immune cells, there will always be the risk of "collateral damage" or toxicity. Given the tremendous redundancy in the human immune system it is unlikely that such a drug or combination of drugs will be developed in the near future. Thus only "immunologic" tolerance can provide the results we strive for: indefinite allograft (or xenograft) function, otherwise normal immune function, without the risks or complications of ongoing immunosuppressive therapy. In the majority of patients, current drug regimens lead to (or allow) some degree of tolerance (as demonstrated by long-term graft function despite decreasing immunosuppressive drug requirements, and the lack of late cellular rejection). However, this tolerance is incomplete (as demonstrated by the ultimate destruction of the graft) and non-durable (as evidenced by the ability to induce acute rejection by decreasing or stopping immunosuppressive drugs or by acute viral infections). While a complete discussion of tolerance is well beyond the scope of this chapter (see Refs [33,34] for more detailed discussions), a few basic concepts are worth noting. Immunologic tolerance has been demonstrated in a variety of non-human transplant models, utilizing a variety of techniques, and based on a variety of immunologic mechanisms. The more commonly invoked mechanisms of tolerance include: chimerism (both macro and micro), clonal deletion, clonal anergy, immune deviation (i.e. Th1:Th2 paradigm), and suppressor and "veto" cells. Unfortunately it seems that different mechanisms (and multiple mechanisms) are operative in the different animal models and with different tolerizing techniques, thus it is unclear which mechanism should be pursued in human heart transplantation.

Chimerism, while allowing a quite durable and complete tolerance, requires lethal irradiation and salvage with allogeneic bone marrow transplantation. Given the current results with non-HLA-identical, allogeneic bone marrow transplantation, this technique has not been applied to human heart transplantation. Based on data from the University of Pittsburgh [35] demonstrating the presence of donor-derived immune cells in patients with long-term graft survival (so-called micro-chimerism), several groups are performing bone-marrow-augmented cardiac transplantation in an attempt to facilitate the development of this micro-chimeric state. However, it is not clear whether the donor-derived cells are actually *responsible for* the long-term graft acceptance or simply are present *because of* the lack of allo-reactivity to the donor (to both the graft and the passenger immune cells). Preliminary results from the University of Pittsburgh [36] suggest a modest improvement in rejection incidence with bone marrow augmentation in heart and lung recipients but no evidence of true tolerance. Attempts at clonal deletion or clonal anergy are arguably the most promising techniques. As discussed in the immuno-biology paragraph above, it has been demonstrated that T-lymphocytes require at least two major signals from the APC to become activated: (1) the TCR/MHC-antigen interaction (often called signal 1 and 2) a co-stimulatory signal involving CD28 on the T-cell and its ligands B7.1/B7.2 (CD80/CD86) (often called signal 2). In addition the interaction between CD154 (CD40 ligand) on the T-cell and its receptor CD40 on the APC is facilitated by signal 1 which then facilitates signal 2. It has been demonstrated in animal models that activation of signal 1 without signal 2 can cause anergy or apoptosis of the T-cell. Interference with signal 2 by administration of antibodies directed at the CD28 or a related receptor CTLA4 while allowing signal 1 to proceed has successfully induced tolerance in animal models. In fact, in one of the most promising animal study to date, Kirk *et al.* [37] treated MHC-mismatched rhesus monkeys undergoing renal transplantation with antibodies against CTLA4 (human CTLA4-Ig) and CD40 ligand (5C8) briefly after transplant without other immunosuppressive drugs. Long-term graft survival without ongoing immunosuppression was demonstrated in several animals. However, this clinical tolerance was not durable as evidenced by late acute rejection episodes in several animals which, interestingly, responded to repeat treatment with these antibodies. In addition, apparently tolerant animals retained normal third-party reactivity as well as donor-reactivity in mixed lymphocyte culture despite the lack of acute rejection. This relatively simple and well-tolerated protocol holds promise for clinical transplantation and human renal transplant trials are currently underway.

A number of other methods have been successful in rodent models including donor-specific transfusions, therapy with peptides of MHC class I and II, intrathymic injection of donor antigen, monoclonal antibodies against a variety of receptors (anti-CD4, anti-CD45, anti-LFA, anti-ICAM1, anti-MHC class I and II antibodies), and increasing Fas-ligand expression in the allograft to cause apoptosis of the infiltrating T-cells.

Unfortunately, memory T-cells are quite difficult to tolerize as compared to naive T-cells, thus tolerizing strategies may not be effective in post-transplant patients already experiencing acute allograft rejection, and potential recipients with HLA-sensitization (especially those with failed grafts).

A very important point is that many of the proposed tolerance mechanism require a competent immune system. In fact, in some models tolerance can be broken by the administration of immunosuppressive agents. Thus our current immunosuppressive regimens, in addition to preventing acute allograft rejection, may also be preventing the development of tolerance. However, it will take a brave investigator and a brave patient to attempt a tolerizing strategy in human heart transplant that includes no long-term immunosuppressive therapy, given the severe consequences of failure. Due to this reality, tolerizing strategies of the (near) future will likely include some degree of underlying immunosuppression.

Cardiac allograft vasculopathy

Cardiac allograft vasculopathy (CAV) is the leading cause of death and a cause of significant morbidity after the first year post-transplant [5,8,10].

Angiographically detectable disease occurs in approximately 50% of recipients by 5 years. Studies utilizing IVUS suggest that the incidence is much greater. Until just recently, the improvements in immunosuppression had not greatly affected the incidence of CAV. The term "CAV" encompasses a wide variety of histologic, physiologic, and temporal findings. Early CAV (within 1–3 years) is usually characterized by diffuse and distal involvement. Late CAV (after 7 years) often is more proximal, focal, and eccentric.

Histologically, CAV is characterized by intense *concentric* and *diffuse* proliferation and migration of smooth muscle cells and macrophages, increased ground substance, foam cells, and lipid clefts, primarily occurring within the intimal layer [38]. Angiographically, several types of lesions have been described, including proximal focal stenoses (Type A), distal tapering of vessels (Type B), and distal obliteration of vessels (Type C) [39].

A variety of immunologic and non-immunologic risk factors have been identified for the development of CAV diagnosed by angiography, IVUS, or angioscopy [5,8,10,40–57]. Not surprisingly older donor hearts are associated with an increased risk for the development of CAV [5,8,10] at 3 years after transplantation. When CAD led to the need for cardiac transplantation, there is a 33% increased risk of developing CAV at 3 years [5,10]. The more common risk factors for atherosclerosis, hypertension, hyperlipidemia, diabetes, smoking, and hyperhomocysteinemia, may be important in the later phase of the disease (>5 years) [44,45]. Rejection history, HLA matching, increased levels of endothelin, the presence of endothelial cell-derived mesenchymal growth factors, CMV infection, the expression of various chemokines, cytokines, and/or, serum cardiac troponin-T concentrations, the quantity of various apolipoproteins, MHC class II expression, gene polymorphisms for plasminogen activation factors, the quantity of various anticoagulation factors, and even race/ethnicity have been associated with increased risk for CAV in small single center studies [46–57].

Diagnosis of CAV

As delayed and incomplete cardiac re-innervation, CAV rarely presents as angina, particularly in the first 5 years. The usual clinical presentations of CAV include acute myocardial infarction (MI), congestive heart failure, arrhythmias, wall motion abnormalities, or sudden death. Most CAV is diagnosed by routinely scheduled yearly surveillance angiography. However, given the often diffuse and distal nature of the disease and the lack of an effective treatment for the disease, some programs have abandoned surveillance angiography. Many have attempted to use noninvasive techniques to decrease the need for invasive testing and identify those patients who may benefit from traditional revascularization techniques [58–60]. Exercise or dobutamine stress echocardiography has been advocated as a useful screening tool to reduce the need for routine surveillance angiography. Dobutamine stress echocardiography may also be able to track the progression of established CAV [58]. A negative dobutamine stress echocardiogram is associated with a low risk of cardiac events. Nuclear techniques, for example, stress thallium scintigraphy and positron emission tomography have also been used [59,60]. Even angiography has its limitations. Due to the often diffuse and concentric nature of the vasculopathy, angiography, which is essentially a "lumen-o-gram," misses even severe disease. IVUS, which directly images the vessel wall is much more sensitive [61,62] and predicts the development of angiographic CAD and subsequent morbidity and mortality [61].

Treatment of CAV

Until recently, augmented immunosuppression has not been conclusively shown to prevent progression, or influence the development of cardiac adverse events. A small, single center study suggests that the conversion from azathioprine or mycophenolate to sirolimus may affect outcomes in patients with advance disease [63]. In a group of 46 patients with angiographic allograft vasculopathy, the 22 patients randomly assigned to rapamycin conversion experienced much fewer subsequent cardiac events (defined as death, MI, need for angioplasty or bypass surgery or >25% worsening of angiographic severity score) (3 points versus 14 points) during follow-up of <2 years [63]. This information, coupled with the results of the everolimus and simolimus trials discussed above, suggest that the addition of sirolimus or everolimus may be reasonable for patients with established CAV. The treatment of established disease is currently limited to re-transplantation and palliative revascularization techniques. Retransplantation is the only option for patients with Type B and C lesions; especially since transmyocardial laser revascularization is unlikely to be beneficial in the long term, using current techniques [64]. Retransplantation for CAV has been disappointing in the past, but currently, if performed more than 2 years after the initial transplantation, can result in survival rates only 5–10% below those of first time transplant recipients [5].

Percutaneous revascularization of proximal vessel lesions when the distal vessels are angiographically normal is associated with primary success and re-stenosis rates similar to those in native vessel interventions. However, because of the aggressive and diffuse nature of the disease, repeated procedures are often necessary to address new lesions. Unfortunately, in the presence of severe distal disease, percutaneous revascularization, even for Type A lesions, is associated with a poor outcome. Coronary artery bypass grafting has been used in rare situations with mixed results. Patients with normal ventricular function, and angiographically normal distal vessels appear to be the best candidates for surgical revascularization. Given the marginal results seen with retransplantation and the current donor/recipient disparity, aggressive use of interventional, and/or surgical techniques to prolong, if possible, the life of the cardiac allograft seems warranted.

Thus given the lack of successful treatment for CAV, strategies to prevent, halt progression or potentially reverse the disease should be a major focus. For both primary prevention and the prevention of progression of established disease, conventional risk factors for coronary disease should be eliminated, minimized, or controlled. While such risk-factor reduction may not affect the early aggressive form associated with intimal hyperplasia, the later form may be impacted. While there is conflicting data on the contribution of lipids in CAV, given the high incidence of glucose intolerance, hypertension, and hyperhomocysteinemia in transplant recipients, it seems reasonable to target low-density lipoprotein (LDL) cholesterol levels below 100 mg/dL even in patients without angiographic CAV.

Immunosuppression-related complications

Infectious complications

Infection is a major cause of morbidity and mortality after organ transplant recipients [8,65,66]. As the varying intensity of immunosuppression post-transplantation, the types of infections expected in cardiac transplant recipients vary relative to the time from transplantation. Although opportunistic fungal and parasitic infections are feared, bacteria, and viruses account for more than 80% of infections after transplantation. In the first 30 days after transplantation, nosocomial bacterial infections are the most common, such as wound infections, infected intravascular catheters/lines, or gram-negative urinary tract or pulmonary infections. The incidence of bacterial infections fall rapidly over the next month but plateaus at a constant level long term and remains a major cause of late infection. The incidence of viral, fungal, and parasitic infections peaks in the first 3–6 months post-transplantation, when therapy against *cell-mediated* immunity is at its greatest. The incidence then decreases slowly and achieves a low but constant level long term. The most common viral infections are caused by the herpes viruses: CMV, herpes zoster, and herpes simplex. In the past, CMV used to be associated with significant morbidity and mortality in heart transplant recipients but the introduction of ganciclovir has significantly improved the prognosis [67,68]. However, gan-ciclovir resistant CMV is occasionally seen. Patients who are CMV seronegative who receive a heart from a seropositive donor are at greatest risk for aggressive disease. Attempts to prevent CMV disease in these mismatched patients have been less disappointing. Many programs use early intravenous ganciclovir followed by a prolonged course of oral ganciclovir or val-ganciclovir often in combination with intravenous CMV-specific immunoglobulin. Many programs now employ a "preemptive" approach to CMV and follow highly sensitive laboratory markers of early infection such as CMV-antigenemia and treat when a certain threshold of CMV replication is found.

Fungi and protozoa account for <15% of infections after transplant, but they are associated with the worst prognosis [69]. Fungal infections often occur in patients who require intensive antibiotic treatment over a prolonged period before or after transplantation or in whom significant rejection occurs which requires intense and prolonged high-dose immunosuppression.

In the current era, the majority of patients remain free of serious infections with an overall incidence of infection of approximately 0.5 infections/patient. The most common site of infection is the lung, accounting for up to one-third of all infections. While most serious infections are successfully treated and despite its low incidence, infection remains a leading cause of death during the first year [66] and long term [8]. However, very often acute infection may be the actual mode of death, but it was severe, acute or chronic rejection that set the stage.

Infection prophylaxis, particularly during the first year post-transplant, is common and has reduced the morbidity and mortality following cardiac transplantation for CMV, *Pneumocystis carinii* pneumonia, and toxoplasmosis [70,71]. Prophylactic regimens are commonly employed against CMV (if either recipient or donor are positive), toxoplasmosis (especially if the recipient is negative and the donor is positive), *Pneumocystis carinii*, *Candida albicans*, and herpes simplex. Prophylactic influenza vaccine is controversial. Concern exists given anecdotal reports of post-vaccine rejection episodes but controlled vaccination trials have failed to document a significant risk [72]. Certainly patients at high risk for influenza and subsequent influenza-related morbidity/mortality should be considered for annual vaccination.

Hypertension

Hypertension occurs in 72% of heart transplant recipients by 1 year and 95% of recipients by 5 years [8]. Hypertension is more common in cyclosporine-treated (70–90%) than in tacrolimus-treated (30–50%) recipients. The role of hypertension in the development of renal dysfunction and CAV in long-term survivors is not known.

ACE-inhibitors and calcium channel blockers in conventional doses are effective monotherapy for many patients [73,74]. The combination of cyclosporine or tacrolimus and ACE inhibition may cause hyperkalemia or worsening renal insufficiency. Due to their inhibition of the hepatic cytochrome p450 enzymes, diltiazem or verapamil will significantly raise cyclosporine and tacrolimus blood levels. Use of both an ACE-inhibitor and a calcium channel blocker is effective in many patients in whom neither class of drugs alone is sufficient. Diuretics are effective in some transplant patients, though rarely as monotherapy. Relative volume depletion should be avoided with the concomitant use of cyclosporine or tacrolimus.

Alpha-blockers, beta-blockers, and direct vasodilators such as hydralazine or minoxidil have all been used successfully in transplant recipients. As the denervated transplant heart relies heavily on circulating catecholamines for its chronotropic response to exercise, beta-blocking agents often severely limit exercise tolerance in these patients and thus are generally reserved for refractory cases or patients with concomitant CAV with infarction. Occasionally, changing from cyclosporine to tacrolimus or minimizing the dose of cyclosporine or prednisone will be helpful.

Malignancy

With the current long-term success of transplantation comes an increasing incidence of late malignancy in these aging, immunosuppressed recipients. Organ transplant recipients have an increased risk of malignancy when compared to the general population. The incidence of malignancy increases steadily each year and by 7 years following transplantation reaches nearly 30% with a fairly linear rate after 2 years of approximately 5%/year [8]. Fortunately, nearly half are skin cancers, occurring predominantly in those who would otherwise be at risk [75] Post-transplant lymphoproliferative disease (PTLD) accounts for approximately 25% of the early malignancies (<1 year) and 12% of the later ones. Overall, however, PTLD occurs in <2% of transplant recipients [76]. PTLD encompasses a wide spectrum of disease, from relatively benign polyclonal B-cell proliferation and mononucleosis-type syndrome to advanced monoclonal or immunoblastic B-cell lymphoma. While early disease may respond to antivirals and reduced immunosuppression, advanced disease often requires intense chemotherapeutics [77]. The Epstein–Barr virus (EBV), a lymphotropic virus that infects >90% of the population by adulthood, is thought to be the etiologic agent responsible for most cases of PTLD [77,78]. As EBV suppression is highly dependent on T-lymphocyte immunity, the incidence of PTLD increased substantially in organ transplantation with the application of potent anti-T-cell agents such as cyclosporine and OKT3. However, the overall degree of immunosuppression is likely a more important risk factor than any particular drug. Recipients who are seropositive for EBV prior to transplantation experience a low (1%) incidence of PTLD; however, recipients who are seronegative for EBV prior to transplant and who receive an organ from an EBV-seropositive donor have a much higher incidence of PTLD (perhaps as high as 50%). In this high-risk group, preemptive antiviral therapy may be indicated [78]. Treatment of PTLD usually involves reduction of immunosuppression, administration of acyclovir, and chemotherapy for widespread disease. More recently, an anti-B-cell antibody, rituximab, has been successfully used to treat PTLD [79]. While other malignancies occur in heart transplant recipients, the behavior of prostate, breast, and colon cancer seems no different than in the general population. The incidence of virally mediated malignancies such as cervical cancer and Kaposi's sarcoma is higher than the general population but still relatively low. Routine cancer screening remains equally important in the follow-up of the cardiac transplant recipient.

Renal insufficiency

By 7 years post-heart transplantation, the cumulative incidence of renal dysfunction (defined as a serum creatinine >2.5 mg/dL) is 36% [8]. In addition, by 5 years post-operatively 2.5% of recipients have progressed to dialysis [8]. Although some renal dysfunction is related to pre-existing renal disease, most is acquired. Cyclosporine and tacrolimus are nephrotoxic and likely account for the majority of the renal problems [80–83]. Minimizing the doses of these and other nephrotoxins, avoidance of dehydration, and a careful search for non-immunosuppression-related reversible causes are warranted [84]. Some individuals may be at greater than usual risk for cyclosporine- or tacrolimus-related nephrotoxicity [82]. Once renal dysfunction occurs, the course is variable. Costs are likely increased and prognosis worsened in

heart transplant patients with significant renal dysfunction [83].

Hyperlipidemia

After cardiac transplantation, hyperlipidemia is common, partly because of pre-existing lipid disorders as well as the known metabolic effects of cyclosporine and corticosteroids [84]. By 1-year post-transplant almost 50% of recipients have hyperlipidemia and the incidence increases to just over 80% by year 5 [8]. All patients are encouraged to limit cholesterol and other fat intake, maintain ideal body weight, and exercise. Minimization or elimination of corticosteroids, when possible, is also helpful. Occasionally changing from cyclosporine to tacrolimus can aid in cholesterol management. While no clear-cut guidelines have been developed for transplant recipients, serum LDL cholesterol <100 mg/dL seems a reasonable target in this high-risk patient population. While gemfibrozil (in doses up to 600 mg twice daily) can be successful is some patients with mild to moderate hyperlipidemia, particularly in the setting of hypertriglyceridemia, moderate to severe hypercholesterolemia generally requires the use of a 3-hydroxy-3-methylglutaryl coenzyme A (HMG-CoA) reductase inhibitor, or "statin", as they are now commonly referred to [84,85]. In fact, two studies [86,87] and a multicenter lipid registry [88] strongly suggest that all transplant recipients should be on statins regardless of their cholesterol levels, reporting less CAV and better long-term survival in cardiac transplant patients routinely receiving statins. Many programs now routinely add statin therapy regardless of lipid levels, beginning early post-operatively. The combination of cyclosporine or tacrolimus and an HMG-CoA reductase inhibitor increases the risk of rhabdomyolysis over that of the HMG-CoA reductase inhibitor alone. When used, HMG-CoA reductase inhibitors should be started at *low* dose and increased slowly while monitoring creatine kinase (CK) and liver enzymes. Combining an HMG-CoA reductase inhibitor with gemfibrozil or nicotinic acid in lipid-lowering doses can also be associated with rhabdomyolysis and these combinations must also be used cautiously in transplant patients. Bile acid sequestrants, probucol, and fish oil (omega-3 free fatty acids) are less used to treat hyperlipidemia post-transplant.

Glucose intolerance

Twenty-four percent of cardiac transplant recipients have diabetes within the first year post-operatively, many of whom had diabetes pre-transplant [8]. By 5 years after transplantation the cumulative incidence has increased to 32% [8], likely due to the chronic effects of post-transplant corticosteroids, weight gain and aging. No evidence exists that cardiac transplant recipients should be treated differently with regard to diabetic control in terms of blood glucose and glycosolated hemoglobin targets and the agents used to treat them. In addition, the lipid abnormalities noted above are difficult to treat in the setting of poorly controlled diabetes.

Osteoporosis

By the time most patients undergo cardiac transplantation, their risk of osteoporosis is high. Prolonged inactivity, age, menopause, and, in some cases, prolonged heparin administration, are all risk factors for osteoporosis. Further bone loss occurs due to high-dose corticosteroid therapy early post-transplant. Bone loss is therefore rapid in the first 6 months after transplantation and is most marked in the lumbar spine. Vertebral compression fractures and aseptic necrosis of the femoral or humoral head (an osteopenia-independent effect of high-dose corticosteroids) are among the most common skeletal problems after heart transplantation. Due to the morbidity associated with osteoporosis, patients at risk are generally treated aggressively [89–91]. For patients at risk, determination of bone mineral density (BMD) is helpful to guide pre- and post-transplant therapy. Post-menopausal women are generally prescribed estrogen replacement. Post-menopausal women and all patients with evidence of pre-transplant osteoporosis receive calcium salts (such as calcium carbonate 1000–1500 mg/day in divided doses) and upwardly titrated doses of calcitriol (beginning at 0.25 g every other day) or ergocalciferol (50,000 units per day) while awaiting transplantation and indefinitely thereafter [89]. Alendronate (10 mg/day or 70 mg/week) effectively increases bone density and should be added to calcium salts and calcitriol in patients with documented osteoporosis [90]. Many programs now treat all transplant patients with alendronate or another bisphosphonate during the high-dose corticosteroid period post-transplant (up to 6–12 months

post-operatively) and those on the waiting list with documented osteoporosis or those at high-risk based on BMD. Treatment of bony complications of the spine is supportive. Clearly, maintaining physical activity and ideal body weight are important measures [91]. Physical therapy is helpful. Joint replacement is successful in the vast majority of post-transplant patients and should be recommended as indicated.

Gastrointestinal complications

High-dose, pulsed corticosteroid therapy and chronic corticosteroid therapy are risk factors for gastric ulceration. Thus most transplant recipients receive either H2-blockers or proton-pump inhibitors during the early post-operative period (up to 6–12 months post-operatively). As noted earlier, CMV can be a major post-operative complication and can cause hepatitis, pancreatitis, gastritis, and colitis. Due to this and the availability of specific treatment, patients with possible CMV enteritis should undergo endoscopy with biopsy of suspicious lesions. The incidence of biliary disease is increased in cardiac transplant recipients when compared with non-transplant patients [92]. The incidence may be as high as 8%, which represents a 17-fold increase over the general population. Cyclosporine increases the risk of cholelithiasis because of its lithogenic and cholestatic properties. Generally, any abdominal symptoms coupled with cholelithiasis warrants surgical intervention. Laparoscopic cholecystectomy is the procedure of choice in uncomplicated situations [93].

Pregnancy

Successful pregnancies after heart transplantation have been reported [94]. Maternal and fetal risk are undoubtedly higher than in the general population and transplant recipients are so counseled. Obviously, the care of a pregnant transplant recipient requires close collaboration with a high-risk obstetrician to avoid teratogenic drugs and manage the pregnancy. Immunosuppressive drug levels require frequent monitoring due to the large plasma volume and metabolic changes that are associated with pregnancy. Radiation exposure can be minimized by performing necessary endomyocardial biopsies using echocardiographic guidance.

Management of the cardiac transplant recipient undergoing surgery

Many of the above noted complications require surgical intervention. The risk associated with non-cardiac surgery depends on the status of the allograft. Patients without ongoing rejection, significant coronary disease, or left ventricular dysfunction are generally at low risk for routine surgical procedures. In fact, because of the necessary frequent endomyocardial biopsies, echocardiograms, and cardiac catheterizations, the typical transplant recipient is much better screened for potential cardiac complications than the average surgical patient. Patients receiving corticosteroids within the preceding 9 months receive stress doses of corticosteroids. If intravenous immunosuppressants are to be needed appropriate dose adjustments must be made.

References

1 Rose EA, Gelijns AC, Moskowitz AJ *et al.* Long-term use of a left ventricular assist device for end-stage heart failure. *N Engl J Med* 2001; **345**: 1435–1443.

2 CIBIS-II Investigators and Committee. The Cardiac Insufficiency Bisoprolol Study II (CIBIS-II): a randomized trial. *Lancet* 1999; **353**: 9–13.

3 The Beta-Blocker Evaluation of Survival Trial Investigators. A trial of the beta-blocker bucindolol in patients with advanced chronic heart failure. *N Engl J Med* 2001; **344**: 1659–1667.

4 Packer M, Coats AJS, Fowler MB, *et al.* Effect of carvedilol on survival in severe chronic heart failure. *N Engl J Med* 2001; **344**: 1651–1658.

5 Hosenpud JD, Bennett LE, Keck BM, Boucek MM, Novick RJ. The Registry of the International Society for Heart and Lung Transplantation: Eighteenth Official Report – 2001. *J Heart Lung Transplant* 2001; **20**: 805–815.

6 Website of United Network for Organ Sharing. http:\\www.unos.org

7 O'Connell JB and Bristow MR. *J Heart Lung Transplant* 1994; **13**: S107–S112.

8 Hertz MI, Taylor DO, Trulock EP *et al.* The Registry of the International Society for Heart and Lung Transplantation: Nineteenth Official Report – 2002. *J Heart Lung Transplant* 2002; **9**: (in press).

9 Miller LW. Criteria for selection of recipients and donors for cardiac transplantation. *Graft* 1999; **2**: S49–S53.

10 Hosenpud JD, Bennett LE, Keck BM, Boucek MM, Novick RJ. The Registry of the International Society for Heart and Lung Transplantation: Seventeenth Official Report –2000. *J Heart Lung Transplant* 2000; **19**: 909–931.

11 Bourge RC, Naftel DC, Costanzo-Nordin MR *et al.* Pretransplantation risk factors for death after heart transplantation: a multiinstitutional study. The Transplant Cardiologists Research Database Group. *J Heart Lung Transplant* 1993; **12**: 549–562.

12 Young JB, Naftel DC, Bourge RC *et al.* Matching the heart donor and heart transplant recipient. Clues for successful expansion of the donor pool: a multivariable, multiinstitutional report. The Transplant Cardiologists Research Database Group. *J Heart Lung Transplant* 1994; **13**: 353–364.

13 Bourge RC, Kirklin JK, Naftel DC, McGiffin DC. Predicting outcome after cardiac transplantation: lessons from the Cardiac Transplant Research Database. *Curr Opin Cardiol* 1997; **12**: 136–145.

14 Costanzo MR, Augustine S, Bourge R *et al.* Selection and treatment of candidates for heart transplantation: a statement for health professionals from the Committee on Heart Failure and Cardiac Transplantation of the Council on Clinical Cardiology, American Heart Association. *Circulation* 1995; **92**: 3593–3612.

15 Mudge GH, Goldstein S, Addonizio LJ *et al.* Bethesda Conference: Cardiac Transplantation: Task Force 3: Recipient guidelines/prioritization. *J Am Coll Cardiol* 1993; **22**: 21–31.

16 Aaronson KD, Eppinger MJ, Dyke DB, Wright S, Pagani FD. Left ventricular assist device therapy improves utilization of donor hearts. *J Am Coll Cardiol* 2002; **39**: 1247–1254.

17 Jaski BE, Kim JC, Naftel DC *et al.* Cardiac transplant outcome of patients supported on left ventricular assist device vs intravenous inotropic therapy. *J Heart Lung Transplant* 2001; **20**: 449–456.

18 Laks H, Scholl FG, Drinkwater DC *et al.* The alternate recipient list for heart transplantation: does it work? *J Heart Lung Transplant* 1997; **16**: 735–742.

19 Lower RR, Shumway NE. Studies of the orthotopic homotransplantation of the canine heart. *Surg Forum* 1960; **11**: 18–23.

20 Dreyfus G, Jebara V, Mihaileanu S, Carpentier AF. Total orthotopic heart transplantation: an alternative to the standard technique. *Ann Thorac Surg* 1991; **52**: 1181–1184.

21 Novitsky D, Cooper DKC, Barnard CN. The surgical technique of heterotopic heart transplantation. *Ann Thorac Surg* 1983; **36**: 476–482.

22 Bainbridge AD, Cave M, Roberts M *et al.* A prospective randomized trial of complete atrioventricular transplantation versus ventricular transplantation with atrioplasty. *J Heart Lung Transplant* 1999; **18**: 407–413.

23 The International Society for Heart Transplantation: Billingham ME, Cary NRB, Hammond ME *et al.* A working formulation for the standardization of nomenclature in the diagnosis of heart and lung rejection: heart rejection study group. *J Heart Transplant* 1990; **9**: 587–593.

24 Pham SM, Kormos RL, Hattler BG *et al.* A prospective trial of tacrolimus (FK506) in clinical heart transplantation: intermediate-term results. *J Thorac Cardiovasc Surg* 1996; **111**: 764–772.

25 Meiser BM, Pfeiffer M, Schmidt D *et al.* Combination therapy with tacrolimus and mycophenole mofetil following cardiac transplantation: importance of mycophenolic acid therapeutic drug monitoring. *J Heart Lung Transplant* 1999; **18**: 143–149.

26 Taylor DO, Barr ML, Radovancevic B *et al.* A randomized, multicenter comparison of tacrolimus and cyclosporine immunosuppressive regimens in cardiac transplantation: decreased hyperlipidemia and hypertension with tacrolimus. *J Heart Lung Transplant* 1999; **18**: 336–345.

27 Reichart B, Meiser B, Vigano M *et al.* European multicenter tacrolimus (FK506) heart pilot study: one-year results – European Tacrolimus Multicenter Heart Study Group. *J Heart Lung Transplant* 1998; **17**: 775–781.

28 Kobashigawa J, Miller L, Renlund D *et al.* A randomized active-controlled trial of mycophenolate mofetil in heart transplant recipients. *Transplantation* 1998; **66**: 507–515.

29 Eisen H, Tuzcu EM, Dorent R *et al.* Everolimus for the prevention of allograft rejection and vasculopathy in cardiac-transplant recipients. *N Engl J Med* 2003; **349**: 847–858.

30 Keogh AM, the Sirolimus Cardiac Trial Group. Sirolimus immunotherapy reduces the rates of cardiac allograft rejection: 6-month results from a phase 2, open-label study. *Am J Transplant* 2002; **2(Suppl 3)**: 246.

31 Keogh AM, the Sirolimus Cardiac Trial Group. Progression of graft vessel disease in cardiac allograft recipients is significantly reduced by sirolimus immunotherapy: 6-month results from a phase 2, open-label study. *Am J Transplant* 2002; **2(Suppl 3)**: 246.

32 Taylor DO, Bristow MR, O'Connell JB *et al.* Improved long-term survival after cardiac transplantation predicted by successful early withdrawal from maintenance corticosteroids. *J Heart Lung Transplant* 1996; **15**: 1039–1046.

33 Rossini AA, Greiner DL, Mordes JP. Induction of immunologic tolerance for transplantation. *Physiol Rev* 1999; **79**: 99–141.

34 Jankowski RA, Ildstad ST. Chimerism and tolerance: from freemartin cattle to neonatal mice to humans. *Human Immunology* 1997; **52**: 155–161.

35 Starzl TE, Demetris AJ. Transplantation milestones viewed with one- and two-way paradigms of tolerance. *J Am Med Assoc* 1995; **273**: 876–879.

36 Pham SM, Rao AS, Zeevi A, *et al.* A clinical trial combining donor bone marrow infusion and heart transplantation: intermediate-term results. *J Thorac Cardiovasc Surg* 2000; **119**: 673–681.

37 Kirk AD, Harlan DM, Armstrong NN *et al.* CTLA4-Ig and anti-CD40 ligand prevent renal allograft rejection in primates. *Proc Natl Acad Sci USA* 1997; **94**: 8789–8794.

38 Johnson DE, Gao SZ, Schroeder JS, DeCampli WM, Billingham ME. The spectrum of coronary artery pathologic findings in human cardiac allografts. *J Heart Transplant* 1989; **8**: 349–359.

39 Gao SZ, Alderman EL, Schroeder JS *et al.* Accelerated coronary vascular disease in the heart transplant patient: coronary arteriographic findings. *J Am Coll Cardiol* 1988; **12**: 334–348.

40 Weis M, von Scheidt W. Cardiac allograft vasculopathy: a review. *Circulation* 1997; **96**: 2069–2077.

41 Costanzo MR, Naftel DC, Pritzker MR *et al.* Heart transplant coronary artery disease detected by coronary angiography: a multiinstitutional study of preoperative donor and recipient risk factors. *J Heart Lung Transplant* 1998; **17**: 744–753.

42 Gao S-Z, Hunt SA, Schroeder JS *et al.* Early development of accelerated graft coronary artery disease: risk factors and course. *J Am Coll Cardiol* 1996; **28**: 673–679.

43 Mehra MR, Ventura HO, Jain SP *et al.* Heterogeneity of cardiac allograft vasculopathy: clinical insights from coronary angioscopy. *J Am Coll Cardiol* 1997; **29**: 1339–1344.

44 Gupta A, Moustapha A, Jacobsen DW *et al.* High homocysteine, low folate, and low vitamin B_6 concentrations: prevalent risk factors for vascular disease in heart transplant recipients. *Transplantation* 1998; **65**: 544–550.

45 Cooke GE, Eaton GM, Whitby G *et al.* Plasma atherogenic markers in congestive heart failure and post-transplant (heart) patients. *J Am Coll Cardiol* 2000; **36**: 509–516.

46 Brunner-La Rocca HP, Schneider J, Kunzli A *et al.* Cardiac allograft rejection late after transplantation is a risk factor for graft coronary artery disease. *Transplantation* 1998; **65**: 538–543.

47 Hornick P, Smith J, Pomerace A *et al.* Influence of acute rejection episodes, HLA matching, and donor/recipient phenotype on the development of "early" transplant-associated coronary artery disease. *Circulation* 1997; **96(Suppl II)**: II-148–II-153.

48 Weis M, Wildhirt SM, Schulze C *et al.* Endothelin in coronary endothelial dysfunction early after human heart transplantation. *J Heart Lung Transplant* 1999; **18**: 1071–1079.

49 Hosenpud JD, Morris TE, Shipley DG *et al.* Cardiac allograft vasculopathy: preferential regulation of endothelial cell-derived mesenchymal growth factors in response to a donor-specific cell-mediated allogeneic response. *Transplantation* 1996; **61**: 939–948.

50 Valantine HA, Gao S-Z, Menon SG *et al.* Impact of prophylactic immediate post-transplant ganciclovir on development of transplant atherosclerosis: a post-hoc analysis of a randomized placebo-controlled trial. *Circulation* 1999; **100**: 61–66.

51 Yun JJ, Fischbein MP, Laks H *et al.* Early and late chemokine production correlates with cellular recruitment

in cardiac allograft vasculopathy. *Transplantation* 2000; **69**: 2515–2524.

52 Faulk WP, Labarrere CA, Torry RJ *et al.* Serum cardiac troponin-T concentrations predict development of coronary artery disease in heart transplant patients. *Transplantation* 1998; **66**: 1335–1339.

53 Lin H, Ignatescu M, Wilson JE *et al.* Prominence of apolipoproteins B, (a), and E in the intimae of coronary arteries in transplanted human hearts: geographic relationship to vessel wall proteoglycans. *J Heart Lung Transplant* 1996; **15**: 1223–1232.

54 Hosenpud JD, Mauck KA, Hogan KB. Cardiac allograft vasculopathy: IgM antibody responses to donor-specific vascular endothelium. *Transplantation* 1997; **63**: 1602–1606.

55 Fredrich R, Toyoda M, Czer LSC *et al.* The clinical significance of antibodies to human vascular endothelial cells after cardiac transplantation. *Transplantation* 1999; **67**: 385–391.

56 Benza RL, Grenett HE, Bourge RC *et al.* Gene polymorphisms for plasminogen activator inhibitor-1/tissue plasminogen activator and development of allograft coronary artery disease. *Circulation* 1998; **98**: 2248–2254.

57 Labarrere CA. Anticoagulation factors as predictors of transplant-associated coronary artery disease. *J Heart Lung Transplant* 2000; **19**: 623–633.

58 Spes CH, Klauss V, Mudra H *et al.* Diagnostic and prognostic value of serial dobutamine stress echocardiography for noninvasive assessment of cardiac allograft vasculopathy: a comparison with coronary angiography and intravascular ultrasound. *Circulation* 1999; **100**: 509–515.

59 Carlsen J, Toft JC, Mortensen SA *et al.* Myocardial perfusion scintigraphy as a screening method for significant coronary artery stenosis in cardiac transplant recipients. *J Heart Lung Transplant* 2000; **19**: 873–878.

60 Allen-Auerbach M, Schoder H, Johnson J *et al.* Relationship between coronary function by positron emission tomography and temporal changes in morphology by intravascular ultrasound (IVUS) in transplant recipients. *J Heart Lung Transplant* 1999; **18**: 211–219.

61 Liang DH, Gao S-Z, Botas J *et al.* Prediction of angiographic disease by intracoronary ultrasonographic findings in heart transplant recipients. *J Heart Lung Transplant* 1996; **15**: 980–987.

62 Wolford TL, Donohue TJ, Bach RG *et al.* Heterogeneity of coronary flow reserve in the examination of multiple individual allograft coronary arteries. *Circulation* 1999; **99**: 626–632.

63 Mancini D, Pinney S, Burkhoff D *et al.* Use of rapamycin slows progression of cardiac transplantation vasculopathy. *Circulation* 2003; **108**: 48–53.

64 Mehra MR, Uber PA, Prasad AK *et al.* Long-term outcome of cardiac allograft vasculopathy treated by transmyocardial

laser revascularization: early rewards, late losses. *J Heart Lung Transplant* 2000; **19**: 801–804.

65 Fishman JA, Rubin RH. Infection in organ-transplant recipients. *N Engl J Med* 1998; **338**: 1741–1751.

66 Miller LW, Naftel DC, Bourge RC *et al.* Infection after heart transplantation: a multiinstitutional study. *J Heart Lung Transplant* 1994; **13**: 381–393.

67 Rubin RH. Prevention and treatment of cytomegalovirus disease in heart transplant patients. *J Heart Lung Transplant* 2000; **19**: 731–735.

68 Barber L, Egan JJ, Lomax J *et al.* A prospective study of a quantitative PCR ELISA assay for the diagnosis of CMV pneumonia in lung and heart-transplant recipients. *J Heart Lung Transplant* 2000; **19**: 771–780.

69 Grossi P, Farina C, Fiocchi R *et al.* Prevalence and outcome of invasive fungal infections in 1,963 thoracic organ transplant recipients. *Transplantation* 2000; **70**: 112–116.

70 Couchoud C, Cucherat M, Haugh M *et al.* Cytomegalovirus prophylaxis with antiviral agents in solid organ transplantation: a meta-analysis. *Transplantation* 1998; **65**: 641–647.

71 Olsen SL, Renlund DG, O'Connell JB *et al.* Prevention of *Pneumocystis carinii* pneumonia in cardiac transplant recipients by trimethoprim/sulfamethoxazole. *Transplantation* 1993; **56**: 359–362.

72 Fraund S, Wagner D, Pethig K *et al.* Influenza vaccination in heart transplant recipients. *J Heart Lung Transplant* 1999; **18**: 220–225.

73 Brozena SC, Johnson MR, Ventura H *et al.* Effectiveness and safety of diltiazem or lisinopril in treatment of hypertension after heart transplantation. *J Am Coll Cardiol* 1996; **27**: 1707–1712.

74 Schwitter J, DeMarco T, Globits S *et al.* Influence of felodipine on left ventricular hypertrophy and systolic function in orthotopic heart transplant recipients: possible interaction with cyclosporine medication. *J Heart Lung Transplant* 1999; **18**: 1003–101380.

75 Lampros TD, Cobanoglu A, Parker F *et al.* Squamous and basal cell carcinoma in heart transplant recipients. *J Heart Lung Transplant* 1998; **17**: 586–591.

76 Mihalov ML, Gattuso P, Abraham K *et al.* Incidence of post-transplant malignancy among 674 solid-organ-transplant recipients at a single center. *Clin Transplant* 1996; **10**: 248–255.

77 Paya CV, Fung JJ, Nalesnik MA *et al.* Epstein-Barr virus-induced posttransplant lymphoproliferative disorders. *Transplantation* 1999; **68**: 1517–1525.

78 Darenkov IA, Marcarelli MA, Basadonna GP *et al.* Reduced incidence of Epstein-Barr virus-associated posttransplant lymphoproliferative disorder using preemptive antiviral therapy. *Transplantation* 1997; **64**: 848–852.

79 Zilz ND, Olson LJ, McGregor CG. Treatment of post-transplant lymphoproliferative disorder with monoclonal

CD20 antibody (rituximab) after heart transplantation. *J Heart Lung Transplant* 2001; **20**: 770–772.

80 Campistol JM, Sacks SH. Mechanisms of nephrotoxicity. *Transplantation* 2000; **69**: SS5–SS1081.

81 MacDonald AS. Management strategies for nephrotoxicity. *Transplantation* 2000; **69**: SS31–SS36.

82 Baan CC, Balk AHMM, Holweg CTJ *et al.* Renal failure after clinical heart transplantation is associated with TGF-B1 Codon 10 gene polymorphism. *J Heart Lung Transplant* 2000; **19**: 866–872.

83 Parry G, Meiser B, Rbago G. The clinical impact of cyclosporine nephrotoxicity in heart transplantation. *Transplantation* 2000; **69**: SS23–SS26.

84 Kobashigawa JA, Kasiske BL. Hyperlipidemia in solid organ transplantation. *Transplantation* 1997; **63**: 331–338.

85 Magnani G, Carinci V, Magelli C *et al.* Role of statins in the management of dyslipidemia after cardiac transplant: randomized controlled trial comparing the efficacy and safety of atorvastatin with pravastatin. *J Heart Lung Transplant* 2000; **19**: 710–715.

86 Kobashigawa JA, Katznelson S, Laks H *et al.* Effect of pravastatin on outcomes after cardiac transplantation. *N Engl J Med* 1995; **333**: 621–627.

87 Wenke K, Meiser B, Thiery J *et al.* Simvastatin reduces graft vessel disease and mortality after heart transplantation: a four-year randomized trial. *Circulation* 1997; **96**: 1398–1402.

88 Ballantyne CM, Short BC, Bourge RC *et al.* Lipid treatment and survival after heart transplantation. *J Am Coll Cardiol* 1998; **31**: 157A.

89 Stempfle H-U, Werner C, Echtler S *et al.* Prevention of osteoporosis after cardiac transplantation: a prospective, longitudinal, randomized, double-blind trial with calcitriol. *Transplantation* 1999; **68**: 523–530.

90 Shane E, Rodino MA, McMahon DJ *et al.* Prevention of bone loss after heart transplantation with antiresorptive therapy: a pilot study. *J Heart Lung Transplant* 1998; **17**: 1089–1096.

91 Braith RW, Mills Jr. RM, Welsch MA *et al.* Resistance exercise training restores bone mineral density in heart transplant recipients. *J Am Coll Cardiol* 1996; 28: 1471–1477.

92 Vega KJ, Pina I, Krevsky B. Heart transplantation is associated with an increased risk for pancreaticobiliary disease. *Ann Intern Med* 1996; **124**: 980.

93 Milas M, Ricketts RR, Amerson JR *et al.* Management of biliary tract stones in heart transplant patients. *Ann Surg* 1996; **223**: 747.

94 Branch KR, Wagoner LE, McGrory CH *et al.* Risks of subsequent pregnancies on mother and newborn in female heart transplant recipients. *J Heart Lung Transplant* 1998; **17**: 698–702.

CHAPTER 14

Perioperative care of the surgical patient with heart failure: from conventional cardiac surgery to mechanical circulatory support

Tiffany Buda & Patrick M. McCarthy

Patients suffering from heart failure (HF) with depressed left ventricular (LV) function are considered high risk candidates for conventional surgical therapies. Surgical therapies include coronary artery bypass grafting (CABG), valve repair or replacement, and correction of LV geometry such as the Dor procedure (or endoventricular circular patch plasty) for LV aneurysm or scarred muscle [1–6]. Finally, for advanced end-stage HF for which conventional surgery is not an option, mechanical circulatory support (MCS) as bridge to transplant (BTT) or permanent support may be options. Ventricular assist devices can be applied to both the LV and right ventricle (RV). Devices available are described in Chapter 12.

A team approach may facilitate smoother recovery of patients with HF from surgery, and this includes the surgical team, cardiology/HF team, nurses, social worker, dietician, exercise physiologist, and outpatient HF healthcare providers for follow-up once discharged from the hospital. Team members are responsible for teaching the patient self-care management to reduce clinical HF events after surgery. Including family in the educational process provides further support to the patient. An attentive nurse can make a difference in the recovery of this sick patient population.

Nurses are integral members of the healthcare team. Nurses identify potential problems preoperatively, assist with recovery, manage intensive care unit (ICU) care, and educate patients in HF self-care management. The purpose of this chapter is to review the care of the patient with HF having cardiac surgery. Throughout the chapter, nursing care, interventions, and helpful "hints" will be incorporated. Care of patients following placement of MCS follows. Specific care issues of MCS will be discussed.

Preoperative evaluation

Candidacy for conventional surgical intervention will be determined by the cardiologist and surgeon after routine preoperative assessment and a discussion of risks and benefits. Coronary angiography is routine. For patients at high risk, surgery may only be performed if the patient meets heart transplantation eligibility and is willing to have left ventricular assist device (LVAD) placement as "back up" therapy as needed. If the HF is too advanced (i.e. when the patient cannot be weaned from continuous intravenous inotropic infusion) transplantation may be the only option clinically indicated.

Objective data of LV function is obtained through multiple diagnostic modalities. Transthoracic echocardiogram (TTE), magnetic resonance imaging (MRI), and positron emission tomography (PET) scanning provide information on LV size and function, wall thickness, valve competency, myocardial viability, hibernating myocardium, LV scar or true aneurysm formation. Complimentary information is obtained from these studies. For example, the PET scan assesses myocardial perfusion and metabolic function and MRI assesses extent and distribution of scar and segmental perfusion as well as valve competence, aneurysm, and LV thrombus [4].

Nursing, medical, and surgical teams must be made aware of the patient's preoperative presentation. Knowledge of the patient's preoperative New York Heart Association (NYHA) functional capacity, ejection fraction (EF), valvular function, and medications provides the background needed to assist the surgical team with optimization of medical management. Each patient is medically optimized prior to surgery. Angiotensin converting enzyme (ACE) inhibitor and vasodilator therapies may prompt hypotension during cardiopulmonary bypass (CPB) or after weaning from CPB. To decrease this risk, if circumstances allow, these medications are held for 1–2 days prior to surgery [7].

Intraoperative care

Patients will be hemodynamically monitored with pulmonary artery and arterial catheters allowing for continuous monitoring of systolic and diastolic blood pressure (BP), mean arterial pressure (MAP), cardiac output (CO), cardiac index (CI), pulmonary artery systolic, diastolic and mean pressures (PAP), and right atrial pressure (RAP). These data provide objective evidence of perfusion and volume status used to guide decisions related to inotropic, vasodilator, vasoconstrictor, and fluid support. If needed, placement of a left atrial (LA) catheter provides additional hemodynamic data. Placement of an LA catheter is routine with LVAD insertion.

In the operating room (OR), a transesophageal echocardiogram (TEE) is performed as baseline to assess LV/RV contractility, valve competency, and the presence of a patent foramen ovale. TEE postsurgical intervention is used to assess LV/RV contractility, intracardiac air, competence of surgical valve repair, and volume reduction. The patient is weaned from CPB after optimizing intravenous vasoactive agents. During the weaning process LV/RV function is monitored by TEE. Patients are carefully observed for need for intra-aortic balloon pump (IABP) or MCS [4,8].

Cardiothoracic ICU management

On admission to the cardiothoracic ICU (CTICU), the surgical and anesthesia team report the patient's medical and surgical history and significant intraoperative events to the receiving nurse. The surgical resident will provide a range of acceptable hemodynamic parameters, such as MAP and CI, on admission so the nursing team can alter intravenous vasoactive drip rates to maintain optimal perfusion status.

Nurses monitor and record heart rate (HR), BP, MAP, PAP, and RAP every 20 min until stable, then every 30 min. Thermodilution CO/CI measurements are obtained and recorded every hour until stable, then every 2 h. A Fick CO/CI may be requested for comparison if the thermodilution CO/CI measurement is inconsistent with the patient's clinical profile. When weaning intravenous inotropic support, assessment of CO/CI is increased and used as a guide to insure optimal cardiac function. Hemodynamic compromise is immediately reported to the surgical team for prompt intervention.

Postoperative care is similar to cardiothoracic surgical patients with normal cardiac function and initially includes assessment of respiratory status and readiness for extubation. Chest X-ray (CXR) and arterial blood gases (ABG) are obtained to determine correct endotracheal placement and determine adequate ventilation. Ongoing assessment of the patient's ventilatory status is monitored via ABG's. The patient is extubated when hemodynamically stable, not bleeding, and has acceptable mechanics for extubation [9].

Pharmacologic intravenous therapy on admission to the CTICU may include inotropic support (epinephrine, milrinone, dobutamine) and either a vasoconstrictor (norepinephrine, vasopressin) or a vasodilator (nitroglycerin or nitroprusside) [8]. Table 14.1 provides a summary of intravenous medications initiated perioperatively and continued in the CTICU as needed. Nursing interventions and considerations are provided as an overview to nursing care. The surgery team writes orders to begin medication weaning when the patient's condition allows. Specific orders are written to wean an inotrope for a specified CI. When patients require multiple vasopressive or inotropic support, one medication is weaned at a time, however, it is possible to wean one vasopressive and one inotropic agent simultaneously. Patients with an EF <20% and NYHA class III to IV HF prior to surgery may require prolonged inotropic support which will be slowly weaned off on the nursing floor. Dopamine

Table 14.1 Intravenous medication administration peri- and post-cardiac surgery in patients with HF.

Medication after Vasoconstrictors for hypotension	Dose	Nursing intervention/consideration
Vasoconstrictor		General for all vasoconstrictors
Norepinephrine	1–20 µg/min	• Monitor BP, RAP, PAP for hemodynamic compromise and notify physician of changes • Assess volume status, H/H (↓H/H may be reason for hypovolemia and need for vasoconstrictor) • Assess perfusion to distal extremities and report signs of decreased perfusion
Dopamine	1–10 µg/kg/min	• Often used when unable to wean norepinephrine • Watch for ectopy and ↑HR • Dose of 3–5 µg/kg/min to aide weaning of norepinephrine • Can be weaned slowly on the nursing floor • Doses higher than 5 µg/kg/min need to remain in CTICU • Infuse via central access
Vasopressin	1–6 units/h	• Use least amount needed for shortest amount of time
Vasodilator		General for all vasodilators
Nitroprusside	10 to > 200 µg/min	• Assess BP, HR, PAP • Keep MAP < 90 mmHg or as specified • Decrease drip rate as BP allows using established parameters for BP established by the surgery team • Assess volume status • Monitor cyanide level if prolonged use (>2 days) for nitroprusside
Nitroglycerin	10–200 µg/min	• Titrate drip rate to maintain BP within established acceptable BP parameters set by the surgery team • Decrease drip rate to off as BP allows after oral vasodilators have been started
Inotrope		General above monitor volume status
Epinephrine	2–12 µg/min	• Monitor volume status (RAP) • Monitor perfusion (CO/CI), BP • Assess for ↑urine output with ↑perfusion • Monitor H/H (↓H/H can lead to hypovolemia and ↓perfusion) • Monitor for atrial or ventricular dysrhythmia as source of ↓CO/CI • Monitor ECG for cardiac ischemia
Dobutamine	3–15 µg/kg/min	• May be added if unable to wean epinephrine in attempt to wean epinephrine • Can be infused on floor via central line at low dose • Monitor ECG for cardiac ischemia, tachycardia
Milrinone Often used for pulmonary hypertension or depressed RV function	0.25–0.75 µg/kg/min	• Milrinone may contribute to hypotension • May be weaned to lowest tolerated dose maintaining adequate perfusion • Monitor ECG for ventricular ectopy, atrial fibrillation, and increase in ventricular response in patients already in atrial fibrillation

RAP: right atrial pressure; BP: blood pressure; PAP: pulmonary artery pressure; H/H: hemoglobin and hematocrit; HR: heart rate; CTICU: cardiothoracic intensive care unit; MAP: mean arterial pressure; CO/CI: cardiac output and cardiac index; ECG: electrocardiogram; RV: right ventricular.

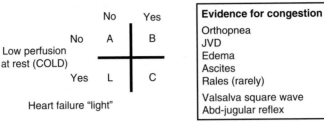

Congestion at rest (WET)

	No	Yes
No	A	B
Yes	L	C

Low perfusion at rest (COLD)

Heart failure "light"

Evidence for congestion
Orthopnea
JVD
Edema
Ascites
Rales (rarely)

Valsalva square wave
Abd-jugular reflex

Evidence for low perfusion
Narrow pulse pressure
Cool extremities
May be sleepy, obtunded
Suspect from ACE1 hypotension and low Na
One cause of worsening renal function

Figure 14.1 Profile A is used to describe a patient that is adequately perfused and free of congestion, warm, and dry. Profile B represents a patient that is adequately perfused but congested, warm, and wet. Profile C represents a patient that is hypoperfused and congested, cold, and wet. Profile L is reserved for patients that are hypoperfused and free of congestion. These profiles were developed to guide medical therapy. In the post surgical patient, this profile can be used to continually assess the patient's response to medical therapy and guide changes in medications during the postoperative course. Reprinted from [10], with permission from the European Society of Cardiology.
JVD: jugular venous distention; Abd: abdominal; ACE1: angiotensin converting enzyme 1; Na: sodium.

(up to $5\,\mu g/kg/min$), dobutamine, and milrinone can be safely managed on the nursing floor, not epinephrine or norepinephrine.

Physical assessment

Healthcare providers must possess keen physical assessment skills to aide interpretation of hemodynamic data. Stevenson described four hemodynamic profiles of acute decompensation in patients with chronic HF (Figure 14.1) [10]. This model evaluates congestion (wet or dry) and perfusion (warm or cold). Laboratory values may reveal worsening renal and/or hepatic function and hyponatremia in patients exhibiting a cold and/or wet hemodynamic profile [10–12]. The postoperative goal is to maintain or achieve a warm and dry hemodynamic profile. Prompt recognition and notification of hemodynamic profile changes will facilitate alterations in the plan of care that preserves end-organ function. Patients in cardiogenic shock who are unresponsive to medication and IABP therapies may need MCS [8].

Postoperative fluid status

Patients with HF are carefully monitored for volume status (RAP, pulmonary artery diastolic pressure) in

an attempt to prevent or minimize hypervolemia, pulmonary edema, and congestive HF. Loop diuretic therapy is initiated soon after return from the OR or the following morning. For patients with decreased urine output and significant volume overload and/or congestion, a continuous infusion loop diuretic (furosemide) drip may be used to increase and optimize urine output. Adding a thiazide diuretic such as metolazone or chlorothiazide may enhance urine output [11]. Low dose spironolactone may be added when patients remain in NYHA class III and IV status and have normal to near normal renal function (i.e. creatinine $< 2\,mg/dL$) [11,13,14]. Once spironolactone is initiated on the nursing floor, routine monitoring of serum potassium, and attention to altering potassium replacement therapy is needed [11,13–16].

Oral medication management for chronic HF

The American College of Cardiology/American Heart Association (ACC/AHA) and the Heart Failure Society of America (HFSA) developed consensus recommendations for the management of patients with chronic systolic HF [15,16]. Routine HF medications include an ACE inhibitor and a β-blocker as core therapy and the addition of diuretics for symptom relief [11–17]. In addition, angiotensin II receptor blocker (ARB), aldosterone inhibitor, combination hydralazine/nitrate, and digoxin are used when criteria are met [15]. After weaning from inotropic and vasopressor support, routine HF medications must be resumed. Additional cardiac medications are prescribed on an individual basis and include agents used in secondary prevention of cardiovascular events (i.e. statin, aspirin, warfarin, nitrate) [15,16].

Postoperatively, special needs may limit the use of core HF medication therapies. Resumption of an ACE inhibitor (i.e. enalapril, captopril) is limited by the patients systolic BP and renal function. Ideally, ACE inhibitor therapy is initiated about 24 h after discontinuation of inotropic therapy. When systolic BP remains low (below 90 mmHg) during the postoperative recovery period, an ACE inhibitor may not be initiated/resumed until after discharge from the hospital. The clinician must assess prior contraindication or intolerance to an ACE inhibitor (i.e. angioedema or severe cough, respectively) and initiate an ARB (i.e. valsartan, or candesartan) or combination of hydralazine and nitrate therapy with isosorbide dinitrate [14–16]. Nursing care includes instructing patients to make position changes slowly, monitoring BP and serum potassium values, and notifying a physician of intolerance to vasodilator medications.

A β-blocker (i.e. metoprolol succinate or carvedilol) should be initiated as soon as possible postoperatively. Patients should be euvolemic without a history of reactive airway pulmonary disease such as asthma, heart block without a pacemaker or unstable class IV HF [13,17]. β-blockers are initiated at the lowest dose and increased as tolerated, usually after hospital discharge. The nurse should monitor the patient's HR and BP after therapy initiation since symptomatic bradycardia can decrease CO and end-organ perfusion. Side effects include lethargy, shortness of breath (SOB), and worsening congestion [10,17].

Low dose digoxin (0.125 mg/day) is used to increase ventricular contraction postoperatively. Nurses should monitor the patient's HR and assess for signs of toxicity that include anorexia, nausea, vomiting, diarrhea, or visual changes. In patient's with poor renal function or in those with limited muscle mass (cachexia), the dose may be decreased to every other day and creatinine clearance should be used to determine the best dose [11,13,16].

General HF medication instructions for the patient include monitoring of their BP, HR, and weight daily. Patients should be given parameters as to acceptable systolic BP and HR specific to their tolerance. Medications are held or the dose is reduced for symptomatic hypotension or bradycardia. For example, an ACE inhibitor is held or the dose decreased if the systolic BP is <85–90 mmHg and the patient developed dizziness or lightheadedness. Nurses should instruct patients to make position changes slowly to avoid orthostatic hypotension and to notify their physician if new or worsening symptoms occur [13]. In addition, patients need to communicate with the healthcare team when they are unable to take their medicine so adjustments can be made.

After cardiac surgery, it is common that patients will be sent home on lower doses of HF medications than their preoperative doses. Up-titration will be continued as tolerated as an outpatient. Careful attention to drug interactions with antiarrhythmic medications must be observed [15,16].

Dysrhythmias and cardiac devices

Postoperatively, patients with HF are at risk for atrial and ventricular dysrhythmias. Atrial tachydysrhythmias may not be well tolerated, especially in patients with postoperative myocardial stunning or those with a low EF. Every attempt is made to return from atrial fibrillation to sinus rhythm. Routine advanced cardiac life support (ACLS) protocols are followed. For patients with depressed EF, amiodarone is the antidysrhythmic agent of choice for supraventricular and ventricular dysrhythmias [15]. Direct current cardioversion (DCC) is attempted if patients failed to convert with an antidysrhythmic agent and after correction of potassium and magnesium deficiencies. While hospitalized after cardiac surgery, DCC is performed within 48 h of the onset of atrial fibrillation. If atrial fibrillation persists, antidysrhythmic therapy is continued and aimed at rate control and anticoagulation is maintained to prevent thromboembolic events [15]. Patients are reassessed in 6 weeks and DCC therapy is repeated if necessary.

Table 14.2 Early complications of the postsurgical patients with HF.

Complication	Findings	Treatment	Nursing care
Hypovolemia	• Decreased BP, RAP, PAP • Decreased CO, CI	• Replace volume	• Monitor and report changes in hemodynamics
Bleeding	• Decreased BP, RAP, PAP • Increased CT output	• Replace volume • Correct coagulopathy with blood, blood products • Protamine may be given	• Monitor and report changes in hemodynamics, CT output • Send coagulation panel and notify any aberrancy • Maintain available blood products • Prepare for return to OR
Cardiac tamponade	• Elevated RAP, LAP, PAP • Decreased CO, CI, BP • CXR reveals ↑cardiac silhouette	• IV inotropic support, vasopressors • TEE may be requested • Return to OR	• Titrate pressor support • Monitor and report changes in hemodynamics • Prepare for return to OR • Have blood products available • Emergency medication available for transfer to OR
Cardiogenic shock	• Elevated RAP, LAP, PAP • Decreased BP, CO, CI	• Add or increase IV inotropic support • Place IABP • Consider LVAD, RVAD, ECMO	• Monitor and report changes in hemodynamics • Prepare for IABP insertion • Maintain inotropic support as ordered • Prepare for MCS if indicated

CT: chest tube; ECMO: extracorporeal membrane oxygenation; OR: operating room; LVAD: left ventricular assist device; RVAD: right ventricular assist device; BP: blood pressure; RAP: right atrial pressure; CO: cardiac output; CI: cardiac index; PAP: pulmonary artery pressure; LAP: left atrial pressure; CXR: chest X-ray; TEE: transesophageal echocardiogram; IV: intravenous; IABP: intra-aortic balloon pump; MCS: mechanical circulatory support.

The electrophysiology (EP) service is consulted postoperatively when patients have a history of or have a new episode of ventricular tachycardia or sudden death to assess the need for an internal cardioverter defibrillator (ICD), with or without cardiac resynchronization therapy (CRT) [15,16,18,19]. Electrophysiology is consulted for all patients having LV reconstructive surgery (Dor procedure) and will have an electrophysiologic study and possible implant of an ICD before discharge [20]. Chapter 5 is dedicated to the discussion of CRT and ICD treatment options for patients with HF.

Permanent LV epicardial pacing leads may be placed in the OR for possible CRT after surgery [18,19]. Initially, temporary external pacing is necessary if bradycardia or heart block occurs [8]. Patients are monitored early in the postoperative period for sinus node recovery. If no recovery after 2–5 days, a permanent pacemaker may be necessary. Appendix 1 provides Cleveland Clinic Foundation websites on patient education topics in HF care.

Complications

The surgical HF patient is a challenge to care for in the postoperative course to prevent both early and late complications. During the early phase of recovery, efforts are aimed at maintaining adequate perfusion and euvolemic status. Sometimes, despite optimal medical therapy, patients continue to require high doses of intravenous vasoactive and inotropic medications and develop cardiogenic shock. In this instance, it is imperative to make decisions early regarding MCS. Prompt MCS intervention helps to protect other vital organs from irreversible damage [8,21]. A list of early complications is summarized in Table 14.2. Prompt recognition and treatment of cardiogenic shock will prevent the potential late complications of renal failure, and hepatic dysfunction [21]. Table 14.3 lists late complications. Specific nursing interventions and considerations are included in each table.

Table 14.3 Late complications of the postsurgical patient with HF.

Complication	Signs and symptoms	Treatment	Nursing care

Neurologic
Encephalopathy
CVA
  Hemorrhagic
  Thromboembolic
	• Decreased mentation
	• Comatose
	• Right or left sided weakness, paralysis
	• Visual changes
		• Correct metabolic derangements
		• Immediate intervention by neurology with possible need for angiogram, intervention
		• Anticoagulate if appropriate
			• Monitor neurologic status, report any changes
			• Prompt recognition allows for prompt intervention, may improve prognosis

Infection Blood Urine Pneumonia Wound infection (Sternum, vein harvest sites, MCS exit site)	• Positive blood, urine, sputum culture • Drainage from surgical sites with positive culture • Erythema, drainage, pus from surgical sites • Fever, hypotension	• All invasive lines to be changed every 7 days • Observe surgical wounds daily; If open wound, pack TID • Prompt recognition and treatment with antibiotics • Infectious disease consult	• Meticulous wound care • Send cultures for temperature >38.3°C • Administer antibiotics • Sterile dressing changes to MCS exit sites
Respiratory failure	• Unable to wean from ventilator • ↑Pulmonary secretions • Pneumonia	• Tracheostomy • Sedation as required to optimize ventilator performance • Appropriate antibiotic coverage specific to organism	• Sedation necessary for comfort • Suction frequently, minimize trauma • Administer antibiotics • Educate patient, family about tracheostomy
Clinical HF	• ↑edema, ↑weight, JVD, SOB, fatigue • Possible ascites or anasarca • ↑congestion on CXR, rales • O$_2$ saturation under 92% • Exercise intolerance • ↓BP, ↑HR • Decreased appetite	• ↑diuretic therapy • Reassess current medications • ↑or ↓dosages as needed based on symptoms • Intravenous inotropic therapy • Hemodynamic monitoring (invasive or non-invasive) as needed to guide treatment (return to ICU)	• Monitor intake, output (I&O) and weight daily • Administer and monitor response to medications ordered • Closely monitor ECG, VS, and signs and symptoms of congestion and perfusion
Gastrointestinal Illeus	• ↓bowel sounds • Abdominal distention • Bowel dilation	• Keep NPO • Consult to GI or colon and rectal surgery	• Strict NPO • Notify of any changes • Obtain KUB as ordered
Hepatic Congestion/failure or shock liver	• ↑bilirubin • ↑transaminases	• Monitor liver enzymes	• Timely lab draws

(Continued)

Table 14.3 (*Continued*)

Complication	Signs and symptoms	Treatment	Nursing care
Renal insufficiency or failure			
	• ↓Urine output • ↑BUN and serum CR • Hypervolemia	• Optimize fluid status • Monitor labs • Consult renal service for dialysis if necessary • Ultrafiltration	• Strict record of intake and urine/other output • Timely lab draws • Administer diuretics as ordered • Monitor RAP, JVD, edema, ascites • Prepare for catheter placement for dialysis as needed

CVA: cerebral vascular accident; MCS: mechanical circulatory support; TID: three times a day; JVD: jugular venous distention; SOB: shortness of breath; CXR: Chest X-ray; BP: blood pressure; HR: heart rate; I/O: intake and output; ECG: electrocardiogram; VS: vital signs; NPO: nothing by mouth; GI: gastrointestinal; BUN: blood urea nitrogen; CR: creatinine; RAP: right atrial pressure; KUB: kidney, ureter, bladder X-ray; ICU: intensive care unit; O_2: oxygenation; GI: gastrointestinal.

Intermediate nursing care

Once transferred to the intermediate care (telemetry) nursing floor, care is aimed at optimizing medication therapies, enhancing functional capacity, and educating the patient on HF and postsurgical self-care actions.

Nurses must have adequate assessment skills to be able to identify patients in one of the four hemodynamic profiles previously described and to recognize signs of decreased perfusion or new/worsening congestion that requires prompt physician notification. Weights are obtained and recorded daily. Close monitoring of response to diuretic therapy by accurate recording of intake and output is imperative. Fluid restriction of 1800–2000 mL/24 h is maintained. Nurses must instruct patients on the steps for daily weight monitoring and the rationale for this behavior.

Nurses must monitor telemetry recordings for HR and rhythm and promptly notify a physician when new or worsening rhythm disturbances are detected. Temporary pacing wires are removed by the surgical team once the patient's rhythm has stabilized, usually the day prior to discharge.

Postoperative discharge and HF self-care education is initiated as soon as possible. Every interaction with patients provides time for education. With every medication given, patients should be instructed on the name of the medication, purpose, dose, frequency, and common side effects.

Cardiac Rehabilitation is consulted for monitoring patient activity during hospitalization. Prior to discharge, the cardiac rehabilitation service provides the patient and family with recommendations for activity immediately after discharge. If patients are suitable candidates, consult to Phase II cardiac rehabilitation will be recommended 6 weeks after recovery. During the early postdischarge period, patients are instructed not to lift anything over 10 lb and not to lift anything over their heads. Patients are instructed to gradually increase their activity as able and allow for rest during the day while recovering. An example of HF exercise guidelines is found at www.clevelandclinic.org/health/health-info/docs. Patients are instructed to follow the recommendations of their physician.

For debilitated patients, consultations with physical and occupational therapy are obtained during the hospitalization. Recommendations may be made for transfer to a rehabilitation facility to gain strength and exercise endurance prior to returning home.

Predischarge testing

Prior to discharge but after weaning of inotropic support, a TTE is performed to assess LV/RV function, wall motion, valve competency, and presence of a pericardial effusion. Patients with an ICD require interrogation of their device prior to discharge. If a CRT device was placed, optimization of device settings is completed with the guidance of a TTE. Depending on the type of surgery performed, additional tests may be recommended such as cardiac MRI or computed tomography (CT) scan.

Discharge teaching

Preparing patients for discharge requires assessing patients preoperative knowledge of heart disease and of HF, including what HF is, consequences, and self-care behaviors [22,23]. Assessing individual learning needs will allow the educational focus to be on new or different material.

Patients receive written educational material to assist with the educational process. Providing written materials reinforces teaching and provides a resource. Nurses should review written materials with patients and family/significant others to advance learning and adaptive potential. No matter what the educational focus, patients will need to understand what is expected postdischarge and what needs to be reported to their healthcare provider [22,23].

Referral to support disciplines provides added resources, a more in depth review of behavior expectations and reinforcement of education already received. The dietician can provide information on food shopping, meal preparation, and dining outside the home to promote adherence to diet modifications. The social worker or financial counselor can assess economic status and barriers to medication and self-care adherence. Many disciplines can assess coping with illness, depression, and level of support available postdischarge.

Specific HF discharge instructions include low sodium diet modification, exercise and activity, medication plan, monitoring fluid status, and identifying worsening HF signs and symptoms to report to health care providers [22,23]. Table 14.4 reviews HF education themes. Other education themes include smoking cessation (if applicable), limiting alcohol and caffeine intake, and warfarin and International Normalization Ratio (INR) testing as needed [23]. With ongoing education and reinforcement of information, patients should experience a better quality of life and fewer hospitalizations if adhere to recommended treatment plan and are able to identify early signs of decompensation [23,24].

Follow-up appointments

Routine surgical follow-up to the Cleveland Clinic occurs within 1–2 weeks after discharge. We have found this decreases visits to the emergency department when the patients are evaluated early and questions can be answered regarding their care. A Nurse Practitioner will assess cardiovascular and respiratory status, incisions, signs and symptoms, activity level and diet, adjust medications, reinforce teaching, and identify learning needs.

Routine cardiac care includes follow-up with the cardiologist within 1–2 weeks of discharge when patients live a long distance from the Cleveland Clinic. If patients would like to continue care at the Cleveland Clinic, they may be placed in the HF Disease Management Program. Advance practice nurses (Nurse Practitioners or Clinical Nurse Specialist) who specialize in HF, provide HF care, and coordinate care with the HF cardiologist and other consultants. Medication adjustment, laboratory values monitoring, physical, psychosocial and emotional assessment, education, and self-care counseling are some of the services offered [25]. (See Chapter 6, Managing an HF Clinic for more information about HF out-patient programs.) Nurses are part of a multidisciplinary team providing care to patients with HF, teaching them to care for themselves by managing diet, exercise, medications, and fluid status.

When patients are followed outside of the Cleveland Clinic, a copy of their operative report and discharge summary are sent to the referring physician. The referring physician is provided other significant details necessary for ongoing care. The frequency of ongoing HF follow-up after the 30-day surgical convalescent period is determined by the cardiologist.

Mechanical Circulatory Support

Evaluation

Candidates for MCS include patients listed for cardiac transplantation from end-stage systolic HF, including post-cardiotomy HF and postacute myocardial infarction cardiogenic shock. Patients described above are labeled bridge to transplant (BTT). MCS can also be used for permanent support, labeled destination therapy (DT). DT applies to

Table 14.4 HF discharge teaching.

Topic	Instructions	Consults/teaching needs	Symptoms to report
Diet	• 2000 mg sodium • Low animal fat diet • Encourage fresh foods	• Dietician • Family members attend teaching sessions • Reading food labels	• Weight gain of 2 lb in 1 day or 5 lb in 1 week • Unusual SOB, DOE, orthopnea, fatigue • Exercise intolerance
Exercise	• No lifting >10 lbs × 6 weeks • No driving × 6 weeks • Progressive ↑in exercise • Cardiac rehabilitation Phase II (6 weeks after DC)	• Cardiac rehabilitation consult • Cardiac rehabilitation Phase II consult at discharge	• Unable to tolerate previous ↑exercise and activity level • ↑SOB, DOE, fatigue
Volume status	• Weigh self daily • Restrict fluid to <2000 mL/day	• Monitor intake and output • Weigh daily	• Report unusual weight gain of 2 lb overnight or 5 lb in 1 week • Abdominal bloating, lower extremity edema, orthopnea, paroxysmal nocturnal dyspnea
Vital signs	• Monitor vital signs (HR, BP)	• Home care consult if patient homebound	• Notify for HR <60 or >120 • Notify for systolic BP <85 or >150
Signs and symptoms	• Notify for new or worsening fatigue, dyspnea, edema, and needing to ↑pillows at night	• Recognize symptoms of CHF early	• Notify ↑HR or ICD shock • Chest pain, dizziness, change in appetite
Medication	• Purpose • Dose • Frequency • Adverse reaction • Normal side effects	• Provide medication list with purpose, dose, frequency • Regular schedule • Skipped doses • Refill of prescriptions • Polypharmacy issues	• Side or adverse reactions • Worsening CHF

SOB: shortness of breath; DOE: dyspnea on exertion; DC: discharge; HR: heart rate; BP: blood pressure; CHF: congestive heart failure; ICD: internal cardioverter-defibrillator.

patients already on maximal medical therapy experiencing NYHA class IV HF without heart transplant as an option. Patients are evaluated and if deemed an appropriate candidate will have MCS placed as DT.

The Heartmate® LVAD and Novacor® left ventricular assist system (LVAS) are implantable, pulsatile devices that can be used outside of a hospital setting. A thorough discussion of available devices and criteria for implantation is found in Chapter 13.

Once the decision is made to place a MCS device, the patient is prepared for surgery. First and foremost is educating the patient and family on the particular device and describing the risks, benefits, and potential complications. When the patient and family can meet a patient currently on support, they will have a

better understanding of what an LVAD is and can learn how patients manage on support. Preoperative education includes seeing the external components, hearing the device, and learning about quality of life after device placement. Showing the patient and family a demonstration pump enhances understanding. For DT patients, preoperative education facilitates full disclosure and aides in making an informed decision about their care.

Routine preoperative orders are written with the addition of specific orders for device placement. Patients with an elevated bleeding time (INR) may be given vitamin K (10 mg intravenous) the evening before and morning of surgery to overcome the liver's inability to make clotting factors due to congestion as a result of HF [26]. Heparin is discontinued 6 h prior to surgery unless contraindicated. Preoperative broad-spectrum antibiotics are given prophylactically to prevent infection. Every effort is made to take patients to surgery in a dry state to prevent intra- and postoperative oxygenation problems.

Intraoperative care

Aprotinin was used routinely to decrease the risk of coagulopathic bleeding until recently [27]. Recent reports indicate a higher rate of renal dysfunction with aprotinin use [28], but the risk of excessive bleeding in this patient population, with subsequent right HF must be weighed when considering which drug to use [27]. In patients with renal impairment aminocaproic acid may be the better choice. Two units of fresh frozen plasma (FFP) are placed in the CPB circuit prior to initiation of CPB to assist clotting and correct prolonged INR. TEE is performed pre-CPB to assess LV/RV function, valve competence (especially aortic insufficiency), condition of the aorta, and presence of a patent foramen ovale. The LVAD is prepared on a back table by the registered nurse (RN) first assistant while the surgical team prepares the pump pocket and places the patient on CPB. If necessary, concomitant procedures will be performed such as valve repair or CABG. Aortic valve repair is performed if aortic insufficiency is >2+ [29]. Once the MCS device is placed, the patient is weaned from CPB by TEE guided de-airing of the heart and device. De-airing the device is accomplished by hand pumping the Heartmate® or providing single strokes to the Novacor® via the LVAS monitor prior to initiation of support. Intravenous inotropic therapy is initiated to assist RV contractility. Once the device is de-aired the patient is weaned from CPB while at the same time activating the device at its lowest fixed setting. Cardiac assessment by TEE continues to monitor RV, valve function, orientation of the inflow cannulae in the LV, LV volume, and reassess for a patent foramen ovale.

During device activation and weaning from CPB, the surgical and anesthesia teams will optimize medical therapy using inotropic, vasopressor, or vasodilator support as previously described. ABG and blood loss are monitored. The anesthesia team will replace volume using leukocyte reduced

Table 14.5 Differential diagnosis of low flow after LVAD.

Hemodynamics	Device flow/ output	Diagnosis
↓BP, RAP, PAP, LAP	↓Flow	Hypovolemia or bleeding
↓BP ↑RAP, LAP, PAP	↓Flow	Tamponade
↑RAP ↓LAP	↓Flow	RV dysfunction/failure
↑RAP, LAP, PAP	↓Flow	Over-ventilation

Note: ↑Flow with ↑Pump rate may be indicative of inflow valve incompetence due to infection or valvular insufficiency after prolonged use.
BP: blood pressure; RAP: right atrial pressure; PAP: pulmonary artery pressure; LAP: left atrial pressure; RV: right ventricular.

red blood cells and other blood products. Platelet transfusion is minimized to help prevent patient sensitization postoperatively for those to receive a heart transplant [27,30]. The chest is closed once bleeding has resolved. Another TEE is performed once the chest is closed to assess inflow conduit position and adequate flow into the device. The patient is then transferred to the CTICU.

Patients' chest may be left open if they received multiple blood products or if they have edema of the heart, wet lungs or unstable hemodynamics. A sterile table is kept at the patient's bedside should urgent exploration be necessary in the CTICU. Closure of the chest occurs 1–2 days later when swelling has diminished and diuresis has occurred.

CTICU care

Once in the CTICU, stabilization of hemodynamics and serum lab values reflecting organ function are focuses of care. Deficient coagulation factors are corrected to minimize bleeding. An FFP drip may be continued until bleeding resolves. Close monitoring of device filling is necessary to assess volume status and RV function. Hemodynamic parameters are monitored assessing for potential early complications found in Table 14.5. Device flows are monitored with other hemodynamic parameters discussed previously.

A few "tricks" have been learned. For patients experiencing decreased volume into the pump and therefore decreased LVAD flows, the ventilator can be removed for about 30 sec to assess for a rise in LVAD flow. If the LVAD flow increases with this maneuver, the decrease in flow may be due to increased intra-thoracic pressure. Decreasing the positive end-expiratory pressure (PEEP) or tidal volume may resolve the problem [31]. Thoratec Corporation has enhanced the software of the Heartmate device to Opti-Fill to allow for 96% pump filling before pump ejection. Therefore, the pump speed does not increase in the automatic mode until the stroke volume is 80 mL or better. As a result, the device is kept in the fixed mode of operation until the patient's cardiac and volume status stabilizes. The automatic mode is used once the clinician identifies consistent pump filling with flows acceptable for perfusion. The change in Heartmate device software was accomplished to increase device durability [32].

Intra and early postoperative medications are the same as those discussed in Table 14.1, with some additions. Milrinone therapy is utilized to assist with depressed RV function since it is a vasodilator as well as an inotropic agent. Milrinone works well but may lead to decreased systemic BP requiring the use of norepinephrine to maintain an adequate BP. If the norepinephrine drip rate is >10 μg/min and the patient remains vasodilated, vasopressin is added [33]. If the patient continues to be vasodilated despite two vasopressive agents, methylene blue may be used although this is rare [34,35]. Methylene blue has been described in the literature for use in refractory hypotension following CPB that is unresponsive to norepinephrine support [34]. It is delivered as a bolus dose followed by a continuous intravenous infusion through a central line, not to exceed 6 h. Serum methemoglobin, bilirubin, and hemoglobin and hematocrit levels must be monitored. Patient responders will have an evident rise in arterial BP. Researchers found no effect on HR, CO, and ABG results [34,35]. Table 14.6 provides details regarding administration of methylene blue.

RV failure

Following LVAD placement, recovery is much like any patient having surgery with HF, except the LVAD will perform the work of the LV. Acceptable LVAD flow/output is determined by how well the RV is functioning or being supported. Close monitoring

Table 14.6 CVICU guidelines for use of intravenous methylene blue for postoperative refractory hypotension [34,35].

Dose/Concentration	Guidelines
Bolus dosing:	Administer via central line over minimum of 15 min
1–2 mg/kg IV	Max dose 250 mg/50 mL or 5 mg/mL
Dilute in 50 mL of 0.9% NaCl	Use actual body weight to calculate dose
	Bolus dose has <4 h effect on hemodynamics
	Assess response to bolus dosing to determine effectiveness
	Do not have to give bolus dose
Continuous Infusion:	Administer via central line
0.25–1.5 mg/kg/h	Adjust dose to maintain prescribed MAP
	Taper other vasopressive agents as able
300 mg/150 mL 0.9% NaCl for total volume (must remove 45 mL of NaCl before adding drug)	Continually monitor BP
	Do not infuse >6 h
	Urine turns bluish-green

IV: intravenous; MAP: mean arterial pressure; BP: blood pressure; NaCl: sodium chloride.

of RV function is imperative. To aide RV function, avoid fluid overload, and hypoxia. Inhaled nitric oxide (NO) may be warranted in combination with intravenous inotropic therapy (most often milrinone) to support the RV without an right ventricular assist device (RVAD) [29,36,37]. Some centers use NO routinely, we use it selectively [31].

Pericardial tamponade

Once bleeding has subsided, patients need to be monitored for pericardial tamponade. Signs of tamponade include decreased LVAD flow (and decreased volume into the pump) and an increase in RAP, LA pressure, and decreased BP. Diagnostic tests include CXR and TTE, but tamponade may not be evident. CXR may reveal an enlarged cardiac silhouette and TEE may reveal compressed RV or LV with hematoma. If tamponade is found, return to the OR is needed [31]. Once the chest is opened, there should be an immediate increase in LVAD flow. If a patient's condition is critical, the chest may be opened at the bedside.

Infection

Efforts to prevent infection are the highest priority in MCS patients. Invasive monitoring lines must be discontinued as soon as the patient's condition allows. All invasive lines to be maintained need to be changed every 7 days or sooner if clinically indicated. Prophylactic broad-spectrum antibiotic therapy is maintained for 48 h unless treating a known infection.

To prevent infection at the device exit site (or driveline exit site), meticulous nursing and patient care is needed. During surgery, a single suture is placed at the driveline exit site to immobilize it, thus promoting wound healing. The suture is removed within 5–7 days of implant. To further immobilize the driveline and prevent local trauma or irritation from the weight of the controller, an abdominal binder or stabilization belt (standard abdominal binder or purchased from LVAD manufacturer) is applied [38,39]. The binder or belt is placed prior to exiting the OR and is maintained at all times except during morning care and dressing changes.

To further prevent infection at the driveline exit site, sterile dressing changes are mandatory. The procedure includes the following steps: (a) the patient and nurse to wear a surgical mask, (b) the nurse performs a 3-min surgical hand wash, and (c) the nurse wears sterile gloves and uses aseptic technique to cleanse the area and apply a dry sterile dressing. Once healing has occurred and no signs of infection exist, the dressing may be changed using a clean technique. The frequency of dressing changes may be as often as three or more times a day to insure a clean and dry site.

Once patients are extubated and are hemodynamically stable, they are transferred to a private room on the intermediate care nursing floor. Patients may continue to require intravenous inotropic therapy for RV support, which will be weaned off when possible.

Intermediate care nursing floor

Once upgraded to the intermediate care unit, cardiac rehabilitation and self-care management are introduced as a focus of care. Nurses need to assess patients' physical and emotional status prior to formalizing a treatment plan.

Consultation with physical and occupational therapy assists patients with rehabilitation as needed. As the patient displays improved strength requiring some assistance, our cardiac rehabilitation team is consulted for monitored ambulation. As part of progressive cardiac rehabilitation, patients initially ambulate in the halls accompanied by a rehabilitation team member. As patient strength increases and ambulation is independent, they are invited to attend treadmill class with a rehabilitation team member who monitors patient tolerance and progress to increased activity. A stationary bike is also available for patient use in the rehabilitation room on the unit.

A nutritional team member assesses the need for and recommends diet supplements to optimize calorie intake for healing. Supplying snacks during the day is necessary as some patients are only able to eat small amounts at a time due to compression of the stomach by the LVAD. A feeding tube may be placed early postoperatively in the CTICU to provide adequate nutrition but placement can be a challenge. Continued tube feedings may be necessary on transfer to intermediate care. Tube feedings are slowly weaned by allowing oral intake during the day and maintaining 12 h nightly infusions. Once oral intake is adequate and oral supplements are tolerated, feeding tubes are removed.

Patients on MCS are treated with core HF medications whenever possible. Keeping the systolic BP below 130 mmHg helps preserve the inflow valve conduit of the device [40]. Use of an ACE inhibitor or ARB when ACE inhibitor is contraindicated, achieves this. β-blockers are restarted as tolerated and diuretics are used for volume overload.

Monitoring and assessing for dysrhthmias continues as with any surgical patient. While ventricular tachycardia is tolerated in patients with devices, ACLS medication protocols rather than DCC are followed if device flow remains stable [29]. When medications are unsuccessful or if the patient is unstable, DCC is indicated. Device manufacturer's have instructions regarding DCC. The Heartmate extended lead vented electric (XVE)® requires the controller be disconnected prior to DCC [31].

Discharge education is an important aspect of care and involves patient (and family) demonstration of expected behaviors. Initially, patients are instructed on monitoring and recording their intake and output daily. Medication education follows with eventual self medication administration while hospitalized. While participating in self medication administration, the patient and family are educated on device self management.

Prior to hospital discharge patients must learn about the device, device components, power supply, alarm conditions, and demonstrate emergency steps and procedures. First, the patient and family are taught how the device operates, the different modes of operation, and the components necessary for proper device function. Second, they learn to change from tethered mode of operation to untethered (battery power). Equipment is available for "hands on" training. Finally, patients and family must demonstrate changing a controller, hand pumping (for Heartmate XVE), identifying alarm conditions, and correction steps. Patients must know how and when to call the LVAD team and demonstrate how to call through the paging system prior to discharge from the hospital [31].

While device education and rehabilitation is ongoing, patients are monitored for late complications (refer to Table 14.3). Infection leads to increased morbidity and the randomized evaluation of mechanical assistance for the treatment of congestive heart failure (REMATCH) trial identified infection as the leading cause of death for DT patients [39]. Infections should always be identified and treated promptly. Other complications include stroke, late bleeding, and tamponade (especially if anticoagulated).

Prior to discharge, a TTE is performed to assess LV unloading in auto mode, RV function, and valve competency. Additionally, to assess patients' response to decreased flow, the pump is switched to the fixed mode of operation and the pump rate is gradually decreased to a rate of 50 beats/min. The LVAD team assesses patient tolerance to the decreased flow and ability to change a controller, should this become necessary.

Patients with MCS receive the same HF guidelines as described in Table 14.4. In addition to monitoring weight, intake and output, and change in urination (decrease in frequency, amount or dark urine), patients are instructed to record their BP, HR, weight, pump flow/output, stroke volume, and pump rate once daily on a flow sheet they maintain. Patients are expected to bring their flow sheet to outpatient department (OPD) appointments. Patients are instructed to call the LVAD team for a decrease in LVAD flows, increased HR, increased weight, and new onset of fever, chills, or signs of infection.

Follow-up appointments

Patients on MCS are followed closely after discharge. A home care nurse visits patients daily to weekly (determined by insurance coverage) to assure optimal adaptation to lifestyle changes and to ensure patients can perform wound care independently. For patients without family support, home care visits may continue for a prolonged period.

Patients are evaluated in the OPD weekly for the first month. During routine appointments, patient and family coping with the complexity of device care is assessed. The social worker assesses patients' need for ongoing support and assistance. In addition to physical examination, laboratory assessment, and device assessment, the driveline exit site is assessed for infection. The MCS device is connected to the monitor to document pump flow/output, rate, and stroke volume. Device related alarms and equipment problems are assessed. Patients are expected to bring their emergency back up equipment with them. Consults are placed to other services as necessary. Routine blood tests are drawn and include a complete metabolic panel, complete blood cell count, prothrombin time, activated prothrombin time, serum free hemoglobin with each visit. Once a month panel reactive antibodies (PRA's) are assessed for patients with BTT status. A CXR and electrocardiogram data are collected as needed. Patients are encouraged to continue Phase II cardiac rehabilitation after discharge [31].

Once patients and families display evidence of adapting to lifestyle changes and device therapy and medical care is stable, OPD visits are decreased to bimonthly then every 4–6 weeks. Patients must demonstrate the ability to call with problems or changes in their condition such as signs and symptoms of infection, weight gain, or SOB. Driveline infections are managed in the OPD for patients able to identify changes in their condition, however, the frequency of visit may need to be increased. Periodic TTE will be done to assess for valve incompetence or to monitor for LV recovery as warranted [32].

If recovery is suspected, the patient will have a "turn off" TTE with BP monitoring. The patient is anticoagulated with heparin and the pump is placed in a fixed mode to a rate of about 10 beats below the patient's intrinsic rate, then decreased by increments of 10 beats to a rate of 50 beats/min. In patients with demonstrated tolerance (maintaining an adequate BP, HR, and no symptoms of dizziness, lightheadedness, or SOB), the device is turned off for 2 min. (Either intermittent hand pumping or single stroke of the device is necessary.) If the patient tolerates the 2 min turn off, they will return for pulmonary artery catheter (or continuous SVO_2) and repeat "turn off" TTE procedure. Hemodynamic assessment is correlated with the TTE data. If remarkable recovery has occurred, the patient may be returned to the OR for device explant, although this is a rare occurrence.

MCS patients have access to the LVAD team 24 h a day. A nurse is on call to manage LVAD questions or problems. The LVAD team is responsible for educating the community in which the patient lives. This is completed prior to the patient returning to their home and includes the local emergency room, local emergency medical system, home health care nurse and local cardiologist, and/or internist. Arrangements are made for emergency return to the implanting facility by ground and air [31].

Patients with DT status living a distance from our institution are eventually followed and managed by their local cardiologist. Patients may need to return to the implanting facility periodically or on the request of their physician. This is center specific.

While patients in BTT and DT status are able to live independently outside of the hospital, healthcare support is ongoing. At the Cleveland Clinic, the social worker established a monthly dinner for patients waiting for transplant in the hospital, those who are postcardiac transplant, and for BTT patients awaiting transplant either in or out of the hospital. Additionally, a transplant education class allows time for HF and transplantation education and a means for patients and families to network with one another.

Summary

Caring for patients with HF after cardiac surgery and/or MCS can be challenging. These patients have complex medical histories and complex care needs. It is imperative for all team members to carefully attend to detail and to collaborate and communicate to promote a successful outcome. A collaborative medical–surgical HF approach facilitates improvement in outcomes and promotes achievement of the ultimate patient goal, to prolong survival, and improve quality of life. Nurses play a vital role in every aspect of care.

Acknowledgment

A special thank you to Nancy Albert for her expert assistance with the writing of this chapter.

References

1 Zeltsman D, Acker MA. Surgical management of heart failure: an overview. *Annu Rev Med* 2002; **53**: 383–391.

2 Kherani AR, Garrido MJ, Cheema FH *et al.* Nontransplant surgical options for congestive heart failure. *Congest Heart Fail* 2003; **9(1)**: 17–24.

3 Miller WL, Tointon SK, Hodge DO *et al.* Long-term outcome and the use of revascularization in patients with heart failure, suspected ischemic heart disease, and large reversible myocardial perfusion defects. *Am Heart J* 2002; **143(5)**: 904–909.

4 Kumpati GS, McCarthy PM, Hoercher KJ. Surgical treatments for heart failure. *Cardiol Clin* 2001; **19(4)**: 669–681.

5 Bolling SF, Smolens IA, Pagani FD. Surgical alternatives for heart failure. *J. Heart Lung Transplant* 2001; **20**: 729–733.

6 Bitran D, Merin O, Klutstein MW *et al.* Mitral valve repair in severe ischemic cardiomyopathy. *J Card Surg* 2001; **16**: 79–82.

7 Pass SE, Simpson RW. Discontinuation and reinstitution of medications during the perioperative period. *Am J Health-Syst Pharm* 2004; **61(9)**: 899–912.

8 Gorman JH, Gorman RC, Milas BC *et al.* Circulatory management of the unstable cardiac patient. *Semin Thorac Cardiovasc Surg* 2000; **12(4)**: 316–325.

9 Savino JS, Hanson CW, Gardner TJ. Cardiothoracic intensive care: operation and administration. *Semin Thorac Cardiovasc Surg* 2000; **12(4)**: 362–370.

10 Stevenson LW. Tailored therapy to hemodynamic goals for advanced heart failure. *Eur J Heart Fail* 1999; **1**: 251–257.

11 Nohria A, Lewis E, Stevenson LW. Medical management of advanced heart failure. *J Am Med Assoc* 2002; **287**: 628–640.

12 Albert NM, Eastwood CA, Edwards ML. Evidenced-based practice for acute decompensated heart failure. *Crit Care Nurse* 2004; **24(6)**: 14–29.

13 Capriotti, T. Current concepts and pharmacologic treatment of heart failure. *Medsurg Nurs* 2002; **11(2)**: 71–83.

14 MacKlin M. Managing heart failure: a case study approach. *Crit Care Nurs* 2001; **21**: 36–48.

15 Hunt SA, Abraham WT, Chin MH *et al.* ACC/AHA 2005 guidelines update for the diagnosis and management of chronic heart failure in the adult-summary article. A report of the American College of Cardiology/American Heart Association task force on practice guidelines (Writing committee to update the 2001 guidelines for the evaluation and management of heart failure): developed in collaboration with the American College of Chest Physicians and the International Society for Heart and Lung Transplantation; endorsed by the Heart Rhythm Society (in process citation). *Circulation* 2005; **112(12)**: 1825–1852.

16 Adams KF, Baughman KL, Dec WG *et al.* Heart failure society of America (HFSA) practice guidelines. HFSA guidelines for management of patients with heart failure caused by left ventricular systolic dysfunction-pharmacological approaches. *J Cardiac Fail* 1999; **5**: 357–382.

17 Meghani SH, Becker D. β-Blockers: a new therapy in congestive heart failure. *Am J Crit Care* 2001; **10**: 417–427.

18 Gregoratos G, Abrams J, Epstein AE *et al.* ACC/AHA/NASPE 2002 guideline update for implantation of cardiac pacemakers and antiarrhythmia devices: summary article. A report of the American College of Cardiology/American Heart Association task force on practice guidelines (ACC/AHA/NASPE committee to update the 1998 pacemaker guidelines). *Circulation* 2002; **106**: 2145–2161.

19 Dressing TJ, Natale A. Congestive heart failure treatment: the pacing approach. *Heart Fail Rev* 2001; **6**: 15–25.

20 O'Neil JO, Starling RC, Khaykin Y *et al.* Residual high incidence of ventricular arrhythmias after left ventricular reconstructive surgery. *J Thorac Cardiovasc Surg* 2005; **130(5)**: 1250–1256.

21 Shinn JA. Implantable left ventricular assist devices. *J Cardiovasc Nurs* 2005; **20(55)**: 522–530.

22 Grady KL, Dracup K, Kennedy G *et al.* AHA scientific statement team management of patients with heart failure. A statement for healthcare professionals from the cardiovascular nursing council of the American Heart Association. *Circulation* 2000; **7**: 2443–2456.

23 Dunbar SB, Jacobson LH, Deaton C. Heart failure: strategies to enhance patient self management. *AACN Clin Issues* 1998; **9(2)**: 244–256.

24 Koelling TM, Johnson ML, Cody RJ *et al.* Discharge education improves clinical outcomes in patients with chronic heart failure. *Circulation* 2005; **111(2)**: 179–185.

25 Albert NM, Young JB. Heart failure disease management: a team approach. *Clev Clin J Med* 2001; **16(1)**: 53–62.

26 Kaplon RJ, Gillinov AM, Smedira NG *et al.* Mechanical and circulatory support vitamin K reduces bleeding in left ventricular assist device recipients. *J Heart Lung Transplant* 1999; **18**: 346–350.

27 Goldstein DJ, Beauford RB. Left ventricular assist devices and bleeding: adding insult to injury. *Ann Thorac Surg* 2003; **75**: S42–S47.

28 Mangano DT, Tudor IC, Dietzel C. The risk associated with aprotinin in cardiac surgery. *N Engl J Med* 2006; **354**: 353–365.

29 Kasirajan V, McCarthy PM, Hoercher KJ *et al.* Clinical experience with long-term use of implantable left ventricular assist devices: indications, implantation, and outcomes. *Semin Thorac Cardiovasc Surg* 2000; **12(3)**: 229–237.

30 Kumpati GS, Cook DJ, Blackstone EH *et al.* HLA sensitization in ventricular assist device recipients: Does type of device make a difference? *J Thorac Cardiovasc Surg* 2004; **127**: 1800–1807.

31 Buda TM, Kendall K. Nursing and psychosocial issues of patients on mechanical support. *J Card Surg* 2001; **16**: 209–221.

32 Poirier VL, Aulenbach CE, Bataille O. Heartmate® VE LVAS Enhancements: The XVE pump clinical perspectives. Thoratec Corporation, Pleasonton, CA, 2002.

33 Morales DL, Gregg D, Helman DN *et al.* Arginine vasopressin in the treatment of 50 patients with postcardiotomy vasodilatory shock. *Ann Thorac Surg* 2000; **69**: 102–106.

34 Leyh RG, Kofidis T, Strüber M *et al.* Methylene blue: the drug of choice for catecholamine-refractory vasoplegia after cardiopulmonary bypass? *J Thorac Cardiovasc Surg* 2003; **125**: 1426–1431.

35 Kirov MY, Evgenov OV, Evgenov NV *et al.* Infusion of methylene blue in human septic shock: a pilot, randomized, controlled study. *Crit Care Med* 2001; **29**: 1860–1867.

36 Oz MC, Ardehali A. Collective review: perioperative uses of inhaled nitric oxide in adults. *Heart Surg Forum* 2004; **7(6)**: E584–E589.

37 Griffiths MJD, Evans TW. Drug therapy. Inhaled nitric oxide therapy in adults. *N Engl J Med* 2005; **353**: 2683–2695.

38 Dembitsky WP, Long JW, Park SJ. Infection control guidelines for the Heartmate® XVE left ventricular assist system (LVAS). Available at: http://www.thoratec.com/ medical-professional/pdf/H017-1103_Infection_Control_Guidelines_English.pdf. Accessed November 19, 2005.

39 Holman WL, Rayburn BK, McGiffin DC *et al.* Infection in ventricular assist devices: prevention and treatment. *Ann Thorac Surg* 2003; **75**: S48–S57.

40 Poirier VL. Inflow valve incompetence. *J Congest Heart Fail Circulat Supp* 2001; **2**: 23–25.

Appendix 1

Cleveland Clinic Websites available on the Care of Patients with Heart Failure

1. http://www.clevelandclinic.org/health/search/show-documents.asp?mediaID=5&topicId=939&sortId=2

You will find links to:

Understanding Heart Failure

Heart Failure Exercise Guidelines

Heart Failure Exercise Precautions

Heart Transplant

Left Ventricular Reconstructive Surgery (Dor procedure)

How Heart Failure is diagnosed

Heart Failure and Nutrition

Potassium Guidelines-Heart Failure

Heart Failure Medications

2. http://www.clevelandclinic.org/heartcenter/pub/guide/disease/heartfailure.asp?firstCat=3&secondCat=246&thirdCat=256

Literature can be found on the topics listed below with many more:

What is Heart Failure

What are the symptoms of heart failure

When to call the doctor about your heart failure symptoms

How heart failure is diagnosed

How is heart failure treated

Understanding heart failure

Surgical procedures to treat heart failure

Learn more about: Biventricular pacemaker

Heart Failure Disease Management Program

Heart Failure Nutritional Guidelines

Left Ventricular Reconstructive Surgery

CHAPTER 15

Biological approaches to heart failure: gene transfer and cell transplantation

Marc S. Penn, Samuel Unzek & Arman T. Askari

Introduction

Congestive heart failure (CHF), primarily as a result of ventricular remodeling in response to myocardial necrosis, remains a leading global cause of morbidity and mortality. Approximately 3.5 million people are presently diagnosed with heart failure in the United States alone, with an expected increase to greater than 6 million people by the year 2030 [1]. Despite an enhanced understanding of the pathophysiologic processes involved in ventricular remodeling [2] and improvements in prevention, diagnosis, and treatment of this disorder, CHF remains a significant therapeutic challenge. Furthermore, although cardiac transplantation may be a definitive therapy for CHF, it remains limited in number.

The limited available therapies and poor prognosis of patients with CHF, coupled with advances in molecular biology and human genomic sciences have resulted in an increased interest in alternative methods that will assist in improving outcomes. Potential targets for this new treatment paradigm may focus on preventing myocardial cell death during myocardial infarction (MI), attenuating pathologic remodeling, and regenerating myocardium. Clinical experience repeatedly demonstrates that two patients can have very different clinical courses despite having "similar" MIs as assessed by location and size. Thus, some of the key molecular processes or pathways involved in left ventricle (LV) remodeling targets may be identified using genomic-population-based strategies focused on identifying patients at highest risk for pathological remodeling following MI. Treatment strategies including gene transfer and autologous cell

transplantation are under active study to determine if they can be used to modulate LV remodeling in the peri-infarct period or augment cardiac performance in the chronically failing heart. This chapter will serve to review the literature on gene transfer and cell transplantation with respect to CHF and will outline potential therapeutic applications of these emerging therapies.

Gene transfer for the treatment of CHF

Although still in its infancy, the utility of gene transfer to enhance myocardial perfusion [3–8] and performance [9–13] has been demonstrated. Along with the identification of a gene of interest, selection of an expression vector and an optimal protocol for gene delivery are all integral components of successful gene transfer. Each of these components must be carefully tailored to the specific pathophysiologic process being targeted.

Mechanisms of gene delivery

The optimal vector for gene delivery would result in (i) the efficient gene expression in a variety of selectable cell types, (ii) allow expression of a reasonably large piece of genetic material including regulatory elements, and (iii) have no adverse effects on the target organ system or the local cellular environment. The ideal gene transfer vector does not exist; however, several viral and non-viral vectors that can be uniquely tailored to specific diseases are available. Of

Table15.1 Vectors for gene transfer: advantages and disadvantages.

Vector		
Synthetic oligonucleotides	Advantages	High transfection efficiency
	Disadvantages	Short half life
		Inability to target-specific cells
		Functions to inhibit gene expression only
Plasmids	Advantages	Non-immunogenic
		Non-pathogenic
		Long-term gene expression
		Able to transfect non-dividing cells
	Disadvantages	Low transduction efficiency
		Delivery via direct injection only
Adeno-associated virus vectors	Advantages	Transduce dividing and non-dividing cells
		Stably transfect cells $\Rightarrow$ long-term gene expression
		Non-pathogenic
		Mild immunogenicity
	Disadvantages	Limited transgene size
		Potential for insertional mutagenesis
		Difficult to produce in large quantities
		Delivery difficulties
Adenovirus vectors	Advantages	Transduce dividing and non-dividing cells
		Facile production
	Disadvantages	Transient gene expression
		Robust inflammatory response
		Not useful for repeat administration
Retroviral vectors	Advantages	Stable transfection within host genome
		Ability to render non-infectious
	Disadvantages	Transduce dividing cells only
		Inefficient gene transfer
		Potential for insertional mutagenesis
		Labile vector *in vivo*
Lentivirus vectors	Advantages	Transduce dividing and non-dividing cells
		Long-term gene expression
		High transduction efficiency
	Disadvantages	Potential for insertional mutagenesis
		Potential for self-replication

the currently available vectors, only a few can achieve efficient, high-level transgene expression in post-mitotic cells such as cardiomyocytes (Table 15.1).

Integral to successful cell and gene transfer strategies is a method that allows adequate delivery to the tissue of interest. Several techniques are being explored including direct myocardial injection [14], catheter-based techniques [15–17], pericardial gene delivery [18], and intravenous infusions [19], each with its own limitations and clinical applicability.

More recently, transplantation of autologous cells that are transfected prior to injection with expression vectors encoding secreted molecules of interest (i.e., vascular endothelial growth factor, VEGF or nitric oxide synthase, NOS) has been studied [20–22]. Thus, the optimal clinical protocol for the delivery of genetic material to the failing myocardium, remains to be determined. That said, it is likely that direct injection into the myocardium either as an adjunct to open-heart surgery, or as a stand-alone procedure via

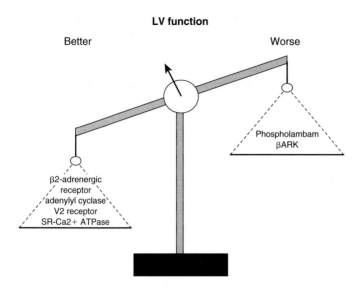

Figure 15.1 Simplified depiction of targets for gene therapy that have been successfully tested. Those targets that have positive inotropic effects (better LV function) have demonstrated benefit with gene over-expression, whereas genetic strategies that inhibit negative inotropic targets (worse LV function) have demonstrated improved LV function.

thorascopy will likely be the earliest techniques associated with consistent clinical benefit.

Candidate genes for the treatment of CHF

Several derangements of myocyte contractile function have been demonstrated within cells isolated from failing hearts. These abnormalities relate in one-way or another to excitation–contraction coupling, and ultimately, ventricular function (Figure 15.1). Abnormalities of intracellular calcium homeostasis, at the level of the sarcoplasmic reticulum (SR) [23,24], the beta-adrenoreceptor (β-AR) [25], and cyclic adenosine monophosphate (cAMP) generation [26]. Other mechanisms have been considered targets for heart failure treatment such as anti-apoptotic signaling (reference is in the text below), angiotensin-converting enzyme (ACE) inhibition (reference is in the text below) as well as others that are further described in this chapter. Arising out of these observations has been a number of *in vitro* and *in vivo* studies that have evaluated the efficacy of gene transfer targeted at these pathways.

Calcium homeostasis

Intracellular calcium (Ca^{2+}) plays an integral role in the contraction and relaxation of cardiac myocytes, and is tightly controlled by mechanisms that regulate its flux within the cytoplasm [27]. In particular, at the completion of a contractile cycle cytosolic Ca^{2+} has to be re-sequestered into the SR by the SR-Ca^{2+}

ATPase (SERCA2a) pump [28]. Cardiomyocytes isolated from human beings with CHF are characterized by contractile dysfunction as evidenced by decreased systolic force generation, prolonged relaxation, and elevated diastolic force [29–31]. The derangements in SERCA2a-mediated Ca^{2+} homeostasis are associated with the contractile dysfunction seen in the failing myocardium [32]. Key components for the development of the abnormalities in contraction and relaxation observed in CHF have been shown to be SERCA2a [23,24,28] and its regulatory protein, phospholamban [10,27,33,34]. SERCA2a controls function of Ca^{2+} re-uptake following myocyte contraction and serves to regulate Ca^{2+} transients initiating diastolic relaxation. Phospholamban exerts an inhibitory effect on SERCA2a reducing its ability to assist in removal of cytosolic Ca^{2+} following contraction, a mechanism felt to contribute to the diastolic dysfunction seen in patients with CHF. The ratio of SERCA2a/phospholamban has been demonstrated to be decreased in these patients, contributing to aberrant force generating and relaxing capabilities [33,34].

Several *in vitro* studies utilizing both animal [33–36] and human [10,37] myocytes have demonstrated the feasibility of gene transfer to normalize the underlying dysfunctional mechanisms and improve myocyte function. Transgenic models of phospholamban over-expression have shown altered Ca^{2+} handling by prolonging Ca^{2+} transients during relaxation, deceasing Ca^{2+} release, and increasing intracellular resting Ca^{2+} concentrations, ultimately resulting in decreased contractile force and impaired relaxation [33,34,38]. In contrast, restoration of the SERCA2a/phospholamban ratio toward normal rectifies the abnormalities of Ca^{2+} handling and contraction in failing myocytes [34,35]. These findings have also been demonstrated in human cardiac myocytes isolated from the LVs of patients with end-stage CHF. Gene transfer of SERCA2a resulted in improvements in contractility to a level comparable in "non-failing" hearts as well as a restoration of Ca^{2+} transients in systole and diastole [37]. Furthermore, gene transfer of antisense oligonucleotides to phospholamban results in improved Ca^{2+} homeostasis and myocyte function [10].

These *in vitro* findings have recently been extended by studies performed in various animal models of decreased cardiac performance. Transgenic over-expression of SERCA2a [39] and phospholamban [33] have resulted in improved and worsened LV systolic and diastolic function, respectively. Recent gene transfer studies have convincingly demonstrated that increasing expression of SERCA2a or inhibiting expression of phospholamban restores ventricular function and improves survival in animal models of dilated cardiomyopathy [11,40,41]. This exciting approach for restoring LV function awaits clinical trails to demonstrate safety and efficacy prior to its expanded use in the clinical arena.

β-AR signaling

Heart failure results in dramatic changes in certain neurotransmitter and hormone receptors that result in alterations in excitation–contraction coupling ultimately contributing to CHF. Derangements in β-adrenergic signaling, including β-AR receptor downregulation, β-AR uncoupling from second messenger systems, and upregulation of β-AR kinase (βARK1) have been demonstrated as significant components of heart failure [25,42,43]. In isolated ventricular myocytes obtained from a rabbit model of heart failure, reversing the depressed levels of β-AR and elevated levels of β-ARK1 to normal with adenoviral gene delivery resulted in restoration of β-AR signaling [43]. Furthermore, β-AR over-expression produced enhanced cardiac function in transgenic mice [44], while over-expression of an inhibitor of β-ARK1 prevented the development of cardiomyopathy in a mouse model of heart failure

[45]. Similarly, adenoviral-mediated over-expression β-AR [45] or an inhibitor of β-ARK1 [46] improved LV contractility. One mechanism for improved contractility seen with β-AR stimulation is an increase in cytosolic cAMP. This could potentially be a double-edged sword as both improved cardiac function *and* increased cardiac mortality has been observed with drugs, such as phosphodiesterase inhibitors, that increase intracellular cAMP levels [47]. In addition, patients with CHF receiving chronic beta agonist therapy have experienced increased mortality [48]. Nevertheless, these data support further work in this area to decipher the optimal mode and timing of gene transfer of the β-AR system in CHF, as well its potential efficacy and safety.

Adenylyl cyclase

The generation of intracellular cAMP, has been tightly linked to excitation–contraction coupling in myocytes [49]. In a transgenic model of cardiomyopathy the over-expression of adenylyl cyclase type VI increased responsiveness to catecholamines and improved LV function [50]. In addition, intracoronary delivery of adenovirus containing adenylyl cyclase typeVI not only resulted in increased adenylyl cyclase protein content and stimulated cAMP levels, but also resulted in a sustained improvement of LV contractility [51]. As mentioned above, further studies are necessary to evaluate the overall safety and efficacy of increasing cAMP levels for the treatment of CHF.

Antiapoptotic signaling

Apoptosis appears to be a universal mechanism by which organisms eliminate damaged or unnecessary cells. It appears that apoptosis is an ongoing process in the failing heart. Mitochondria by the way of cytochrome *c* and several other factors down the ladder as caspases, a family of cysteine proteases, are intimately related in apoptosis. The previous is relevant because of Bcl-2, an antiapoptotic factor, can prevent the opening of the mitochondrial transition pores that leaks cytochrome *c* producing apoptosis. Chatterjee *et al.* administered a replication deficient adenoviral vector containing the transgene encoding human Bcl-2 in an ischemia–reperfusion rabbit model. The animals that received the gene maintained higher ejection fractions at 2, 4, and 6 weeks as well as preservation of LV geometry with less ventricular dilation than the control rabbits (empty vector adeno null) [52].

ACE inhibition

ACE inhibitors have demonstrated an immense benefit in the treatment of these patients. ACE is the same enzyme as kinase II, a kinin-degradating enzyme, therefore inhibition of ACE not only results in reduced angiotensin II levels but also decreases kinin breakdown resulting in high concentration in the tissues. When kinin binds to the kinin β_2 receptor, it activates second messengers such as nitric oxide/cGMP and prostacyclin/cAMP attenuating the cascade of events that progress to CHF. *Agata et al.* demonstrated that by injecting adenovirus containing human tissue kallikrein gene under the control of a cytomegalovirus promoter in the tail vein of mice 1 week after MI prevents progression of heart failure by several mechanisms: (1) by decreasing myocardial apoptosis through the Akt-mediated pathway, (2) improving endothelial function by reducing vascular resistance, increasing LV blood flow and cardiac nitric oxide levels, and (3) attenuating cardiac hypertrophy and fibrosis by decreasing collagen density, cardiomyocyte size, and LV internal perimeter [53].

Other intracellular abnormalities leading to heart failure

V2 vasopressin receptor

Systemic levels of arginine vasopressin (AVP) are increased in CHF, resulting in vasoconstriction and reduced cardiac contractility via V1 vasopressin receptors. V2 vasopressin receptors (V2Rs), which promote activation of adenylyl cyclase, are physiologically expressed only in the kidney and are absent in the myocardium; however, one could postulate improved LV contractility in response to V2R expression in the myocardium. Consistent with this hypothesis, adenoviral gene transfer of the V2R into myocardium, improved cardiac contractility when stimulated with 1-deamino-8-D-arginine vasopressin (DDAVP) [54].

Despite significant achievements in our understanding of the molecular mechanisms responsible for decreased cardiac performance in animals and patients with CHF, numerous hurdles remain before targeting these pathways with gene transfer contributes significantly to treatment of clinical

populations with CHF, as well as expansion of their use to patients with ischemic cardiomyopathy.

Hepatocyte growth factor

Hepatocyte growth factor (HGF) concentrations in the myocardium in cardiomyopathic hamsters are decreased compared to normal hamsters at 12 weeks of age. The decrease in local HGF production in the myocardium might be caused by angiotensin II or transforming growth factor-β (TGF-β), which are known to suppress HGF production. It is postulated that heart failure is related to blood flow and collagen synthesis. HGF, a mesenchyme-derived pleiotropic factor is known to regulate cell growth, motility, and morphogenesis of various types of cells but it has also been shown to regress fibrosis in animal injury models of liver and lung. Taniyama and cols proved that HGF has angiogenesis and antifibrotic effects in hamsters transfected with an HGF-gene. HGF gene or control vector was injected in the heart of cardiomyopathic hamsters once per week (8 times in total). Blood flow and capillary density were measured and found to be increased, and the fibrotic area was reduced in the HGF group by the way of activating MMP-1 [55].

Cell therapy for the treatment of CHF

The goal of cell-based therapies for the treatment of CHF, is not simply to improve cardiac performance through the optimization of cardiac myocyte contractility, but rather re-engineering of myocardial tissue through either (i) differentiated cell transplantation for the replacement of scarred tissue with living cells, or (ii) regeneration of contractile myocardial tissue through the introduction of pluripotent stem cells. Excitingly, clinical trials evaluating the safety and efficacy of autologous skeletal myoblast transplantation in patients as an adjunct to coronary artery bypass grafting (CABG) have begun [56]. In addition, emerging data reveals the feasibility of treating ischemic heart disease with the delivery of autologous bone-marrow stem cells [57,58].

Prior to cell transplantation becoming "common place" therapy, several scientific issues surrounding this therapy need to be optimized. The cell types utilized must possess the capacity to incorporate into the recipient myocardium. In addition, these cells must be able to survive, mature, and electro-mechanically couple with each other and the native myocardium, in order to decrease the arrhythmo-genic risk and optimize the overall benefit to cardiac function. Several cell types have been or are being considered for cell transplantation in the peri-infarct period including differentiated cells such as fetal car-diac myocytes [59,60], skeletal myoblasts [61–63], fibroblasts [64], and smooth muscle cells [65], as well as stem cells [66,67]. Cell therapy at or near the time of MI has been shown to attenuate ventricular remodeling following MI by engrafting into the scarred myocardium and increasing ventricular wall thickness, and decreasing LV end-diastolic dimen-sion. However, the ultimate goal of this therapy, to regenerate functional myocardium and its associated blood supply, appears to be most achievable with the use of pluripotent stem cells mobilized from the bone marrow.

The use of differentiated cells for transplantation

The utility of differentiated cell transplantation as a means to improve ventricular function following MI has been assessed in several studies using various ani-mal models. These cell types include fully differenti-ated cells, such as smooth muscle cells, fibroblasts, and skeletal muscle cells, as well as those committed to differentiation along a specific pathway, such as skeletal myoblasts. The value of differentiated cell types arises out of their accessibility, and their ability to be expanded *in vitro* and potential for being genet-ically altered prior to transplantation [20,21].

Cardiac myocytes and skeletal myoblasts

Initial studies assessed the feasibility of cell trans-plantation in normal hearts. The ability of both car-diac myocytes and skeletal myoblasts to engraft and survive for at least several months has been demon-strated when injected into syngeneic myocardium [59,68]. However, "functional" engraftment, with the visualization of intercalated disks, has only been demonstrated in hearts transplanted with fetal cardiomyocytes [60].

Cell engraftment fetal of cardiomyocytes or skeletal myoblasts has been demonstrated when transplantation occurs 1 week following MI, with evidence of improved ventricular function mea-sured by echocardiography at 1 month following

transplantation [69,70]. Similarly, other groups have demonstrated an improved LV hemodynamics fol-lowing differentiated cell transplantation [63,71,72]. Interestingly, no significant difference in functional improvement was observed between transplan-tation with skeletal myoblasts and fetal cardiac myocytes [70].

Despite the utility of cardiac myocytes in integrat-ing with native cardiac myocytes and augmenting heart function following MI, the limited availability of these cells coupled with ethical issues regarding the use of fetal tissues has essentially eliminated them from clinical consideration at this time. In contrast to cardiac myocytes, skeletal myoblasts maintain their regenerative capacity. In addition, when provoked by a stress such as ischemia, skeletal myoblasts may proliferate, leading to the formation of new muscle fibers capable of contraction [73]. Additionally, skele-tal muscle possesses a greater resistance to ischemia than cardiac muscle and is able to withstand many hours of ischemia without sustaining irreversible injury [74]. Coupled with their accessibility and ease of handling, these properties may prove to promote skeletal myoblasts as the differentiated cell type of choice for the treatment of CHF.

Proposed mechanism of action

Depending on the timing of differentiated cell trans-plantation relative to the MI, potential benefits of differentiated cell transplantation may include increasing the mass of contracting cells within the myocardium, thickening of the infarct zone and attenuation of post-infarct remodeling leading to improved wall stress and ventricular performance [75–77]. Thus, the use of differentiated cells for the treatment of ischemic heart disease may be most beneficial when transplantation can occur within days to weeks of MI, prior to the development of sig-nificant pathologic ventricular remodeling.

Limitations of differentiated cell transplantation

Several limitations of differentiated cell transplan-tation exist which may preclude the possibility of these cells achieving their therapeutic potential for the treatment of CHF. First, the harvesting and expanding of these cell types prior to transplanta-tion requires 3–4 weeks. Thus, a potential candidate would need to be identified early following a MI in order to prepare the cells for delivery and to realize the benefits of altered remodeling. Second, despite the improvements of ventricular function as a result of altered remodeling, these cells do not lead to the regeneration of blood vessels or cardiac myocytes [22,76,78]. Given these limitations, the search for a cell type that could improve LV systolic function through the regeneration myocardium, as well as reestablish local coronary perfusion has led many investigators to study the potential of autologous stem cells to regenerate myocardial tissue.

The potential for myocardial regeneration

Recent studies have revealed the presence of proliferating myocytes in human hearts following MI [79]. A plausible explanation for the presence of proliferating myocytes in the human hearts is that the cells identified as cardiac myocytes were in fact proliferating and differentiating stem cells that originated from the bone marrow and were mobilized as part of the naturally occurring repair process. This evolution in thinking has spawned great interest in utilizing the plasticity of stem cells for the treatment of ischemic heart disease and its manifestation, CHF.

The widespread enthusiasm surrounding the use of stem cells for the treatment of ischemic heart disease is based on their unique biological properties along with their capacity to self-renew and to regenerate tissue and organ systems [80–84]. Pertinent to this patient population, both mesenchymal and hematopoietic stem cells possess the ability to differentiate into cardiomyocytes [85,86] and vascular structures [84,87], respectively. Moreover, recent studies have shown that part of the normal physiologic response to MI involves mobilization of stem cells, "homing" of these cells to the damaged myocardium, and differentiation of at least some of these stem cells into cardiac myocytes [79,88,89]. Similarly, "homing" of stem cells originating from transplant recipients to donor hearts has also been demonstrated [84]. Unfortunately, present data reveals that stem cell engraftment and differentiation into the essential components of functional myocardium, cardiac myocytes (0.02%) and endothelial cells (3.3%), is an infrequent event [89], precluding any meaningful regeneration of the damaged myocardium. However, the data suggests that if this natural repair mechanism can be potentiated,

clinically relevant myocardial regeneration may be achievable.

Routes for delivery

Intramyocardial injection

This modality may require fewer cells to achieve engraftment compared to intracoronary or intravenous administration. There is one study that reports a success rate of 40% due to intraoperative and postoperative risks associated with the cardiac surgery [67]. The other downside is that targets can sometimes be difficult to map. To overcome this obstacle a group of investigators use a percutaneous catheter-based myocardial injection approach with the use of electromechanical mapping which can help to guide the surgeon where the scarred and viable myocardium is located [90].

Intracoronary injection

This modality can deliver the maximum concentration of cells to the site of the damaged myocardium. It is known that cells distribute homogenously in the infarct zone in contrast to intramyocardial injection where "islands" of cells can form, making this tissue more propense to electrical instability [91]. The downside to this intervention is coronary flow impairment and myocardial cell necrosis if the duration and quantity of cells infused are not well determined. In current human studies $10–40 \times 10^6$ cells have been used with good results.

Intravenous injection

It is practical and less invasive than the other modalities. A key element for success of this modality is the homing signal which can sometimes be non-specific making cells home into other organs than the one desired. This route seems to be the least effective delivery method since it requires multiple coronary circulation passages to deliver enough cells to populate the damaged tissue [92].

Autologous stem cell transplantation

One potential technique of harnessing the pluripotent capacity of stem cells is to transplant these cells either locally or systemically. This strategy of delivering stem cells offers several advantages. Specific populations of stem cells can be isolated via the use of flow cytometry prior to transplantation. Moreover, the number and timing of cell delivery can be tailored to the specific clinical situation. Notably, the efficacy of both hematopoietic and mesenchymal stem cell transplantation has been demonstrated for the treatment of acute MI [66,67,93,94]. Using isolated mesenchymal stem cells Tomita *et al.* demonstrated that transplanted cells engrafted and differentiated into cardiac tissue 3 weeks following cryoinjury in a rat myocardial injury model [94]. An improvement in LV function was also seen in a proportion of the treated animals. In addition, it appeared transplantation of these stem cells-induced angiogenesis within the injured myocardium.

The regenerative capacity of bone-marrow-derived stem cells was also demonstrated in a mouse MI model [67]. Direct transplantation of a specific sub-population of stem cells (Lin⁻c-kit^{POS}) from a mouse whose cells express green fluorescent protein into the border zone of an MI 3–5 h following left anterior descending artery (LAD) ligation resulted in almost complete regeneration of the infarcted anterior wall. Consistent with regeneration of functional myocardium, transplanted hearts demonstrated improved hemodynamics with a lower diastolic pressure and an increased force generating capacity 9 days after MI compared with control animals [67].

Expanding upon the above studies, systemically delivered human bone-marrow-derived CD34+ hematopoietic stem cells nude rats 2 days following LAD ligation resulted in improved LV function [66]. This may have resulted from enhanced neovascularization of the infarct zone with a significant reduction in the amount of scar tissue in the LV of treated rats. Notably, this study demonstrated the ability of circulating stem cells to "home" to the infarct zone. That stem cells can home to injured myocardium suggests the possibility that transplantation of stem cells may not be necessary, but rather, mobilization of endogenous stem cells could lead to the same effect.

Stem cell mobilization

The potential efficacy of stem cell mobilization as a non-invasive therapeutic strategy for the regeneration of the myocardium following MI has been demonstrated [93]. Mobilized bone-marrow stem cells using Granulocyte-colony stimulating factor (G-CSF), stem cell factor, and splenectomy *prior* to LAD ligation resulted in decreased infarct size (40%) and LV cavity dilation (26%). Ejection fraction and

hemodynamics significantly improved as a consequence of the formation of new myocytes and vasculature. Enthusiasm for this therapy must be tempered until these results are reproduced in a more clinically relevant situation such as following MI and until safety of this therapy can be more definitively demonstrated in additional pre-clinical models.

In addition to G-CSF, the effects of other endogenous (growth factors) and exogenous (pharmacologic) mediators on stem cell mobilization are becoming more evident. For example, VEGF administration has been demonstrated to mobilize CD34+ hematopoietic stem cells in mice [95]. Interestingly, the peak in the number of CD34+ cells released from the bone marrow following MI correlates with the peak in plasma VEGF levels [88]. Surprisingly, initiation of 3-hydroxy-3-methylglutaryl coenzyme A (HMG CoA) reductase inhibitor (statins) therapy induces stem cell mobilization [96]. This finding could offer one potential mechanism by which patients may receive early benefits of statin therapy immediately following MI. Similarly, statin therapy in patients with stable coronary artery disease (CAD) has been shown to augment the level of circulating endothelial progenitor cells in patients with enhanced functional activity [97]. Despite the encouraging results revealed in the studies above, enhanced knowledge of the safety and efficacy of various stem cell mobilization techniques needs to be obtained before this therapy can become a reality. Furthermore, we need to establish if simply increasing the number of circulating progenitor cells is sufficient, or whether we need to optimize the regenerative capacity of the tissue in the target organ prior to mobilizing stem cells. That said, it appears that stem cell mobilization for the regeneration of damaged myocardium reveals the potential of cardiovascular cell therapy.

It is important to note that the studies to date focusing of stem cell transplantation or mobilization for the treatment of ischemic heart disease have been limited to the peri-infarct period and leave unanswered the question of efficacy in the CHF population. Stem cell mobilization is obviously the least invasive of the cell therapies under study; thus, an enhanced understanding of the mechanisms involved in mobilization, homing of these cells to target organs, and differentiation of these cells is imperative. The time course and

(a)

(b)

(c)

(d)

(e)

(f)

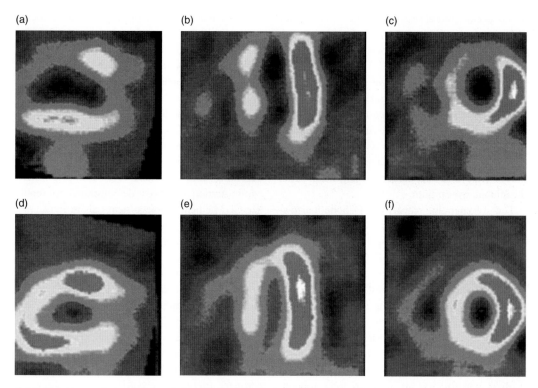

Figure 15.2 Improved myocardial perfusion of infarcted anterior wall 3 months after intracoronary cell transplantation subsequent to an acute anterior wall infarction detected by [201]thallium scintigraphy. The images on the left (a, d, sagittal) and in the middle (b, e) show the long axis, whereas those on the right (c, f, frontal) show the short axis of the heart. Initially the anterior wall, with green-colored apical and anterior regions, had reduced myocardial perfusion (a, b, c). Three months after cell transplantation the same anterior wall, now yellow in color, revealed a significant improvement in myocardial perfusion (d, e, f). All illustrations depict the exercise phase (*Source*: [99]).

level of expression of the signaling pathways involved in the above processes would also need to be better outlined, mainly since it appears that stem cell homing to damaged myocardium occurs for only a finite period following MI [98]. In addition, which specific sub-populations of bone-marrow-derived stem cells may be better suited for therapy in specific situations, such as acute MI versus chronic ischemic heart disease needs to be evaluated.

Clinical experience with stem cells

The translation of these emerging therapies from pre-clinical promise to clinical reality is still in its infancy. However, the feasibility of stem cell transplantation, via percutaneous delivery or direct injection during bypass surgery, has recently been demonstrated in a number of studies in patients with ischemic heart disease [58,90,91,99]. A Phase 1 trial in ten patients within days of MI suggested that intracoronary delivery of bone-marrow-derived mononuclear cells resulted in improved LV contractility (Figure 15.2(a) and (b)) and improved perfusion (Figure 15.2(c) and (d)) of the infarct zone [99]. Expanding upon these data, Assmus *et al.* demonstrated that intracoronary delivery of both bone-marrow-derived and peripheral blood mononuclear cells resulted in improved regional LV function (Figure 15.3(a) and (b)) and viability (Figure 15.3(c) and (d)) within the infarct zone [91]. Similar improvements in LV perfusion and function have also been seen with direct myocardial injection, either percutaneously or surgically, of bone-marrow cells in patients with stable ischemic heart disease, further exhibiting the clinical possibility of harnessing these cells for the treatment of the manifestations of CAD [58,90]. Most importantly, not only was feasibility demonstrated, safety was also revealed as no untoward effects were experienced in any of these studies.

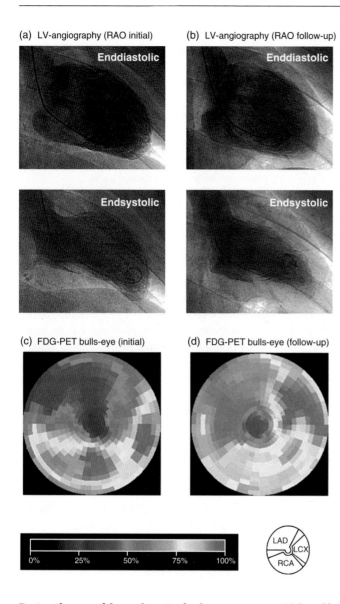

(a) LV-angiography (RAO initial)

Enddiastolic

Endsystolic

(b) LV-angiography (RAO follow-up)

Enddiastolic

Endsystolic

(c) FDG-PET bulls-eye (initial)

(d) FDG-PET bulls-eye (follow-up)

0%   25%   50%   75%   100%

LAD
LCX
RCA

Figure 15.3 Left ventriculogram before injection of circulating blood-derived progenitor cells (a: left panels) and at 4 months follow-up (b: right panels). The figures (c) and (d), corresponding to FDG-PET bulls-eye views of the LV of the patient depicted in figures (a) and (b).
LAD: left anterior descending artery; LCX: left circumflex artery; and RCA: right coronary artery (*Source*: [91]).

Detection and imaging techniques

For labeling in animal experiments, retroviral transduction with a marker gene or labeling with thymidine or bromodeoxyuridine have been used.

Several methods have been used to detect the transplanted cells. Cardiac magnetic resonance imaging (MRI) has been used to identify mesenchymal stem cells by magnetically labeling the cell of interest. It also allows to assess the size of the injection as well as the targets [100,101]. Another technique to identify these cells has been scintigraphy. Several models have used human endothelial progenitor cells labeled with 111-indium oxine with success [102].

Side effects

It is difficult to assess the clinical safety of these interventions since animal studies are short term and human studies have been scant in number. A potential problem of using undifferentiated cells is that implanted stem cells may differentiate into fibroblasts rather than myocytes producing more scar formation resulting in worsening myocardial contraction and propensity for cardiac arrhythmias [103]. The cells can also home into other tissues like lungs, liver, brain, and many other organs which can potentiate problems. They can home into the regenerating myocardium and result in non-cardiac tissues hindering its effect. It is proven that endothelial progenitor cells and multipotent adult progenitor cells can incorporate into tumors (specifically in the angiogenic vasculature system).

Up to now, there has been no significant acute toxicity when autologous or allogenic mesenchymal stem cells are injected in human beings.

Combined gene transfer and cell therapy for the treatment of CHF

As demonstrated above, gene transfer as a therapeutic modality for the treatment of myocardial ischemia and/or infarction has been proposed as a revolutionary approach to improve collateral circulation, enhance myocardial viability, optimize the healing process, and potentially restore the failing heart. However, direct gene transfer into infarcted myocardium, while being the most feasible approach, is limited by low transfection efficiency and a vigorous inflammatory response to the current vectors available for clinical use [104]. A potential significant advancement could be the combination of gene transfer and cell transplantation. Such protocols would involve engineering cells to secrete soluble factors prior to transplantation. In its simplest form, cells being expanded in culture could be transfected with already established viral vectors that encode growth factors or enzymes such as VEGF or eNOS. Additional molecular strategies will need to be developed and studied before being able to deliver relevant transcription factors and intracellular enzyme systems [105–107]. With this approach, we should be able to (i) minimize the host inflammatory response, (ii) know exactly which cells receive the vectors of interest, (iii) avoid transfection of other cell types, and (iv) be able to stably or transiently express the molecules of interest.

Support for this approach of combining cell and gene therapy are studies that have shown that skeletal myoblasts stably transfected with expression vectors encoding genes of interest including TGFβ-1 or VEGF have been successfully engrafted into the myocardium and have lead to neovascularization [20,108]. In addition, Yau et al. assessed the efficacy of cell transplantation using skeletal myoblasts stably transfected with VEGF-165, 3 weeks following cryoinjury and demonstrated enhanced neovascularization within the damaged myocardium [21]. Using an ischemic cardiomyopathy model, we recently demonstrated that the transplantation of skeletal myoblasts transfected with an adenovirus encoding VEGF-165 resulted in significantly greater angiogenesis and recovery of LV function than either direct AdVEGF-165 injection or skeletal myoblast transplantation alone [22]. Despite these encouraging results, further evaluation of this "designer" cell approach is necessary before expanding this therapeutic modality into the clinical arena.

Future directions

The past decade has seen an explosion in our understanding of the pathophysiology of cardiovascular diseases ranging from hypertensive heart disease to the acute coronary syndromes and CHF. This understanding, coupled with recent "cracking" of the genetic code and an enhanced understanding of cellular cardiomyoplasty, has paved the way for novel therapeutic techniques such as gene transfer and cell therapy to achieve clinical reality. Despite promising results in animal models, many significant hurdles must be overcome before these techniques become clinically meaningful to patients with CHF.

Gene transfer for CHF would conceptually need to be targeted to the underlying pathophysiology of the disease processes resulting in CHF. As demonstrated in the above discussion, elucidating the underlying myopathic processes leading to LV dysfunction can result in improvements in muscle function and, ultimately, clinical outcome. On the other hand, targeting vascular cells with other gene products may prove beneficial in post-MI CHF. This strategy could cause favorable LV remodeling following myocardial ischemia and necrosis, leading to improved LV function despite decreased cardiac myocyte number [109–111]. Additionally, the timing of gene transfer needs to be studied in order for this therapy to achieve its full potential. Gene transfer late following an MI, once irreversible damage to the LV myocardium has taken place, could focus on restoration of deranged metabolic and contractile mechanisms, inhibition of apoptosis or homing and differentiation of circulating stem cells. The demonstration that differentiated cells can engraft and improve function early following an MI and that stem cells can actually regenerate functional myocardium has set the stage for future treatment of CHF. However, many significant challenges remain.

Integral to assessing the quality of cell therapy with or without concomitant gene transfer within the clinical sector will be a non-invasive method of quantifying cell engraftment *in vivo*. Cell engraftment has to be determined in an *in vivo* system, and to date, quantifying engraftment requires ending the experiment. Furthermore, no clinical or experimental system for the quantification of cell engraftment in a human population exists. As we begin to plan to test the efficacy of autologous cell transplantation in clinical populations, having the ability to correlate the level of cell engraftment with clinical outcome will likely decrease the number of patients required in clinical trial, and further our assessment of the benefits of this strategy.

Conclusions

Despite the significant achievements in the area of gene transfer and cell therapy over the past decade, numerous hurdles still need to be overcome before these techniques can contribute significantly to the therapy for CHF. Currently, gene transfer functions mainly as an important tool to better understand the processes that result in and maintain CHF. Cell-based therapies may facilitate myocardial regeneration, therapies that could revolutionize current understanding, approach, and prognosis of CHF. The encouraging experiences to date regarding combined gene transfer and cell transplantation provide a new paradigm for future studies. However, further improvements in technique as well as expansion into larger animal models of CHF are still required before these techniques become innovative weapons in our armamentarium to improve the morbidity and mortality of this ever increasingly prevalent syndrome.

References

1 Robbins MA, O'Connell JB. Economic impact of heart failure. In: Rose EA & Stevenson LW, eds. *Management of End-Stage Heart Disease*. Lippincott-Raven, Philadelphia, 1998: 3–13.

2 Fuster V, Badimon L, Badimon JJ, Chesebro JH. The pathogenesis of coronary artery disease and the acute coronary syndromes (1). *N Engl J Med* 1992; **326**: 242–250.

3 Baumgartner I, Pieczek A, Manor O, Blair R, Kearney M, Walsh K, Isner JM. Constitutive expression of phVEGF165 after intramuscular gene transfer promotes collateral vessel development in patients with critical limb ischemia. *Circulation* 1998; **97**: 1114–1123.

4 Losordo DW, Vale PR, Symes JF, Dunnington CH, Esakof DD, Maysky M, Ashare AB, Lathi K, Isner JM. Gene therapy for myocardial angiogenesis: initial clinical results with direct myocardial injection of phVEGF165 as sole therapy for myocardial ischemia. *Circulation* 1998; **98**: 2800–2804.

5 Vale PR, Losordo DW, Milliken CE, McDonald MC, Gravelin LM, Curry CM, Esakof DD, Maysky M, Symes JF, Isner JM. Randomized, single-blind, placebo-controlled pilot study of catheter-based myocardial gene transfer for therapeutic angiogenesis using left ventricular electromechanical mapping in patients with chronic myocardial ischemia. *Circulation* 2001; **103**: 2138–2143.

6 Vale PR, Losordo DW, Milliken CE, Maysky M, Esakof DD, Symes JF, Isner JM. Left ventricular electromechanical mapping to assess efficacy of phVEGF(165) gene transfer for therapeutic angiogenesis in chronic myocardial ischemia. *Circulation* 2000; **102**: 965–974.

7 Losordo DW, Vale PR, Hendel RC, Milliken CE, Fortuin FD, Cummings N, Schatz RA, Asahara T, Isner JM, Kuntz RE. Phase 1/2 placebo-controlled, double-blind, dose-escalating trial of myocardial vascular endothelial growth factor 2 gene transfer by catheter delivery in patients with chronic myocardial ischemia. *Circulation* 2002; **105**: 2012–2018.

8 Grines CL, Watkins MW, Helmer G, Penny W, Brinker J, Marmur JD, West A, Rade JJ, Marrott P, Hammond HK et al. Angiogenic Gene Therapy (AGENT) trial in patients with stable angina pectoris. *Circulation* 2002; **105**: 1291–1297.

9 Beeri R, Guerrero JL, Supple G, Sullivan S, Levine RA, Hajjar RJ. New efficient catheter-based system for myocardial gene delivery. *Circulation* 2002; **106**: 1756–1759.

10 Del Monte F, Harding SE, Dec GW, Gwathmey JK, Hajjar RJ. Targeting phospholamban by gene transfer in human heart failure. *Circulation* 2002; **105**: 904–907.

11 Del Monte F, Williams E, Lebeche D, Schmidt U, Rosenzweig A, Gwathmey JK, Lewandowski ED, Hajjar RJ. Improvement in survival and cardiac metabolism after gene transfer of sarcoplasmic reticulum Ca(2+)-ATPase in a rat model of heart failure. *Circulation* 2001; **104**: 1424–1429.

12 Hoshijima M, Ikeda Y, Iwanaga Y, Minamisawa S, Date MO, Gu Y, Iwatate M, Li M, Wang L, Wilson JM et al. Chronic suppression of heart-failure progression by a pseudophosphorylated mutant of phospholamban via *in vivo* cardiac rAAV gene delivery. *Nat Med* 2002; **8**: 864–871.

13 Ikeda Y, Gu Y, Iwanaga Y, Hoshijima M, Oh SS, Giordano FJ, Chen J, Nigro V, Peterson KL, Chien KR et al. Restoration

of deficient membrane proteins in the cardiomyopathic hamster by *in vivo* cardiac gene transfer. *Circulation* 2002; **105**: 502–508.

14 Guzman RJ, Lemarchand P, Crystal RG, Epstein SE, Finkel T. Efficient gene transfer into myocardium by direct injection of adenovirus vectors. *Circ Res* 1993; **73**: 1202–1207.

15 Barr E, Carroll J, Kalynych AM, Tripathy SK, Kozarsky K, Wilson JM, Leiden JM. Efficient catheter-mediated gene transfer into the heart using replication-defective adenovirus. *Gene Ther* 1994; **1**: 51–58.

16 Hajjar RJ, Schmidt U, Matsui T, Guerrero JL, Lee KH, Gwathmey JK, Dec GW, Semigran MJ, Rosenzweig A. Modulation of ventricular function through gene transfer *in vivo*. *Proc Natl Acad Sci USA* 1998; **95**: 5251–5256.

17 Svensson EC, Marshall DJ, Woodard K, Lin H, Jiang F, Chu L, Leiden JM. Efficient and stable transduction of cardiomyocytes after intramyocardial injection or intracoronary perfusion with recombinant adeno-associated virus vectors. *Circulation* 1999; **99**: 201–205.

18 Fromes Y, Salmon A, Wang X, Collin H, Rouche A, Hagege A, Schwartz K, Fiszman MY. Gene delivery to the myocardium by intrapericardial injection. *Gene Ther* 1999; **6**: 683–688.

19 Stratford-Perricaudet LD, Makeh I, Perricaudet M, Briand P. Widespread long-term gene transfer to mouse skeletal muscles and heart. *J Clin Invest* 1992; **90**: 626–630.

20 Suzuki K, Murtuza B, Smolenski RT, Sammut IA, Suzuki N, Kaneda Y, Yacoub MH. Cell transplantation for the treatment of acute myocardial infarction using vascular endothelial growth factor-expressing skeletal myoblasts. *Circulation* 2001; **104**: I207–I212.

21 Yau TM, Fung K, Weisel RD, Fujii T, Mickle DA, Li RK. Enhanced myocardial angiogenesis by gene transfer with transplanted cells. *Circulation* 2001; **104**: I218–I222.

22 Askari A, Goldman CK, Forudi F, Ellis SG, Thomas JD, Penn MS. VEGF-expressing skeletal myoblast transplantation induces angiogenesis and improves left ventricular function late after myocardial infarction. *Mol Ther* 2002; **5**: S162.

23 Mercadier JJ, Lompre AM, Duc P, Boheler KR, Fraysse JB, Wisnewsky C, Allen PD, Komajda M, Schwartz K. Altered sarcoplasmic reticulum Ca(2+)-ATPase gene expression in the human ventricle during end-stage heart failure. *J Clin Invest* 1990; **85**: 305–309.

24 Schmidt U, Hajjar RJ, Helm PA, Kim CS, Doye AA, Gwathmey JK. Contribution of abnormal sarcoplasmic reticulum ATPase activity to systolic and diastolic dysfunction in human heart failure. *J Mol Cell Cardiol* 1998; **30**: 1929–1937.

25 Bristow MR, Minobe W, Rasmussen R, Larrabee P, Skerl L, Klein JW, Anderson FL, Murray J, Mestroni L, Karwande SV *et al.* Beta-adrenergic neuroeffector abnormalities in the failing human heart are produced by local rather than systemic mechanisms. *J Clin Invest* 1992; **89**: 803–815.

26 Feldman MD, Copelas L, Gwathmey JK, Phillips P, Warren SE, Schoen FJ, Grossman W, Morgan JP. Deficient production of cyclic AMP: pharmacologic evidence of an important cause of contractile dysfunction in patients with end-stage heart failure. *Circulation* 1987; **75**: 331–339.

27 Morgan JP. Abnormal intracellular modulation of calcium as a major cause of cardiac contractile dysfunction. *N Engl J Med* 1991; **325**: 625–632.

28 Arai M, Matsui H, Periasamy M. Sarcoplasmic reticulum gene expression in cardiac hypertrophy and heart failure. *Circ Res* 1994; **74**: 555–564.

29 Gwathmey JK, Copelas L, MacKinnon R, Schoen FJ, Feldman MD, Grossman W, Morgan JP. Abnormal intracellular calcium handling in myocardium from patients with end-stage heart failure. *Circ Res* 1987; **61**: 70–76.

30 Gwathmey JK, Slawsky MT, Hajjar RJ, Briggs GM, Morgan JP. Role of intracellular calcium handling in force-interval relationships of human ventricular myocardium. *J Clin Invest* 1990; **85**: 1599–1613.

31 Arai M, Alpert NR, MacLennan DH, Barton P, Periasamy M. Alterations in sarcoplasmic reticulum gene expression in human heart failure: a possible mechanism for alterations in systolic and diastolic properties of the failing myocardium. *Circ Res* 1993; **72**: 463–469.

32 Whitmer JT, Kumar P, Solaro RJ. Calcium transport properties of cardiac sarcoplasmic reticulum from cardiomyopathic Syrian hamsters (BIO 53.58 and 14.6): evidence for a quantitative defect in dilated myopathic hearts not evident in hypertrophic hearts. *Circ Res* 1988; **62**: 81–85.

33 Kadambi VJ, Ponniah S, Harrer JM, Hoit BD, Dorn GW, Walsh RA, Kranias EG. Cardiac-specific overexpression of phospholamban alters calcium kinetics and resultant cardiomyocyte mechanics in transgenic mice. *J Clin Invest* 1996; **97**: 533–539.

34 Hajjar RJ, Schmidt U, Kang JX, Matsui T, Rosenzweig A. Adenoviral gene transfer of phospholamban in isolated rat cardiomyocytes. Rescue effects by concomitant gene transfer of sarcoplasmic reticulum Ca(2+)-ATPase. *Circ Res* 1997; **81**: 145–153.

35 Giordano FJ, He H, McDonough P, Meyer M, Sayen MR, Dillmann WH. Adenovirus-mediated gene transfer reconstitutes depressed sarcoplasmic reticulum Ca(2+)-ATPase levels and shortens prolonged cardiac myocyte Ca2+ transients. *Circulation* 1997; **96**: 400–403.

36 He H, Meyer M, Martin JL, McDonough PM, Ho P, Lou X, Lew WY, Hilal-Dandan R, Dillmann WH. Effects of mutant and antisense RNA of phospholamban on SR Ca(2+)-ATPase activity and cardiac myocyte contractility. *Circulation* 1999; **100**: 974–980.

37 del Monte F, Harding SE, Schmidt U, Matsui T, Kang ZB, Dec GW, Gwathmey JK, Rosenzweig A, Hajjar RJ.

Restoration of contractile function in isolated cardiomyocytes from failing human hearts by gene transfer of SERCA2a. *Circulation* 1999; **100**: 2308–2311.

38 Bristow MR, Minobe W, Rasmussen R, Hershberger RE, Hoffman BB. Alpha-1 adrenergic receptors in the nonfailing and failing human heart. *J Pharmacol Exp Ther* 1988; **247**: 1039–1045.

39 He H, Giordano FJ, Hilal-Dandan R, Choi DJ, Rockman HA, McDonough PM, Bluhm WF, Meyer M, Sayen MR, Swanson E *et al*. Overexpression of the rat sarcoplasmic reticulum Ca2+ ATPase gene in the heart of transgenic mice accelerates calcium transients and cardiac relaxation. *J Clin Invest* 1997; **100**: 380–389.

40 Miyamoto MI, Del Monte F, Schmidt U, DiSalvo TS, Kang ZB, Matsui T, Guerrero JL, Gwathmey JK, Rosenzweig A, Hajjar RJ. Adenoviral gene transfer of SERCA2a improves left-ventricular function in aortic-banded rats in transition to heart failure. *Proc Natl Acad Sci USA* 2000; **97**: 793–798.

41 Hoshijima M, Ikeda Y, Iwanaga Y, Minamisawa S, Date MO, Gu Y, Iwatate M, Li M, Wang L, Wilson JM *et al*. Chronic suppression of heart-failure progression by a pseudophosphorylated mutant of phospholamban via *in vivo* cardiac rAAV gene delivery. *Nat Med* 2002; **8**: 864–871.

42 Bristow MR, Ginsburg R, Minobe W, Cubicciotti RS, Sageman WS, Lurie K, Billingham ME, Harrison DC, Stinson EB. Decreased catecholamine sensitivity and beta-adrenergic-receptor density in failing human hearts. *N Engl J Med* 1982; **307**: 205–211.

43 Akhter SA, Skaer CA, Kypson AP, McDonald PH, Peppel KC, Glower DD, Lefkowitz RJ, Koch WJ. Restoration of beta-adrenergic signaling in failing cardiac ventricular myocytes via adenoviral-mediated gene transfer. *Proc Natl Acad Sci USA* 1997; **94**: 12100–12105.

44 Liggett SB, Tepe NM, Lorenz JN, Canning AM, Jantz TD, Mitarai S, Yatani A, Dorn GW. Early and delayed consequences of beta(2)-adrenergic receptor overexpression in mouse hearts: critical role for expression level. *Circulation* 2000; **101**: 1707–1714.

45 Shah AS, Lilly RE, Kypson AP, Tai O, Hata JA, Pippen A, Silvestry SC, Lefkowitz RJ, Glower DD, Koch WJ. Intracoronary adenovirus-mediated delivery and overexpression of the beta(2)-adrenergic receptor in the heart: prospects for molecular ventricular assistance. *Circulation* 2000; **101**: 408–414.

46 Shah AS, White DC, Emani S, Kypson AP, Lilly RE, Wilson K, Glower DD, Lefkowitz RJ, Koch WJ. *In vivo* ventricular gene delivery of a beta-adrenergic receptor kinase inhibitor to the failing heart reverses cardiac dysfunction. *Circulation* 2001; **103**: 1311–1316.

47 Mann DL, Kent RL, Parsons B, Cooper G. Adrenergic effects on the biology of the adult mammalian cardiocyte. *Circulation* 1992; **85**: 790–804.

48 O'Connor CM, Gattis WA, Uretsky BF, Adams Jr. KF, McNulty SE, Grossman SH, McKenna WJ, Zannad F, Swedberg K, Gheorghiade M, *et al*. Continuous intravenous dobutamine is associated with an increased risk of death in patients with advanced heart failure: insights from the Flolan International Randomized Survival Trial (FIRST). *Am Heart J* 1999; **138**: 78–86.

49 Gao MH, Lai NC, Roth DM, Zhou J, Zhu J, Anzai T, Dalton N, Hammond HK. Adenylylcyclase increases responsiveness to catecholamine stimulation in transgenic mice. *Circulation* 1999; **99**: 1618–1622.

50 Roth DM, Gao MH, Lai NC, Drumm J, Dalton N, Zhou JY, Zhu J, Entrikin D, Hammond HK. Cardiac-directed adenylyl cyclase expression improves heart function in murine cardiomyopathy. *Circulation* 1999; **99**: 3099–3102.

51 Lai NC, Roth DM, Gao MH, Fine S, Head BP, Zhu J, McKirnan MD, Kwong C, Dalton N, Urasawa K *et al*. Intracoronary delivery of adenovirus encoding adenylyl cyclase VI increases left ventricular function and cAMP-generating capacity. *Circulation* 2000; **102**: 2396–2401.

52 Chattarjee S, Stewart AS, Bish LT, Jayasankar V, Kim EM, Pirolli T, Burdick J, Woo YJ, Gardner TJ, Sweeney HL. Viral gene transfer of the antiapoptotic factor Bcl-2 protects against chronic postischemic heart failure. *Circulation* 2002; **106(Suppl 1)**: 1212–1217.

53 Agata J, Chao L, Chao J. Kallikrein gene delivery improves cardiac reserve and attenuates remodeling after myocardial infarction. *Hypertension* 2002; **40**: 653–659.

54 Weig HJ, Laugwitz KL, Moretti A, Kronsbein K, Stadele C, Bruning S, Seyfarth M, Brill T, Schomig A, Ungerer M. Enhanced cardiac contractility after gene transfer of V2 vasopressin receptors *in vivo* by ultrasound-guided injection or transcoronary delivery. *Circulation* 2000; **101**: 1578–1585.

55 Taniyama Y, Morishita R, Aoki M, Hiraoka K, Yamasaki K, Hashiya N, Matsumoto K, Nakamura T, Kaneda Y, Ogihara T. Angiogenesis and antifibrotic action by hepatocyte growth factor in cardiomyopathy. *Hypertension* 2002; **40**: 47–53.

56 Menasche P, Hagege AA, Scorsin M, Pouzet B, Desnos M, Duboc D, Schwartz K, Vilquin JT, Marolleau JP. Myoblast transplantation for heart failure. *Lancet* 2001; **357**: 279–280.

57 Hamano K, Nishida M, Hirata K, Mikamo A, Li TS, Esato K, Harada A, Miura T. Preliminary results of clinical trials of therapeutic angiogenesis achieved by the implantation of self bone marrow cells for ischemic heart disease. *Circulation* 2001; **104**: II-69.

58 Stamm C, Westphal B, Kleine HD, Petzsch M, Kittner C, Klinge H, Schumichen C, Nienaber CA, Freund M, Steinhoff G. Autologous bone-marrow stem-cell transplantation for myocardial regeneration. *Lancet* 2003; **361**: 45–46.

59 Koh GY, Soonpaa MH, Klug MG, Field LJ. Long-term survival of AT-1 cardiomyocyte grafts in syngeneic myocardium. *Am J Physiol* 1993; **264**: H1727–H1733.

60 Soonpaa MH, Koh GY, Klug MG, Field LJ. Formation of nascent intercalated disks between grafted fetal cardiomyocytes and host myocardium. *Science* 1994; **264**: 98–101.

61 Koh GY, Klug MG, Soonpaa MH, Field LJ. Differentiation and long-term survival of C2C12 myoblast grafts in heart. *J Clin Invest* 1993; **92**: 1548–1554.

62 Taylor DA, Atkins BZ, Hungspreugs P, Jones TR, Reedy MC, Hutcheson KA, Glower DD, Kraus WE. Regenerating functional myocardium: improved performance after skeletal myoblast transplantation. *Nat Med* 1998; **4**: 929–933.

63 Jain M, DerSimonian H, Brenner DA, Ngoy S, Teller P, Edge AS, Zawadzka A, Wetzel K, Sawyer DB, Colucci WS *et al.* Cell therapy attenuates deleterious ventricular remodeling and improves cardiac performance after myocardial infarction. *Circulation* 2001; **103**: 1920–1927.

64 Sakai T, Li RK, Weisel RD, Mickle DA, Jia ZQ, Tomita S, Kim EJ, Yau TM. Fetal cell transplantation: a comparison of three cell types. *J Thorac Cardiovasc Surg* 1999; **118**: 715–724.

65 Li RK, Jia ZQ, Weisel RD, Merante F, Mickle DA. Smooth muscle cell transplantation into myocardial scar tissue improves heart function. *J Mol Cell Cardiol* 1999; **31**: 513–522.

66 Kocher AA, Schuster MD, Szabolcs MJ, Takuma S, Burkhoff D, Wang J, Homma S, Edwards NM, Itescu S. Neovascularization of ischemic myocardium by human bone-marrow-derived angioblasts prevents cardiomyocyte apoptosis, reduces remodeling and improves cardiac function. *Nat Med* 2001; **7**: 430–436.

67 Orlic D, Kajstura J, Chimenti S, Jakoniuk I, Anderson SM, Li B, Pickel J, McKay R, Nadal-Ginard B, Bodine DM *et al.* Bone marrow cells regenerate infarcted myocardium. *Nature* 2001; **410**: 701–705.

68 Koh GY, Soonpaa MH, Klug MG, Pride HP, Cooper BJ, Zipes DP, Field LJ. Stable fetal cardiomyocyte grafts in the hearts of dystrophic mice and dogs. *J Clin Invest* 1995; **96**: 2034–2042.

69 Scorsin M, Hagege AA, Marotte F, Mirochnik N, Copin H, Barnoux M, Sabri A, Samuel JL, Rappaport L, Menasche P. Does transplantation of cardiomyocytes improve function of infarcted myocardium? *Circulation* 1997; **96**: II-93.

70 Scorsin M, Hagege A, Vilquin JT, Fiszman M, Marotte F, Samuel JL, Rappaport L, Schwartz K, Menasche P. Comparison of the effects of fetal cardiomyocyte and skeletal myoblast transplantation on postinfarction left ventricular function. *J Thorac Cardiovasc Surg* 2000; **119**: 1169–1175.

71 Pouzet B, Vilquin JT, Hagege AA, Scorsin M, Messas E, Fiszman M, Schwartz K, Menasche P. Factors affecting functional outcome after autologous skeletal myoblast transplantation. *Ann Thorac Surg* 2001; **71**: 844–850.

72 Rajnoch C, Chachques JC, Berrebi A, Bruneval P, Benoit MO, Carpentier A. Cellular therapy reverses myocardial dysfunction. *J Thorac Cardiovasc Surg* 2001; **121**: 871–878.

73 Campion DR. The muscle satellite cell: a review. *Int Rev Cytol* 1984; **87**: 225–251.

74 Jennings RB, Reimer KA. Lethal myocardial ischemic injury. *Am J Pathol* 1981; **102**: 241–255.

75 Etzion S, Battler A, Barbash IM, Cagnano E, Zarin P, Granot Y, Kedes LH, Kloner RA, Leor J. Influence of embryonic cardiomyocyte transplantation on the progression of heart failure in a rat model of extensive myocardial infarction. *J Mol Cell Cardiol* 2001; **33**: 1321–1330.

76 Murry CE, Wiseman RW, Schwartz SM, Hauschka SD. Skeletal myoblast transplantation for repair of myocardial necrosis. *J Clin Invest* 1996; **98**: 2512–2523.

77 Atkins BZ, Hueman MT, Meuchel JM, Cottman MJ, Hutcheson KA, Taylor DA. Myogenic cell transplantation improves *in vivo* regional performance in infarcted rabbit myocardium. *J Heart Lung Transplant* 1999; **18**: 1173–1180.

78 Murry CE, Kay MA, Bartosek T, Hauschka SD, Schwartz SM. Muscle differentiation during repair of myocardial necrosis in rats via gene transfer with MyoD. *J Clin Invest* 1996; **98**: 2209–2217.

79 Beltrami AP, Urbanek K, Kajstura J, Yan SM, Finato N, Bussani R, Nadal-Ginard B, Silvestri F, Leri A, Beltrami CA *et al.* Evidence that human cardiac myocytes divide after myocardial infarction. *N Engl J Med* 2001; **344**: 1750–1757.

80 Wobus AM, Wallukat G, Hescheler J. Pluripotent mouse embryonic stem cells are able to differentiate into cardiomyocytes expressing chronotropic responses to adrenergic and cholinergic agents and Ca2+ channel blockers. *Differentiation* 1991; **48**: 173–182.

81 Pittenger MF, Mackay AM, Beck SC, Jaiswal RK, Douglas R, Mosca JD, Moorman MA, Simonetti DW, Craig S, Marshak DR. Multilineage potential of adult human mesenchymal stem cells. *Science* 1999; **284**: 143–147.

82 Brazelton TR, Rossi FM, Keshet GI, Blau HM. From marrow to brain: expression of neuronal phenotypes in adult mice. *Science* 2000; **290**: 1775–1779.

83 Lagasse E, Connors H, Al Dhalimy M, Reitsma M, Dohse M, Osborne L, Wang X, Finegold M, Weissman IL, Grompe M. Purified hematopoietic stem cells can differentiate into hepatocytes *in vivo*. *Nat Med* 2000; **6**: 1229–1234.

84 Quaini F, Urbanek K, Beltrami AP, Finato N, Beltrami CA, Nadal-Ginard B, Kajstura J, Leri A, Anversa P. Chimerism of the transplanted heart. *N Engl J Med* 2002; **346**: 5–15.

85 Maltsev VA, Wobus AM, Rohwedel J, Bader M, Hescheler J. Cardiomyocytes differentiated *in vitro* from embryonic

stem cells developmentally express cardiac-specific genes and ionic currents. *Circ Res* 1994; **75**: 233–244.

86 Makino S, Fukuda K, Miyoshi S, Konishi F, Kodama H, Pan J, Sano M, Takahashi T, Hori S, Abe H *et al.* Cardiomyocytes can be generated from marrow stromal cells *in vitro. J Clin Invest* 1999; **103**: 697–705.

87 Takahashi T, Kalka C, Masuda H, Chen D, Silver M, Kearney M, Magner M, Isner JM, Asahara T. Ischemia- and cytokine-induced mobilization of bone marrow-derived endothelial progenitor cells for neovascularization. *Nat Med* 1999; **5**: 434–438.

88 Shintani S, Murohara T, Ikeda H, Ueno T, Honma T, Katoh A, Sasaki K, Shimada T, Oike Y, Imaizumi T. Mobilization of endothelial progenitor cells in patients with acute myocardial infarction. *Circulation* 2001; **103**: 2776–2779.

89 Jackson KA, Majka SM, Wang H, Pocius J, Hartley CJ, Majesky MW, Entman ML, Michael LH, Hirschi KK, Goodell MA. Regeneration of ischemic cardiac muscle and vascular endothelium by adult stem cells. *J Clin Invest* 2001; **107**: 1395–1402.

90 Tse HF, Kwong YL, Chan JK, Lo G, Ho CL, Lau CP. Angiogenesis in ischaemic myocardium by intramyocardial autologous bone marrow mononuclear cell implantation. *Lancet* 2003; **361**: 47–49.

91 Assmus B, Schachinger V, Teupe C, Britten M, Lehmann R, Dobert N, Grunwald F, Aicher A, Urbich C, Martin H *et al.* Transplantation of Progenitor Cells and Regeneration Enhancement in Acute Myocardial Infarction (TOPCARE-AMI). *Circulation* 2002; **106**: 3009–3017.

92 Strauer BE, Kornowsky R. Stem cell therapy in perspective. *Circulation* 2003; **107**: 929–934.

93 Orlic D, Kajstura J, Chimenti S, Limana F, Jakoniuk I, Quaini F, Nadal-Ginard B, Bodine DM, Leri A, Anversa P. Mobilized bone marrow cells repair the infarcted heart, improving function and survival. *Proc Natl Acad Sci USA* 2001; **98**: 10344–10349.

94 Tomita S, Li RK, Weisel RD, Mickle DA, Kim EJ, Sakai T, Jia ZQ. Autologous transplantation of bone marrow cells improves damaged heart function. *Circulation* 1999; **100**: II247–II256.

95 Asahara T, Masuda H, Takahashi T, Kalka C, Pastore C, Silver M, Kearne M, Magner M, Isner JM. Bone marrow origin of endothelial progenitor cells responsible for postnatal vasculogenesis in physiological and pathological neovascularization. *Circ Res* 1999; **85**: 221–228.

96 Dimmeler S, Aicher A, Vasa M, Mildner-Rihm C, Adler K, Tiemann M, Rutten H, Fichtlscherer S, Martin H, Zeiher AM. HMG-CoA reductase inhibitors (statins) increase endothelial progenitor cells via the PI 3-kinase/Akt pathway. *J Clin Invest* 2001; **108**: 391–397.

97 Vasa M, Fichtlscherer S, Adler K, Aicher A, Martin H, Zeiher AM, Dimmeler S. Increase in circulating endothelial progenitor cells by statin therapy in patients with stable coronary artery disease. *Circulation* 2001; **103**: 2885–2890.

98 Caparelli DJ, Cattaneo SM, Shake JG, Flynn EC, Meyers J, Baumgartner WA, Martin DM. Cellular cardiomyoplasty with allogeneic mesenchymal stem cells results in improved cardiac performance in a swine model of myocardial infarction. *Circulation* 2001; **104**: II-599.

99 Strauer BE, Brehm M, Zeus T, Kostering M, Hernandez A, Sorg RV, Kogler G, Wernet P. Repair of infarcted myocardium by autologous intracoronary mononuclear bone marrow cell transplantation in humans. *Circulation* 2002; **106**: 1913–1918.

100 Kraitchman DL, Heldman AW, Atalar E, Amado LC, Martin BJ, Pittenger MF *et al. In vivo* magnetic resonance imaging of mesenchymal stem cells in myocardial infarction. *Circulation* 2003; **107**: 2290–2293.

101 Lederman RJ, Guttman MA, Peters DC, Thompson RB, Sorger JM, Dick AJ *et al.* Catheter-based endomyocardial injection with real-time magnetic resonance imaging. *Circulation* 2002; **105**: 1282–1284.

102 Becker W, Meller J. The role of nuclear medicine in infection and inflammation. *Lancet Infect Dis* 2001; **1**: 326–333.

103 Zhang YM, Hartzell C, Narlow M, Dudley Jr. SC. Stem cell-derived cardiomyocytes demonstrate arrhythmic potential. *Circulation* 2002; **106**: 1294–1299.

104 Leor J, Patterson M, Quinones MJ, Kedes LH, Kloner RA. Transplantation of fetal myocardial tissue into the infarcted myocardium of rat. A potential method for repair of infarcted myocardium? *Circulation* 1996; **94**: II332–II336.

105 Roy I, Holle L, Song W, Holle E, Wagner T, Yu X. Efficient translocation and apoptosis induction by adenovirus encoded VP22-p53 fusion protein in human tumor cells *in vitro. Anticancer Res* 2002; **22**: 3185–3189.

106 Cashman SM, Sadowski SL, Morris DJ, Frederick J, Kumar-Singh R. Intercellular trafficking of adenovirus-delivered HSV VP22 from the retinal pigment epithelium to the photoreceptors-implications for gene therapy. *Mol Ther* 2002; **6**: 813–823.

107 Zender L, Kock R, Eckhard M, Frericks B, Gosling T, Gebhardt T, Drobek S, Galanski M, Kuhnel F, Manns M *et al.* Gene therapy by intrahepatic and intratumoral trafficking of p53-VP22 induces regression of liver tumors. *Gastroenterology* 2002; **123**: 608–618.

108 Koh GY, Kim SJ, Klug MG, Park K, Soonpaa MH, Field LJ. Targeted expression of transforming growth factor-beta 1 in intracardiac grafts promotes vascular endothelial cell DNA synthesis. *J Clin Invest* 1995; **95**: 114–121.

109 Askari AT, Brennan ML, Zhou X, Thomas JD, Topol EJ, Hazen SL, Penn MS. Myeloperoxidase and plasminogen activator inhibitor-1 play a central role in ventricular remodeling after myocardial infarction. *J Exp Med* 2003; **197**: 615–624.

110 Ducharme A, Frantz S, Aikawa M, Rabkin E, Lindsey M, Rohde LE, Schoen FJ, Kelly RA, Werb Z, Libby P *et al.* Targeted deletion of matrix metalloproteinase-9 attenuates left ventricular enlargement and collagen accumulation after experimental myocardial infarction. *J Clin Invest* 2000; **106**: 55–62.

111 Heymans S, Luttun A, Nuyens D, Theilmeier G, Creemers E, Moons L, Dyspersin GD, Cleutjens JP, Shipley M, Angellilo A *et al.* Inhibition of plasminogen activators or matrix metalloproteinases prevents cardiac rupture but impairs therapeutic angiogenesis and causes cardiac failure. *Nat Med* 1999; **5**: 1135–1142.

CHAPTER 16

Ethical issues in cardiothoracic medicine

Katrina A. Bramstedt

Introduction

The current technological offerings of both cardiology and cardiothoracic surgery provide numerous benefits to heart failure patients, yet they are not without clinical risk. Some technologies have the potential for ethical dilemmas due to their scarcity, materials, and methods, for example. Future technologies pose possible benefit that makes clinical trial participation enticing for patients with untreatable heart failure; yet, the uncertainties of these experimental technologies raises ethical concerns. The next sections describe and analyze the ethical dilemmas associated with current and future cardiac technology in light of the goals of medicine and clinical research.

Heart transplantation

Organ donation

A glance at the United Network for Organ Sharing (UNOS) web page (www.unos.org) provides visitors with statistical insight into transplantation and organ donation. Trending of the heart donation data finds a consistent shortfall of organs available for patients on the heart transplant waiting list. It is estimated that while approximately 4500 patients are waiting for a heart in the United States, only 2200 hearts are donated each year, and 25% of those waiting for a heart will die before getting a transplant [1]. While it is true that many people refuse to give advance consent for their organs to be used for transplant in the event of their death, others do give this advance consent but it is overridden by family members at the time of death [2]. It is estimated

that yearly, 11,000 people die as potential organ donors and consent for organ donation is obtained for less than half of these individuals [3].

While organ procurement organizations are not obligated to accept this "override", most do out of fear of litigation by family members. A new concept of "first-person consent" (Table 16.1) is active in several states including Colorado, Ohio, Pennsylvania, and Virginia [2]. Under this plan, an individual's advance decision to be an organ donor is respected even in the face of family dissention. In general, these plans work by individuals registering their preference to be an organ donor at their State Motor Vehicle Registration Facility. This organ donation preference is registered in a computer, and also on the individual's vehicle driver's license. There is no legal requirement to make a formal decision to register or not register into the system, and no additional permission from the patient's family, guardian, or estate is required for organ procurement to be pursued in the case of registered individuals. These

Table 16.1 Summary of strategies to increase organ donation.

- Educate the public about the continuing organ shortfall
- Educate the public about the organ donation process
- "First-person consent"
- "Presumed consent"
- Payment for organs (very ethically problematic)
- Financial incentives for organ donation (e.g., contribution toward funeral expenses)
- Commendation award
- "Give–receive bundle"

programs are very new in the United States thus it is too soon to tell if they are effective in increasing organ donation; nonetheless, these plans do respect the autonomy of individuals in that their choice about organ donation will be respected and not overridden by others who ascribe to different values.

Other methods of attempting to increase organ donation include education campaigns by UNOS, organ procurement organizations, and special interest groups. In general, the focus of these educational efforts is to enlighten people regarding the organ donation process and de-bunk the myths of both donation and transplantation. Public concerns include the fear that physicians will do less than their medical best for patients known to be willing to donate their organs; death will be declared prematurely so that organs can be retrieved; and the body will be mutilated due to organ retrieval [4]. These fears can only be allayed through education of the public as to the realities of organ donation, thus it is ethically imperative that these educational efforts continue.

Presumed consent is another method proposed for increasing organ donation. Though not used in the United States, some countries such as Belgium and Spain employ a presumed consent policy for organ donation in which individuals are required to opt-out of organ donation in advance, or be presumed to have opted-in. According to the Presumed Consent Foundation, Inc. (New York, USA), the opt-out rate is approximately 2% in countries using presumed consent policy [5]. According to data presented at the *XIX International Congress of the Transplantation Society* [6], the nations with the highest per capita organ donation rates in the world are Spain, Austria, and Belgium (all operating under presumed consent policies). While Spain's donor rate is 32.5 donors per million, the US donation rate is 21.4 donors per million [6]. From an ethics perspective, presumed consent forces individuals to make a choice or be presumed to have made a choice. Some people may not want to think about their future death and thus avoid making a decision about organ donation. When these people die, their "decision" not to make a choice will result in a choice being forced upon them; namely, they will be considered to have opted-in for donation because they did not make a choice before death to opt-out. This can be viewed by some as ethically problematic.

Presumed consent would be more ethically palatable if the following measures were in place:
1 the individual's identifying information and their opt-out decision must be securely stored, yet readily accessible when needed;
2 documentation of the opt-out decision should be able to be made by a process that is simple and conducive for those who may lack the means to present themselves at a designated data recording facility;
3 lacking a documented opt-out decision, the patient's family should be contacted to gather information on possible verbal expressions made by the patient with regard to not wanting to be an organ donor;
4 the public should be educated regarding the policy and procedures of presumed consent using methods that facilitate a widespread distribution of the information in a manner that is easy to comprehend.

Financial incentives for organ donation (e.g., funeral expense contributions) can be viewed as ethically problematic and it is unclear that these measures would increase organ donation. In fact, the monetary association may cast a negative shadow on transplant medicine and have the effect of decreasing donation [4]. In the United States, the National Organ Transplant Act prohibits the sale or purchase of human organs [7]. Organs are generally understood as the "gift of life" and as such, they are given to patients without requirement of payment. Payment and financial incentives could be viewed as tarnishing the altruism of organ donation – a value generally held by the US society.

Two other options for potentially increasing organ donation are (1) commendation and (2) the give–receive bundle. In 2001, the United States House of Representatives and Senate introduced the "Gift of Life Congressional Medal Act S. 325/H. R. 708" for consideration. This legislation would create a commemorative bronze medal to honor organ donors and their survivors. Senator Frist, a heart and lung transplant surgeon, was one of the authors. The program to design, manufacture, and distribute the medals is planned to be self-supporting through charitable donations and is currently pending before the Senate Banking, Housing, and Urban Affairs Committee and the House Committee on Energy and Commerce. Such a medal would represent a non-financial acknowledgement of the donor's generosity to society. Further, this form of thanks does not jeopardize the altruistic nature of organ donation and thus would be ethically permissible.

The give–receive bundle policy, also called reciprocal-duties [8], would operate by way of the concept that those willing to receive an organ for transplant should also be willing to donate organs for transplant. The argument is that considering oneself as willing to take from the donor organ pool should require the reciprocal obligation of registering oneself as a potential organ donor. Transplant eligibility is thus bundled with organ donor status. Ethical arguments against this approach include the fact that there may be people who are morally opposed to being an organ donor but yet not opposed to receiving an allograft (e.g., those who believe their body must be fully intact after death). The question becomes should this "special value" (which may seem irrational by some) be respected as is done for certain religious values that seem to conflict with the logic of medicine? Also there may be those who are physically unable to be an organ donor, but suitable as an allograft recipient. Problems with the give–receive bundle policy will also be met by transplant surgeons who encounter patients who have refused to enlist themselves on the donor registry and yet present as "great" candidates for transplantation. These surgeons will likely feel obligated to offer beneficent medicine by way of an allograft without regard to the patient's donor status.

Heart transplantation and the elderly

Alternate recipient list[1]

Due to the ongoing shortfall of allografts, some hospitals have engaged the strategy of an alternate recipient list (ARL) for heart transplantation, yet examination of their outcome data alone is not enough to justify its use as an ethical practice. Specifically, issues regarding using age as a transplant eligibility criterion must be explored (Table 16.2).

An ARL for heart transplantation functions by attempting to match donor organs for which the

Table 16.2 Ethical issues with marginal hearts and ARL.

- Inability to predict lifespan of marginal hearts
- Clinical issues with marginal hearts (e.g., increased ischemic time, coronary artery disease, reduced ejection fraction)
- Allowing older patients to receive heart transplantation enlarges the pool of patients waiting for a heart transplant, potentially affecting the waiting times of younger patients
- Giving marginal hearts (instead of standard hearts) to older people can be viewed as age discrimination
- Determining the donor age cut off for marginal hearts versus standard hearts
- Marginal hearts may be wasted if not used by the elderly

long-term outcome is unknown with recipients who are elderly. Generally, these patients are over age 60, however age criteria vary among transplant centers. The use of the term "alternate" can carry with it emotionally charged visions of organs that are defective or recipients who are "second class". These perceptions are both unfortunate and inaccurate. Organs allocated through an alternate list program are those for which the long-term clinical outcome is uncertain due to variables such as increased donor age, the presence of coronary artery disease, prolonged ischemic time, elevated central venous pressure, elevated inotrope exposure, and reduced ejection fraction [9]. Data have shown that these variables do not *necessarily* impart statistically significant negative impact on the short- or medium-term outcomes of recipients, nor do they significantly impact ejection fraction, the number of rejection episodes, or the length of post-transplant hospitalization when compared to "standard" donor heart transplantation [10,11]. However, because ARLs have been used in only a few transplant centers for approximately 7 years, the long-term outcome of these transplants is not known.

There have been reports of older donor hearts transmitting coronary artery disease [12] and prostate cancer [13]. Not all centers evidence similar atherosclerosis results, and it may be that this is related to variables such as organ screening, donor/recipient risk screening, donor recipient viral screening, and immunosuppressive regimen. Some older hearts also evidence chronotropic incompetence after implantation and require placement of a pacemaker

---

[1]Portions reprinted by permission, from [24] © 2001 University of Otago.

for treatment of the conduction abnormality [14]. The combination of positive and negative clinical findings (some treatable or screenable), as well as an unclear long-term outcome, creates a unique dilemma in determining the criteria for recipient selection. Some have suggested donor testing, balancing the resulting risk with the risk of dying without a heart transplant [15].

The University of California, Los Angeles is one of the largest volume users of marginal hearts in older recipients, reporting a 4-year survival of 78%. They report no significant difference in early mortality or actuarial survival between patients on the ARL and patients on the standard waiting list [11]. The University of Padova, Italy reports a 4-year survival of 81% for older patients receiving a marginal heart and 80% for older patients receiving non-marginal hearts [16]. International transplantation registry data (1991–1997) indicates a 4-year survival rate of 68% for patients receiving a marginal heart [17]. Several centers report that the use of standard hearts and marginal hearts has not shown significant difference with regards to the incidence of post-transplant acute rejection or infection, however, older recipients are more likely to die of infection or malignant disease. Many older patients receiving a marginal heart have shown significant reduction in their New York Heart Association (NYHA) score that can be correlated to an improved quality of life (QOL) due to less pain and fatigue, and more mobility that can facilitate independence [11,16].

Accepting that these "marginal" hearts are indeed clinically effective (with or without pre-implantation revascularization) it could be problematic *not* to use them due to the fact that their potential benefit (though possibly time limited) will be discarded along with the organ. Probing further it could also be problematic to give a marginal heart to a patient who would optimally benefit from a long-term implant due to their anticipated life expectancy. While each patient's life span is unknown because humans can theoretically die at any moment, it is nonetheless easily posed that the potential quantity of years remaining for a young person is greater than that remaining for an elderly person. If there is reason to believe that long-term transplant outcomes might be reduced with marginal hearts, then these organs should be offered to a patient pool that includes those of advanced age as they have a shorter span of life ahead of them as part of their baseline presentation. Patients, who are likely candidates for a long-term result, should be in line for a long-term organ, and transplant centers may have to adjust their ARL entry criteria as further morbidity and survival data is gained while using these protocols.

There is no discrimination against the potential elderly recipients as they are offered organs that have the potential for the most practical life span match. An ARL allocation strategy respects a patient's capacity to benefit from transplantation regardless of their age, prevents the discard of usable organs, and overall, represents transplant medicine's strive toward ethical technology stewardship. Restated, alternate recipients make use of hearts that will go to waste if not used by those on the standard list. It gives them a chance they would otherwise not have because their age automatically sets them aside from the Status I UNOS list.

In light of ethical technology stewardship, and the structure and function of an ARL, it appears that age-based exclusions to transplantation are unnecessary. The same reasons which make such an exclusion unnecessary (the inability to determine each potential recipient's life span, the potential diminution of capacity to benefit toward the end of an elderly patient's life when they have clinical exclusion factors or elevated surgical risks, the availability of marginal organs that will go unused or be placed in patients who are unsuitably matched for potential long-term outcome) are the same reasons which render aged-based categorical limits unethical. Further, instead of making transplantation age based, using capacity to benefit (with the organ matching concept espoused by an ARL) is more just because it defines eligibility at a non-arbitrary level. At the Cleveland Clinic, an ARL is not used; however, a patient's age value is not a rigid criterion for heart transplant candidacy.

Certainly there will be those who will argue that ARL programs are ethically troublesome because while potentially allowing transplant eligibility for the elderly and reducing organ wastage, there is no economic mechanism to increase the financial resources to pay for these additional surgical procedures (and their related medical expenses). The number of geriatric patients receiving a heart transplant is growing each year with 174 recipients in 2003, up from 104 recipients in 1993. It is unknown how many clinically eligible patients are not placed on this waiting list due to hospitals deterring patients from transplantation based on age value alone; however, the ethical acceptance of ARLs could change practice patterns.

Retransplantation

For a small percentage of heart transplant patients, chronic rejection or primary graft failure can lead to the consideration of retransplantation. Approximately 50 heart transplants are recorded yearly in the Registry of the International Society for Heart and Lung Transplantation as retransplants [18]. At the Cleveland Clinic, 13 patients (out of 1002) have been retransplanted since the inception of the heart transplant program in 1984. Although these numbers are small, the ethical complexities of retransplantation loom large. As allografts are scarce resources, it is ethically imperative to allocate them fairly. Retransplantation is ethically problematic because it allows some patients to receive multiple heart transplants while others are still waiting for their first one. Further concern is added when patient's non-compliance is determined to be contributory to primary graft rejection.

Some have argued that it is ethically irrelevant that some patients may receive multiple retransplants while others still wait for their first allograft [19]. However, allografts are not "off-the-shelf" spare body parts to facilitate immortality. The fairest distribution of any limited resource would preclude multiple distributions to the same patients while excluding others who have equal or greater capacity to benefit from that particular resource. This does not mean that retransplantation is never justified; however, retransplantation as a practice should follow ethical guidelines.

It has been shown that with regard to primary heart transplants, pre-transplant non-compliance can predict post-transplant non-compliance [20]. It is also possible that non-compliance post-primary heart transplantation will also predict non-compliance with retransplantation, although there is no published data to this effect. As non-compliance can impact post-transplant QOL and mortality [21], ethical stewardship of scarce resources would preclude retransplantation in non-compliant patients due to the potential for patient-induced negative outcomes. Participating in transplantation means more than receiving an organ. The clinical duty to provide beneficent medicine has a co-joined patient responsibility to be compliant with medical regimens that are critical to the efficacy of the technology. This patient responsibility is due out of respect for others who are also waiting and in need of the technology, and out of respect for the personnel resources needed to implement the technology. The doctor–patient relationship is a partnership requiring both the doctor and the patient to do their best, and physicians should not be held captive by patients who are not promoting their own health via compliance [22]. Physicians are under no ethical obligation to provide retransplantation to patients who jeopardize the success of their transplants with non-compliant behavior.

Also critical to the concept of fairness in retransplantation is the matter of clinical efficacy. The largest cardiac retransplantation study to-date concluded that retransplantation is a higher risk procedure than primary transplantation, especially when the elapsed time between transplants is 6 months or less [23]. This study examined the Joint International Society for Heart and Lung Transplantation/UNOS Registry data from 514 cardiac retransplant patients (1987–1998) and concluded that retransplant patients fare worse than primary transplant patients and they tend to have a greater incidence of renal dysfunction (likely due to their increased time on cyclosporin therapy). Only retransplantation due to coronary allograft vasculopathy has survival rates approaching that of primary transplantation. Due to the poorer outcomes of retransplantation, it can be argued that patients awaiting their first allograft should receive priority allograft allocation. Also, those waiting for their first transplant should not have to compete with people who have already experienced life extension through transplantation. Organs declined by these primary waiting patients should then be referred to patients awaiting retransplantation. Another option is the use of "marginal hearts" for retransplantation [24]. Although ethically controversial, "marginal hearts" could be used as allografts for retransplantation as it appears from Registry data that patient outcomes would be better matched to organs with potentially shorter lifespans (see above section, "ARL").

Transplantation in HIV positive patients

"Nothing short of unbelievable" and "medically unjustifiable" were 1990 comments to the concept of organ transplantation in human immunodeficiency virus positive (HIV+) patients [25]. Similar views are also held by numerous organ transplant coordinators [26]. While the American Medical Association (AMA) argues it is unethical for a physician to refuse to treat an HIV+ patient solely because the patient is seropositive [27], and UNOS policy does not permit HIV status alone as a categorical exclusion criterion for transplantation [28], to our knowledge, only two US hospitals perform heart transplantation for HIV+ patients; namely, The Cleveland Clinic and Columbia Presbyterian Medical Center (New York, NY). As far as we know, only three heart transplants have been performed in the United States on patients for whom their HIV status was known to be positive at the time of transplant [29–31]. There have been other cases in which heart transplants have been performed on patients who were not known to be HIV+ prior to transplantation and subsequent post-transplant serology indicated positive reactivity (either due to perioperatively acquired HIV or likely existing HIV seropositivity prior to the advent of HIV testing) [32,33].

As a result of highly active antiretroviral therapy (HAART), HIV+ patients are living longer and with less comorbidity [34]. Nonetheless, many arguments against organ transplantation in HIV+ patients have been made [35], including: (1) protease inhibitor therapy may increase the risk for coronary heart disease and myocardial infarction; (2) cardiac surgery may accelerate the progression from HIV to acquired immunodeficiency syndrome (AIDS); (3) transplant required immunosuppression may increase the risk of infection in HIV+ individuals; (4) survival rates and QOL may be lower for HIV+ transplant patients and thus not the "best" allocation of scarce allografts; (5) the risk of HIV transmission to the surgical team does not justify organ transplantation in HIV+ patients; (6) HIV+ individuals are not morally worthy of an organ transplant; (7) adding HIV+ individuals to the organ transplant waiting list will further swell the pool of those waiting for an organ and thus

Table 16.3 Ethical issues in transplantation of HIV+ patients.

- Possible negative cardiovascular effects of protease inhibitor therapy
- Transplantation possibly increasing the progression of HIV to AIDS
- Immunosuppression possibly increasing the risk of infection in HIV+ patients
- Possible lower QOL and lifespan of HIV+ transplant recipients
- Risk of HIV transmission to transplant team
- The moral "worthiness" of HIV+ patients
- Giving organs to HIV+ patients may make HIV− patients wait longer for their transplants
- Organ donation may decrease if HIV+ patients are allowed to receive transplants

lengthen the waiting times for people on the list who are HIV negative; and (8) organ donation may decrease if HIV+ individuals are allowed to receive organ transplants (summary presented in Table 16.3).

With regard to protease inhibitor exposure, the largest study to-date concluded that the risk of coronary heart disease was associated with duration of protease inhibitor use, but they were unable to find a similar association with myocardial infarction [36]. Everson et al. followed 19 HIV+ patients for an average of 33 months and argue that there is no conclusive evidence that cardiac surgery accelerates HIV into AIDS [37]. Regarding transplant required immunosuppression, several studies have concluded that such therapy does not increase susceptibility to opportunistic infections or malignancy in HIV+ patients [38,39]. Regarding the Cleveland Clinic's patient, at 2-year status post-transplantation, the development or reactivation of opportunistic infection has been negative, and he continues to work full-time and exercise regularly [30]. Lastly, with regard to the risk of HIV transmission to the surgical team, this risk is lower than that of the patient–surgeon transmission of hepatitis C virus and these patients are frequently operated upon [40].

The ethics-related arguments are more difficult to address because ethical dilemmas are generally not solved via empirical methods. In addressing the ethically problematic nature of organ transplants in HIV+ patients, beneficence requires that the clinical good that can be provided be maximized; while non-malfeasance requires that harm to the patient be minimized. Justice requires that patients be treated fairly without preference to a particular social or economic class, for example. Thus, the argument that HIV+ patients are not morally worthy of a heart transplant is not supported by the principle of justice. HIV status does not correspond to the morality of an individual. Clearly, any patient behavior that risk compromising an allograft should be screened for during the transplant patient selection process; however, categorically excluding HIV+ patients do not accomplish this task. Further, a categorical exclusion of this nature denies HIV+ patients the chance at a therapeutic intervention which could bring them clinical benefit.

Adding HIV+ patients to the heart transplant waiting list will indeed swell the already large waiting pool of patients; however, lacking data that heart transplantation is not clinically successful in HIV+ patients, there is no ethical justification for banning this group of patients from the list. Transplant lists are currently "swelled" with patients who are diabetic, aged, and obese, as well as those with prior alcohol and tobacco use, thus there is no ethical justification for a categorical exclusion of HIV+ individuals unless science determines a significant correlation between HIV seropositivity and post-transplant morbidity, QOL, and mortality. Examining morbidity, QOL and mortality, and determining that transplantation can benefit appropriate HIV+ patients is ethical justification for making such technology available to these patients through the waiting list process, even if allografts cannot be allocated to everyone on the waiting list due to the ongoing organ shortfall. Thus said, caution is warranted at this early stage of heart transplantation in HIV+ patients. The Cleveland Clinic believes careful patient selection and continued data monitoring are essential.

In response to the argument that heart transplantation in HIV+ patients will result in a decrease in organ donation, this is speculative. There is no indication that liver donation is lower than it could be due to the presence of recovering alcoholics on the UNOS liver transplant waiting list. Similarly, there is no indication that lung donation is lower

than it could be due to the presence of former tobacco users on the UNOS lung transplant waiting list. Even if such data did exist, it would not justify denying transplantation to patients agreeing to a pre- and post-transplant regimen that is free of risk factors that significantly jeopardize successful transplantation. As discussed, valid ethical arguments against heart transplantation in HIV+ patients must be based on clinical evidence that such a procedure is significantly less effective in HIV+ patients in terms of post-transplant morbidity, QOL, and mortality. Although ethically controversial, "marginal hearts" could be used as allografts for HIV+ patients if it is determined that patient outcomes would be better matched to organs with potentially shorter lifespans (see above section, "ARL") [24]. Further, the use of marginal hearts through an ARL does not foster arbitrary categorical limits on the number of retransplants that patients can have because the allocation of organs is based on each patient's capacity to benefit from the transplant.

Xenotransplantation

Xenotransplantation (cross-species transplantation) may be on the medical horizon either as bridge or destination therapy. While xenograft research has been more secretive since the famous baboon to human transplant at Loma Linda University Medical Center (USA) in 1984 [41], research in this area has not abated, and neither has the ethical uproar. In addition to the technical challenges (e.g., rejection, zoonosis), there is a wide range of ethical opinion regarding the whole-organ xenotransplantation. Interestingly, the reasons for viewing such as ethically impermissible often do not seem to relate to the general clinical use of animal tissue but rather to the use of whole organs for transplant [42], although some are vehemently opposed to any use of animal tissue for medical therapy or otherwise [43]. As animal molecules, cells, and tissues are currently used for human therapy, and organs are tissues integrated to perform a specific function, an ethical distinction allowing animal cell and tissue transplantation, and disallowing whole-organ transplantation is difficult to make. It seems "drawing the line" at whole-organ transplants, yet allowing transplants of animal cells and tissues (such as heart valves) is arbitrary. If xenotransplantation becomes clinical reality, one could argue that using only animal cells and tissues, and not using whole organs is potentially wasteful of medical resources.

The use of non-transgenic animals presents the dilemma of hyperacute rejection; however, transgenic animals may be able to address this challenge. Companies such as Baxter (Princeton, NJ) and Alexion Pharmaceuticals (Chesire, CT) currently have porcine breeding farms in which they produce animals, which have modified genomes intended to reduce the risk of complement activation and xenorejection when the organs are transplanted into humans. In 1991, pigs in which the alpha 1,3 galactosyl transferase gene had been knocked out were born, preventing the addition of alpha 1,3 galactose to the cell surface (which would trigger an immune response in humans, leading to hyperacute rejection of transplanted organs or cells) [44]. Theoretically, transgenic manipulation would provide a predictable availability of organs from a carefully selected single strain of pigs, unlike human allografts where availability is limited and sudden, and matching rarely perfect.

In terms of human genetics and manipulation of the human genome, the intent is nearly always to correct a defect (with the aim of curing or preventing disease). With regard to the genetic manipulation of animals, the focus is generally the enhancement of a "healthy" genome. In this latter case, there are no defects to be cured or prevented in the animal, but rather the animal is being modified for human use. Whether manipulating the human genome to cure or prevent disease, or manipulating an animal genome to enhance it with human proteins, the motivation of both technologies is ultimately therapeutic and the ability of both technologies to provide clinical therapy is directly related to the ethical principle of beneficence [45].

With the technology of xenotransplantation still emerging, the risk of human infection via zoonosis is unclear. Endogenous retroviruses in porcine tissue have shown the capacity to infect human cells *in vitro* [46], with the Food and Drug Administration (FDA) requiring retrovirus testing on xenotransplant recipients [47]. In addition to the possible risk of animal-to-human infection, there is also the possible risk of human-to-human infection, with the route of infection also currently unknown. Not only could the transplant recipient be risking infection, but he/she might also be risking infection to the immediate family, and possibly even society at large. Here the discussion then switches from autonomy to justice. Along with considering the possible benefits to oneself, the obligation to protect society from the spread of infection cannot be ignored. If significant zoonosis theories are proved, the intended healing of the transplant community, would in fact be only temporary, and the technology would then be harmful to both the patient and others – thus making xenotransplantation ethically impermissible.

Due to the undeterminable moral claim of animals, it is unrealistic to use this concept as an argument against utilizing animals for medical therapy, even if it means modifying their genome. Nonetheless, it is important for society to make an ethical assessment of technologies as they develop. Emerging technologies need emergent ethical evaluation, as well as evaluation in the post-market phase in order to ensure an appropriate balance of risks and benefits to both individual patients and society at large.

Cell transplantation and gene therapy

Cell transplantation has been posed as a potential adjunctive treatment for heart failure. The theory of this experimental technology is that infarction scar tissue can be engrafted with cells to either return kinesis to the area, or to create a cellular scaffold to prevent expansion of the infarct [48] as infarct size is related to the degree of impaired heart function [49]. Combining cell transplantation with gene therapy (see below) may also be an option for heart failure therapy.

As cell therapy is an emerging technology, there are many unknowns including the optimal type of cell for transplantation, the mode of delivery of the cells, the dosage of cells, and the timing of cell transplantation with respect to infarct onset. Human embryonic and fetal cells remain ethically contentious, thus the search for other sources continues. Cells chosen should have limited proliferation potential so as to reduce the likelihood of tumor formation [50]. The invasiveness of the mode of cell delivery should be reflected upon in light of the possible need for multiple transplants. Cell transplantation dosage can potentially facilitate arrhythmias, possibly generating the need for automated cardioverter defibrillator implantation [51]. Techniques to enhance cell survival and optimize dose volume could be beneficial to reducing the number of transplant sessions required to reach clinical efficacy.

The highly complex nature of cell transplantation technology poses ethical dilemmas in terms of clinical trial design, research subject selection, and informed consent. The risk level of the clinical trial should reflect upon the number of dosing interventions required for research subjects, the level of invasiveness of the mode of cell delivery, the possibility of cell proliferation, as well as the risk of arrhythmias. In an effort to facilitate comprehension and informed decision-making, the consent process should involve the explanation of cell transplantation technology in a manner that is commensurate with the educational and technological sophistication of each research subject.

Although currently experimental, gene therapy for the treatment of cardiac dysfunction may prove safe and effective upon completion of clinical trials. Hypotheses pose gene therapy as a remedy for abnormalities in calcium homeostasis [52], derangements in β-adrenergic signaling [53], and cardiac cell apoptosis [54]. Gene therapy is also posed as a mechanism to facilitate myocardial angiogenesis [55]. As gene therapy is experimental at this point in time, there are many unknowns, especially with regard to identification of appropriate gene vectors, methods of gene delivery, as well as timing and frequency of gene delivery. Issues of host immune response and mutagenesis are critical, as evidenced by the death of a research subject enrolled in a study of gene transfer in partial ornithine transcarbamylase deficiency [56]. In this study, researchers discovered that some side effects of therapy were not predicted by pre-clinical models, and some aspects of the toxicity were not proportional to the vector dose.

As with cell transplantation, the highly complex nature of gene therapy technology poses ethical dilemmas in terms of clinical trial design, research subject selection, and informed consent. For studies using gene delivery methods that are invasive and require general anesthesia (e.g., thoracotomy), placebo controls are ethically inappropriate due to

the level of risk. Risk level should also be reflected upon in terms of the number of dosing interventions required for research subjects, and the possibility that the delivery method may expose non-intended sites to the gene and its vector.

To date there is limited data on informed consent for cardiac gene therapy, yet the highly technological nature of gene therapy does add complexity to the dilemma of obtaining "truly" informed consent for trial participation. A recent study of patient attitudes about gene therapy for cardiac disease found that 17% of those interviewed were not able to understand the basic principles of gene therapy [57]. Most of these individuals were older, lived in rural areas, and were less educated compared to those who were able to understand basic principles of gene therapy. According to this study, individuals had various conceptualizations of genes including, "has something to do with cloning", "has something to do with paternity", "important for growth", and "very small element that can control the whole body". Of those deemed to have a correct understanding of genes, 94% would agree to catheter-based gene transfer and 80% would agree to surgically delivered gene transfer. Regarding a prophylactic gene transfer to prevent future heart disease, 54% would agree to such therapy. Risks were clearly on their mind, with the unpredictability and potentially irreversible side effects of gene therapy as their main concerns. They viewed "properly designed" studies that were regulated by an institutional review board as important to human safety. Clearly, the informed consent process for gene therapy should include educating potential recipients about the concept of gene therapy in a manner that is commensurate with their level of educational and technological sophistication.

Mechanical and electronic cardiac technology

Mechanical circulatory support

Mechanical heart technology in the form of ventricular assist devices is standard of care for certain patients requiring hemodynamic support. Currently, these devices are used in both inpatient and outpatient settings as a bridge to transplant, although in November 2002, the US FDA approved one device, the HeartMate SNAP-VE Left Ventricular Assist System (Thoratec Corporation, Pleasanton, CA) for

Table 16.4 Ventricular assist device (VAD) versus total artificial heart (TAH).

VAD	TAH
The use of VADs as bridging devices swells the pool of patients waiting to receive a heart transplant. The use of VADs as permanent implants shrinks the pool of patients waiting for a heart transplant.	If clinically safe and effective, the use of TAHs as permanent implants would shrink the pool of patients waiting for a heart transplant.
VADs can be mass produced	TAHs can be mass produced
Very expensive technology	Very expensive technology
No immunosuppression required	No immunosuppression required
Device "rejection" not possible	Device "rejection" not possible
VADs can pose comfort issues for recipients	Device can pose comfort issues for recipients
Battery power must be supplied	Battery power must be supplied
Risk of stroke, infection, device malfunction	Risk of stroke, infection, device malfunction
With VAD use, the native heart remains in place; thus, if the VAD is stopped or removed the native heart is still available.	With TAH use, the native heart is explanted; thus, the TAH must function flawlessly.
VADs can facilitate repair of the native heart	TAH technology has no effect on improving the human heart

permanent cardiac support in lieu of heart transplantation. These devices have been empirically proven to improve the contractile properties of myocytes in the resting ventricle [58], improve pre-transplantation QOL [59], and increase both pre-and post-transplant survival time [60]. As ventricular assist device patients are automatically added to the Status I heart transplant waiting list, this raises ethical concern about swelling the pool of waiting patients for a limited amount of organs (Table 16.4) [61].

While ventricular assist technology does nothing to increase the pool of potential donors, a study by the Cleveland Clinic concluded that patients who received pre-transplant left ventricular assist devices waited longer for their transplant than did non-assist device patients on the Status I list [62]. Another study has reported similar findings [60]. Wait times increased due to rehabilitation and recovery time after the device implant procedure, and the difficulty in finding a suitable allograft for human leukocyte antigen (HLA) sensitized patients. While Status I non-device patients are not exposed to longer wait times, Status II patients likely are as organs will continue to be referred to Status I patients before they are referred to those in the Status II category. Those on the Status II list are indeed less sick to start with, but prolonged waiting in the Status II category may result in further cardiac

decompensation, making these patients sicker at the time of transplant (which could affect post-transplant outcomes) or requiring upgrade to the Status I list with the insertion of an assist device (and the additional associated medical expenses). Longer wait times do not usually adversely affect assist device patients because they hemodynamically and functionally improve while on device therapy, making them healthier at the time of allograft transplant. Ventricular assist devices do thus allow more people eligibility for a transplant; however, because the number of available allografts remains relatively the same from year to year, some waiting patients may further suffer as their waiting time lengthens. In light of the benefits of assist device technology, the need is elevated for increased organ donation and/or devices that can be used for permanent cardiac support or replacement.

Total artificial heart (TAH) technology is again being considered as a possible solution to the ongoing shortfall of donor organs. Between July 2001 and May 2004, 14 completely self-contained TAH devices were implanted in the United States [63]. This after an 11-year moratorium on such implants after the FDA stopped the Jarvik-7 TAH clinical trial in 1990. While the Jarvik-7 trial implanted nearly 200 TAH devices, issues of hemorrhage, stroke, and sepsis were prominent [64]. Even with the data from the Jarvik-7 trial, TAH data from various animal studies, and the extensive pool of data from the long-term use of ventricular assist devices, further human trials of TAH technology are not without significant risk, and it is not enough to argue that these device might save lives. The known and potential risks of TAH technology must be weighed in light of the potential harm to research participants (Table 16.4). Further, psychological and social variables must also be reflected upon in the course of selecting research subjects for trial participation. Also trial participation should not be the result of social or financial pressure. Ethical principles and scientific goals should guide the selection of research subjects, not convenience, privilege, or arbitrary age limits [65].

Obtaining informed consent for TAH trial participation will likely be made difficult by the complex nature of the technology and the general lack of technological sophistication of many patients. The consent process will be further impacted by the level of desperation of those seeking to participate in such a trial [66,67]. Knowing the scarcity of allografts, some individuals may feel an artificial heart is their only hope, and thus be eager to participate in the trial without reflecting on its risks. (see "Clinical trials and the ethical conduct of research" below). As mechanical cardiac technologies evolve, such permanent support and replacement devices could be viewed as safer than transplantation due to its issues of immunosuppression and rejection; however, the safety and efficacy profile of such permanent devices are significant unknowns. At this time, the Cleveland Clinic feels that cardiac replacement technology is not optimal in part because the removal of the native heart makes TAH technology one that must perform perfectly – a likely difficult task to accomplish.

Inactivating electronic and circulatory support therapy in cases of futility

Implanted cardiac therapies such as pacemakers, cardioverter defibrillators, and ventricular assist devices are clearly designed with the intent of clinical benefit for the recipient; however, the time may come when termination of such therapy is ethically

warranted [68]. As with total artificial organs, no assistive therapy should be viewed as a means of immortality for patients. Further, physicians are under no ethical obligation to provide futile care (offering no benefit or a high likelihood of no success) [69]. When the burdens of a therapy are more than its benefits, this is the time to consider therapy withdrawal. When therapy is futile, it is clinically and ethically appropriate to no longer offer it. Importantly, patients should be appraised of the situations that would warrant device inactivation during the device implantation informed consent process so that they and their families are aware of the concept in advance [70].

From both an ethics and legal perspective, it is generally accepted that patients with decision-making capacity can make informed choices to have life-sustaining therapies terminated [71]. In the case of implanted cardioverter defibrillators, shocks provided by the device can be painful, and even the anticipatory anxiety of possible future shocks can be stressful for the patient [72]. When the device is no longer positively influencing QOL and is no longer clinically indicated from the standpoint of palliative care, device inactivation should be considered [73]. The same can be said for ventricular assist devices [70]. Pump dependence is theoretically possible when patients are receiving implant therapy but then determined to be ineligible for heart transplantation. Such a situation may result, for example, due to neurological devastation (e.g., stroke, permanent vegetative state). Physicians and families must assess the benefits and burdens of the treatment in light of the goal of the intervention and the values and preferences of the patient, especially when the patient cannot speak for him/herself. When the values and preferences of the patient are unknown, physicians should make recommendations based on the best interest of the patient.

It is highly advantageous for implant device recipients to reflect upon their device status and denote their treatment preferences in an Advance Directive that also names surrogate decision-makers in the event that they lose decision-making capacity [73]. Cardiologists following such implant patients should recommend that both a primary and an alternate decision-maker be appointed who know the patient's values and who will recommend actions that are in accordance with the patient's personal wishes. While contemplating device inactivation may be emotionally difficult for patients, it is critical that they conceptualize the actions of these devices as a form of life support that may indeed need to be withdrawn under certain clinical situations. In reality, it is no different than considering the possible withdrawal of other forms of invasive medical therapy such as artificial ventilation and dialysis. At the Cleveland Clinic, bioethicists are available to assist patients, their families, and the medical team in discussions of this nature.

Clinical trials and the ethical conduct of research

In the setting of untreatable heart failure and the potential hope of cell transplantation, gene therapy, and other experimental technologies, the expectations of clinical trial research subjects may run high (Table 16.5). Research subject selection should reflect upon the vulnerability of individuals who possibly "have no other hope" and may view clinical trial participation as a form of health care when in fact, the goal of clinical research is to gain knowledge that is generalizable for the benefit of future patients [74]. Until the risks and benefits of these technologies are fully understood, research investigators must strive to anticipate the therapeutic misconception that clinical trial participation will provide direct benefit to the research subjects, aiming toward an informed consent process that clearly denotes the experimental nature of the technology and its known and potential risks. Accepting that many of these technologies are complex, the informed consent process should be geared to reflect the intellectual capacity of potential research subjects, and should incorporate tools to aid their comprehension of the study technology, its risks, and its benefits. Tools to assist the informed consent process include videos, brochures, diagrams, and flowcharts. Potential research subjects should be encouraged to discuss the trial with those currently enrolled to get a first-person account of research participation.

Placebo controls are ethically problematic in studies that use highly invasive methods (e.g., open surgery with anesthesia) due to the risks imposed on an individual who will get no benefit. Placebo controls are also ethically problematic for individuals who are critically ill for in the face of no therapeutic

Table 16.5 Research ethics issues.

- Recruitment of critically ill research subjects
- Obtaining informed consent from critically ill individuals (e.g., issues of mental status, understanding of complex technology, desperation of patients)
- Randomization
- Placebos
- Unknown risks and benefits of experimental technology
- Therapeutic misconception
- Conflict of interest issues (e.g., research investigator is also the patient's treating physician; research investigator has financial ties to the technology/study sponsor)
- Determination of authorship
- Timely publication of research results

intervention, these subjects are "a means to an end", and depending upon the nature of the placebo intervention, they are potentially at risk of incurring further disability or even dying sooner as a result of trial participation. These arguments are still valid in the setting of clinical trials which have shown positive effects for surgical placebo recipients [75], and also less bias and more objectivity in research data analysis [76]. This is because the overall balance of risks and benefits to the research subjects is unacceptable in the situations posed. Unless the risks to the research subject are ascertained to be less than his/her direct benefit from the sham surgery, such surgery is ethically inappropriate for both clinical practice and clinical research.

Also important to the ethical conduct of research is disclosure of actual and perceived conflicts of interest. This is especially important when the principal investigator is also the personal physician of the enrolled research subjects. Conflicts of interest come in a variety of forms including equity interest in the clinical trial sponsor, and consultant or paid spokesperson positions for the sponsor. Even if such conflicts cannot be avoided, their disclosure is critical to the trust relationship between the research team and the research subjects. Undisclosed conflicts of interest can harm the integrity of the research project, as well as the integrity of the research team, its host institution, and the study sponsor. These negative effects can also seep into society's constructions of science and research, and the view of such may become distorted with visions of financially motivated researchers who disregard the welfare of research subjects. The best approach is for researchers to avoid conflicts of interest; and for those that cannot be avoided, they must be disclosed.

Reporting of study data should be timely, especially for trials that are publicly funded. Corporate policies which micromanage data analysis and reporting are generally ethically inappropriate as they poise studies for bias and impaired objectivity. Data fabrication and falsification are also ethically inappropriate for numerous reasons, including the fact they represent poor stewardship of the resources that funded and supported the study. Also, such manipulation of data can potentially harm future research participants or patients, in that technology risks and benefits are not "truly" understood because of false information. "Honorary authorship" is unethical. Authorship should be accorded only to those who directly and substantially contributed to the conception, methodology, data analysis, and/or writing of the manuscript. Further, all those taking credit for the manuscript must also bear responsibility for its contents [77]. At the Cleveland Clinic, bioethicists and the Institutional Review Board are available to assist research investigators with such research ethics matters.

References

1 2003 Annual Report of the U.S. Organ Procurement and Transplantation Network and the Scientific Registry for Transplant Recipients: Transplant Data 1993–2002. Department of Health and Human Services, Health Resources and Services Administration, Office of Special Programs, Division of Transplantation, Rockville, MD; United Network for Organ Sharing, Richmond, VA; University Renal Research and Education Association, Ann Arbor, MI, 2003.

2 Sokohl K. First person consent. *UNOS Update* 2002; September–October: 1, 3.

3 Center for Organ Recovery and Education. It's a Fact. Available on-line at http://www.core.org/itsafact.html. Accessed 03 January 2005.

4 1993 Public Attitudes toward Organ and Tissue Donation Gallup Poll.

5 The Presumed Consent Foundation, Inc. Solutions. Available on-line at http://www.presumedconsent.org/solutions. htm. Accessed 03 January 2005.

6 Transplant Procurement Management International Registry of Organ Donation and Transplantation. Available on-line at http://www.tpm.org

7 National Organ Transplant Act 1984: 98–507 (Title III prohibition of organ purchase).

8 Rackoff J. A reciprocity obligation to donate cadaveric organs: re-visioning opting in. *ASBH Exchange* 2002; **5**: 1, 10.

9 Laks H, Marelli D. The alternate recipient list for heart transplantation: a model for expansion of the donor pool. *Adv Cardiac Surg* 1999; **11**: 233–244.

10 Livi U, Caforio ALP, Tursi V *et al.* Donor age greater than 50 years does not influence mid-term results of heart transplantation. *Transpl Proc* 1996; 28: 91–92.

11 Laks H, Scholl FG, Drinkwater DC *et al.* The alternate recipient list for heart transplantation: does it work? *J Heart Lung Transpl* 1997; **16**: 735–742.

12 Livi U, Caforio ALP. Heart donor management and expansion of current donor selection criteria. *J Heart Lung Transpl* 2000; **19(Suppl 8)**: S43–S48.

13 Loh E, Couch FJ, Hendricksen C *et al.* Development of donor-derived prostate cancer in a recipient following orthotopic heart transplantation. *J Am Med Assoc* 1997; **277**: 133–137.

14 Chau EM, McGregor CG, Rodeheffer RJ *et al.* Increased incidence of chronotropic incompetence in older donor hearts. *J Heart Lung Transpl* 1995; **14**: 743–748.

15 Detry O, Honore P, Hans MF *et al.* Organ donors with primary central nervous system tumor. *Transplantation* 2000; **70**: 244–248.

16 Luciani GB, Livi U, Faggian G *et al.* Clinical results of heart transplantation in recipients over 55 years of age with donors over 40 years of age. *J Heart Lung Transpl* 1992; **11**: 1177–1183.

17 Hosenpud JD, Bennett LE, Keck BM *et al.* The Registry of the International Society for Heart and Lung Transplantation: 14th Official Report-1997. *J Heart Lung Transpl* 1997; **16**: 691–712.

18 Hosenpud JD, Bennett LE, Keck BM *et al.* The Registry of the International Society for Heart and Lung Transplantation Fifteenth Official Report-1998. *J Heart Lung Transpl* 1998; **17**: 656–668.

19 Ubel PA, Arnold RM, Caplan AL. Rationing failure: the ethical lessons of the retransplantation of scarce vital organs. *J Am Med Assoc* 1993; **270**: 2469–2474.

20 Paris W, Muchmore J, Pribil A *et al.* Study of the relative incidences of psychosocial factors before and after heart transplantation and the influence of posttransplantation psychosocial factors on heart transplantation outcome. *J Heart Lung Transpl* 1994; **13**: 424–432.

21 Bunzel B, Laederach-Hofmann K. Solid organ transplantation: are there predictors for posttransplant non-compliance? A literature overview. *Transplantation* 2000; **70**: 711–716.

22 Draper H, Sorell T. Patients' responsibilities in medical ethics. *Bioethics* 2002; **16**: 335–352.

23 Srivastava R, Keck BM, Bennett LE *et al.* The results of cardiac retransplantation: an analysis of the Joint International Society for Heart and Lung Transplantation/

United Network for Organ Sharing Thoracic Registry. *Transplantation* 2000; **70**: 606–612.

24 Bramstedt KA. Why an alternate recipient list for heart transplantation is not a form of ageism. *N Zeal Bioethics J* 2001; **2**: 27–31.

25 Boyd AS. Organ transplantation in HIV-positive patients. *N Engl J Med* 1990; **323**: 1492.

26 Corley MC, Westerberg N, Elswick Jr. RK *et al*. Rationing organs using psychosocial and lifestyle criteria. *Res Nurs Health* 1998; **21**: 327–337.

27 American Medical Association. Code of Ethics Opinion E-9.131, HIV-Infected Patients and Physicians, June 1998. Available on-line at http://www.ama-assn.org/ama/pub/category/2498.html. Accessed 03 January 2005.

28 United Network for Organ Sharing. Policy 4.2.1, HIV-Ab Sero-positive Transplant Candidates, June 1992. Available on-line at www.unos.org. Accessed 03 January 2005.

29 Ragni MV, Bontempo FA, Lewis JH. Organ transplantation in HIV-positive patients with hemophilia. *N Engl J Med* 1990; **322**: 1886–1887.

30 Calabrese LH, Albrecht M, Young J *et al*. Successful cardiac transplantation in an HIV-1 infected patient with advanced disease. *N Engl J Med* 2003; **348**: 2323–2328.

31 Bisleri G, Morgan JA, Deng MC *et al*. Should HIV-positive recipients undergo heart transplantation? *J Thorac Cardiovasc Surg* 2003; **126**: 1639–1640.

32 Calabrese F, Angelini A, Cecchetto A *et al*. HIV infection in the first heart transplantation in Italy: fatal outcome. Case report. *APMIS* 1998; **106**: 470–474.

33 Anthuber M, Kemkes BM, Heiss MM *et al*. HIV infection after heart transplantation: a case report. *J Heart Lung Transplant* 1991; **10**: 611–613.

34 Palella FJ, Delaney KM, Moorman AC *et al*. Declining morbidity and mortality among patients with advanced human immunodeficiency virus infection. *N Engl J Med* 1998; **338**: 853–860.

35 Halpern SD, Ubel PA, Caplan AL. Solid-organ transplantation in HIV-infected patients. *N Engl J Med* 2002; **347**: 284–287.

36 Klein D, Hurley L, Quesenberry Jr. C *et al*. Hospitalization for coronary heart disease and myocardial infarction among Northern California men with HIV-1 infection: additional follow-up. In: *Abstracts of the 10th Conference on Retroviruses and Opportunistic Infections*, Boston, February 10–14, 2003; **326** [Abstract #739].

37 Everson ZR, Sabbaga AM, Varejao STM *et al*. Significance of the human immunodeficiency virus infection in patients submitted to cardiac surgery. *J Cardiovasc Surg* 1999; **40**: 477–479.

38 Ragni MV, Dodson SF, Hunt SC *et al*. Liver transplantation in a hemophilia patient with acquired immunodeficiency syndrome. *Blood* 1999; **93**: 1113–1114.

39 Prachalias AA, Pozniak A, Taylor C *et al*. Liver transplants in adults coinfected with HIV. *Transplantation* 2001; **72**: 1684–1688.

40 Goldberg D, Johnston J, Cameron S *et al*. Risk of HIV transmission from patients to surgeons in the era of post-exposure prophylaxis. *J Hosp Infect* 2000; **44**: 99–105.

41 Bailey LL, Nehlsen-Cannarella SL, Concepcion W *et al*. Baboon-to-human cardiac xenotransplantation in a neonate. *J Am Med Assoc* 1985; **254**: 3321–3329.

42 Bramstedt, KA. Ethics and the clinical utility of animal organs. *Trends Biotechnol* 1999; **17**: 428–429.

43 Singer P. *Animal Liberation*. Avon Books, New York, 1990.

44 Dai Y, Vaught TD, Boone J *et al*. Targeted disruption of the alpha1,3-galactosyltransferase gene in cloned pigs. *Nat Biotechnol* 2002; **20**: 251–255.

45 Bramstedt KA. Arguments for the ethical permissibility of transgenic xenografting. *Gene Ther* 2000; **7**: 633–634.

46 Patience C, Takeuchi Y, Weiss R. Infection of human cells by an endogenous retrovirus of pigs. *Nature Med* 1997; **389**: 681–682.

47 Public Health Service Guideline on Infectious Disease Issues in Xenotransplantation. Washington, DC, January 2001, pp 35–38. Available on-line at http://www.fda.gov/cber/gdlns/xenophs0101.pdf. Accessed 03 January 2005.

48 Menasche P. Cell transplantation for the treatment of heart failure. *Sem Thorac Cardiovasc Surg* 2002; **14**: 157–166.

49 Pfeffer MA, Braunwald E. Ventricular remodeling after myocardial infarction. Experimental observations and clinical implications. *Circulation* 1990; **81**: 1161–1172.

50 MacLellan WR. Mending broken hearts one cell at a time. *J Mol Cell Cardiol* 2002; **34**: 87–89.

51 Menasche P, Hagege AA, Vilquin JT *et al*. Autologous skeletal myoblast transplantation for severe postinfarction left ventricular dysfunction. *J Am Coll Cardiol* 2003; **41**: 1078–1083.

52 del Monte F, Harding SE, Schmidt U *et al*. Restoration of contractile function in isolated cardiomyocytes from failing human hearts by gene transfer of SERCA2a. *Circulation* 1999; **100**: 2308–2311.

53 Akhter SA, Skaer CA, Kypson AP *et al*. Restoration of beta-adrenergic signaling in failing cardiac ventricular myocytes via adenoviral-mediated gene transfer. *Proc Natl Acad Sci USA* 1997; **12100**–12105.

54 Matsui T, Li L, del Monte F *et al*. Adenoviral gene transfer of activated phosphatidylinositol 3′-kinase and Akt inhibits apoptosis of hypoxic cardiomyocytes in vitro. *Circulation* 1999; **100**: 2373–2379.

55 Losordo DW, Vale PR, Symes JF *et al*. Gene therapy for myocardial angiogenesis: initial clinical results with direct myocardial injection of phVEGF$_{165}$ as sole therapy for myocardial ischemia. *Circulation* 1998; **98**: 2800–2804.

56 Raper SE, Yudkoff M, Chirmule N *et al.* A pilot study of *in vivo* liver-directed gene transfer with an adenoviral vector in partial ornithine transcarbamylase deficiency. *Hum Gene Ther* 2002; **13**: 163–175.

57 Bonatti J, Haeusler C, Klaus A *et al.* Acceptance of gene therapy by the heart surgery patient. *Eur J Cardiothorac Surg* 2002; **21**: 981–986.

58 Dipla K, Mattiello JA, Jeevanandam V *et al.* Myocyte recovery after mechanical circulatory support in humans with end-stage heart failure. *Circulation* 1998; **97**: 2316–2322.

59 Grady KL, Meyer P, Mattea A *et al.* Predictors of quality of life at 1 month after implantation of a left ventricular assist device. *Am J Crit Care* 2002; **11**: 345–352.

60 Frazier OH, Rose EA, McCarthy P *et al.* Improved mortality and rehabilitation of transplant candidates treated with a long-term implantable left ventricular assist system. *Ann Surg* 1995; **22**: 327–338.

61 Bramstedt KA. Left ventricular assist devices: an ethical analysis. *Sci Eng Ethics* 1999; **5**: 89–96.

62 Massad MG, McCarthy PM, Smedira NG *et al.* Does successful bridging with the implantable left ventricular assist device affect cardiac transplantation outcome? *J Thorac Cardiovasc Surg* 1996; **112**: 1275–1283.

63 ABIOMED Inc. News. Available on-line at www.abiomed.com/news/press_releases.cfm. Accessed 03 January 2005.

64 DeVries WC. The permanent artificial heart: four case reports. *J Am Med Assoc* 1988; **259**: 849–859.

65 Bramstedt KA. Ethical issues associated with the determination of patient selection criteria for total artificial heart technology. *Cardiovasc Eng* 2001; **6**: 58–61.

66 Bramstedt KA. Informed consent documentation for total artificial heart technology. *J Artif Organs* 2001; **4**: 273–277.

67 Burling S. Widow sues artificial-heart maker. *Philadephia Inquirer*, October 17, 2002: B1.

68 Rhymes JA, McCullough LB, Luchi RJ *et al.* Withdrawing very low-burden interventions in chronically ill patients. *J Am Med Assoc* 2000; **283**: 1061–1063.

69 Jonsen AR, Siegler M, Winslade WJ. *Clinical Ethics: A Practical Approach to Ethical Decisions in Clinical Medicine.* McGraw-Hill, New York, 1992: 25.

70 Bramstedt KA, Wenger NS. When withdrawal of life-sustaining care does more than allow death to takes its course: the dilemma of left ventricular assist devices. *J Heart Lung Transpl* 2001; **20**: 544–548.

71 President's Commission for the Study of Ethical Problems in Medicine and Biomedicine and Behavioral Research. Deciding to Forego Life-Sustaining Treatment: Ethical, Medical and Legal Issues in Treatment Decisions. US Government Printing Office, Washington, DC, 1983: 89–90.

72 Fricchione G, Olson L, Vlay S. Psychiatric syndromes in patients with automatic internal cardioverter defibrillator: anxiety, psychological dependence, abuse and withdrawal. *Am Heart J* 1989; **117**: 1411–1414.

73 Bramstedt KA. The use of advance directives and do not resuscitate orders when considering the inactivation of implantable cardioverter-defibrillators in terminal patients. *Cardiovasc Rev Rep* 2001; **22**: 175–176.

74 United States Title 45 Code of Federal Regulations Section 46.102(d).

75 Stolberg S. Sham Surgery Returns as a Research Tool. *New York Times*, April 25, 1998.

76 Clark PA. Placebo surgery for Parkinson's disease: do the benefits outweigh the risks? *J Law Med Ethics* 2002; **30**: 58–68.

77 National Academy of Sciences. *On Being a Scientist: Responsible Conduct in Research.* National Academy of Science, Washington, DC, 1995: 13–15.

Disclosure Statements

Nancy M. Albert
Consultations: GlaxoSmithKline and Medtronic; Speakers Bureau: GlaxoSmithKline, Medtronic, NitroMed.

Arman T. Askari
Dr Askari does not have any disclosures.

Mandeep Bhargava
The Cleveland Clinic does research funded by Medtronic, Boston Scientific, St Jude Medical and Biotronik.

Katrina A. Bramstedt
Dr Bramstedt does not have any disclosures.

Tiffany Buda
Ms Buda does not have any disclosures.

Gary S. Francis
Advisory Boards: Novartis, Medtronic, Neurocrine, BI, Nitromed, SKF, and Otsuka; Stock Options: CardoMems; Grants: Pfizer.

Bruce W. Lytle
Dr Lytle does not have any disclosures.

Patrick M. McCarthy
Dr. Patrick M. McCarthy was the inventor of the Edwards MC³ Tricuspid Valve Repair Ring; the Myxo ETLogix Mitral Repair Ring; and Co-inventor of the Carpentier-McCarthy-Adams IMR ETLogix Mitral Ring and receives royalties on those products. He is a consultant to Edwards Lifesciences, Myocor, Terumo Heart, and AtriCure.

Edwin C. McGee Jr.
Dr. Edwin C. McGee, Jr. does not have any disclosures.

Raymond Q. Migrino
Dr Migrino does not have any disclosures.

José Luis Navia
Consulting, teaching and speaking: Guidant; teaching and speaking: Medtronic; research development: Johnson & Johnson and CryoLife.

Marc S. Penn
Dr Penn does not have any disclosures.

Randall C. Starling
Research and honorarium: Thoratec, Acorn Cardiovascular, World Heart, Myocor, Scios, Medtronic, Novartis, Roche. Employee of the Cleveland Clinic.

David O. Taylor
Dr Taylor does not have any disclosures.

W. H. Wilson Tang
Dr. Tang serves as a consultant for Medtronic Inc, Boston-Scientific Inc, Neurocrine Biosciences Inc, F-Hoffman La Roche Inc, Otsuka Pharmaceuticals, CV Therapeutics, Amylin Pharmaceuticals, NovaCardia Inc and Amgen Inc. He is a member in the Speakers' Bureau for Takeda Pharmaceuticals. He receives research support from the American Heart Association, National Institute of Health, CV Therapeutics, GlaxoSmithKline Pharmaceuticals (drug supplies only), and Abbott Diagnostics Inc.

Samuel Unzek
Dr Unzek does not have any disclosures.

Richard D. White
Dr White receives research support from Siemens Medical Solutions.

Bruce L. Wilkoff

Dr Wilkoff is a Consultant and Clinical Investigator for Medtronic, Boston Scientific (Guidant) and St. Jude Medical. The Cleveland Clinic does clinical research supported by Medtronic, Boston Scientific (Guidant), St. Jude Medical and Biotronik.

Mohamad Yamani

Dr Yamani does not have any disclosures.

James B. Young

Dr. Young, since 2004, has received research grants from or been a consultant to Abbott, Amgen, Artesion Therapeutics, AstraZeneca, Biomax Canada, Biosite, Boehringer Ingelheim, CoTherix, GlaxoSmithKline, Guidant, Medtronic, National Institute of Health, Protemix, Savacor, Scios, Sunshine, Transworld Medical Corporation, Vasogen, World Heart.

Index